Seminars in Clinical Psychopharmacology

Second edition

College Seminars Series

Series Editors

Professor Anne Farmer Professor of Psychiatric Nosology, Institute of Psychiatry and Honorary Consultant Psychiatrist, South London and Maudsley NHS Trust, London

Dr Louise Howard Wellcome Trust Research Fellow, Institute of Psychiatry, London

Dr Elizabeth Walsh Clinical Senior Lecturar, Institute of Psychiatry, London

Professor Greg Wilkinson Professor of Liaison Psychiatry and Honorary Consultant Psychiatrist, University of Liverpool

---

Praise for the first editions of books in the series

This very reasonably priced textbook should improve knowledge and stimulate interest in a common and challenging topic.

BMJ

The editors state that this book is not intended to be a substitute for supervised clinical practice. It is, however, the next best thing.

Psychological Medicine

...this book joins others in the series in being both readily understandable and accessible. ... should be on every psychiatrist's bookshelf...

Journal of Psychopharmacology

...an excellent, up-to-date introductory text. It can be strongly recommended for residents, clinicians, and researchers....

American Journal of Psychiatry

Every chapter informs, but also pleases. This is expert teaching by skilled and committed teachers.

Journal of the Royal Society of Medicine

Congratulations are due to the editors for the breadth of their vision and to the authors for the thoroughness and liveliness of their contributions.

Psychological Medicine

...an excellent teaching and revision aid for psychiatric trainees...

Criminal Behaviour and Mental Health

Seminars in Clinical Psychopharmacology

Second edition

Edited by David J. King

Gaskell

© The Royal College of Psychiatrists 2004
First edition © The Royal College of Psychiatrists 1995

Gaskell is an imprint of the Royal College of Psychiatrists, 17 Belgrave Square, London SW1X 8PG
http://www.rcpsych.ac.uk

British Library Cataloguing-in-Publication Data.
A catalogue record for this book is available from the British Library.
ISBN 1-904671-08-X

Distributed in North America by Balogh International Inc.

The views presented in this book do not necessarily reflect those of the Royal College
of Psychiatrists, and the publishers are not responsible for any error of omission or fact.

The Royal College of Psychiatrists is a registered charity (no. 228636).
Printed by Bell & Bain Limited, Thornliebank, Glasgow.

Contents

Figures

Tables

Boxes

Contributors

Dr N. Adrian, Department of Psychological Medicine, Great Ormond Street Hospital for Children, London WC1N 3JH, UK

Dr M. J. Arranz, Department of Clinical Neuropharmacology, Institute of Psychiatry, London SE5 8AF, UK

Professor C. M. Bradshaw, Department of Psychopharmacology, B Floor, Queen's Medical Centre, Nottingham NG7 2UH, UK

Dr S. J. Cooper, Department of Mental Health, Queen's University Belfast, Whitla Medical Building, 97 Lisburn Road, Belfast BT9 7BL, UK

Professor S. Curran, Calder Unit, Fieldhead Hospital, Wakefield WF1 3SP, UK

Dr J. G. Edwards, Emeritus Consultant Psychiatrist, West Hampshire NHS Trust, Royal South Hants Hospital, Southampton SO14 0YG; Visiting Professor, Khon Kaen University, Khon Kaen, and Prince of Songkla University, Hat Yai, Thailand

Dr P. Harrison-Read, Department of Psychiatry, Royal Free Hospital, London NW3 2QG, UK

Professor P. Hill, Department of Psychological Medicine, Great Ormond Street Hospital for Children, London WC1N 3JH, UK

Professor I. Hindmarch, Human Psychopharmacology Research Unit, University of Surrey, Egerton Road, Guildford, Surrey GU2 7XP, UK

Dr C. B. Kelly, Department of Psychiatry, Windsor House, Belfast City Hospital, Lisburn Road, Belfast BT9 7AB, UK

Professor R. W. Kerwin, Department of Clinical Neuropharmacology, Institute of Psychiatry, London SE5 8AF, and Consultant Psychiatrist, Holywell Hospital, Antrim BT41 2RJ, UK

Professor D. J. King, Department of Therapeutics and Pharmacology, Queen's University Belfast, Whitla Medical Building, 97 Lisburn Road, Belfast BT9 7BL, UK

Professor B. E. Leonard, Emeritus Professor of Pharmacology, National University of Ireland, Galway, Republic of Ireland

Professor G. R. McClelland, Postgraduate Medical School, University of Surrey, Surrey Research Park, Guildford, Surrey GU2 7DJ, UK

Professor R. J. McClelland, Department of Mental Health, Queen's University Belfast, Whitla Medical Building, 97 Lisburn Road, Belfast BT9 7BL, UK

Dr J. I. Morrow, Department of Neurology, Royal Victoria Hospital, Grosvenor Road, Belfast BT12 6BA, UK

Dr R. K. Shelley, Consultant Psychiatrist, St John of God Hospital, Stillorgan, County Dublin, Republic of Ireland

Dr G. S. Stein, Farnborough Hospital, Orpington, Kent BR6 8ND, UK

Professor E. Szabadi, Section of Psychopharmacology, Division of Psychiatry, B Floor, Queen's Medical Centre, Nottingham NG7 2UH, UK

Professor P. Tyrer, Department of Psychological Medicine, Imperial College Faculty of Medicine, London W6 8RP, UK

Professor J. L. Waddington, Department of Clinical Pharmacology, Royal College of Surgeons in Ireland, Dublin 2, Republic of Ireland

Professor J. P. Wattis, School of Human and Health Sciences, University of Huddersfield, Huddersfield HD1 3DH, UK

Foreword

Series Editors

We are very pleased to introduce the second editions of *College Seminars*, now updated to reflect changes in the understanding, treatment and management of psychiatric illness and mental health, as well as changes in the MRCPsych examination and the need for continuing professional development. These titles represent a distillation of the collective wisdom of hundreds of individuals, but written in approachable, tutorial-style prose.

As the body responsible for maintaining professional standards and developing the MRCPsych curriculum, the Royal College of Psychiatrists has a duty to assist trainees in psychiatry as well as all practising psychiatrists throughout their careers. The first of the *College Seminars*, a series of textbooks covering the breadth of psychiatry, were published by the College in 1993. Widely acclaimed as essential and approachable texts, they were each written and edited to the brief of 'all the College requires the trainee to know about a sub-specialty, and a little bit more'.

Anne Farmer
Louise Howard
Elizabeth Walsh
Greg Wilkinson

Preface

I was delighted when the Royal College of Psychiatrists invited me in April 2000, 5 years after the appearance of the first edition of this little book on clinical psychopharmacology, to edit a second edition. Although in this new electronic age books are not yet obsolete, they do age rather quickly and the first edition is sadly now very much out of date. Nevertheless, I underestimated how long it was going to take all of us to put together a revised and updated edition. Unfortunately textbooks have become one of the casualties of the UK Research Assessment Exercise, which has undervalued scholarship at the expense of original research.

In terms of its scope and focus, the book's reviews seemed to agree that the strength of the first edition was in the integration of theoretical pharmacology with clinical practice. After reviewing John Cookson's fifth edition of *Use of Drugs in Psychiatry*, I decided that the second edition of *Seminars in Clinical Psychopharmacology* should move a little away from clinical guidelines and practical prescribing (which are done very well by Cookson *et al*), to include more of the recent scientific developments in psychopharmacology in a way that is accessible to trainees and practising clinicians.

All the chapters have been updated, some have been virtually rewritten and three are completely new. Of our 22 contributors, nine are new, and I am indebted to all of them for their commitment, hard work and forbearance. We have not produced a very homogeneous product and, as before, there are a variety of styles and extent of referencing. Nevertheless, we have tried to remain true to our aim of providing a text that is relevant to prescribing clinicians and trainees and that provides a flavour of the basic neuroscientific underpinings of our rapidly expanding discipline.

Although the science changes, our patients' conditions do not, and I hope our book will help towards a better understanding of what is known, an awareness of how great is our ignorance and an enthusiasm for clinical research. We also hope it will help towards prescribing that is more rational, appropriate and safe.

David J. King
September 2002

Part I
General principles

CHAPTER 1

Introduction to neuropharmacology

Brian E. Leonard

Neurons and synapses

It has been estimated that the mammalian brain comprises several billion neurons, which, together with their surrounding glial cells, form a unique network of connections that is ultimately responsible for all thoughts and actions. While the glial cells may play a critical role in brain development, their main function in the mature brain is to maintain the structure and metabolic homoeostasis of the neurons which they surround.

A typical neuron (Fig. 1.1) consists of a cell body and an axonal projection; information in the form of an action potential passes from the cell body to the axonal terminal. Information is received by the cell body via a complex array of dendrites, which make contact with adjacent neurons. The structural complexity and the number of dendritic processes vary according to the type of nerve cell and its physiological function. For example, the granule cells in the dentate gyrus of the hippocampus (a region of the brain that plays a role in short-term memory) receive and integrate information from up to 10 000 other cells in the vicinity.

The majority of the inputs to the granule cells are excitatory and each provides a small depolarising current to the membrane of the cell body. The point of contact between the axonal projection from the neuron and an adjacent cell is termed the synapse. Under the electron microscope, the synapse appears as a swelling at the end of the axon. Most synapses are excitatory and are usually located along the dendritic branches of the neuron. The contributions of the individual excitatory synapses are additive and, as a result, when an excitatory stimulus occurs a wave of depolarising current travels down the axon to stimulate the adjacent cell body. However, some synapses are inhibitory; for most cell types these are fewer in number than excitatory synapses and are strategically located near the cell body. These synapses, when activated,

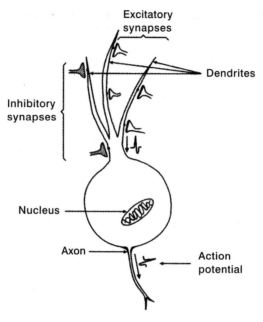

Fig. 1.1 A single neuron, represented by a dentate granule cell, receives numerous synaptic contacts, which are of either excitatory or inhibitory type (Leonard, 2003: p. 17. © 2003 John Wiley & Sons Ltd. Reproduced with permission).

inhibit the effects of any excitatory currents which may travel down the dendritic processes, and thereby block their actions on the neuron.

The nerve impulse

Action potentials are the means by which information is passed from one neuron to an adjacent neuron. The balance between the excitatory and inhibitory impulses determines how many action potentials will reach the axonal terminal and, by releasing a specific type of neuro-transmitter from the terminal, influence the adjacent neuron. Thus, in summary, chemical information – in the form of small neurotransmitter molecules released from axonal terminals – is responsible for changing the membrane potential at the synaptic junctions, which may occur on the dendrites or directly on the cell body. The action potential then passes down the axon to initiate the release of the neurotransmitter from the axonal terminal and thereby pass information on to any adjacent neurons.

The concept of chemical transmission in the nervous system arose in the early years of the twentieth century, when it was discovered that the functioning of the autonomic nervous system was largely dependent on the secretion of acetylcholine and noradrenaline from the para-sympathetic and sympathetic nerves, respectively. The physiologist Sherrington proposed that nerve cells communicate with one another, and with any other type of adjacent cell, by liberating the neuro-transmitter into the space, or synapse, in the immediate vicinity of the nerve ending. He believed that transmission across the synaptic cleft was unidirectional and, unlike conduction down the nerve fibre, was delayed by some milliseconds because of the time it takes the transmitter to diffuse across the synapse and activate a specific neurotransmitter receptor on the cell membrane.

While it was generally assumed that the brain also contains acetylcholine and noradrenaline as transmitters, it was only in the early 1950s that experimental evidence for this accumulated, along with evidence that there are also many other types of transmitters in the brain.

A summary of the neurotransmitters and neuromodulators that have been identified in the mammalian brain are listed in Table 1.1. The term neuromodulator is applied to those substances that may be released with a transmitter but which do not produce a direct effect on a receptor; a neuromodulator seems to work by modifying the responsiveness of the receptor to the action of the transmitter.

The metabolic unity of the neuron requires that the same transmitter is released at all its synapses. This is known as Dale's law (or principle), which Sir Henry Dale proposed in 1935. Dale's law applies only to the presynaptic portion of the neuron, not the postsynaptic effects that the transmitter may have on other target neurons. For example, acetylcholine released at motor neuron terminals has an excitatory action at the motor neuron junction, whereas the same transmitter released at vagal nerve terminals has an inhibitory action on the heart.

In addition to the diversity of action of a single transmitter released from a neuron, it has become well established that among invertebrates up to four different transmitters can occur in the same neuron (see Cotransmission, below). In the vertebrate there is also increasing evidence, from the seminal studies of Höckfelt and colleagues in Stockholm, that some neurons in the central nervous system can also contain more than one transmitter (see Höckfelt et al, 1986). Such neurons appear to contain a peptide within monoamine-containing terminals. The peptide transmitters (usually referred to as neuro-peptides) are contained in specific types of storage vesicles. Thus Dale's law has to be modified to allow for the presence of neuropeptides in amine-containing nerve terminals, whose function is to act as a neuromodulator of the amine when it acts on the postsynaptic receptor.

There are several criteria that must be fulfilled for a substance to be considered as a transmitter. These are given in Box 1.1.

Table 1.1 Some of the neurotransmitters and neuromodulators that have been identified in the mammalian brain

Transmitter/ modulator	Distribution in the brain	Physiological effect	Involvement in disease
Noradrenaline	Most regions: long axons project from pons and brain-stem	α_1-receptors – inhibitory β_1-receptors – inhibitory β_2-receptors – excitatory?	Depression Mania
Dopamine	Most regions: short, medium and long axonal projections	D_1/D_5 receptors – stimulatory D_2 receptors – inhibitory D_3/D_4 receptors – ?	Schizophrenia Mania?
Serotonin	Most regions: project from pons and brain-stem	5-HT$_{1A}$ receptors – inhibitory 5-HT$_2$ receptors – ? 5-HT$_3$ receptors – ?	Depression Schizophrenia? Anxiety
Acetylcholine	Most regions: long and short axonal projections from basal forebrain	M_1 receptors – excitatory M_2 receptors – inhibitory N receptors – excitatory	Dementias Mania?
Adrenaline	Midbrain and brain-stem	Possibly same as for noradrenaline	Depression?
GABA	Supraspinal interneurons	A-receptors – hyperpolarise membranes (inhibitory) B-receptors – inhibitory	Anxiety Seizures, epilepsy
Glycine	Spinal interneurons; modulates NMDA amino acid receptors in brain	Hyperpolarise membranes Strych-sensitive receptors – inhibitory Strych-insensitive receptors – excitatory	Seizures? Learning and memory Seizures?
Glutamate and aspartate	Long neurons	Quisqualate – depolarises membranes NMDA – depolarises membranes Kainate – depolarises membranes	Seizures Schizophrenia?

Substances with a neuromodulatory effect on brain neurotransmitters by direct actions of specific receptors that modify the actions of the transmitters listed include: prostaglandins, adenosine, enkephalines, substance P, cholecystokinin, endorphins, endogenous benzodiazepine receptor ligands, and possibly histamine. NMDA, N-methyl-D-aspartate. Strych, strychnine.

Box 1.1 Criteria that must be fulfilled for a substance to be considered a neurotransmitter

- It should be present in a nerve terminal and in the vicinity of the area of the brain where it is thought to act.
- It should be released from the nerve terminal (this is generally by a calcium-dependent process) following stimulation of the nerve.
- The enzymes concerned in its synthesis and metabolism should be present in the nerve ending, or in the proximity of the nerve ending.
- It should produce a physiological response following its release by activating a postsynaptic receptor site. Such changes should be identical to those seen following the local application of the transmitter (e.g. by micro-ionophoresis).
- Its effects should be selectively blocked by a specific antagonist and mimicked by a specific agonist.

Note that these criteria should be regarded as general guidelines, not specific rules.

Neurotransmitter receptor mechanisms

Ion channels in nerve conduction

Ion channels are pores through the neuronal membrane that are formed by large proteins. The precise structure of the ion channels depends on their physiological function and distribution along the dendrites and cell body. For example, some are specialised neurotransmitter-sensitive receptor channels, and others are activated by specific metal ions such as sodium or calcium. The voltage-dependent sodium channel has been shown to consist of a complex protein with both a hydrophilic and a hydrophobic domain: the former domain occurs within the neuronal membrane, while the latter domain occurs both inside and outside the neuronal membrane (Fig. 1.2).

Four regions containing the hydrophilic units are arranged in the membrane in the form of a pore, with two units forming the remaining sides of the pore. This allows the sodium ions to pass in a regulated manner as the diameter of the pore, and the electrical charges on the amino acids that comprise the proteins lining the pore, determines the selectivity of the ion channel for sodium.

The DNA sequences that code for the proteins that make up the ion channels can be modified by point mutations, and these will alter the protein structure. Such a change to the structure of the protein – by even a single amino acid – can alter the properties of the ion channel; for example, the channel might open and close for longer or shorter periods, or it might carry larger or smaller currents. As a consequence

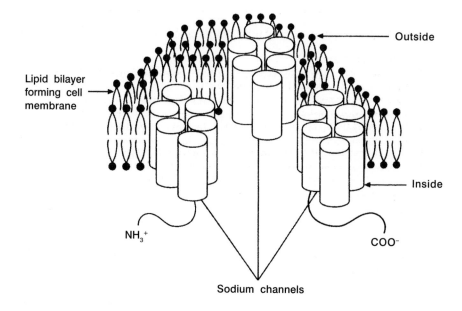

Outside

Lipid bilayer
forming cell
membrane

Inside

NH_3^+

COO^-

Sodium channels

Fig. 1.2 Diagram of a voltage-activated sodium channel protein. The channel is composed of a long chain of amino acids interconnected by peptide bonds. The amino acids perform specific functions within the ion channel. The cylinders represent amino acid assemblies located within the membrane of the nerve cell; these are responsible for the foundation of the ion pore (Leonard, 2003: p. 21. © 2003 John Wiley & Sons Ltd. Reproduced with permission).

of molecular biological studies, it is now recognised that most ion channels of importance in neurotransmission are composed of three to five protein subunits. Their identification and characterisation have now made it possible to map their location on specific neurons and to correlate their location with their specific function.

Synaptic transmission

The sequence of events that results in neurotransmission of information from one nerve cell to another across the synapses (see Box 1.2) begins with a wave of depolarisation which passes down the axon and results in the opening of the voltage-sensitive calcium channels in the axonal terminal. These channels are frequently concentrated in areas that correspond to the active sites of neurotransmitter release. A large (up to 100 µmol/l) but brief rise in the calcium concentration within the nerve terminal triggers the movement of the synaptic vesicles, which contain the neurotransmitter, towards the synaptic membrane. By means of specific membrane-bound proteins (such as synaptobrevin

Box 1.2   Stages of neurotransmission in the brain

1   Action potential depolarises the axonal terminal
2   Depolarisation produces opening of voltage-dependent calcium channels
3   Calcium ions diffuse into the presynaptic nerve terminal and bind with specific proteins on the vesicular and neuronal membranes
4   Vesicles move towards the presynaptic membrane and fuse with it
5   Neurotransmitter is released into the synaptic cleft by a process of exocytosis
6   Neurotransmitter activates receptors on adjacent neurons
7   The postsynaptic receptors respond either rapidly (ionotropic type) or slowly (metabotropic type), depending on the nature of the neuro-transmitter

from the neuronal membrane and synaptotagrin from the vesicular membrane) the vesicles fuse with the neuronal membrane and release their contents into the synaptic gap by a process of exocytosis. Thereafter the vesicle membrane is reformed and recycled within the neuronal terminal. The cycle is completed when the vesicles have accumulated more neurotransmitter by means of an energy-dependent transporter on the vesicle membrane.

The neurotransmitters diffuse across the synaptic cleft in a fraction of a millisecond. On reaching the postsynaptic membrane on an adjacent neuron, they bind to specific receptor sites and trigger appropriate physiological responses.

Two main types of receptor are activated by neurotransmitters. These are the ionotropic and metabotropic receptors. The former receptor type is illustrated by the amino acid neurotransmitter receptors for glutamate, gamma-aminobutyric acid (GABA) and glycine, and the acetylcholine receptors of the nicotinic type. These are examples of fast transmitters, in that they rapidly open and close the ion channels in the neuronal membrane. Peptides are often co-localised with these fast transmitters but act more slowly and modulate the excitatory or inhibitory actions of the fast transmitters. In contrast to the amino acid neurotransmitters, the biogenic amine transmitters, such as noradrenaline, dopamine and serotonin, and the non-amine transmitter acetylcholine acting on the muscarinic type of receptor, activate metabotropic receptors. Metabotropic receptors are linked to intracellular second messenger systems by means of G (guanosine triphosphate dependent) proteins. These comprise the slow transmitters, so-called because of the relatively long time required for their physiological response to occur. It must be emphasised, however, that a number of metabotropic receptors have recently been identified that are activated by fast transmitters, so that a rigid separation of these receptor types cannot be maintained in these terms.

9

Over 50 different types of neurotransmitter have so far been identified in the mammalian brain and these may be categorised according to their chemical structure.

Presynaptic mechanisms

Another important mechanism whereby the release of a neurotransmitter may be altered is by presynaptic inhibition. Initially this mechanism was thought to be restricted to noradrenergic synapses, but it is now known also to occur at GABA-ergic, dopaminergic and serotonergic terminals.

In brief, it has been shown that at noradrenergic synapses the release of noradrenaline may be reduced by high concentrations of the transmitter in the synaptic cleft. Conversely, some adrenoceptor antagonists, such as phenoxybenzamine, have been found to enhance the release of the amine. It is now known that the subclass of adrenoceptors involved in this process of autoinhibition are distinct from the α_1-adrenoceptors, which are located on blood vessels, on secretory cells and in the brain. These autoinhibitory receptors, or α_2-adrenoceptors, can be identified by the use of specific agonists and antagonists, for example clonidine and yohimbine, respectively. Drugs acting as specific agonists or antagonists on α_1-receptors, for example the agonist methoxamine and the antagonist prazosin, do not affect noradrenaline release by this mechanism.

The inhibitory effect of α_2-agonists on noradrenaline release involves a hyperpolarisation of the presynaptic membranes by the opening potassium ion channels. The reduction in the release of noradrenaline following the administration of an α_2-agonist is ultimately due to a reduction in the concentration of free cytosolic calcium, which is an essential component of the mechanism whereby the synaptic vesicles containing noradrenaline fuse to the synaptic membrane before their release.

There is evidence that a number of closely related phosphoproteins associated with the synaptic vesicles, called synapsins, are involved in the short-term regulation of neurotransmitter release. These proteins also appear to be involved in the regulation of synapse formation, which allows the nerve network to adapt to the long-term passage of nerve impulses.

Experimental studies have shown that the release of a transmitter from a nerve terminal can be decreased or increased by a variety of other neurotransmitters. For example, stimulation of serotonin receptors on noradrenergic terminals can lead to an enhanced release of noradrenaline. While the physiological importance of such a mechanism is unclear, it could be a means whereby drugs produce some of their effects. Such receptors have been termed heteroceptors.

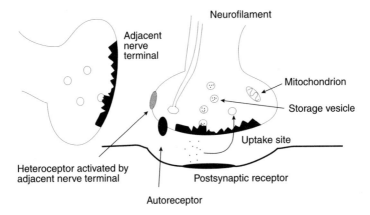

Fig. 1.3 Relationship between pre- and postsynaptic receptors. Storage vesicles for the neurotransmitter are formed from the neurofilament network, which projects from the cell body to the nerve terminal. Following the reuptake of the transmitter by an energy-dependent, active transport process, the transmitter may be re-stored in empty vesicles or metabolised in the case of biogenic amines by monoamine oxidase. The enzyme is associated with mitochondria, which also may act as a source of energy in the form of adenosine triphosphate (ATP).

In addition to the physiological process of autoinhibition, another mechanism of presynaptic inhibition has been identified in the peripheral nervous system, although its precise relevance to the brain is unclear. In the dorsal horn of the spinal cord, for example, the axon terminal of a local neuron makes axo–axonal contact with a primary afferent excitatory input, which leads to a reduction in the neurotransmitter released. This is due to the local neuron partly depolarising the nerve terminal, so that when the axon potential arrives, the change induced is diminished, thereby leading to a smaller quantity of transmitter being released. In the brain, it is possible that GABA can cause presynaptic inhibition in this way.

Summary

It seems that the release of a transmitter from its nerve terminal is dependent not only on the passage of an action potential but also on the intersynaptic concentration of the transmitter and the modulatory effects of other neurotransmitters that act presynaptically on the nerve terminal. The interrelationship between these different processes is illustrated in Fig. 1.3.

Postsynaptic mechanisms

Neurotransmitters can either excite or inhibit the activity of a cell with which they are in contact. When an excitatory transmitter such as acetylcholine, or an inhibitory transmitter such as GABA, is released from a nerve terminal it diffuses across the synaptic cleft to the postsynaptic membrane, where it activates the receptor site. Some receptors, such as the nicotinic receptor, are directly linked to sodium ion channels, so that when acetylcholine stimulates the nicotinic receptor, the ion channel opens to allow an exchange of sodium and potassium ions across the nerve membrane. Such receptors are called ionotropic receptors and they consist of a relatively small group responsible for fast synaptic transmission at neuromuscular junctions, autonomic ganglia and central synapses. Glutamate, GABA, acetylcholine, serotonin, glycine and adenosine triphosphate (ATP) are known to activate specific ionotropic receptors. As a general principle, only a relatively few transmitters are used in neurotransmission and the diversity of physiological effect is achieved by utilising a diversity of receptors. Thus, except for glycine, all fast transmitters activate both ionotropic and metabotropic receptors. Within each receptor class there are usually several subtypes.

The generation of action potentials by nerve axons and muscle fibres was first described by the German physiologist Emil DuBois-Reymond in 1849. However, it was not until over a century later that the underlying mechanism was explained in terms of the properties of the specific membrane proteins forming the voltage-gated ion channels of sodium and potassium ions.

Second messenger system

When receptors are directly linked to ion channels, fast excitatory or inhibitory postsynaptic potentials occur. However, it is well established that slow potential changes also occur and that such changes are due to the receptor being linked to the ion channel indirectly, via a second messenger system.

For example, the stimulation of β-adrenoceptors by noradrenaline results in the activation of adenylate cyclase on the inner side of the nerve membrane. This enzyme catalyses the breakdown of ATP to the very labile, high-energy compound cyclic 3,5-adenosine monophosphate (cyclic AMP). Cyclic AMP then activates a protein kinase which, by phosphorylating specific membrane proteins, opens an ion channel to cause an efflux of potassium and an influx of sodium ions. Such receptors are termed metabotropic receptors.

Many monoamine neurotransmitters are now thought to work by this receptor-linked second messenger system. In some cases, however, stimulation of the postsynaptic receptors can cause the inhibition of adenylate cyclase activity. For example, D_2 dopamine receptors inhibit, while D_1 receptors stimulate, the activity of the cyclase. Such differences have been ascribed to the fact that the cyclase is linked to two distinct

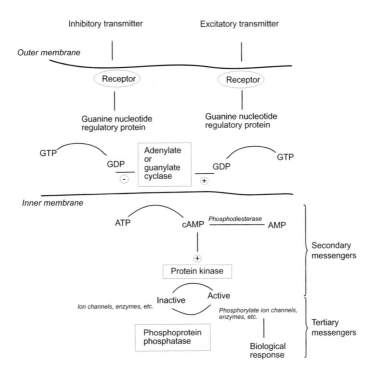

Fig. 1.4 Relationship between the postsynaptic receptor and the second messenger system. GTP and GDP, guanosine tri- and diphosphate; ATP and cAMP, adenosine triphosphate and cyclic adenosine monophosphate.

guanosine triphosphate (GTP) binding proteins in the cell membrane, termed Gi and Gs. The former protein inhibits the cyclase, possibly by reducing the effects of the Gs protein, which stimulates the cyclase.

The relationship between the postsynaptic receptor and the second messenger system is illustrated in Fig. 1.4.

Recently there has been much interest in the possible role of the family of protein kinases that translate information from the second messenger to the membrane proteins. Many of these kinases are controlled by free calcium ions within the cell. It is now established that some serotonin receptors, for example, are linked via G-proteins to the phosphatidyl inositol pathway, which, by mobilising membrane-bound diacylglycerol and free calcium ions, can activate a specific protein kinase C. This enzyme affects the concentration of calmodulin, a calcium-sequestering protein that plays a key role in many intra-cellular processes.

Structurally, G-proteins are composed of three subunits, termed alpha, beta and gamma. The alpha subunits are structurally diverse, so

---

Box 1.3 The role of G-proteins in neurotransmission

1 An excitatory neurotransmitter, such as noradrenaline or serotonin, acts on its receptor and activates the intermembrane G-protein by converting guanosine diphosphate (GDP) to guanosine triphosphate (GTP), thereby linking the receptor to the second messenger system, usually adenylate cyclase.
2 The second messenger, for example cyclic adenosine monophosphate (cAMP), then activates cAMP-dependent protein kinase, which modulates the function of a broad range of membrane receptors, intracellular enzymes, ion channels and transcription factors.
3 An inhibitory neurotransmitter activates an inhibitory G-protein, thereby leading to a reduction in cAMP synthesis.
4 The termination of signal transduction results from the hydrolysis of GTP to GDP by GTPase, thereby returning the G-protein to its inactive form.

---

that each member of the G-protein super-family has a unique alpha subunit. Thus the variability of the alpha, and to a lesser extent the beta and gamma, subunits provides for the coupling of a variety of receptors to different second messenger systems. In this way, different receptor types are able to interact and regulate each other, thereby allowing for greater signal divergence, convergence or filtering than could be achieved solely on the basis of receptor diversity.

The role of G-proteins in neurotransmission is summarised in Box 1.3.

Changes in receptor sensitivity

The functional response of a nerve cell to a transmitter can change as a result of the receptor becoming sensitised or desensitised following a decrease or increase, respectively, in the concentration of the trans- mitter at the receptor site. Among those receptors that are directly coupled to ion channels, receptor desensitisation is often rapid and pronounced.

Most of the experimental evidence came initially from studies of the frog motor end-plate, where it was shown that the desensitisation of the nicotinic receptor caused by continuous short pulses of acetyl- choline was associated with a slow conformational change, in that the ion channel remained closed despite the fact that the transmitter was bound to the receptor surface.

A similar mechanism has also been shown to occur in brain cells. For example, continuous exposure to noradrenaline of α-adrenoceptors on rat glioma cells *in vitro* results in a rapid reduction in their responsiveness. This is followed by a secondary stage of desensitisation, whereby the number of α-receptors decreases. It seems likely that the receptors are not lost but move into the cell and are therefore no longer accessible to the transmitter. The importance of the changes in receptor sensitivity to our understanding of the chronic effects of psychotropic drugs is discussed in Chapter 15.

It must be emphasised that there is considerable integration and modulation between the various second messenger systems and these interactions lead to cross-talk between neurotransmitter systems. Such cross-talk between the second messenger systems may account for changes in the sensitivity of neurotransmitter receptors following prolonged stimulation by an agonist, whereby a reduction in the receptor density is associated with a reduced physiological response (also termed receptor down-regulation).

Summary

Neurotransmitters can control cellular events by two basic mechanisms. First, they may be linked directly to sodium (e.g. acetylcholine acting on nicotinic receptors, or excitatory amino acids such as glutamate acting on glutamate receptors) or chloride (as exemplified by GABA) ion channels, thereby leading to the generation of fast excitatory or inhibitory postsynaptic potentials, respectively. Second, the receptor may be linked to a second messenger system that mediates slower postsynaptic changes. These different mechanisms, whereby neuro-transmitters may change the activity of a postsynaptic membrane by fast, voltage-dependent mechanisms, or slower mechanisms mediated by second messengers, provide functional plasticity within the nervous system.

Cotransmission

During the mid-1970s studies on such invertebrates as the mollusc *Aplysia* showed that at least four different types of transmitters could be liberated from the same nerve terminal. This was the first evidence that Dale's law does not always apply. Extensive histochemical studies of the mammalian peripheral and central nervous systems followed, and it was shown that transmitters such as acetylcholine, noradrenaline and dopamine can coexist with such peptides as cholecystokinin, vasoactive intestinal peptide, and gastrin-like peptides.

It is now evident that nerve terminals in the brain may contain different types of storage vesicles for peptide cotransmitters. Following their release, these peptides activate specific pre- or postsynaptic receptors, and thereby modulate the responsiveness of the membrane to the action of the traditional neurotransmitters, such as acetylcholine or noradrenaline. In the mammalian (including human) brain, acetyl-choline has been found to localise with vasoactive intestinal peptide, dopamine with cholecystokinin-like peptide, and serotonin with

---

Box 1.4 Similarities and differences between the peptide transmitters/cotransmitters

- Both neurotransmitters and peptides show high specificity for their specific receptors.
- Neurotransmitters produce physiological responses in nano- or micromolar (10^{-9} to 10^{-6}) concentrations, whereas peptides are active in picomolar (10^{-12}) concentrations.
- Neurotransmitters bind to their receptors with high affinity but low potency, whereas peptides bind with very high affinity and high potency.
- Neurotransmitters are synthesised at a moderate rate in the nerve terminal, whereas the rate of synthesis of peptides is probably very low.
- Neurotransmitters are generally of low molecular weight (200 or below), whereas peptides are of intermediate molecular weight (1000–10 000 or occasionally more).

---

substance P. In addition, there is increasing evidence that some peptides may act as neurotransmitters in their own right in the mammalian brain. These include the enkephalins, thyrotrophin-releasing hormone, angiotensin II, vasopressin, substance P, neurotensin, somatostatin and corticotropin, among many others. With the advent of specific and sensitive immunocytochemical techniques, several more peptides are being added to this list every year.

The similarities and differences between the peptide transmitters/cotransmitters and the 'classical' transmitters such as acetylcholine are summarised in Box 1.4.

The peptide transmitters form the largest group of neurotransmitters in the mammalian brain, at least 40 different types having been identified so far. The mechanism governing their release differs from those of the non-peptide transmitters. Thus peptides are stored in large, dense core vesicles, which appear to require more prolonged and widespread diffusion of calcium into the nerve terminal before they can be released. In general, the peptide transmitters form part of the slow transmitter group, as they activate metabotropic receptors.

Classification of neurotransmitter receptors

The British physiologist Langley, in 1905, was first to postulate that most drugs, hormones and transmitters produce their effects by interacting with specific sites on the cell membrane, which we now call receptors. Langley's postulate was based on his observation that drugs can mimic both the specificity and potency of endogenous hormones and neurotransmitters, while others appear to be able selectively to antagonise the actions of such substances. Thus, substances that stimulate the receptor, or mimic the action of natural ligands for the receptor, are called *agonists*, while those substances blocking the receptor are called *antagonists*. This revolutionary hypothesis was later extended by Hill, Gaddum and Clark, who quantified the ways in which agonists and antagonists interacted with receptors both *in vitro* and *in vivo*.

More recently the precise structure of a large number of different types of transmitter receptors has been determined using cloning and other techniques, so that it is now possible to visualise precisely how an agonist or antagonist interacts with certain types of receptor. To date, different types of cholinergic, β-adrenergic and serotonergic receptors have been cloned, and their essential molecular features identified. In addition, a number of peptide receptors – such as the insulin, gonadotrophin, angiotensin, glucagon, prolactin and thyroid stimulating hormone receptors – have also been identified and their key structures determined.

The location and possible functional importance of the different types of neurotransmitter receptors which are of relevance to the psychopharmacologist are summarised below. It must be emphasised that the list is by no means complete and that many of these receptor types are likely to be further subdivided as a result of the development of highly selective ligands.

Cholinergic receptors

Sir Henry Dale noticed that the different esters of choline elicited responses in isolated organ preparations that were similar to those seen following the application of either of the natural substances muscarine (from a poisonous toadstool) or nicotine. This led Dale to conclude that, in the appropriate organs, acetylcholine could act on either muscarinic or nicotinic receptors. Later it was found that the effects of muscarine and nicotine could be blocked by atropine and tubocurarine, respectively. Further studies showed that these receptors differed not only in their molecular structure but also in the ways in which they brought about their physiological responses once the receptor had been stimulated by an agonist. Thus nicotinic receptors were found to be linked directly to an ion channel and their activation always caused a rapid increase in cellular permeability to sodium and potassium ions. Conversely, the responses to muscarinic receptor stimulation were slower and involved the activation of a second messenger system, which was linked to the receptor by G-proteins.

Muscarinic receptors

To date, five subtypes of these receptors have been cloned. However, initial studies relied on the pharmacological effects of the muscarinic antagonist pirenzepine, which was shown to block the effect of several muscarinic agonists. These receptors were termed M_1 receptors, to distinguish them from those receptors for which pirenzepine had only a low affinity (termed M_2 receptors). More recently, M_3, M_4 and M_5 receptors have been identified which, like the M_1 and M_2 receptors, occur in the brain. Recent studies have shown that M_1 and M_3 are located postsynaptically in the brain, whereas the M_2 and M_4 receptors occur presynaptically, where they act as inhibitory autoreceptors that inhibit the release of acetylcholine. The M_2 and M_4 receptors are coupled to the inhibitory Gi protein, which (as mentioned above) reduces the formation of cyclic AMP within the neuron. By contrast, the M_1, M_3 and M_5 receptors are coupled to the stimulatory Gs protein, which stimulates the intracellular hydrolysis of the phosphoinositide messenger within the neuron.

Use of cholinomimetic drugs in the treatment of Alzheimer's disease

The cholinergic system has the capacity to adapt to changes in the physiological environment of the brain. Thus the density of the cholinergic receptors is increased by antagonists and decreased by agonists. The reduction in the density of these receptors is a result of their rapid internalisation into the neuronal membrane (receptor sequestration), followed by their subsequent destruction. This phenomenon may have a bearing on the long-term efficacy of the administration cholinomimetic drugs and anticholinestersases for the symptomatic treatment of Alzheimer's disease. Although it is widely believed that the relapse in the response to treatment is due to the continuing neurodegenerative changes in the brain, which are unaffected by cholinomimetic drugs, it is also possible that such treatments could impair cholinergic function by causing an increased sequestration and destruction of muscarinic receptors.

The possible detrimental effect of cholinergic agonists on memory is supported by the observation that the chronic administration of physostigmine or oxotremorine to rats decreases the number of muscarinic receptors and leads to an impairment of memory when the drugs are withdrawn. Conversely, chronic treatment with a cholinergic antagonist such as atropine increases the number of cholinergic receptors and leads to a memory improvement when the drug is withdrawn. Whether these effects in experimental animals are relevant to the clinical situation in which cholinomimetic agents are administered for several months is unknown.

Although other transmitters, such as noradrenaline, serotonin and glutamate, are involved, there is now substantial evidence to suggest that muscarinic receptors play a key role in learning and memory. It is well established that muscarinic antagonists, such as atropine and scopolamine, impair memory and learning in man and that their effects can be reversed by anticholinesterases. Conversely, muscarinic agonists such as arecholine improve some aspects of learning and memory. However, some cholinomimetic drugs, such as carbachol, stimulate the inhibitory autoreceptors and thereby impair memory by blocking the release of acetylcholine in the hippocampus and cortex. Conversely, the selective autoreceptor antagonist secoverine enhances acetylcholine release and thereby improves memory.

In addition to the accumulation of senile plaques (abnormal beta amyloid containing proteins) and neurofibrillary tangles (modified microtublar associated proteins) which characterise Alzheimer's disease, the most consistent neuropathological finding is a degeneration of the projections from the main cholinergic cell body which comprise the nucleus basalis of Meynert. The degenerative changes involve the loss of cholinergic neurons containing M_1 and M_2 receptors, and a reduction in the activity of choline acetyltransferase (CAT), the rate-limiting enzyme for the synthesis of acetylcholine. The reduction in CAT and the associated neuronal loss in the basal forebrain are the most consistent correlates of cognitive impairment seen in Alzheimer's disease.

The treatment strategies are primarily aimed at increasing cholinergic transmission. These include the centrally acting reversible inhibitors of acetylcholinesterase, such as tacrine, donepezil, galanthamine and metrofinate. Physostigmine has also been used but its efficacy and peripheral side-effects have limited its widespread clinical use. Such drugs have beneficial effects in about 40% of patients; the patients show an improved score on several tests of cognitive function. However, even in those patients who do show some improvement following the administration of these drugs at an early stage in the development of the disease, the benefit is limited to approximately 18 months. Furthermore, gastrointestinal side-effects are often problematic.

Nicotinic receptors

Following studies of the actions of specific agonists and antagonists on the nicotinic receptors from skeletal muscle and sympathetic ganglia, it soon became apparent that not all nicotinic receptors are the same. The heterogeneity of the nicotinic receptors was further revealed by the application of molecular cloning techniques. This has led to the classification of nicotinic receptors into N-m receptors and N-n receptors, the former being located in the neuromuscular junction, where activation causes end-plate depolarisation and muscle contraction, while the latter are found in the autonomic ganglia (involved in ganglionic transmission), adrenal medulla (where activation causes catecholamine release) and in the brain, where their precise physiological importance is currently unclear. Of the specific antagonists that block these receptor subtypes, and which have clinical application, tubocurarine and related neuromuscular blockers inhibit the N-m type receptor, while the antihypertensive agent trimetaphan blocks the N-n receptor.

In contrast to the more numerous muscarinic receptors, much less is known about the function of nicotinic receptors in the brain. In addition to their distribution in the neuromuscular junction, ganglia and adrenal medulla, nicotinic receptors occur in a high density in the neocortex.

Nicotinic receptors are of the ionotropic type, which, on stimulation by acetylcholine, nicotine or related agonists, open to allow the passage of sodium ions into the neuron. There are structural differences between the peripheral and central receptors, the former being pentamers composed of two alpha and one beta, one gamma and one delta subunit, while the latter consist of single alpha and beta subunits. It is now known that there are at least four variants of the alpha and two of the beta subunits in the brain. In Alzheimer's disease it would appear that there is a selective reduction in the nicotinic receptors that contain the alpha 3 and 4 subunits.

Unlike the muscarinic receptors, repeated exposure of the neuronal receptors to nicotine, both *in vivo* and *in vitro*, results in an increase in the number of receptors; similar changes are reported to occur after physostigmine is administered directly into the cerebral ventricles of rats. These changes in the density of the nicotinic receptors are accompanied by an increased release of acetylcholine. Following the chronic administration of physostigmine, however, a desensitisation of the receptors occurs.

Functionally, nicotinic receptors appear to be involved in memory formation; in clinical studies it has been shown that nicotine can reverse the effects of scopolamine on short-term working memory and both nicotine and arecholine have been shown to have positive, though modest, effects on cognition in patients with Alzheimer's disease.

Adrenergic receptors

Ahlquist, in 1948, first proposed that noradrenaline could produce its diverse physiological effects by acting on different populations of adrenoceptors, which he termed α- and β-receptors. This classification was based upon the relative selectivity of adrenaline for the α-receptors and isoprenaline for the β-receptors; drugs such as phentolamine were found to be specific antagonists of the α-receptors, and propranolol for the β-receptors.

The adrenergic receptors have been purified and their genes cloned. They have seven membrane-spanning units, which are involved in binding the selective agonists and antagonists.

Alpha receptors

It later became possible to separate these main groups of receptors further, into α_1 and α_2, based on the selectivity of the antagonists prazosin (the antihypertensive agent that blocks α_1-receptors) and yohimbine (which is an antagonist of α_2-receptors).

At one time it was thought that α_1-receptors were postsynaptic and the α_2 type were presynaptic and concerned with the inhibitory control of noradrenaline release. Indeed, novel antidepressants like mianserin, and more recently the highly selective α_2-receptor antagonist idazoxan, were thought to act by stimulating the release of noradrenaline from central noradrenergic synapses. It is now established, however, that the α_2-receptors also occur postsynaptically, and that their stimulation by such specific agonists as clonidine leads to a reduction in the activity of the vasomotor centre, thereby leading to a decrease in blood pressure.

The α_1-receptors are excitatory in their action, while α_2-receptors are inhibitory, owing to the different types of second messengers or ion channels to which they are linked. Thus, α_2-receptors hyperpolarise presynaptic membranes by opening potassium ion channels, and thereby reduce noradrenaline release. Conversely, stimulation of α_1-receptors increases intracellular calcium via the phosphatidyl inositol cycle, which causes the release of calcium from its intracellular stores; protein kinase C activity is increased as a result of the free calcium, which then brings about further changes in the membrane activity.

Both types of receptor occur in the brain as well as in vascular and intestinal smooth muscle: α_1-receptors are found in the heart, whereas the α_2-receptors occur on the platelet membrane (where stimulation induces aggregation) and nerve terminals (where stimulation inhibits release of the transmitter). There are several subtypes of α_1- and α_2-receptors but their precise function is unclear.

Beta receptors

So far three subtypes of β-receptors have been identified and cloned. They differ in their distribution, the β_1 type being found in the heart, the β_2 in the lungs, smooth muscle, skeletal muscle and liver, while the β_3 type occurs in adipose tissue. There are β_2-adrenoceptors on the lymphocyte membrane but their precise function is presently unknown.

The antihypertensive drug metoprolol is a clinically effective example of a β_1 antagonist. All the β-receptor subtypes are linked to adenylate cyclase as the second messenger system. It seems that both β_1- and β_2-receptor types occur in the brain and that their activation leads to excitatory effects. Of particular interest to the psychopharmacologist is the finding that chronic antidepressant treatment leads to a decrease in the functional responsiveness of the β-receptors in the brain, and in the density of these receptors on lymphoctyes. Moreover, the timing of these changes coincides with the time necessary for the therapeutic effects of the drugs to be manifest. Such changes have been ascribed to the drugs affecting the activity of the G-proteins that couple the receptor to the cyclase subunit.

Dopamine receptors

Two types of dopamine receptors have been characterised in the mammalian brain, and these have been termed D_1 and D_2. This subtyping largely arose in response to the finding that while all types of clinically useful neuroleptics inhibit dopaminergic transmission in the brain, there is a poor correlation between reduction in adenylate cyclase activity, believed to be the second messenger linked to dopamine receptors, and the clinical potency of the drugs. This was particularly true for the butyrophenone series (e.g. haloperidol), members of which are known to be potent neuroleptics and yet are relatively poor at inhibiting adenylate cyclase.

Detailed studies of the binding ^{3}H-labelled haloperidol to neuronal membranes showed that there was a much better correlation between the therapeutic potency of a neuroleptic and its ability to displace this ligand from the nerve membrane. This led to the discovery of two types of dopamine receptor: the D_1 receptor which is positively linked to adenylate cyclase, and the D_2 receptor which is negatively linked to it. It was also shown that the D_1 receptor is approximately 15 times more sensitive to the action of dopamine than the D_2 receptor; conversely, the D_1 receptor has a low affinity for the butyrophenones and atypical neuroleptics such as clozapine, whereas the D_2 receptor appears to have a high affinity for most therapeutically active antipsychotics.

There is still some controversy over the precise anatomical location of the dopamine receptor subtypes, but there is now evidence that the D_2 receptors are located presynaptically on the corticostriatal neurons and postsynaptically in the striatum and substantia nigra. Conversely, the D_1 receptors are found presynaptically on nigrostriatal neurons, and postsynaptically in the cortex. It is possible to differentiate these receptor types on the basis of their agonist and antagonist affinities.

In addition to these two subtypes, there is also evidence that the release of dopamine is partially regulated by feedback inhibition operating via the dopamine autoreceptor.

With the development of D_1 and D_2 agonists, however, emphasis has become centred on the pharmacological characteristics of the specific drug in order to determine whether an observed effect is mediated by D_1 or D_2 receptors. It is now apparent that dopamine receptors with the same pharmacological characteristics do not necessarily produce the same functional responses at the same receptor. For example, D_2 receptors are present in both the striatum and the nucleus accumbens, but cause an inhibition of adenylate cyclase only in the striatum.

Furthermore, recent studies indicate that dopamine receptors can influence cellular activities through mechanisms other than that involving adenylate cyclase. These may include direct effects on potassium and calcium channels, as well as modulation of the phosphatidyl inositol cycle. To complicate the picture further, D_1 and D_2 receptors have opposite effects on some behaviours (e.g. chewing in rats) but are synergistic in causing other behaviours (e.g. locomotor activity and some types of stereotypy). The precise clinical importance of these interactions is unclear.

The densities and functional activities of dopamine receptors have been shown to change in response to chronic drug treatment and in disease. Thus, an increase in dopamine receptor density in the nigro-striatal pathway appears to be related to the behavioural supersensitivity observed following unilateral destruction of the dopaminergic system in the striatum. Dopamine receptor antagonists, such as the 'classical' antipsychotics like chlorpromazine, are also known to increase the density (number) of dopamine receptors in the striatal region. This contributes to the extrapyramidal side-effects of such drugs, which frequently follow their prolonged use and reflect the drug-induced functional deficit of dopamine in the brain. Abrupt withdrawal of a neuroleptic after its prolonged administration is frequently associated with tardive dyskinesia, a disorder that may be partly due to the sudden activation of an increased number of dopamine receptors, thereby leading to an increased receptor response. Despite the appeal of this hypothesis, it should be emphasised that many other factors, such as brain damage and prior exposure to tricyclic antidepressants, may also predispose patients to this condition.

With regard to the change in dopamine receptor activity in disease, there is some evidence from post-mortem studies that the density of D_2 receptors is increased in the mesocortical areas of the schizophrenic brain, and in the putamen and caudate nucleus in neuroleptic-free patients. Positron emission tomography of people with schizophrenia has, however, failed to confirm these findings. There is also evidence that the link between the D_1 and D_2 receptors is defective in some patients with diseases in which the dopaminergic system might be involved. Thus the well-known loss of dopaminergic function in patients with Parkinson's disease is associated with a compensatory rise in the density of postsynaptic D_1 and D_2 receptors. The long-term treatment of Parkinson's disease with L-dopa reduces the receptor density to normal (so-called receptor 'down-regulation'). Similarly, the densities of D_1 and D_2 receptors are reduced in the striata of patients with Huntington's chorea, as is the linkage between these receptors.

Dopamine has been implicated in a number of psychiatric conditions, of which schizophrenia and the affective disorders are the most widely established.

Five major subtypes of dopamine receptors have now been cloned. These are divided into two main groups, D_1 and D_2, respectively. The D_1 group of receptors consist of the D_1 and D_5 types and are positively linked to the adenylate cyclase second messenger system, while the D_2 group consist of the D_2, D_3 and D_4 receptors, which are negatively linked to the adenylate cyclase system.

The D_1 receptors have been subdivided into the D_{1A} and D_{1B} types and are coded by genes located on chromosomes 5 and 4, respectively. Several selective antagonists of the D_1 receptors have been developed (e.g. SCH 31966, SCH 23390 and SKF 83959), none of which has so far been developed for therapeutic use.

Apomorphine is an agonist at both D_1 and D_2 receptors. From the pathological viewpoint, a malfunction of the D_1 receptors has been implicated in the negative symptoms of schizophrenia, but as there is a close interaction between these receptor types it is difficult to conclude whether the primary changes seen in schizophrenia are attributable to a primary decrease in D_1 receptor function or an increase in D_2 receptor function. The function of the D_5 receptors is unclear; these receptors, although widely distributed in the brain, are present at a low density in comparison with the other dopamine receptor types.

The D_2 receptor types, besides being subdivided in D_3 and D_4 types, are further divided into the D_2-long and D_2-short forms. D_2 antagonists, in addition to virtually all therapeutically active neuroleptics, also include such novel drugs as raclopride, eticlopride and sniperone, while quinpirole is an example of a specific D_2 receptor agonist. These drugs are not available for therapeutic use. A malfunction of the D_2 receptors has been associated with psychosis, extrapyramidal side-effects and with hyperprolactinaemia.

The human D_3 gene has produced two variants, D_3 and D_{3S}. So far there do not appear to be any selective agonists or antagonists of the D_3 receptor that enable the function of this receptor to be clearly distinguished from that of the D_2 receptor. The D_3 receptors are located in the ventral and limbic regions of the brain but are absent from the dorsal striatum. This suggests that specific antagonists of the D_3 receptors may be effective antipsychotics but without causing extra-pyramidal side-effects.

The D_4 receptor has eight polymorphic variants in the human. However, even though several specific antagonists of this receptor type have been developed and shown to have antipsychotic activity in animal models of schizophrenia, the clinical findings have been disappointing. Because of the high density of the D_4 receptors in the limbic cortex and hippocampus, and its absence from the motor regions of the brain, it was anticipated that such drugs would show antipsychotic efficacy without causing motor side-effects. In support of this view, it has been shown that the atypical antipsychotic clozapine has a high affinity for

D_4 receptors; other studies have also indicated that many of the atypical, and some of the typical, antipsychotics have similar affinities for these receptors.

In addition to the postsynaptic receptors, dopamine autoreceptors also exist on the nerve terminals, dendrites and cell bodies. Experimental studies have shown that stimulation of the autoreceptors in the somatodendritic region of the neuron slows the firing rate of the dopaminergic neuron, while stimulation of the autoreceptors on the nerve terminal inhibits both the release and the synthesis of the neurotransmitter. Structurally, the autoreceptor appears to be of the D_2 type. While several experimental compounds have been developed that show a high affinity for the autoreceptors, to date there is no convincing evidence for their therapeutic efficacy.

Serotonin receptors

Gaddum and Picarelli, in 1957, were the first investigators to provide evidence for the existence of two types of serotonin (5-hydroxytryptamine, 5-HT) receptor in peripheral smooth muscle (see Gaddum, 1954). These receptors were termed D (for dibenzyline, an α_1-adrenoceptor antagonist which also blocks serotonin receptors) and M (for morphine, which blocks the contractile response mediated through the myenteric plexus in the intestinal wall). Studies undertaken in the 1980s revealed the existence of multiple binding sites for serotonin receptors. The D receptor was shown to have the characteristics of the 5-HT$_2$ receptor, while the M receptor was shown to be identical to the 5-HT$_3$ receptor in the brain and gastrointestinal tract.

Serotonin contributes to the regulation of a variety of psychological phenomena, including mood, arousal, attention, impulsivity, aggression, appetite, pain perception and cognition. In addition, it plays a crucial role in regulating the sleep–wake cycle and in the control of brain maturation. It is therefore understandable that a dysfunction of the serotonergic system has been implicated in a variety of psychiatric disorders, such as schizophrenia, depression, alcoholism and phobic states. Undoubtedly, interest in the role of the serotonergic system in psychiatry has been stimulated by the therapeutic success of the selective serotonin reuptake inhibititors (SSRIs), which have proved to be effective in alleviating the symptoms of many of these disorders.

The complexity of the serotonergic system lies in the number of different serotonin receptors within the brain. These are classified into seven distinct types, which are heterogeneously distributed in the brain, and each of which has a specific physiological function, as a consequence of its structure. For example, 5-HT$_3$ receptors are ionotropic in nature (and therefore directly linked to the ion-conducting channel on the neuronal membrane), whereas the remainder are metabotropic, are coupled to specific G-proteins and share a common seven-membrane domain structure.

Serotonin receptors have been cloned and their physiological activity shown to be associated with the activation of either phospholipase C (5-HT$_{2A-C}$ receptors) or adenylate cyclase (5-HT$_{4-7}$). The 5-HT$_{1A}$, 5-HT$_{1B}$ and 5-HT$_{1D}$ receptors are also coupled to adenylate cyclase but they inhibit the function of this second messenger system. It should be noted that 5-HT$_{1C}$ receptors have been reclassified as 5-HT$_{2C}$ on the grounds of their structure and function.

Although the precise physiological activity of the different serotonin receptors is still the subject of ongoing studies, links between specific receptor subtypes and their possible involvement in specific neurological and psychiatric disorders have been identified. For example, the antimigraine drug sumatriptan decreases headache by activating the inhibitory 5-HT$_{1B}$-receptors located presynaptically on perivascular nerve fibres. This blocks the release of pain-causing neuropeptides and conduction in the trigeminal vascular neurons.

With regard to the 5-HT$_{1A}$ receptors, agonists such as buspirone and ipsapirone act as anxiolytics, while the antidepressant effects of the SSRIs have been associated with an indirect reduction in the activity of this receptor subtype. Conversely, the sexual side-effects of the SSRIs is attributed to their indirect action on 5-HT$_{2C}$ receptors, which follows the enhanced serotonergic function; these receptors may also be involved in the regulation of food intake, which could help to explain the antibulimic action of the SSRIs.

Several types of serotonin receptor (e.g. 5-HT$_{1A}$, 5-HT$_{2A}$, 5-HT$_{2C}$, 5-HT$_{1B/1D}$) have been associated with the motor side-effects of the SSRIs, which may arise if these drugs are administered in conjunction with a monoamine oxidase inhibitor.

The 5-HT$_3$ receptor is an example of a non-selective cation channel receptor which is permeable to both sodium and potassium ions, and because both calcium and magnesium ions can modulate its activity, it resembles the glutamate N-methyl-D-aspartate (NMDA) receptor (on which, see below). Antagonists of the 5-HT$_3$ receptor, such as ondansetron, are effective anti-emetics and are particularly useful when nausea is associated with the administration of cytotoxic drugs or some anaesthetic agents. However, they are ineffective against the nausea of motion sickness or that induced by apomorphine, which suggests that 5-HT$_3$ receptors function at the level of the vomiting centre in the brain. In addition, there is evidence from experimental studies that these receptors are involved in anxiety and in cognition. 5-HT$_3$ antagonists have both anxiolytic and cognitive enhancing properties but it still remains to be proven that such properties are therapeutically relevant.

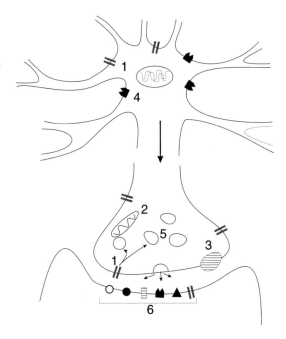

Fig. 1.5 Sites of action of various types of psychotropic drugs on the cell body, neuronal terminal and synaptic sites in the brain.

(1) Amine reuptake site, including the binding site for tricyclic antidepressants, where tricyclic antidepressants, SSRI antidepressants and dual-action antidepressants (e.g. venlafaxine) act.

(2) Monoamine oxidase, the site of action of MAO inhibitors.

(3) Autoreceptor, which, when activated by excessive amine concentration in the synaptic cleft, reduces the mobilisation of calcium ions in the neuronal terminal and reduces the release of neurotransmitter from the terminal.

(4) 5-HT$_{1A}$ receptors located on the cell body. These are the site of action of novel anxiolytics such as buspirone. Stimulation of these receptors results in a reduction in the release of serotonin from the neuronal terminal. The 5-HT$_{1A}$ receptors are desensitised following the chronic administration of SSRI antidepressants, thereby enhancing the release of serotonin.

(5) Synaptic vesicles that store the biogenic amine neurotransmitter. On activation, the vesicles move to the terminal and in the presence of calcium ions fuse to the synaptic membrane and release their contents into the synaptic cleft.

(6) Second messenger and tertiary messenger systems are linked to the array of postsynaptic receptors. Tertiary messengers link the second messenger signals (cAMP, cGMP, etc.) to other enzymes (such as phosphokinases) that phosphorylate membrane proteins to open ion channels, activate gene transcription factors, etc. On activation by the different types of neurotransmitters, the activation of these messengers results in the phosphorylation of the membrane-linked ion channels that result in the depolarisation of the postsynaptic membrane. The tertiary messengers also activate the synthesis of nerve growth factors (e.g. brain-derived neurotropic factor), leading to neuronal sprouting, repair and possibly synaptogenesis.

The precise function of the 5-HT$_{4-7}$ receptors is less certain. All of these receptors have been cloned and their distribution in the brain determined. There is some evidence that 5-HT$_4$ receptors act as heteroreceptors on cholinergic terminals and thereby modulate the release of acetylcholine. While the physiological role of the 5-HT$_{5-7}$ receptors is unclear, it is of interest to note that several atypical antipsychotics, such as clozapine, and several antidepressants have a good affinity for these receptors. There is also evidence that selective agonists and antagonists, such as zacopride, ergotamine, methysergide and LSD, have a high affinity for the 5-HT$_4$ and 5-HT$_5$ receptors, but how these effects relate to their pharmacological actions is presently unknown.

Fig. 1.5 summarises the possible sites of action of different classes of psychotropic drugs on the serotonin receptors in the brain.

Clearly, much remains to be learned about the distribution and functional activity of these receptor subtypes before their possible roles in mental illness can be elucidated. A summary of the distribution of the different types of serotonin receptors and their agonists is shown in Table 1.2.

Amino acid receptors

There are two amino acid neurotransmitters, namely GABA and glutamate, which have been of major interest to the psychopharmacologist because of the potential therapeutic importance of their agonists and antagonists. The receptors upon which GABA and glutamate act to produce their effects differ from the 'classical' transmitter receptors in that they seem to exist as receptor complexes that contain separate sites for agonists, in addition to sites for the amino acid transmitters; these sites for agonists, when occupied, modulate the responsiveness of the receptor to the amino acid. For example, the benzodiazepines have long been known to facilitate inhibitory transmission, and their therapeutic properties as anxiolytics and anticonvulsants are attributable to this. It is now apparent that benzodiazepines occupy a site on the GABA receptor complex which enhances that receptor's responsiveness to the inhibitory action of GABA. Similarly, it has recently been shown that the inhibitory transmitter glycine can act on a strychnine-insensitive site on the NMDA receptor and thereby modify its responsiveness to glutamate.

Knowledge of the mechanisms whereby the amino acid transmitters produce their effects has been valuable in the development of psychotropic drugs that may improve memory, reduce anxiety, or even counteract the effects of post-stroke hypoxia on brain cell survival. Some of these aspects are considered below.

Table 1.2 Summary of the properties of serotonin receptor subtypes in the mammalian brain

Receptor subtype	Second messenger	Location	Ligands	Physiological/pathological effects
5-HT$_{1A}$	Cyclic AMP?	Hippocampus, raphé, cortex	8-OH-DPAT, ipsapirone, gepirone, buspirone*, pindolol*	Anxiety, depression appetite, aggression, pain, sexual behaviour
5-HT$_{1B}$ [a]	Cyclic AMP?			?
5-HT$_{1C}$ [b]	PI?	Choroid plexus	Methiopin*, mesulergine*, ritanserin* Metergoline*	Appetite, anxiety, mood
5-HT$_{1D}$ [c]	Cyclic AMP?	Cortex, olfactory system, claustrum	DOI, DOM, LSD, ketanserin, sergolexole	Vasoconstriction, appetite
5-HT$_2$ [c]	PI?			
5-HT$_3$	Ion channel	Area postrema; cortex (low-density) vagal efferents	M-chlorophenylbiguanide, ondansetron, granisetron, raclopride	Emesis, anxiety, pain, cognition?
5-HT$_4$	Cyclic AMP?	Superior colliculi, hippocampus	ICS 205-930, renzapride, cisapride, metoclopramide*, 5-methoxytryptamine	Arrhythmia, atrial fibrillation, cognition?
5-HT$_5$	?	Cortex, hippocampus, olfactory bulb, cerebellum	2-bromo-LSD, ergotamine, methysergide	Similar to 5-HT$_{1D}$
5-HT$_{5B}$	?	Habenula, hippocampus	LSD, dihydrolergotamine, methysergide, methiothepin	?
5-HT$_6$	Cyclic AMP	Striatum, amygdala, cortex	Clozapine, amoxapine, clomipramine, amitriptyline	?
5-HT$_7$	Cyclic AMP	Hypothalamus, hippocampus cortex, olfactory bulb	LSD, clozapine, loxapine, amitriptyline	?

a 5-HT$_{1B}$ and 5-HT$_{1D}$ receptors are structurally and functionally similar and act as inhibitory presynaptic receptors. 5-HT$_{1B}$ receptors occur in most mammalian brains, whereas 5-HT$_{1D}$ receptors are located in primates and the guinea pig brain.
b Now classified as 5-HT$_{2C}$.
c Now classified as 5-HT$_{2A}$.
*Indicates ligand is non-selective and also acts on other 5-HT, and possibly non-5-HT, receptors.
Italic indicates compounds in therapeutic use.
PI, phosphatidyl inositol; DOI, (2,5-dimethoxy-1-iodophenyl)-2-aminopropane; DOM, dimethoxy-methamphetamine; AMP, adenosine monophosphate.

Inhibitory amino acid receptors: GABA receptors

The major amino acid neurotransmitters in the brain are GABA, an inhibitory transmitter, and glutamic acid, an excitatory transmitter. GABA is widely distributed in the mammalian brain and has been calculated to be present in over 40% of the synapses in the cortex alone. While it is evident that a reduction in GABAergic activity is associated with seizures, and that most anticonvulsant drugs either directly or indirectly facilitate GABAergic transmission, GABA also has a fundamental role in the brain by shaping, integrating and refining information transfer generated by the excitatory transmitters. Indeed, because of its wide anatomical distribution, GABA may be involved in such diverse functions as vigilance, consciousness, arousal, thermo-regulation, learning, food consumption, hormonal control, motor control and pain control.

At the cellular level, GABA is located in the interneurons. GABAergic neurons project both locally and, by long axons, to more distant regions of the brain. For example, GABAergic neurons project from the neostriatum to the substantia nigra.

As with the biogenic amine neurotransmitters, the synthesis of GABA is highly regulated. GABA is synthesised from glutamate by an enzyme, glutamate decarboxylase. This enzyme is involved in the rate-limiting step, as its activity is dependent on the pyridoxal phosphate cofactor; it has been estimated that at least 50% of glutamate decarboxylase present in the brain is not bound to cofactor and is therefore inactive.

Newly synthesised GABA is stored in vesicles in the nerve terminal and, following its release, its action is terminated by a reuptake mechanism into the glial cells which surround the neuron, and also into the nerve terminal. GABA is then metabolised by GABA trans-aminase to succinic semialdehyde (a component of what is termed the GABA-shunt pathway), and thence to the tricarboxylic acid cycle to generate metabolic energy. Thus GABA differs substantially from the conventional biogenic amine transmitters in that it is largely metabolised once it has been released during neurotransmission.

Of the many drugs that have been developed which modulate GABA function, the inhibitors of GABA transaminase have been shown to be effective anticonvulsants. These are derivatives of valproic acid that not only inhibit the metabolism of GABA but may also act as antagonists of the GABA autoreceptor and thereby enhance the release of the neurotransmitter. GABA uptake inhibitors have been developed (e.g. derivatives of nipecotic acid, guvacine) which also have anti-convulsant activity, at least in experimental animals. However, the major development in the pharmacology of the GABAergic system has been in drugs that facilitate the functioning of the $GABA_A$ receptors. These are discussed below.

There are three types of GABA receptor, A, B and C. Unlike the ionotropic $GABA_A$ receptors, the $GABA_B$ receptors are metabotropic and are coupled via inhibitory G-proteins to adenylate cyclase. Not only do the $GABA_B$ receptors inhibit the second messenger but they also modulate potassium and calcium channels in the neuronal membrane. Baclofen, the antispastic drug, owes it therapeutic efficacy to its agonistic action on these receptors, while phaclofen, an experimental drug, acts as an antagonist. Unlike drugs that act on $GABA_A$ receptors, $GABA_B$ receptor agonists have antinociceptive properties, which may account for the efficacy of drugs like baclofen in the treatment of trigeminal neuralgia. Experimental studies suggest that $GABA_B$ antagonists may have anti-epileptic activity. $GABA_B$ receptors are widely distributed throughout the brain and in several peripheral organs. Their distribution differs from that of $GABA_A$ receptors. In the cortex and several other brain regions, $GABA_B$ receptors occur on the terminals of both GABA and non-GABA neurons, where they modulate neurotransmitter release.

The $GABA_C$ receptors have only recently been identified and their function is still uncertain. There is evidence that, besides GABA, the GABA receptor agonists muscimol and isoguvacine have a high affinity for these receptors. A high density of $GABA_C$ receptors has been detected in the retina, where they appear to be involved in the development of retinal rod cells. In the brain, there is evidence that $GABA_C$ receptors are concentrated in the superior colliculus, where they have a disinhibitory role. There is also evidence that they play an important role in some aspects of neuroendocrine regulation, both in the gastrointestinal tract and in the secretion of thyroid-stimulating hormone.

The $GABA_A$ receptors have been cloned and the structures of some of the 10 subtypes of this receptor have been described. As these subtypes appear to be heterogeneously distributed throughout the brain, it may ultimately be possible to develop drugs that will affect only one specific species of $GABA_A$ receptor, thereby optimising the therapeutic effect and reducing the possibility of non-specific side-effects. It seems likely that this will be an important area for psychotropic drug development in the near future.

The $GABA_A$ receptor is directly linked to chloride ion channels, activation of which results in an increase in the membrane permeability to chloride ions, and thereby the hyperpolarisation of cell bodies. $GABA_A$ receptors are also found extrasynaptically, where, following activation, they can depolarise neurons. The convulsant drug bicuculline acts as a specific antagonist of GABA on its receptor site, while the convulsant drug picrotoxin binds to an adjacent site on the $GABA_A$ receptor complex and directly decreases chloride ion flux; barbiturates have the opposite effect on the chloride channel and lock the channel open.

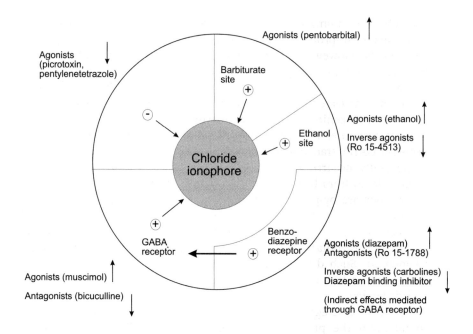

Fig. 1.6 Diagrammatic representation of the GABA–benzodiazepine supramolecular complex. Compounds that increase inhibitory transmission may do so either by directly activating the GABA receptor site (e.g. muscimol) or by acting directly on the chloride ionophore (e.g. barbiturates). Benzodizepines (e.g. diazepam) enhance the sensitivity of the GABA$_A$ receptor to GABA. Compounds that decrease inhibitory transmission may do so by activating the picotoxin site, which closes the chloride ionophore, or by blocking the GABA$_A$ receptor.

The inhibitory effect of GABA is mediated by the chloride ion channel (Fig. 1.6). When the GABA$_A$ receptor is activated by GABA or a specific agonist such as muscimol, the frequency of opening of the channel is increased and the cell is hyperpolarised. Barbiturates such as phenobarbitone, and possibly alcohol, also facilitate the chloride ion influx, but these drugs increase the duration rather than the frequency of channel opening. Recently, novel benzodiazepine receptor ligands have been produced which, like the typical benzodiazepines, increase the frequency of chloride channel opening. The cyclopyrrolone sedative/hypnotic zopiclone is an example of such a ligand. Some glucocorticoids are also known to have sedative effects, which may be ascribed to their ability to activate specific steroid receptor facilitatory sites on the GABA$_A$ receptor.

In addition to the benzodiazepine receptor agonists, which, depending on the dose administered, have anxiolytic, anticonvulsant, sedative and amnestic properties, benzodiazepines have also been developed which block the action of agonists on this receptor. Such antagonists may be exemplified by flumazenil. Other compounds have a mixture of agonist and antagonist properties and are termed partial agonists or partial antagonists. However, the complexity of the benzodiazepine receptor became fully apparent only recently, when a series of compounds was discovered that had the opposite effects of the 'classical' benzodiazepines when they activated the receptor. These inverse agonists were found to have anxiogenic, proconvulsant, stimulant, spasmogenic and pro-mnestic properties in man and animals. Such compounds were found to decrease GABA transmission.

Naturally occurring inverse agonists called the β-carbolines have been isolated from human urine, but it now seems probable that these compounds are by-products of the extraction procedure.

Thus, the benzodiazepine receptor is unique in that it has a bidirectional function. This may be of considerable importance in the design of benzodiazepine ligands which act as partial agonists (see Chapter 5). Such drugs may combine the efficacy of the conventional agents with a lack of unwanted side-effects, such as sedation, amnesia and dependence.

Partial inverse agonists have also been described. Such drugs appear to maintain the promnestic properties of the full inverse agonists without causing excessive stimulation and convulsions, which can occur with full inverse agonsits.

The presence of a specific benzodiazepine site in the mammalian brain also raises the possibility that endogenous substances are present that modulate the activity of the site. While the precise identity of such natural ligands remains an enigma, there is evidence that substances like tribulin, nephentin and a peptide called the diazepam-binding inhibitor could have a physiological and pathological function. There is also evidence that trace amounts of benzodiazepines (such as nordiazepine and lorazepam) occur in human brain, human breast milk and also in many plants, including the potato. Such benzodiazepines have been found in post-mortem examinations of brains from the 1940s and 1950s, before the discovery of the benzodiazepine anxiolytics.

Modulation of GABA$_A$ receptors

During brain development, the RNA expression of the subunits that comprise the GABA$_A$ receptor change, so that each subunit exhibits a unique regional and temporal profile. Such changes may reflect the increase in the sensitivity of the foetal brain to GABA, and its decreased sensitivity to the benzodiazepines which indirectly enhance GABA$_A$ receptor function. Thus, during the later stages of development of the foetal brain, at a stage when the synapses are present, GABA acts as a neurotrophic factor that promotes neuronal growth and differentiation, synaptogenesis and the synthesis of GABA$_A$ receptors. This may account for the increased sensitivity of these receptors to the actions of GABA, as the concentration of the transmitter in the developing brain is relatively low. GABA has to diffuse to receptors that are relatively far from the neurons from which it is released, and the increased sensitivity of the GABA$_A$ receptors ensures that they are activated even by a low concentration of the transmitter.

Changes have also been reported to occur in the subunit composition of the GABA$_A$ receptor following chronic exposure to barbiturates, neurosteroids, alcohol and benzodiazepine agonists. These changes may underlie the development of tolerance, physical dependence and the problems that are associated with the abrupt withdrawal of such drugs.

Excitatory amino acid receptors: glutamate receptor

It has long been recognised that glutamic and aspartic acids occur in uniquely high concentrations in the mammalian brain and that they can cause excitation of nerve cells. However, these amino acids have only recently been identified as excitatory neurotransmitters, as a result of both microdialysis and micro-iontophoretic techniques, by which release of these agents and the effect of their local application could be demonstrated, and the synthesis and isolation of specific agonists for the different types of excitatory amino acid receptor (e.g. quisqualic, ibotenic and kainic acids).

Glutamate is uniformly distributed throughout the mammalian brain. Unlike the biogenic amine transmitters, glutamate has an important metabolic role as well as a neurotransmitter role in the brain (which made its identification as a neurotransmitter the more difficult). For example, glutamate is an important component of brain proteins and peptides, and is a precursor of GABA. In addition, it is metabolised to alpha-ketoglutaric acid as part of the the tricarboxylic acid cycle. In nerve terminals, glutamate is stored in vesicles and released by calcium-dependent exocytosis. Specific glutamate transporters move the amino acid from the synaptic cleft to both the nerve terminals and the surrounding glial cells.

Four main types of glutamate receptor have been identified and cloned. These are the three ionotropic receptor types – the NMDA, alpha-amino-3-hydroxy-5-methylisoxazole (AMPA) and kainate ones – and a group of metabotropic receptors, of which eight subtypes have been discovered. Of the ionotropic group, AMPA and kainate receptors are involved in fast excitatory transmission, whereas the NMDA receptors (unlike other ionotropic receptors) mediate slower excitatory responses and play a more complex role in mediating synaptic plasticity.

The NMDA receptors are heteromeric pentamers composed of at least one NR1 subunit and one or more of the four different NR2 subunits: NR2A, NR2B, NR2C and NR2D. The different isoforms of the NR2 subunits give rise to structurally different glutamate receptors in the brain. The functional significance of these different receptor

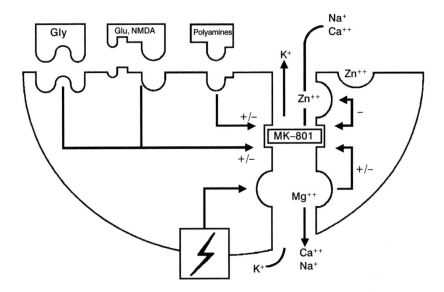

Fig. 1.7 Schematic model of the NMDA receptor. The flow of ions through the channel of the NMDA receptor can be regulated by a variety of factors. Glycine (Gly) and glutamate (Glu) must both bind to the NMDA receptor to cause opening of the ion channel. Polyamines bind to a distinct recognition site on the receptor to regulate the opening of the ion channel. Compounds such as MK-801 appear to bind in the open channel. At physiological concentrations of Mg^{++}, the channel is blocked unless the membrane is depolarised. Zn^{++} also regulates the opening of the ion channel (Leonard, 2003: p. 58. © 2003 John Wiley & Sons Ltd. Reproduced with permission).

subtypes is presently unclear. The subunits comprising the AMPA and kainate receptors, termed GluR1–7 and KA1,2, are closely related.

The NMDA receptors are unique among the ligand-gated cation channel receptors in that they are permeable to calcium but blocked by magnesium, the latter acting at a specific receptor site within the ion channel (Fig. 1.7). The purpose of the voltage-dependent magnesium blockade of the ion channel is to permit the summation of excitatory postsynaptic potentials. Once these have reached a critical point, the magnesium blockade of the ion channel is terminated and calcium flows into the neuron, to activate the calcium-dependent second messengers. Such a mechanism would appear to be particularly important for the induction of long-term potentiation, a process which underlies short-term memory in the hippocampus.

With regard to the action of psychotropic drugs on NMDA receptors, there is evidence that one of the actions of the anticonvulsant lamotrigine is to modulate glutamatergic function; the antidementia drug memantine has a similar action. Thus, the therapeutic efficacy of some of the newer drugs used to treat epilepsy and Alzheimer's disease arises from their ability to modulate a dysfunctional glutamatergic system.

Some of the hallucinogens related to the dissociation anaesthetic ketamine, such as phencyclidine, block the ion channel of the NMDA receptor. Whether the hallucinogenic actions of phencyclidine are primarily due to this action is uncertain, as the putative anticonvulsant dizocilpine (MK–801) is also an NMDA ion channel inhibitor but is not a notable hallucinogen. Presumably the ability of phencyclidine to enhance dopamine release, possibly by activating NMDA heteroceptors on dopaminergic terminals, and also its action on σ receptors, which it shares with benzomorphan-like hallucinogens, contribute to its hallucinogenic activity. The σ receptors are thought to modulate NMDA receptor function by activating the glycine-sensitive site on the NMDA receptor. Three types of σ receptor have been identified, of which σ_1 and σ_2 types occur in the brain. Dystonic side-effects of some SSRI antidepressants may be due to activation of the σ_2 receptors in the rubro-cerebellar area of the brain.

In contrast to the ionotropic receptors, the metabotropic receptors are monomeric in structure and are unique in that they show no structural similarity to the other neurotransmitter receptors coupled to G-protein. They are located both pre- and postsynaptically and there is experimental evidence that they are involved in synaptic modulation and excitotoxicity, functions that are also shared with the NMDA receptors. To date, no drugs have been developed for therapeutic use that are based on the modulation of these receptors.

The NMDA receptor complex has been extensively characterised and its anatomical distribution in the brain has been determined. The NMDA receptor is analogous to the $GABA_A$ receptor in that it contains several binding sites, in addition to the glutamate site, whereby the movement of sodium and calcium ions into the nerve cell can be modulated.

These sites include a regulatory site that binds glycine, a site which is insensitive to the antagonistic effects of strychnine. This contrasts with the action of glycine on glycine receptors in the spinal cord, where strychnine, on blocking the receptor, causes the characteristic tonic seizures.

In addition to the glutamate and glycine sites on the NMDA receptor, there are also polyamine sites, which are activated by the naturally occurring polyamines spermine and spermidine. Specific divalent cation sites are also associated with the NMDA receptor, namely the voltage-dependent magnesium site and the inhibitory zinc site. In addition to the excitatory amino acids, the natural metabolite of brain tryptophan, quinolinic acid, can also act as an agonist of the NMDA receptor and may contribute to nerve cell death at high concentrations.

Interest in the therapeutic potential of drugs acting on the NMDA receptor has risen with the discovery that epilepsy and related convulsive states may occur as a consequence of a sudden release of glutamate. Sustained seizures of the limbic system in animals result in brain damage that resembles the changes seen in glutamate toxicity. Similar changes are seen at autopsy in patients with intractable epilepsy. It has been shown that the non-competitive NMDA antagonists, such as phencyclidine and ketamine, can block glutamate-induced damage. The novel anti-epileptic drug lamotrigine would also appear to act by this mechanism, in addition to its ability to block sodium channels, in common with many other types of anti-epileptic drugs.

In addition to epilepsy, neuronal death due to the toxic effects of glutamate has also been implicated in cerebral ischaemia associated with multi-infarct dementia and possibly Alzheimer's disease. With the plethora of selective excitatory amino acid receptor antagonists which are currently undergoing development, some of which are already in clinical trials, one may expect definite advances in the drug treatment of neurodegenerative disorders in the near future.

Substance P and related neurokinins

Substance P was discovered in 1931, but its physiological role has only recently become apparent. Substance P, and the neurokinins A and B, exert their physiological actions by activating the neurokinin receptor NK_1, NK_2 or NK_3 respectively. Preclinical studies have suggested the therapeutic potential of neurokinin antagonists for the treatment of pain, migraine, schizophrenia, depression and anxiety disorder. In preclinical trials NK_1 receptor antagonists have shown limited efficacy as antidepressants and antiemetics. More detailed studies of NK antagonists are essential before any conclusions can be made on their therapeutic value.

Nitric oxide – an important gaseous neurotransmitter

The discovery that mammalian cells generate nitric oxide (NO) – until recently considered solely in its gaseous state and as an atmospheric pollutant – is providing new insights into a number of regulatory processes in the nervous system. There is evidence that it is synthesised in the vascular epithelium, where it is responsible for regulating the vascular tone of the blood vessels. When released from neurons in the brain, nitric oxide acts as a novel transmitter, one of whose functions is in memory formation. In the periphery, the non-adrenergic, non-cholinergic nerves synthesise and release nitric oxide, which is responsible for neuro-genic vasodilatation and for the regulation of various gastrointestinal, respiratory and genito-urinary tract functions. Nitric oxide is also involved in platelet aggregation. These numerous actions are attributed to its direct stimulatory action on soluble guanylate cyclase, which enables it to act as a modulator of conventional neurotransmitters.

In all tissues, it is synthesised by the action of nitric oxide synthase on the amino acid arginine. Nitric oxide synthase activity has been detected in all brain regions, the highest activity being located in the cerebellum.

One of the main physiological roles of nitric oxide is in memory formation. There is evidence that in the hippocampus it is released from postsynaptic sites to act on presynaptic neurons as a retrograde transmitter to release glutamate. This leads to a stable increase in synaptic transmission and forms the basis of long-term potentiation and the initiation of memory formation. Inhibition of nitric oxide synthase activity has been shown experimentally to impair memory formation.

Other roles for nitric oxide include the development of the cortex and in vision, where it assists in the transduction of light signals in the retinal photoreceptor cells, as well as feeding behaviour, nociception and olfaction. Recent evidence suggests that the microglia cells in the brain, which form part of the monocyte/macrophage system, express an inducible form of nitric oxide synthase. Overactivity of these cells has been implicated in the pathogenesis of a number of neurological diseases, including multiple sclerosis, Alzheimer's disease and Parkinson's disease. Presumably drugs will be developed in the near future to counteract the degenerative effects of nitric oxide.

Conclusions

In this chapter, no attempt has been made to give a complete overview of neurotransmission. Those wishing to obtain a fuller account of this rapidly growing area are recommended to consult the key review articles and monographs listed below. This brief discourse on the nature of the adrenergic, cholinergic, serotonergic, dopaminergic and amino acid receptors should provide the reader with the basis upon which the actions of the various drugs mentioned in subsequent chapters may be better understood.

Bibliography

Bowery, N. G. (1989) GABA$_B$-receptors and their significance in mammalian pharmacology. *Trends in Pharmacological Science*, **10**, 401–407.

Davis, K. L., Charney, D., Coyle, J. T., et al (2002) (eds) *Neuropsychopharmacology: The Fifth Generation of Progress*. Philadelphia, PA: Lippincott, Williams & Wilkins.

Deneris, E. S., Connolly, J., Rodgers, S. W., et al (1991) Pharmacological and functional diversity of neuronal nicotinic acetylcholine receptors. *Trends in Pharmacological Science*, **12**, 34–40.

Gaddum, J. H. (1954) Drug antagonists to 5-hydroxytryptamine. In *Ciba Foundation Symposium on Hypertension, Humoral and Neurogenic Factors*, pp. 75–77. Boston: Little, Brown.

Höckfelt, F., Fuxe, K. & Penow, B. (eds) (1986) Co-existence of neuronal messengers – a new principle in chemical transmission. In *Advances in Brain Research, 68*. New York: Elsevier Science.

Leonard, B. E. (2003) *Fundamentals of Pharmacology* (3rd edn). Chichester: John Wiley & Sons.

Olsen, R. W. & Tobin, A. J. (1990) Molecular biology of GABA$_A$ receptors. *FASEB Journal*, **4**, 1469–1480.

Sedvall, G. (1990) PET imaging of dopamine receptors in human basal ganglia: relevance to mental illness. *Trends in Neuroscience*, **13**, 302–308.

Sibley, D. R. & Monsma, F. J. (1992) Molecular biology of dopamine receptors. *Trends in Pharmacological Sciences*, **13**, 61–68.

TIPS (1990) The pharmacology of excitatory amino acids – a TIPS special report. *Trends in Pharmacological Sciences*, **11**, 1–20.

Further reading

Books

Baskys, A. & Remmington, G. (eds) (1996) *Brain Mechanisms and Psychotropic Drugs*. Boca Raton: CRC Press.

Feigner, J. P. & Boyer, W. F. (eds) (1991) *Selective Serotonin Reuptake Inhibitors*. Chichester: John Wiley & Sons.

Leonard, B. E. (2003) *Fundamentals of Psychopharmacology* (3rd edn). Chichester: John Wiley & Sons.

Nahas, G. G., Sutin, K. M., Harvey, D. J., *et al* (eds) (1999) *Marihuana and Medicine*. Totowa, NJ: Humana Press.

Riederer, P., Kipp, N. & Pearson, J. (eds) (1990) *An Introduction to Neurotransmission in Health and Disease*. Oxford: Oxford University Press.

Schatzberg, A. F. & Nemesoff, C. B. (1998) *Textbook of Psychopharmacology*. Washington, DC: American Psychiatric Press.

Smith, C. U. M. (1996) *Elements of Molecular Neurobiology* (2nd edn). Chichester: John Wiley & Sons.

Stahl, S. M. (1996) *Essential Psychopharmacology*. Cambridge: Cambridge University Press.

Webster, R. A. (2001) (ed.) *Neurotransmitters, Drugs and Brain Function*. Chichester: John Wiley & Sons.

Review papers

Bourne, H. R., Sanders, D. A. & McCormick, F. (1991) The GTP'ase superfamily: conserved structure and molecular mechanism. *Nature*, **349**, 117–127.

Changeux, J. P., Devillers-Thiery, A. & Galzi, J. L. (1992) New mutants to explore nicotinic receptor functions. *Trends Pharmacological Science*, **13**, 299–301.

Charney, D. S., Krystal, J. D., Delgado, P. L., *et al* (1990). Serotonin specific drugs for anxiety and depressive disorders. *Annual Review of Medicine*, **41**, 437–446.

Chuang, D. (1989) Neurotransmitter receptors and phosphoinositide turnover. *Annual Review of Pharmacological Toxicology*, **29**, 71–110.

Garattini, S. (1992) Pharmacology of second messengers: a critical appraisal. *Drug Metabolism Reviews*, **24**, 125–194.

Haefely, W. (1990) The GABA–benzodiazepine interaction – 15 years later. *Neurochemical Research*, **15**, 169–174.

Krupinski, J. (1992) The adenylyl cyclase family. *Molecular and Cellular Biochemistry*, **104**, 73–79.

McGreer, E. G. (1989) Neurotransmitters. *Current Opinion in Neurology and Neuro-surgery*, **2**, 520–531.

Meldrum, B. S. (1989) Gaba-ergic mechanisms in the pathogenesis and treatment of epilepsy. *British Journal of Clinical Pharmacology*, **27**, 35–113.

Schmidt, H. W. & Walter, O. (1994) NO at work. *Cell*, **78**, 919–925.

Schuman, E. M. & Madison, D. V. (1994) Nitric oxide and synaptic function. *Annual Review of Neuroscience*, **17**, 153–184.

Seeman, P. (1995) Dopamine receptors and psychosis. *Scientific American*, September/October, 2–11.

Siever, I. J., Khan, R. S. & Lawlor, B. A. (1991) Critical issues in defining the role of serotonin in psychiatric disorders. *Pharmacological Reviews*, **43**, 509–525.

CHAPTER 2

Pharmacogenomics and pharmacogenetics in psychopharmacology

Robert W. Kerwin and Maria J. Arranz

Pharmacogenetic research, the study of variability in drug response, is more than 50 years old. The first landmark finding of pharmacogenetics was the discovery by Kalow and collaborators that adverse reactions to the muscle relaxant succinylcholine are caused by inactive forms of the enzyme serum cholinesterase, which is responsible for drug metabolism (Kalow, 1962). During the 1960s and 1970s, Harris matched structural gene mutations with physiological and pathological data in haemoglobinopathies and enzymopathies (Weber, 1997). Since then, numerous studies have reported adverse or toxic reactions to drug treatment that have been caused by genetic alterations in metabolic enzymes.

In particular, cytochrome P450 (CYP) enzymes, responsible for phase I metabolic reactions, have been extensively studied and consequently several naturally occurring mutations with functional effects have been described. CYP polymorphisms are likely to play an important role in variability to psychiatric treatment, since they are responsible for the biotransformation of the majority of psychiatric drugs currently available.

Thus, while the term 'pharmacogenetics' was initially associated with the investigation of genetic alterations of metabolic activity, the field has since expanded to the investigation of pharmacodynamic as well as pharmacokinetic factors. Recent findings suggest that genetic alterations in the site of action of drugs also contribute to response variability. The completion of the human genome sequence also opens the possibility of finding further genes related to drug response. A new term, 'pharmacogenomics', was coined to express this wider approach and will be used preferentially in this chapter. Although the use of genetic information for the estimation of response is still at an early stage of development, pre-treatment determination of patients' metabolic status to prevent adverse reactions is slowly being introduced in clinical laboratories and, in the near future, prediction of treatment response is expected. It is probably now, when the benefits of the clinical applications of pharmacogenomics are beginning to be appreciated, that interest in the science is at its highest.

Pharmacogenomic research and psychopharmacology

The variability observed in individuals treated with psychotropic drugs suggests that therapeutic response is a complex trait influenced by several genes. Genetic alterations at both the metabolic level and the site of action of a particular drug are likely to contribute to the overall response, although the extent of this contribution is yet unknown. That there is a genetic influence on metabolic traits has been proved in twin studies: a much higher concordance in isoniazide elimination was observed among monozygotic (MZ) than among dizygotic (DZ) twins ($n = 73$ pairs, $P < 0.0001$) (Weber, 1997). Similar observations have been reported for the metabolism of antipyrine, aspirin, ethanol, lithium and other therapeutic agents (Weber, 1997). However, no systematic epidemiological study has investigated the heritability of response to psychiatric treatment. Only a few observations of similar response, weight gain and incidence of agranulocytosis in MZ twins treated with an antipsychotic drug have been reported (Vojvoda *et al*, 1996; Horacek *et al*, 2001; Mata *et al*, 2001). One can imagine that negative reports of the same sort (MZ twins presenting differences in treatment response) would be less likely to be accepted for publication, and therefore the validity of these findings cannot be established until a systematic epidemiological study of response to psychiatric drugs is performed.

In spite of the lack of epidemiological evidence, pharmacogenomic research has tried to identify genetic factors that influence response to psychopharmacological treatment. In this chapter, we summarise the most important findings. Association studies, the comparison of genotype and allele frequencies between groups of unrelated patients presenting variable responses, are the preferred strategy for the identification of genes with moderate effects on clinical outcome. Because they are prone to type I errors (false positive results), association studies should be carefully planned for pharmacogenomic research. Clinical differences may play an important part in discrepant findings and may hinder the confirmation of interesting results.

Initially, genetic studies investigated the influence of metabolic polymorphisms on drug response but more recently research was extended to drug-targeted neurotransmitter systems. The next two sections review these areas.

Metabolic pathways

Exactly how many genes in the human genome are related to metabolic pathways is not known. Potentially, many of them may have a major or minor input in drug activity. However, we concentrate here on genes that code for metabolic enzymes already known to be involved in the biotransformation of psychotropic compounds. Drugs are transformed during phase I (hydrolysis and oxidation reactions) and phase II (conjugation reactions) processes before elimination. Alterations in the genes coding for enzymes controlling these processes may have a disruptive effect on drug metabolism, with direct implications for treatment response. Toxic responses can be the result of drug accumulation in individuals possessing inactive or slow enzymes. Alternatively, lack of treatment efficacy in patients possessing ultrarapid metabolic variants may be the result of drug elimination before a therapeutic effect has been obtained. Gene mutations related to such metabolic alterations have already been identified for phase I enzymes (i.e. CYP enzymes) (see Table 2.1). However, although genetic variants of phase II enzymes (N-acetyltransferases, UDP-glucuronosyltransferases, and thiopurine methyltransferases) have been detected, their relation to treatment response is still unclear.

The metabolism of most psychotropic drugs is started by CYP enzymes; in particular, by the CYP1–CYP4 families. Several subtypes are known in each family; the most extensively studied are CYP1A2, CYP2C9, CYP2C19, CYP2D6 and CYP3A4. Numerous genetic variants of these subtypes have been detected in human populations (see http://www.imm.ki.se/CYPalleles/ for an updated list). Their distribution varies among different populations and may explain some of the heterogeneity observed in treatment response.

CYP1A2

CYP1A2 constitutes the main metabolic pathway of antipsychotics such as clozapine, olanzapine and haloperidol (Ring et al, 1996; Jerling et al, 1997). Allelic variants with functional effect and a potential influence on metabolic rates have been described in the promoter region (determinant of gene expression) of the CYP1A2 gene (Nakajima et al, 1999). The population frequency of CYP1A2 poor metabolisers ranges from 10% to 5% (Ou-Yang et al, 2000).

Interestingly, impaired variants of CYP1A2 have been associated with tardive dyskinesia (Ozdemir et al, 2001), although this finding has yet to be confirmed by independent investigators.

CYP2C9

The CYP2C subfamily metabolises approximately 20% of clinically used drugs (Goldstein, 2001). There are four subtypes in this group: CYP2C8, CYP2C9, CYP2C18 and CYP2C19. CYP2C9 and CYP2C19 are of clinical importance for psychotropic drugs. Three CYP2C9 variants are known to have a markedly reduced activity (CYP2C9*2, *3 and *5), and therefore result in increased drug levels in blood (Crespi & Miller, 1997). Additional functional mutations have recently been described in the promoter region of the gene (Shintani et al, 2001).

Table 2.1 List of mutations in CYP enzymes with a known effect on metabolic rates

Polymorphism	Enzyme activity[a]	Reference
CYP1A2*1C	Decreased	Nakajima et al (1999)
CYP2A6*6	Decreased	Kitagawa et al (2001)
CYP2A6*	Decreased	Ariyoshi et al (2001)
CYP2A6*9	Decreased	Pitarque et al (2001)
CYP2C9*2	Decreased	Crespi & Miller (1997)
CYP2C9*3	Decreased	Sullivan-Klose et al (1996)
CYP2C9*5	Decreased	Dickmann et al (2001)
CYP2C19*8	Decreased	Ibeanu et al (1999)
CYP2D6*1XN	Increased	Dahl et al (1995)
CYP2D6*2XN	Increased	Dahl et al (1995)
CYP2D6*9	Decreased	Marez et al (2000)
CYP2D6*10B	Decreased	Ingelman-Sundberg et al (1994)
CYP2D6*17	Decreased	Oscarson et al (1997)
CYP2D6*18	Decreased	Nakajima et al (1999)
CYP2D6*35X2	Increased	Griese et al (1998)
CYP2D6*36	Decreased	Leathart et al (1998)
CYP2D6*41	Decreased	Raimundo et al (2000)
CYP8A1*1D	Increased	Chevalier et al (2001)
CYP8A1*1E	Increased	Chevalier et al (2001)
CYP8A1*1F	Increased	Chevalier et al (2001)

[a]In comparison with wild type.

Blood levels of the anti-epileptic drug phenytoin are affected by these polymorphisms, and so individuals carrying a CYP2C9 mutant allele may require lower doses of the drug (Spear, 2001; van der Weide et al, 2001). As in other metabolic polymorphisms, large differences have been observed within ethnic groups and may result in discrepancies in therapeutic results among populations (Wilson et al, 2001).

CYP2C19

Alterations in CYP2C19 activity, revealed by deficient metabolism of the anticonvulsant drug mephenytoin, are related to genetic impairment (Ibeanu et al, 1999). Poor and extensive metabolising variants have been identified in populations at different frequencies: poor metabolisers represent 3–5% of Caucasians and Africans, although a much higher frequency has been described in Asian populations (Dandara et al, 2001; Goldstein, 2001).

CYP2C19 participates in the metabolism of antidepressants such as paroxetine, clomipramine and amitriptyline (Tanaka & Hisawa, 1999) and may contribute to variation in response to these drugs.

CYP2D6

The existence of CYP2D6 polymorphisms was first discovered when individuals treated with debrisoquine who suffered a drastic fall in blood pressure were found to possess a defective enzyme (Eichelbaum & Evert, 1996). Individuals possessing slow CYP2D6 variants are classified as poor metabolisers, and three other phenotypes – normal or extensive metabolisers, intermediate metabolisers and ultrarapid metabolisers – have been described (Bertilsson & Dahl, 1996). Important inter-ethnic differences exist in the frequencies of these phenotypes: 7–10% of Caucasians are poor metabolisers, in comparison with 1–2% of Asians; extreme variation can also be found in Black populations (between 0% and 19% of whom have been classified as poor metabolisers) (Bradford & Kirlin, 1998). These geographic/ethnic differences are particularly important as it has been reported that 20% of drugs are metabolised by the CYP2D6 subtype.

Several studies have failed to find a relation between CYP2D6 variants and therapeutic response (Arranz et al, 1995; Spina et al, 1997), although there are clear indications that genetically impaired CYP2D6 metabolism is related to the incidence of drug-induced side-effects (Scordo et al, 2000).

CYP3A4

The CYP3A4 enzyme is the most abundant form of CYP in the liver and is involved in the metabolism of a variety of antipsychotic drugs (including ziprasidone, clozapine, risperidone, chlorpromazine and haloperidol) (Ring et al, 1996; Tanaka & Hisawa, 1999) and anti-depressant drugs (paroxetine, mirtazapine, trazodone and amitriptyline) (Tanaka & Hisawa, 1999; Timmer et al, 2000). Numerous allelic variants have been reported in the coding and promoter region of the CYP3A4 gene, although none of them completely inactivates the enzyme (Evans & Johnson, 2001). Additional enzyme variants have been described with altered catalytic activity (Hsieh et al, 2001).

Phase II enzymes

Phase II enzymes metabolise the conjugation of external compounds. Several of these enzymes, including N-acetyltransferase (NAT), thio-purine methyltransferase (TPMT) and UDP-glucurunosyltransferase (UGT), are known to exist in several forms in the population. However, relatively little research has been done into their influence on drug therapy.

The enzyme NAT catalyses the acetylation of drugs and their metabolites during phase II reactions. Two NAT subtypes, NAT1 and NAT2, have been described, and several allelic variants of these are known (de Leon *et al*, 2000; Wikman *et al*, 2001). NAT2 slow-acetylation variants have been related to lung, bladder and hepatic forms of cancer (Miller *et al*, 2001; Wikman *et al*, 2001). There are large differences in the geographic/ethnic distribution of NAT2 polymorphisms: more than 40% of Caucasians but less than 10% of Japanese and 30% of Asian populations are slow acetylators (Lin *et al*, 1993). Although slow acetylation can potentially cause cytotoxic reactions due to accumulation of drug metabolites, there is no evidence as yet of the influence of NAT variants on the outcome of treatment with psychotropic drugs.

Other phase II enzymes, such as TPMT and UGT, have also been reported to present altered activity in association with genetic mutations (Ciotti *et al*, 1997; Clarke *et al*, 1997). In addition, polymorphisms in drug transporters, such as glycoproteins (e.g. MDR1 and SPGP), may also play a role in drug therapy. However, as in the case of acetylator enzymes, their relation to psychiatric drug treatment requires elucidation. Future research on drug safety should investigate the influence of these polymorphisms on toxic reactions.

Drug interactions

Drug interactions can also result in toxic reactions; concomitant treatment with drugs metabolised by the same subtype of a particular enzyme may result in competition for it, and consequently reduced metabolism and enzyme saturation (Vandel *et al*, 2000). Numerous cases of metabolic interactions have been reported in individuals with normal metabolic rates (Caraco, 1998; Kosuge *et al*, 2001). These interactions can be aggravated by deficient metabolic enzymes. Consideration should be given to metabolic status and possible drug interactions when concomitant treatment is prescribed.

Summary

Metabolic polymorphisms are important factors for treatment success. Genetic association studies comparing the frequency of metabolic polymorphisms between groups of patients designated responders and non-responders to treatment have failed to produce clear results. Nevertheless, several studies have confirmed the hypothesis that metabolic variants are related to drug-induced side-effects such as tardive dyskinesia (Arthur *et al*, 1995; Ozdemir *et al*, 2001). Metabolic alterations may have minor clinical effects on patients receiving drugs with a broad therapeutic index or with several metabolic pathways (Evans & Johnson, 2001), when deficiencies can be compensated for through other enzymes. Nevertheless, interactions between drugs can lead to enzyme saturation and toxic accumulations, and so produce similar effects to genetic enzymatic deficiencies. Consequently, population and individual variation in drug metabolism should be considered when prescribing treatment with psychotropic drugs. Dose adjustment according to the patient's metabolic status (Kirchheiner *et al*, 2001) or the selection of alternative treatment could reduce adverse reactions. Reliable and simple methods for the identification of metabolic variants of CYP1A2, CYP2C19 and CYP2D6 already exist (Persidis, 1998) and it is to be hoped that their use in clinical laboratories will increase in the near future.

Drug-targeted neurotransmitter systems

Therapeutic success is not guaranteed even in individuals presenting normal metabolic rates. Aside from metabolic reactions, therefore, additional events must contribute to determine treatment response. Pharmacokinetic and pharmacodynamic processes are both hypothesised to contribute to response heterogeneity. Pharmacogenomic research in psychiatry is searching for gene factors in neurotransmitter systems that may contribute to this. This search serves several purposes: the validation of therapeutic targets, the identification of new putative sites of action for psychotropic drugs, and, in combination with metabolic polymorphisms, the identification of genetic determinants of treatment response. The search has focused on brain receptors and neurotransmitter transporter systems with high drug-binding affinities (see Table 2.2). Dopaminergic and serotonergic receptors have been extensively studied as candidates for involvement in mental disorders and as therapeutic targets, but the adrenergic, histaminergic and muscarinic receptors are also hypothesised to contribute to the success of psychiatric treatment.

Dopaminergic system

Dopamine receptor polymorphisms have been extensively investigated in relation to response to antipsychotic drugs. Alterations in the dopaminergic system of patients with schizophrenia are well documented and dopaminergic receptors were chosen as primary targets for the first generation of antipsychotics. Recent investigations suggest that moderate blockade of dopamine receptors together with rapid dissociation are determinants of successful treatment and a low incidence of extrapyramidal symptoms (Kapur & Seeman, 2001). Genetic research has investigated mutations in proteins in the dopaminergic

Table 2.2 Binding affinities of commonly used antipsychotic drugs (in K_i, nmol/l)

Drug	Receptor subtype															
	D_1	D_2	D_3	D_4	5-HT$_{1A}$	5-HT$_{2A}$	5-HT$_{2C}$	5-HT$_3$	5-HT$_6$	H1	M1	M2	M3	M4	α_1	α_2
Haloperidol	120	1.4	2.5	3.3	>1000	120	>1000	>1000	6000	440	>1000				46	360
Clozapine	290	130	240	54	140	8.9	17	95	11	1.8	1.8	48	20	11	3.9	33
Risperidone	580	2.2	9.6	8.5	210	0.29	10	>1000	2000	19	>1000	>1000		>1000	2	3
Olanzapine	52	20	45	60	>1000	3.3	10.2	57	10	2.8	4.7	13	10	6	54	170
Ziprasidone	130	3.1	7.2	32	2.5	0.39	0.72	76	76	47	5100		>1000		13	310
Quetiapine	1300	180	320	2200	230	220	>1000	>1000	4100	8.7	100	705	225	>1000	15	1000

receptor that, by affecting expression, binding or functioning, may influence their interaction with drugs.

There are five types of dopamine receptors (D_1-D_5), of which D_2 receptors are thought to mediate the antipsychotic activity of most conventional antipsychotics (Kerwin & Osborne, 2000). However, association studies investigating D_2 genetic variants and antipsychotic drug response have failed to provide definitive evidence – several studies have supported the hypothesis but others have not (see Wong *et al*, 2000). A recent study that related D_2 polymorphisms to early treatment response (Schafer *et al*, 2001) may explain some of the discrepancies between studies: certain neurotransmitter systems may be more important in the early stages of treatment, whereas other systems may intervene later, when saturation processes have influenced their regulation mechanism. Studies on D_3 and D_4 genetic variants have also failed to provide clear evidence of their mediation of antipsychotic activity (Wong *et al*, 2000). These contradictory findings may be the result of false positives or false negatives, or may have been caused by differences in the clinical characteristics of the samples investigated.

Being a complex trait, the response to antipsychotic drugs is likely to result from the combined action of several systems. Dopamine polymorphisms may still play an important role in determining specific response phenotypes or side-effects. In support of this hypothesis, several studies have recently reported an increased frequency of mutations in D_2 and D_3 receptor genes among patients with tardive dyskinesia (Inada *et al*, 1999; Liao *et al*, 2001), which suggests there is a genetic predisposition to the development of side-effects. We have detected in pilot studies a relationship between D_3 polymorphisms and improvement in positive symptoms (unpublished data). If confirmed, these results would provide evidence of the involvement of the dopaminergic system in the positive symptoms of schizophrenia.

Serotonergic system

The serotonergic system is involved in sleep, appetite, pain perception and sexual behaviour. Its dysfunction has been implicated in mental disorders such as depression, obsessive–compulsive disorder and affective disorder. Serotonin (5-HT) receptors are strongly targeted by a second generation of antipsychotic drugs that are termed 'atypical' (Meltzer, 1999). 5-HT_2 receptors are strongly targeted by clozapine, the most successful atypical antipsychotic, but also by olanzapine, risperidone and ziprasidone, among others (Schmidt *et al*, 2001). This serotonergic affinity is hypothesised to be the reason for the superior improvement in negative symptoms obtained by atypical antipsychotics (Meltzer, 1999).

Polymorphisms in 5-HT_2 receptors seem to influence the response to clozapine in particular (Arranz *et al*, 1998; Masellis *et al*, 1998) and to antipsychotic drugs in general (Joober et al, 1999), confirming the importance of this system as a therapeutic target. Their relevance to negative symptoms has to be investigated in appropriate samples. Recent investigations have studied the influence of other serotonin receptors on antipsychotic response: several naturally occurring mutations have been detected in 5-HT_3 and 5-HT_5 genes after sequence analysis but were not found to affect treatment response. 5-HT_6 polymorphisms have been investigated in relation to clozapine response, with conflicting results (Yu et al, 1999; Masellis et al, 2001). As in the case of dopaminergic variants, it is likely that stronger associations are found with specific symptoms or drug-induced side-effects. Association studies indicate that 5-HT_2 polymorphism may be related to tardive dyskinesia (Segman et al, 2000; Tan et al, 2001) and, to a minor extent, with drug-induced weight gain (Basile et al, 2001).

Adrenergic system

Adrenergic transmission is involved in cognitive and emotional functioning, and dysfunction of the system contributes to disorders such as depression, cognitive disorders and schizophrenia. Adrenergic receptors, in particular the α_{1A}- and α_{2A}-receptors, are a target for psychiatric treatment. Several variants of the α_{2A} gene are known to exist in the population, although none of them has been observed to be associated with mental disorders (Feng et al, 2001). The α_{1A} and α_{2A} variants were investigated in relation to clozapine response, but no significant association was found (Bolonna et al, 2000; Tsai et al, 2001). However, a trend of association was observed between α_{1A} alleles and clozapine-induced weight gain (Basile et al, 2001). Further studies investigating the influence of mutant adrenergic receptors on mental disorders and drug response are currently in progress and should determine their real value as pharmacological targets.

Histaminergic system

Malfunctioning of the histaminergic system has been hypothesised to contribute to the aetiology of schizophrenia (Arnold & Trojanowski, 1996). Symptoms of mental disorder, such as apathy and social withdrawal, are thought to be influenced by high activity of the histaminergic system. Histamine receptors, in particular the H_1 subtype, are strongly targeted by atypical antipsychotics, such as clozapine. Although several polymorphic variants have been described in the genes coding for histaminergic receptors, none has been found to have a major influence on treatment response (Mancama et al, 2000a), with the exception of a rare polymorphism in the promoter region of the H_2 gene that contributes to clozapine response (Arranz et al, 2000; Schumacher et al, 2000). The effect of histaminergic antagonism and genetic variation on improvement of specific symptoms has yet to be investigated in adequate samples. Histaminergic polymorphisms are also proposed to influence treatment reactions such as weight gain, but there is no empirical evidence to support this hypothesis (Basile *et al*, 2001).

Muscarinic system

The five muscarinic receptor subtypes (M1–M5) have been screened for disease-related mutations (Mancama *et al*, 2000*b*). Antipsychotic drugs act mainly as antagonists of muscarinic receptors, in particular of the M1 and M2 receptors. Several mutations in the coding region were identified, but were not associated with response or disease (Mancama *et al*, 2000*b*). Failure to find mutants associated with response suggests that the receptor does not play an important role in therapeutic efficacy. However, this assumption can be confirmed only if all receptor mutations have been investigated and functional mutations are found not to influence response. Mutation screening of muscarinic receptors has yet to be completed for the genetic studies to be fully informative.

Neurotransmitter transporters

Neurotransmitter transporters control the availability of neurotrans-mitter proteins in the brain and play an important role in the regulation of transmission mechanisms. For instance, a variant of the serotonin transporter (5-HTT), associated with decreased expression levels of the transporter protein (Collier *et al*, 1996), is related to blunted serotonin function (Reist *et al*, 2001). Genetic alterations in transporters are likely to influence the mechanisms of regulation and to play a role in the success of psychiatric treatment. An example of this is the selective serotonin reuptake inhibitors (SSRIs), which target the 5-HTT; their efficacy may be influenced by mutations in the transporter protein. For instance, subjects with a copy of the long allele in the promoter region of the 5-HTT gene were found to be more likely to respond to the SSRI drug fluvoxamine than were individuals who were homozygotes for the short variant (Smeraldi *et al*, 1998). 5-HTT variants have also been associated with antidepressant-induced mania in subjects with bipolar disorders (Mundo *et al*, 2001). Mutations in the dopamine transporter (DAT1) have been reported to influence behavioural response to methylphenidate, a drug used for the treatment of attention-deficit hyperactivity disorder (Joober *et al*, 2000*b*).

Related genes

Other genes, including those encoding for methylenetetrahydro-folate reductase (MTHR), brain-derived neurotrophic factor (BDNF), G-protein beta 3 and catechol-O-methyltransferase (COMT), have been reported to be associated with variation in treatment response (Joober et al, 2000a; Krebs et al, 2000; Zill et al, 2000; Lee et al, 2001). Although the proteins coding for these genes may not have a direct relation with the mechanisms of action of antipsychotic drugs or with metabolic enzymes, they may control general processes in the systems within which the drugs act and, therefore, may have an indirect effect on response.

Genetic influences on symptoms and side-effects

The complexity of treatment response impedes the identification of determining factors. However, the dissection of treatment response in terms of symptoms or other response traits can facilitate the task. Neurotransmitter systems may be directly responsible for certain disease symptoms and side-effects. For example, D_2 antagonism is related to the efficacy of antipsychotic drugs and is also associated with their production of extrapyramidal side-effects (Kerwin & Osborne, 2000). In addition, it has been hypothesised that the dopaminergic system is related to the positive symptoms of schizophrenia and the serotonergic system to negative symptoms (Meltzer, 1999). It is likely that mutations in these receptors influence the development of symptoms and the production of side-effects. The reports of association between dopamine and serotonin receptor polymorphisms and tardive dyskinesia illustrate the utility of this strategy (Inada et al, 1999; Eichhammer et al, 2000; Segman et al, 2000; Liao et al, 2001). Recent evidence also suggests that D_2 mutant variants are related to the neuroleptic malignant syndrome (Suzuki et al, 2001). This strategy of investigating particular symptoms or effects is very likely to produce reliable results with strong associations between clinical traits and genetic changes, and it is a clear way forward for pharmacogenomic studies. In addition, prediction of adverse reactions is as valuable for psychiatric treatment as prediction of general response.

Association studies: false positives or true findings?

It is important to remind the reader that for nearly every positive finding mentioned in this chapter, there are negative studies that have failed to replicate the initial findings. The reasons behind replication failure can be several, the most obvious being that the initial report was a false positive. However, replication failure can be also caused by insufficient sample size (lack of power to detect the initial finding), ethnic differences, population stratification, trait heterogeneity or clinical characteristics – including type of drug, duration of treatment, method of diagnosis and response assessment. True associations of genetic polymorphisms with general response are as difficult to find as associations with disease: both are complex traits that are influenced by several genes to a greater or lesser extent. However, to maximise the reliability of pharmacogenomic research using association studies, a series of conditions have been recommended by experts in the area (Rietschel *et al*, 1999; Masellis *et al*, 2000). These recommendations will facilitate the replication of findings by different groups of investigators and improve the reliability of results.

Combining pharmacogenetic information to predict treatment response

Association studies help to identify genes with major or minor effects on treatment response. However, individual findings have little or no clinical value: the effect of one particular polymorphism is too small to have any practical use. Most psychiatric drugs display affinity for a variety of neurotransmitter receptors, and it is likely that several of these neurotransmitter systems mediate their therapeutic activity. Alterations in the drug availability caused by metabolic polymorphisms may contribute to response variability. The use of genetic information to predict complex traits has proved difficult in the past and there is no epidemiological study supporting or refuting the heritability of treatment response. Nevertheless, the anticipated benefits of response prediction justify the attempt.

We recently reported that a combination of six polymorphisms in drug-targeted receptors resulted in the correct prediction of response to long-term treatment with clozapine in 76% of cases (Arranz *et al*, 2000). In a study on patients with Alzheimer's disease, it was shown that a combination of polymorphisms in the APOE, PS1 and PS2 genes might be useful for the prediction of treatment variability (Cacabelos *et al*, 2000). Although awaiting replication, these results show the feasibility of using a genetic approach for the prediction of response to psychiatric drugs.

Easier than predicting response will be the prediction of particular phenotypes or side-effects, which has been achieved in several of the studies cited above. This strategy of dissecting response phenotypes is likely to be more successful in the detection of response-related polymorphisms that, in combination with others, may give a clear idea of treatment response. The identification of the genes controlling or determining positive and negative symptoms, hallucinations, weight gain, movement disorders and other response reactions may greatly contribute to the final goal of predicting a patient's response before the treatment is started, thereby facilitating the drug selection for each individual.

Future direction of pharmacogenomic research

New high-technology methods are already being used to improve the results of pharmacogenomic research. The rapidly developing microarray technology is being used to compare large numbers of gene sequences and expression levels between treatment responders and non-responders, and will help to identify response-related genetic factors and new targets of putative therapeutic value. Genotyping in phase I clinical trials will be extended to phases II, III and IV (for definitions see Chapter 3). In addition to those encoding for metabolic enzymes, other genes that may be related to the effects of psychotropic drugs are being investigated. Information gathered from clinical trials can be used to select groups of patients likely to respond positively to treatment and will improve drug safety.

Although pharmacogenomic research has concentrated mainly on DNA mutations, more attention is required on gene regulation and environmental interactions. The human genome mapping project showed that there were a surprisingly small number of genes (about 35 000, when 70 000–100 000 had been expected) (Lander *et al*, 2001). A human being has approximately twice the number of genes of a fly (Rubin, 2001). Therefore, gene number alone cannot explain differences among species, and gene regulation mechanisms may play an important part in the complexity of brain processes. New research in this field will help us to understand the mechanisms and processes of psychiatric treatment.

All this information will undoubtedly help us to obtain the ultimate goal: to predict which drug will be more successful and safer for each individual. The first attempts to combine genetic information to predict treatment response have proven the feasibility of the project and it is expected that in the next few years there will be improved methods of response prediction available for clinical use.

References

Ariyoshi, N., Sawamura, Y. & Kamataki, T. (2001) A novel single nucleotide polymorphism altering stability and activity of CYP2a6. *Biochemical and Biophysical Research Communications*, **281**, 810–814.

Arnold, S. E. & Trojanowski, J. Q. (1996) Recent advances in defining the neuropathology of schizophrenia. *Acta Neuropatholigica (Berlin)*, **92**, 217–231.

Arranz, M. J., Dawson, E., Shaikh, S., *et al* (1995) Cytochrome P4502D6 genotype does not determine response to clozapine. *British Journal of Clinical Pharmacology*, **39**, 417–420.

Arranz, M. J., Munro, J., Sham, P., *et al* (1998) Meta-analysis of studies on genetic variation in 5-HT$_{2A}$ receptors and clozapine response. *Schizophrenia Research*, **32**, 93–99.

Arranz, M. J., Munro, J., Birkett, J., *et al* (2000) Pharmacogenetic prediction of clozapine response. *Lancet*, **355**, 1615–1616.

Arthur, H., Dahl, M. L., Siwers, B., *et al* (1995) Polymorphic drug metabolism in schizophrenic patients with tardive dyskinesia. *Journal of Clinical Psychopharmacology*, **15**, 211–216.

Basile, V. S., Masellis, M., McIntyre, R. S., *et al* (2001) Genetic dissection of atypical antipsychotic-induced weight gain: novel preliminary data on the pharmacogenetic puzzle. *Journal of Clinical Psychiatry*, **62** (suppl. 23), 45–66.

Bertilsson, L. & Dahl, M. L. (1996) Polymorphic drug oxidation – relevance to the treatment of psychiatric disorders. *CNS Drugs*, **5**, 220–223.

Bolonna, A. A., Arranz, M. J., Munro, J., *et al* (2000) No influence of adrenergic receptor polymorphisms on schizophrenia and antipsychotic response. *Neuroscience Letters*, **280**, 65–68.

Bradford, L. D. & Kirlin, W. G. (1998) Polymorphism of CYP2D6 in black populations: implications for psychopharmacology. *International Journal of Neuropsychopharmacology*, **1**, 173–185.

Cacabelos, R., Alvarez, A., Fenandez-Novoa, L., *et al* (2000) A pharmacogenomic approach to Alzheimer's disease. *Acta Neurologica Scandinavica*, suppl. 176, 12–19.

Caraco, Y. (1998) Genetic determinants of drug responsiveness and drug interactions. *Therapeutic Drug Monitoring*, **20**, 517–524.

Chevalier, P., Rey, J., Pasquier, O., *et al* (2001) Multiple-dose pharmacokinetics and safety of two regimens of quinupristin/dalfopristin (Synercid) in healthy volunteers. *Journal of Clinical Pharmacology*, **41**, 404–414.

Ciotti, M., Marrone, A., Potter, C., *et al* (1997) Genetic polymorphism in the human UGT1A6 (planar phenol) UDP-glucuronosyltransferase: pharmacological implications. *Pharmacogenetics*, **7**, 485–495.

Clarke, D. J., Moghrabi, N., Monaghan, G., *et al* (1997) Genetic defects of the UDP-glucuronosyltransferase-1 (UGT1) gene that cause familial non-haemolytic unconjugated hyperbilirubinaemias. *Clinica Chimica Acta*, **266**, 63–74.

Collier, D. A., Stober, G., Li, T., *et al* (1996) A novel functional polymorphism within the promoter of the serotonin transporter gene: possible role in susceptibility to affective disorders. *Molecular Psychiatry*, **1**, 453–460.

Crespi, C. L. & Miller, V. P. (1997) The R144C change in the CYP2C9*2 allele alters interaction of the cytochrome P450 with NADPH: cytochrome P450 oxidoreductase. *Pharmacogenetics*, **7**, 203–210.

Dahl, M. L., Johansson, I., Bertilsson, L., *et al* (1995) Ultrarapid hydroxylation of debrisoquine in a Swedish population – analysis of the molecular genetic basis. *Journal of Pharmacology and Experimental Therapeutics*, **274**, 516–520.

Dandara, C., Masimirembwa, C. M., Magimba, A., *et al* (2001) Genetic polymorphism of CYP2D6 and CYP2C19. *European Journal of Clinical Pharmacology*, **57**, 11–17.

de Leon, J. H., Vatsis, K. P. & Weber, W. W. (2000) Characterization of naturally occurring and recombinant human N-acetyltransferase variants encoded by NAT1. *Molecular Pharmacology*, **58**, 288–299.

Dickmann, L. J., Rettie, A. E., Kneller, M. B., *et al* (2001) Identification and functional characterization of a new CYP2C9 variant (CYP2C9*5) expressed among African Americans. *Molecular Pharmacology*, **60**, 382–387.

Eichelbaum, M. & Evert, B. (1996) Influence of pharmacogenetics on drug disposition and response. *Clinical and Experimental Pharmacology and Physiology*, **23**, 983–985.

Eichhammer, P., Albus, M., Borrmann-Hassenbach, M., *et al* (2000) Association of dopamine D_3-receptor gene variants with neuroleptic induced akathisia in schizophrenic patients: a generalization of Steen's study on DRD3 and tardive dyskinesia. *American Journal of Medical Genetics*, **96**, 187–191.

Evans, W. E. & Johnson, J. A. (2001) Pharmacogenomics: the inherited basis for interindividual differences in drug response. *Annual Review of Genomics and Human Genetics*, **2**, 9–39.

Feng, J., Zheng, J., Gelernter, J., *et al* (2001) An in-frame deletion in the alpha(2C) adrenergic receptor is common in African-Americans. *Molecular Psychiatry*, **6**, 168–172.

Goldstein, J. A. (2001) Clinical relevance of genetic polymorphisms in the human CYP2C subfamily. *British Journal of Clinical Pharmacology*, **52**, 349–355.

Griese, E. U., Zanger, U. M., Brudermanns, U., *et al* (1998) Assessment of the predictive power of genotypes for the in-vivo catalytic function of CYP2D6 in a German population. *Pharmacogenetics*, **8**, 15–26.

Horacek, J., Libiger, J., Hoschl, C., *et al* (2001) Clozapine-induced concordant agranulocytosis in monozygotic twins. *International Journal of Psychiatry in Clinical Practice*, **5**, 71–73.

Hsieh, K. P., Lin, Y. Y., Cheng, C. L., *et al* (2001) Novel mutations of CYP3A4 in Chinese. *Drug Metabolism and Disposition*, **29**, 268–273.

Ibeanu, G., Blaisdell, J., Ferguson, R. J., *et al* (1999) A novel transversion in the intron 5 donor splice junction of CYP2C19 and a sequence polymorphism in exon 3 contribute to the poor metabolizer phenotype for the anticonvulsant drug S-mephenytoin. *Journal of Pharmacology and Experimental Therapeutics*, **290**, 635–640.

Inada, T., Arinami, T. & Yagi, G. (1999) Association between a polymorphism in the promoter region of the dopamine D_2 receptor gene and schizophrenia in Japanese subjects: replication and evaluation for antipsychotic-related features. *International Journal of Neuropsychopharmacology*, **2**, 181–186.

Ingelman-Sundberg, M., Johansson, I., Persson, I., *et al* (1994) Genetic polymorphism of cytochrome P450. Functional consequences and possible relationship to disease and alcohol toxicity. *EXS*, **71**, 197–207.

Jerling, M., Merle, Y., Mentre, F., *et al* (1997) Population pharmacokinetics of clozapine evaluated with the nonparametric maximum likelihood method. *British Journal of Clinical Pharmacology*, **44**, 447–453.

Joober, R., Benkelfat, C., Brisebois, K., *et al* (1999) T102C polymorphism in the 5HT$_{2A}$ gene and schizophrenia: relation to phenotype and drug response variability. *Journal of Psychiatry and Neuroscience*, **24**, 141–146.

Joober, R., Benkelfat, C., Lal, S., *et al* (2000a) Association between the methylene-tetrahydrofolate reductase 677C/T missense mutation and schizophrenia. *Molecular Psychiatry*, **5**, 323–326.

Joober, R., Toulouse, A., Benkelfat, C., *et al* (2000b) DRD3 and DAT1 genes in schizophrenia: an association study. *Journal of Psychiatric Research*, **34**, 285–291.

Kalow, W. (1962) *Pharmacogenetics: Heredity and the Response to Drugs*. Philadelphia, PA: W. B. Saunders.

Kapur, S. & Seeman, P. (2001) Does fast dissociation from the dopamine d(2) receptor explain the action of atypical antipsychotics? A new hypothesis. *American Journal of Psychiatry*, **158**, 360–369.

Kerwin, R. W. & Osborne, S. (2000) Antipsychotic drugs. *Medicine*, **28**, 23–25.

Kirchheiner, J., Brosen, K., Dahl, M. L., *et al* (2001) CYP2D6 and CYP2C19 genotype-based dose recommendations for antidepressants: a first step towards subpopulation-specific dosages. *Acta Psychiatrica Scandinavica*, **104**, 173–192.

Kitagawa, K., Kunugita, N., Kitagawa, M., *et al* (2001) CYP2A6*6, a novel polymorphism in cytochrome p450 2A6, has a single amino acid substitution (R128Q) that inactivates enzymatic activity. *Journal of Biological Chemistry*, **276**, 17830–17835.

Kosuge, K., Jun, Y., Watanabe, H., *et al* (2001) Effects of CYP3A4 inhibition by diltiazem on pharmacokinetics and dynamics of diazepam in relation to CYP2C19 genotype status. *Drug Metabolism and Disposition*, **29**, 1284–1289.

Krebs, M. O., Guillin, O., Bourdel, M. C., *et al* (2000) Brain derived neurotrophic factor (BDNF) gene variants association with age at onset and therapeutic response in schizophrenia. *Molecular Psychiatry*, **5**, 558–562.

Lander, E. S., Linton, L. M., Birren, B., *et al* (2001) Initial sequencing and analysis of the human genome. *Nature*, **409**, 860–921.

Leathart, J. B., London, S. J., Steward, A., *et al* (1998) CYP2D6 phenotype–genotype relationships in African-Americans and Caucasians in Los Angeles. *Pharmacogenetics*, **8**, 529–541.

Lee, M. S., Lyoo, C. H., Ulmanen, I., *et al* (2001) Genotypes of catechol-O-methyltransferase and response to levodopa treatment in patients with Parkinson's disease. *Neuroscience Letters*, **298**, 131–134.

Liao, D. L., Yeh, Y. C., Chen, H. M., *et al* (2001) Association between the Ser9Gly polymorphism of the dopamine D_3 receptor gene and tardive dyskinesia in Chinese schizophrenic patients. *Neuropsychobiology*, **44**, 95–98.

Lin, H. J., Han, C. Y., Lin, B. K., *et al* (1993) Slow acetylator mutations in the human polymorphic N-acetyltransferase gene in 786 Asians, blacks, Hispanics, and whites: application to metabolic epidemiology. *American Journal of Human Genetics*, **52**, 827–834.

Mancama, D., Arranz, M. J., Munro, J., *et al* (2000*a*) The histamine 1 and histamine 2 receptor genes – candidates for schizophrenia and clozapine response. *GeneScreen*, **1**, 29–34.

Mancama, D., Munro, J., Arranz, M. J., *et al* (2000*b*) Association analysis of muscarinic acetylcholine receptor polymorphisms in clozapine treated schizophrenics. *American Journal of Medical Genetics*, **96**, 269.

Marez, D., Legrand, M., Sabbagh, N., *et al* (2000) Polymorphims of the cytochrome P450 CYP2D6 gene in a European population: characterization of 48 mutations and 53 alleles, their frequencies and evolution. *Pharmacogenetics*, **7**, 193–202.

Masellis, M., Basile, V. S., Meltzer, H. Y., *et al* (1998) Serotonin subtype 2 receptor genes and clinical response to clozapine in schizophrenia patients. *Neuropsychopharmacology*, **19**, 123–132.

Masellis, M., Basile, V. S., Ozdemir, V., *et al* (2000) Pharmacogenetics of antipsychotic treatment: lessons learned from clozapine. *Biological Psychiatry*, **47**, 252–266.

Masellis, M., Basile, V. S., Meltzer, H. Y., *et al* (2001) Lack of association between the T–C267 serotonin 5-HT_6 receptor gene (HTR6) polymorphism and prediction of response to clozapine in schizophrenia. *Schizophrenia Research*, **47**, 49–58.

Mata, I., Madoz, V., Arranz, M. J., *et al* (2001) Olanzapine: concordant response in monozygotic twins with schizophrenia (Letter). *British Journal of Psychiatry*, **178**, 86.

Meltzer, H. Y. (1999) The role of serotonin in antipsychotic drug action. *Neuropsychopharmacology*, **21**, s106–s115.

Miller, M. C., III, Mohrenweiser, H. W. & Bell, D. A. (2001) Genetic variability in susceptibility and response to toxicants. *Toxicology Letters*, **120**, 269–280.

Mundo, E., Walker, M., Cate, T., *et al* (2001) The role of serotonin transporter protein gene in antidepressant-induced mania in bipolar disorder: preliminary findings. *Archives of General Psychiatry*, **58**, 539–544.

Nakajima, M., Yokoi, T., Mizutani, M., *et al* (1999) Genetic polymorphism in the 5'-flanking region of human CYP1A2 gene: effect on the CYP1A2 inducibility in humans. *Journal of Biochemistry*, **125**, 803–808.

Oscarson, M., Hidestrand, M., Johansson, I., *et al* (1997) A combination of mutations in the CYP2D6*17 (CYP2D6Z) allele causes alterations in enzyme function. *Molecular Pharmacology*, **52**, 1034–1040.

Ou-Yang, D. S., Huang, S. L., Wang, W., *et al* (2000) Phenotypic polymorphism and gender-related differences of CYP1A2 activity in a Chinese population. *British Journal of Clinical Pharmacology*, **49**, 145–151.

Ozdemir, V., Basile, V. S., Masellis, M., *et al* (2001) Pharmacogenetic assessment of antipsychotic-induced movement disorders: contribution of the dopamine D_3 receptor and cytochrome P450 1A2 genes. *Journal of Biochemical and Biophysical Methods*, **47**, 151–157.

Persidis, A. (1998) Pharmacogenomics and diagnostics. *Nature Biotechnology*, **16** (suppl.), 20–21.

Pitarque, M., von Richter, O., Oke, B., *et al* (2001) Identification of a single nucleotide polymorphism in the TATA box of the CYP2A6 gene: impairment of its promoter activity. *Biochemical and Biophysical Research Communications*, **284**, 455–460.

Raimundo, S., Fischer, J., Eichelbaum, M., *et al* (2000) Elucidation of the genetic basis of the common 'intermediate metabolizer' phenotype for drug oxidation by CYP2D6. *Pharmacogenetics*, **10**, 577–581.

Reist, C., Mazzanti, C., Vu, R., *et al* (2001) Serotonin transporter promoter polymorphism is associated with attenuated prolactin response to fenfluramine. *American Journal of Medical Genetics*, **105**, 363–368.

Rietschel, M., Kennedy, J. L., Macciardi, F., *et al* (1999) Application of pharmacogenetics to psychotic disorders: the first consensus conference. *Schizophrenia Research*, **37**, 191–196.

Ring, B. J., Catlow, J., Lindsay, T. J., *et al* (1996) Identification of the human cytochromes P450 responsible for the in vitro formation of the major oxidative metabolites of the antipsychotic agent olanzapine. *Journal of Pharmacology and Experimental Therapeutics*, **276**, 658–666.

Rubin, G. M. (2001) The draft sequences. Comparing species. *Nature*, **409**, 820–821.

Schafer, M., Rujescu, D., Giegling, I., *et al* (2001) Association of short-term response to haloperidol treatment with a polymorphism in the dopamine D(2) receptor gene. *American Journal of Psychiatry*, **158**, 802–804.

Schmidt, A. W., Lebel, L. A., Howard, H. R., Jr, *et al* (2001) Ziprasidone: a novel antipsychotic agent with a unique human receptor binding profile. *European Journal of Pharmacology*, **425**, 197–201.

Schumacher, J., Schulze, T. G., Wienker, T. F., *et al* (2000) Pharmacogenetics of the clozapine response. *Lancet*, **356**, 506–507.

Scordo, M. G., Spina, E., Romeo, P., *et al* (2000) CYP2D6 genotype and antipsychotic-induced extrapyramidal side effects in schizophrenic patients. *European Journal of Clinical Pharmacology*, **56**, 679–683.

Segman, R. H., Heresco-Levy, U., Finkel, B., *et al* (2000) Association between the serotonin 2C receptor gene and tardive dyskinesia in chronic schizophrenia: additive contribution of 5-HT2Cser and DRD3gly alleles to susceptibility. *Psychopharmacology (Berlin)*, **152**, 408–413.

Shintani, M., Ieiri, I., Inoue, K., *et al* (2001) Genetic polymorphisms and functional characterization of the 5'-flanking region of the human CYP2C9 gene: in vitro and in vivo studies. *Clinical Pharmacology and Therapeutics*, **70**, 175–182.

Smeraldi, E., Zanardi, R., Benedetti, F., *et al* (1998) Polymorphism within the promoter of the serotonin transporter gene and antidepressant efficacy of fluvoxamine. *Molecular Psychiatry*, **3**, 508–511.

Spear, B. B. (2001) Pharmacogenetics and epileptic drugs. *Epilepsia*, **42** (5), 31–34.

Spina, E., Gitto, C., Avenoso, A., *et al* (1997) Relationship between plasma desipramine levels, CYP2D6 phenotype and clinical response to desipramine: a prospective study. *European Journal of Clinical Pharmacology*, **51**, 395–398.

Sullivan-Klose, T. H., Ghanayem, B. I., Bell, D. A., *et al* (1996) The role of the CYP2C9-Leu359 allelic variant in the tolbutamide polymorphism. *Pharmacogenetics*, **6**, 341–349.

Suzuki, A., Kondo, T., Otani, K., *et al* (2001) Association of the TaqI A polymorphism of the dopamine D(2) receptor gene with predisposition to neuroleptic malignant syndrome. *American Journal of Psychiatry*, **158**, 1714–1716.

Tan, E. C., Chong, S. A., Mahendran, R., *et al* (2001) Susceptibility to neuroleptic-induced tardive dyskinesia and the T102C polymorphism in the serotonin type 2A receptor. *Biological Psychiatry*, **50**, 144–147.

Tanaka, E. & Hisawa, S. (1999) Clinically significant pharmacokinetic drug interactions with psychoactive drugs: antidepressants and antipsychotics and the cytochrome P450 system. *Journal of Clinical Pharmacy and Therapeutics*, **24**, 7–16.

Timmer, C. J., Sitsen, J. M. A. & Delbressine, L. P. (2000) Clinical pharmacokinetics of mirtazapine. *Clinical Pharmacokinetics*, **38**, 461–474.

Tsai, S. J., Wang, Y. C., Yu Younger, W. Y., *et al* (2001) Association analysis of polymorphism in the promoter region of the alpha$_{2a}$-adrenoceptor gene with schizophrenia and clozapine response. *Schizophrenia Research*, **49**, 53–58.

van der Weide, J., Steijns, L. S., van Weelden, M. J., *et al* (2001) The effect of genetic polymorphism of cytochrome P450 CYP2C9 on phenytoin dose requirement. *Pharmacogenetics*, **11**, 287–291.

Vandel, P., Haffen, E., Vandel, S., *et al* (2000) Drug extrapyramidal side-effects or not: is there a dextromethorphan phenotype difference? *Therapie*, **55**, 349–353.

Vojvoda, D., Grimmell, K. & Sernyak, M. (1996) Monozygotic twins concordant for response to clozapine. *Lancet*, **347**, 61.

Weber, W. W. (1997) *Pharmacogenetics* (1st edn). New York: Oxford University Press.

Wikman, H., Thiel, S., Jager, B., *et al* (2001) Relevance of N-acetyltransferase 1 and 2 (NAT1, NAT2) genetic polymorphisms in non-small cell lung cancer susceptibility. *Pharmacogenetics*, **11**, 157–168.

Wilson, J. F., Weale, M., Smith, A. C., *et al* (2001) Population genetic structure of variable drug response. *Nature Genetics*, **29**, 265–269.

Wong, A. H. C., Buckle, C. E. & Van Tol, H. H. M. (2000) Polymorphisms in dopamine receptors: what do they tell us? *European Journal of Pharmacology*, **410**, 183–203.

Yu, Y. W. Y., Tsai, S.-J., Lin, C.-H., *et al* (1999) Serotonin-6 receptor variant (C267T) and clinical response to clozapine. *Neuroreport*, **10**, 1231–1233.

Zill, P., Baghai, T. C., Zwanzger, P., *et al* (2000) Evidence for an association between a G-protein beta 3-gene variant with depression and response to antidepressant treatment. *Neuroreport*, **11**, 1893–1897.

Further reading

Arranz, M. J. & Kerwin, R. W. (2000) Neurotransmitter-related genes and antipsychotic response: pharmacogenetics meets psychiatric treatment. *Annals of Medicine*, **32**, 128–133.

Arranz, M. J., Collier, D. A. & Kerwin, R. W. (2001) Pharmacogenetics for the individualization of psychiatric treatment. *American Journal of Pharmacogenomics*, **1**, 3–10.

McGuffin, P., Owen, M. J., O'Donovan, M. C., *et al* (1994) *Seminars in Psychiatric Genetics*. London: Gaskell.

McLeod, H. L. & Evans, W. E. (2001) Pharmacogenomics: unlocking the human genome for better drug therapy. *Annual Review of Pharmacological Toxicology*, **41**, 101–121.

Nebert, D. W. & Dieter, M. Z. (2000) The evolution of drug metabolism. *Pharmacology*, **61**, 124–135.

CHAPTER 3

Pharmacokinetics, pharmaco-dynamics and drug development

Ian Hindmarch and Graham R. McClelland

Clinical pharmacokinetics can be simplistically defined as the study of what the human body does to a drug, whereas pharmacodynamics is the study of what a drug does to the body. In this chapter the basic principles of pharmacokinetics and pharmacodynamics are explained together with their application in the development of new medicines, in particular drugs intended for the treatment of psychiatric diseases.

The effects of any drug in any individual will depend on three interrelated factors:

(1)   the dose, which will determine
(2)   the concentration of drug in the body, which will determine
(3)   the magnitude of effect in the individual cells/tissue/organ.

Principles of pharmacokinetics

There are four critical phases in what happends to a drug after it has been administered to someone – absorption, distribution, metabolism and excretion. Each of these phases relies upon different body processes and organs, as depicted in Fig. 3.1. These processes can be quantified by measurement of the concentrations of drug, and any metabolite(s), in urine and blood, in particular blood plasma. Drug concentrations in faeces can be determined, but the data will be sparse and, although they can be of qualitative value, are usually of little quantiative use. It is fortunate that plasma is the medium by which most drugs are distributed throughout the body and delivered to the tissues where the drug exerts its pharmacological effect, and also to those tissues and organs responsible for metabolism and excretion.

At any one time there may be drug at the absorption site, drug in the plasma (being distributed throughout the body), metabolites in the body, and drug that has been excreted. This is represented in diagrammatically in Fig. 3.2 and graphically in Fig. 3.3.

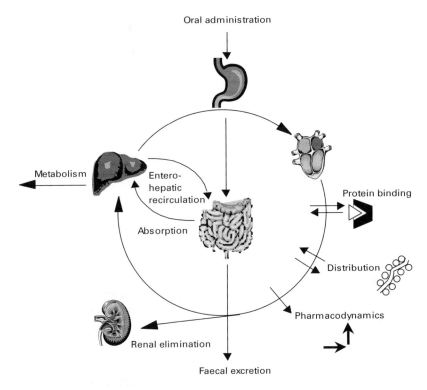

Fig. 3.1 Diagrammatic representation of the passage of a drug through the body.

Rapid intravenous injection

The simplest mode of administration to describe pharmacokinetically is the intravenous route, as it avoids the absorption phase. Also, with a rapid intravenous injection we can assume that the distribution phase is avoided since the drug is rapidly distributed throughout the body via the blood. This is known as a 'well stirred' or one-compartment model. If

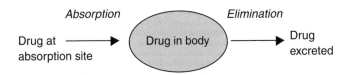

Fig. 3.2 Simplified (one-compartment) model of drug handling.

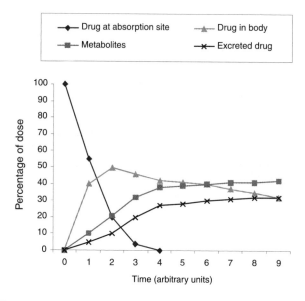

Fig. 3.3 Example of material balance accounting for a dose of a drug over time.

plasma samples are taken and the concentration of drug measured, the results can be plotted graphically, against time, both arithmetically and with logarithmically transformed concentrations, as shown in Fig. 3.4.

The concentration declines in an exponential fashion, obeying first-order kinetics, that is, where the rate of elimination is proportional to the concentration remaining. First-order kinetics is the most common

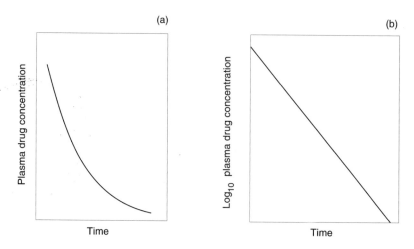

Fig. 3.4 Arithmetic (a) and semi-logarithmic (b) plots of plasma drug concentration following the administration of a single intravenous dose.

characteristic of drug elimination. This is observed because the processes of elimination (uptake and metabolism in the liver, secretion in the bile, and elimination in the urine by glomerular filtration and tubular secretion) are all first-order processes. Since the decline in concentration is exponential, a semi-logarithmic plot of the data produces a straight line, and this is the usual method by which plasma concentration data are presented.

As with all generalisations, there are exceptions to first-order elimination kinetics, with drugs whose rate of elimination is linearly related to concentration. Such drugs follow zero-order kinetics (i.e. the exponent of the function is zero). Examples of such drugs include alcohol and phenytoin, which both rapidly saturate their metabolising enzymes and then follow zero-order elimination. Such non-linear kinetics can have major implications for therapy, since a small increase in dose can lead to a large increase in plasma concentration. Barbiturates also show non-linearity in the part of the toxic range that is encountered clinically.

Single oral dose

Drugs can be administered by many routes, including oral, sublingual, buccal, intramuscular, subcutaneous, pulmonary, rectal, transdermal, as well as intravenous, each of which has different absorption character-istics. Because the most common route of administration is oral, it is the one that is the focus in this chapter.

A single oral dose results in a rising plasma concentration, until the point occurs when the rate of elimination exceeds the rate of absorption; thereafter concentrations progressively fall, as shown in Fig. 3.5.

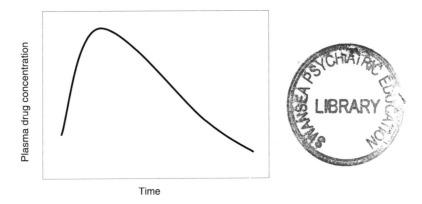

Time

Fig. 3.5 The plasma drug concentration profile after the administration of a single oral dose.

Absorption

Bioavailability

Drugs must cross cell membranes to reach the systemic circulation unless they are administered intravenously. The ability to cross membranes is determined by the lipid solubility of the drug and the area of the membrane available for absorption (the area of the ileum is very large because of the villi and microvilli). Small lipid-insoluble drugs are able to penetrate the membranes via aqueous channels and some drugs can be absorbed by specific, active, carrier-mediated transport processes.

A number of factors slow absorption from the gastrointestinal tract – for example, the presence of food in the stomach will delay gastric emptying, drugs formulated pharmaceutically in a slow-release form, or the presence of other drugs that might have a pharmacological effect on the gastrointestinal tract or compete for active absorption sites. Fig. 3.6 shows the effect on plasma concentration of different rates of absorption.

Fig. 3.6 illustrates that a lower absorption rate results in a peak concentration that is both later in time (later T_{max}) and lower in amplitude (lower C_{max}). The area under the curve (AUC) is directly proportional to the total amount of drug in the body, and thus can be used to determine the fraction of dose that has been absorbed (F). Intravenous administration inherently produces 100% bioavailability; 0% bioavailability implies that no drug has entered the systemic circulation. The bioavailability of a different formulation or different routes of administration of a drug are compared with the bioavailability obtained after intravenous administration of the drug, to establish absolute bioavailability.

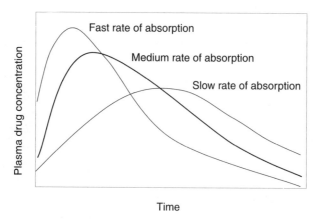

Fig. 3.6 The effects on plasma concentration of three different rates of absorption of single oral doses.

It is important to be aware that two dosage forms with equal bioavailability are not necessarily bioequivalent. Bioequivalence refers to equal biological effect (efficacy and toxicity), which is a function of plasma concentration. A dosage form that is rapidly absorbed may produce a higher peak effect, which could result in greater adverse effects. Conversely, a more slowly absorbed drug form may produce a lower peak concentration, which will fail to produce the desired therapeutic effects.

It also important to remember that different people have different characteristics that will produce different plasma concentration profiles, and that different circumstances (e.g. whether the stomach is empty) will result in different plasma concentration profiles within the same individual on different occasions.

First-pass effect

Even if a drug is completely absorbed, not all of the dose may reach the systemic circulation. Some of the dose may be metabolised in the gut wall or in the main site of metabolism in the body, the liver, which can extract drug from the portal blood before it reaches the systemic circulation via the hepatic vein. This pre-systemic metabolism is termed the 'first-pass effect'.

A wide range of drugs exhibit a first-pass effect. Notable psycho-tropic examples include the tricyclic antidepressants nortriptyline and desipramine, L-dopa, chlorpromazine, and the analgesics pentazocine and morphine. A large first-pass effect often explains why some drugs have a potent effect when administered intravenously but are ineffective when administered orally.

Entero-hepatic recirculation

Some drugs are secreted by the liver into bile. This results in the drug re-entering the gastrointestinal tract and being again available to be absorbed. Thus the same chemical molecule can repeatedly be absorbed, secreted and reabsorbed. This is known as entero-hepatic recirculation (Fig. 3.1), and results in a flattening, or prolonging, of the peak plasma concentration (C_{max}).

Distribution

Once a drug has been absorbed and reaches the bloodstream, it begins to be distributed to the tissues of the body. The rate and extent to which this process occurs depend on: how well each tissue is perfused (i.e. regional blood flow), the degree of binding of the drug to plasma proteins, and the ability of the drug to penetrate tissue membranes.

Apparent volume of distribution

A useful indication of the distribution characteristics of a drug can be obtained from its apparent volume of distribution (V_d). This can be defined as the volume of fluid required to contain the total amount of the drug in the body at the same concentration as that present in the plasma. A depiction of volume of distribution immediately after an intravenous dose is shown in Fig. 3.7, where if the initial dose (D) administered to a 'barrel' of water is known and the concentration of a sample taken from the barrel determined, then the volume of the barrel can be determined. This can be written in the form of an equation, where C is the plasma concentration:

$$V_d = D/C$$

In humans, it is an *apparent* volume of distribution, as it does not necessarily reflect the literal volume of fluid in which the drug is located (the volume of body water in a person is approximately 0.55 l/kg). To continue the barrel analogy, it is possible that drug will be adsorbed onto the wooden slats of the barrel, and this will reduce the concentration of drug measured in the water, resulting in a calculation that greatly overestimates the volume of the barrel. In humans, the less well perfused tissues equate to adsorption onto the wood barrel slats, and can be depicted as shown in Fig. 3.8. This is known as a two-compartment model.

The term V_d can give useful information on the distribution characteristics of drugs. Phenylbutazone and aspirin have V_d values which are close to the plasma volume, because these drugs show high

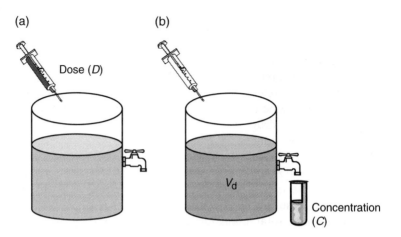

Fig. 3.7 Depiction of the ability to determine the volume of distribution (V_d) from knowledge of the dose administered (a) and concentration in a sample (b).

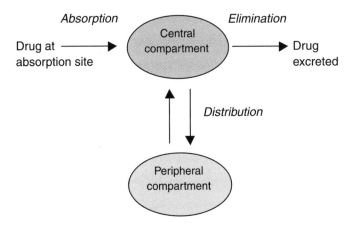

Fig. 3.8   A two-compartment drug distribution model.

plasma protein binding. Conversely, morphine, haloperidol and nor-triptyline have V_d values from 2 to 10 l/kg, because they have high affinity for tissues containing little body water, such as fat cells. Drugs with large volumes of distribution will invariably cross membranes and reach regions such as the brain and foetus.

Plasma protein binding

In the blood, a proportion of the drug is bound to plasma proteins, mainly albumin (in the case of acidic drugs) and alpha-1-glycoprotein (in the case of basic drugs). Only the free, unbound drug distributes to the tissues, because the protein–drug complex is too big to pass through membrane. It is therefore only the free drug that produces a pharmacodynamic effect. Movement of the drug between the blood and the tissues proceeds until an equilibrium between the free drug in the plasma and in the tissues is achieved.

Drug–drug interactions caused by protein binding displacement are rarely clinically relevant. Following the initial addition of a new second drug there may be a transient increase in the free concentrations of an existing (first) drug. However, equilibrium is rapidly re-established, with the free concentration of the first drug returning to levels comparable to those proir to the addition of the second drug. But it is likely that the bound concentration of the first drug will be lower (as both the first and the second drugs will be binding to the same protein receptors), resulting in lower total concentrations. So if the drug assay is measuring total concentrations, this can be misleading for the clinican.

A further example of how the results from total concentration assays of drugs with high protein binding can mislead is phenytoin concentrations in patients with hypoalbuminaemia and renal impairment, in whom the free drug fraction can be up 40% (and bound drug 60%), as opposed to 10% free drug (and 90% bound) in normal patients. So with the same total concentrations as in normal patients, their effective (free) concentrations could be four times higher.

Single-compartment and multiple-compartment models

We initially assumed that drugs distribute rapidly throughout the body: the body is assumed to behave as a single compartment, as illustrated in Fig. 3.2. However, different parts of the body, such as the brain, body fat and muscle, differ in their blood supply and partition coefficient for drugs. It is better, in the case of most drugs, to consider the body as comprising two interconnecting compartments, with reversible transfer occurring between the two. The central compartment is generally regarded as consisting of the blood plasma, and the peripheral compartment as consisting of more slowly equilibrating tissues, as illustrated in Fig. 3.8.

When a drug is intravenously injected (into the central compartment) the drug concentration in the plasma falls biphasically in a two-compartment model (Fig. 3.9), rather than linearly, as happens in a one-compartment model (Fig. 3.4). The initial rapid fall in plasma concentration is called the alpha phase and mainly reflects distribution from the central compartment to the peripheral compartment, although elimination will have started from the moment a drug enters the body. The second phase begins once equilibrium between the central and peripheral compartments has been achieved. The second phase is termed the beta phase, and mainly represents elimination of drug from the body.

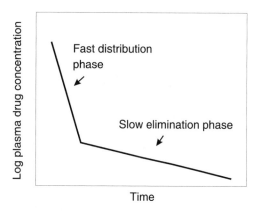

Fig. 3.9 Drug disappearance from plasma, following a single intravenous dose, in a two-compartment model.

Blood–brain barrier

In the two-compartment model, the brain is invariably considered to be within the peripheral compartment, and this is clearly an important consideration with psychotropic drugs. In order for drugs to act upon the brain, they must first enter it by penetrating the blood–brain barrier. This barrier, which surrounds the central nervous system (CNS), behaves as an extreme form of lipid membrane; that is, it is highly selective for lipid-soluble molecules. Lipophilic drugs pass in both directions between plasma water and the brain, usually by passive diffusion, and equilibrium between them is relatively rapidly achieved because the brain is highly perfused with blood. Elimination of drug from the plasma results in movement of drug out of the brain into the plasma to maintain the equilibrium between the central and peripheral compartments.

The rapid and short-acting nature of the barbiturate thiopentone is explained by its distribution characteristics. Administered intravenously to induce anaesthesia, thiopentone is highly lipophilic and rapidly distributes to the brain, where it acts. The lipophilicity of thiopentone results in a high affinity for fat cells and as the blood circulates to the less well perfused body fat stores drug is removed from the circulation. This is turn results in diffusion of drug out of the brain to the blood, resulting in a reduction in the pharmacodynamic effect.

In contrast to thiopentone, barbitone is a more polar, less lipophilic molecule, which does not rapidly distribute to the brain compartment, resulting in a slower onset of sedation and anaesthesia. Another example of the importance of the blood–brain barrier is in the treatment of parkinsonism. Unlike dopamine, L-dopa is able to cross the blood–brain barrier, where it is converted to dopamine and is able to produce the beneficial effects.

Metabolism and elimination

During the distribution phase, the concentrations of drug in the plasma primarily reflect movement of drug within the body, rather than elimination. Once distribution equilibrium is reached, and the elimination phase begins, the body acts kinetically as a single compartment.

The liver and the kidney are the principal routes by which drugs are eliminated. The liver is primarily concerned with metabolism and the kidney is the major route of excretion. The lungs play a major role in the excretion of some drugs, notably gaseous anaesthetics.

Hepatic metabolism

In recent years there have been major advances in our understanding of the mechanisms by which drugs are metabolised in the liver. There are two phases to the metabolism of lipid-soluble drugs by the liver to more water-soluble molecules, which are more easily excreted by the kidney. The first phase of metabolism is mainly oxidation (or sometimes reduction or hydrolysis) to a more polar compound. The second phase involves conjugation, usually with glucuronic acid or sulphate.

Most drugs are oxidised in the liver by a family of microsomal cytochrome P450 isoenzymes. Induction or inhibition of the cytochrome P450 system is a mechanism for drug interaction. These enzymes can be induced by drugs and dietary constituents such as carbamazepine, alcohol and Brussels sprouts, and inhibited by drugs and dietary constituents such as cimetidine, fluoxetine and grapefruit juice.

Elimination half-life

During elimination, the plasma concentration falls exponentially to zero. On a semi-logarithmic plot the rate of decline is defined as the elimination rate constant (K_{el}). Another important pharmacokinetic parameter that can be derived from such a graphical plot is the elimination half-life ($t_{1/2}$), which is the time taken for the plasma concentration to fall by one half. Fig. 3.10 illustrates the estimation of half-life following a single intravenous injection.

The value of knowing a drug's half-life is that it allows a prediction of the drug's duration of action and therefore for an optimal dosing regimen to be planned. However, care has to be taken not to overemphasise

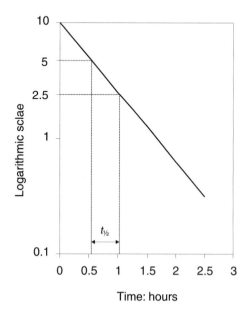

Fig. 3.10 Plot of plasma concentration against time after a single intravenous dose of a drug with a $t_{1/2}$ of around 0.5 h.

the importance of half-life, since the value shows significant inter-subject variation and can be greatly affected by altered hepatic and renal function brought on by disease or old age. Also, recent improvements to assay methodology have dramatically increased sensitivity, such that very low plasma concentrations can now be quantified. This has led to the determination of longer terminal elimination half-lives, but such values derive from deep peripheral compartments that account for very little of the total drug and therefore have little impact upon overall drug pharmacodynamic effects.

Clearance

While the half-life can be important to the understanding of elimin-ation, clearance concepts have greater value in this respect and have greater potential for clinical application. Clearance from plasma (Cl_p) is usually defined in terms of the volume of plasma cleared of a drug in unit time. Volume per unit time is essentially a constant for any one drug, regardless of the concentration of the drug in the body. In the barrel analogy used in Fig. 3.7, clearance is the equivalent of how far open is the tap. Regardless of the concentration in the barrel, this is a constant rate. Clearance, therefore, encompasses both metabolic and renal clearance. Usually, as the concentration of drug in the body rises, the rate of elimination correspondingly increases, and so clearance remains constant.

Multiple doses and steady-state kinetics

We have so far limited our consideration to the case of single-dose administration; however, most drugs are administered as a course of treatment of multiple doses. In multiple-dose administration, the amount absorbed from each dose is added to any drug remaining in the body from previous doses. If the interval between doses is much greater than the half-life, little, if any, accumulation occurs, as shown in Fig. 3.11.

When the dosing interval is less than the half-life, accumulation does occur, until the rate of elimination equals the rate of adminis-tration, resulting in a saw-tooth plasma concentration profile that reaches a plateau, as illustrated in Fig. 3.12.

Steady-state concentration

Consider the case of a drug intravenously injected repeatedly, every half-life. Immediately before the second dose is administered, 50% of the drug from the first dose still remains in the body. Immediately before the third dose, there will be 25% of the first dose and 50% of the second dose remaining in the body. This progression continues until after the fifth dose the average concentration achieves 96.875% of the maximum average steady-state concentration.

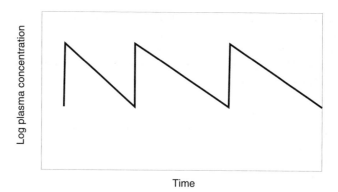

Fig. 3.11 Absence of drug accumulation with repeated administration at a frequency significantly longer than the drug's $t_{1/2}$.

Clinical trials during drug development usually establish the steady-state concentrations required to produce the desired therapeutic effect. The steady-state concentrations that are achieved within a patient vary with both the dose and the frequency of administration. Also, conditions that can bring about a decrease in clearance, such as old age and renal disease, result in an increase in steady-state concentrations.

Therapeutic index

The range of plasma concentrations that yield therapeutic success is termed the therapeutic range, or therapeutic window. The size of the therapeutic window – the therapeutic index – is the ratio of the maximum tolerated concentration to the minimum effective concentration.

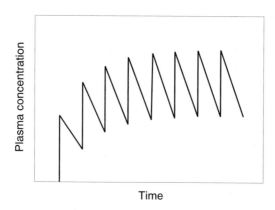

Fig. 3.12 Drug accumulation with repeated administration at a frequency equal to the duration of the drug's $t_{1/2}$.

Caution needs to be exercised in relying upon the therapeutic index as a guide to clinical usefulness, since a particular dosage regimen will result in a wide range of individual responses within the total patient population. The therapeutic index therefore indicates a relatively imprecisely defined dose range and represents a compromise between beneficial and unwanted effects.

Even though some drugs, such as digoxin, may have a very narrow therapeutic window (low therapeutic index), they are of considerable clinical value. In some respects the therapeutic index is of more relevance as a measure of a drug's general safety. One of the main reasons that benzodiazepines replaced barbiturates was that their therapeutic index was substantially higher, as benzodiazepines are less toxic in overdose.

Therapeutic drug monitoring

If a dose of a drug is prescribed to a number of patients, the plasma concentrations can be quite variable, owing to differences in absorption, distribution, metabolism, excretion, gastrointestinal, hepatic, renal or cardiac disease, drug interactions, or poor compliance. The monitoring of plasma drug concentrations in patients helps the clinician to achieve concentrations within the therapeutic window for that individual patient.

Therapeutic drug monitoring is especially useful with drugs that have a narrow therapeutic range. Plasma concentration monitoring is recommended for several psychotropic drugs, including lithium (accepted therapeutic range 0.4–1.0 mmol/l), phenytoin (40–80 mmol/l) and carbamazepine (20–50 mmol/l).

Pharmacokinetics of benzodiazepines

The benzodiazepines are a class of drugs that are often used to exemplify pharmacokinetics, as their pharmacodynamic effects are similar. The onset and duration of the actions of benzodiazepines and their metabolites are dependent upon absorption, distribution, metabolism and elimination. A relatively rapid rate of absorption is a prerequisite for hypnotic activity, while a slower rate of absorption avoids the initial high peak plasma concentration, and is more appropriate for an anxiolytic effect.

The pharmacodynamic consequences of the pharmacokinetic properties of benzodiazepines can be followed by tracking impairment of psychomotor performance. Diazepam is rapidly absorbed and a single 10 mg oral dose produces peak impairment after just 30 minutes, and recovery is rapid. In contrast, oxazepam is more slowly absorbed and a single 30 mg oral dose produces peak impairment after about 3 hours, and recovery is slower.

Table 3.1 Pharmacokinetic classification of benzodiazepines

Short acting	Long acting
Short elimination half-life	Long elimination half-life
High volume of distribution	Low volume of distribution
Minimal accumulation	Accumulation
No active metabolites	Active metabolites
No/minimal residual effects	Residual effects

The duration of pharmacodynamic activity of a psychotropic drug is generally determined by its concentration in the brain, with sedative actions of benzodiazepines ceasing when concentrations fall below a certain threshold. If this threshold is passed during the distribution phase, then the pharmacodynamic effect will be short. If the threshold is passed during the elimination phase, then the effect should parallel the elimination half-life.

Differences in elimination are important for considering daily dosages. The half-life of diazepam is 20–95 hours; daily administration therefore leads to accumulation and may produce residual daytime sedation. As the pharmacodynamic effects of benzodiazepines are similar, they have been classified according to their elimination half-life. The essential characteristics of short- and long-acting drugs are summarised in Table 3.1. Such a classification can be useful, but must be used be care, since aspects of absorption and distribution can be important, and there are pharmacodynamic differences between some benzodiazepines; for instance, midazolam has a half-life of 3 hours, but memory function has been shown to remain impaired 18 hours after a single dose (Subhan & Hindmarch, 1983).

In general, benzodiazepines with a shorter half-life, such as temazepam ($t_{1/2}$ = 15–20 hours) are used for the treatment of insomnia, and those with a longer half-life, such as diazepam, are used for the treatment of anxiety.

Active metabolites of benzodiazepines

The benzodiazepines illustrate the importance of pharmacodynamically active metabolites. Active metabolites can have a major impact upon the duration of pharmacodynamic effect, and hence classification as either short or long acting. If appreciable amounts of an active metabolite, with a relatively long elimination half-life, are formed, then the drug is likely to be long acting, even if the half-life of the parent compound is short.

Benzodiazepines that contain nitrogen-substituted groups, such as diazepam and flurazepam, undergo N-dealkylation to form active metabolites with a long half-life. However, benzodiazepines that contain a hydroxyl group, such as temazepam and lorazepam, are readily conjugated to inactive products, and so have a short-acting clinical effect.

Principles of pharmacodynamics

The biological activity of drugs occurs at target sites that are pharmacologically defined as receptors. Drug receptors may be specific macromolecular proteins or glycoprotein sites in the cell membrane or cytoplasm that have a natural, or endogenous, mediator, as with benzodiazepines and gamma-aminobutyric acid (GABA). Alternatively, drugs may exert their effect by combining with an enzyme, transport protein or other cellular macromolecule (such as DNA), and interfering with its function, such as with the monoamine oxidase inhibitors (used in the treatment of depression and parkinsonism). For the purpose of this chapter, the term 'receptor' is used to encompass both types of physiological target.

Dose and response

A graphical plot of the measured biological response to a drug (e.g. blood pressure) against the logarithm of the dose produces a sigmoid dose–response curve (Fig. 3.13). The linear portion usually lies between 20% and 80% of the maximal response, with sigmoidal tails above and below the linear range. This plot illustrates the concentrations required

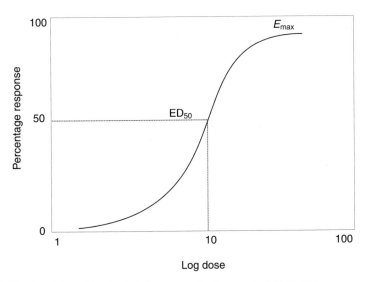

Fig. 3.13 Semi-logarithmic plot of a concentration–response curve.

to produce the maximal effect (E_{max}) and can be used to estimate the dose that elicits 50% of the maximal response (ED_{50}).

Agonists and antagonists

Drugs that are capable of stimulating receptors to produce their maximal effect are termed full agonists. Agonists produce their effect by combining with the receptor and activating the signal conduction pathway to which the receptor is linked. The biological effect may be excitatory, such as the increase in cardiac contractility produced by adrenaline, or inhibitory, as with the smooth muscle relaxation produced by dopamine.

Antagonists are drugs that reduce or wholly block the effects of agonists. Partial agonists are drugs which do stimulate receptors, but to a lesser extent than full agonists, and will act as an antagonist in the presence of a full agonist (buprenorphine is a partial agonist of the morphine µ-receptor).

Competitive antagonists usually bind to the same receptor as an agonist, but presumably do not produce the conformational changes in the receptor that lead to signal transduction. Consequently, in the presence of an antagonist, higher concentrations of an agonist are required to produce the same effect as in the absence of that antagonist. This can be represented as a parallel shift in the dose–response curve (Fig. 3.14a), with an increase in the ED_{50}, but no change in the E_{max}. Non-competitive antagonists bind to a site distant from that occupied by an agonist, and irreversible inhibitors bind to the same site as an agonist – both produce an increase in the ED_{50} *and a lowering of the* E_{max} (Fig. 3.14b).

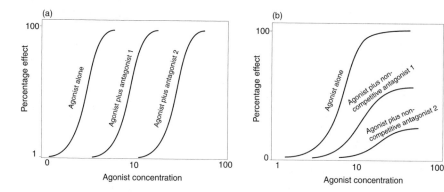

Fig. 3.14 Illustration of the dose–response curves to an agonist alone, and in the presence of two different (a) competitive antagonists, and (b) non-competitive antagonists.

Different drugs that produce the same maximal effect (E_{max}) will have equal efficacy, provided that they equally arrive at the receptor sites. However, drugs that produce their maximal effect at lower doses are said to have greater potency.

Receptor binding

Dose–response curves represent the biological response to a drug. However, these data alone cannot provide estimates of the affinity of individual molecules for a particular receptor for two main reasons: first, knowledge of the dose administered does not directly reflect drug concentrations at the receptor site; and second, the relationship between receptor occupancy and biological response is not necessarily linear. Information on drug receptor affinity and receptor dynamics is derived from ligand binding affinities and measurement of receptor occupancy.

Ligand binding

The reversible binding of a drug with a receptor can be expressed as:

D + R = DR

where D reresents the drug, R the receptor and DR the receptor–drug complex (i.e. bound drug). At equilibrium, the association rate constant K_{-1} must equal the dissociation rate constant K_1. Thus, the above equation can be rearranged to derive the equilibrium binding constant K_D, which will be constant for any concentration of drug:

$$\frac{[D]\,[R]}{[DR]} = \frac{K_1}{K_{-1}} = K_D$$

Using radiolabelled ligands, it is possible to measure accurately the concentrations of bound drug [DR] and free drug [D] and thereby to derive a value for K_D.

This radiolabelled-ligand binding technique can also be used to measure how well competitive antagonists can displace agonist ligands and to derive a value for the concentration required to displace 50% of the ligand, the IC_{50}. The IC_{50} value depends on the concentration of agonist in the assay; however, it can be used to derive the equilibrium dissociation constant (K_I), which will be constant for any given concentration of drug.

Brain receptor occupancy

The use of positron emission tomography (PET) has made possible the measurement of drug receptor dynamics in the living human brain. Using PET, Farde *et al* (1988) studied 11 different antipsychotics in patients with schizophrenia, and were able to show between 65% and

77

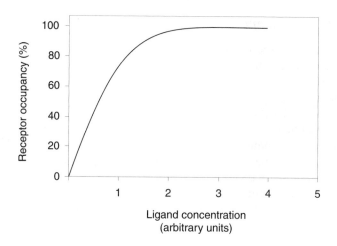

Fig. 3.15 Curvilinear relationship between ligand concentration and receptor occupancy.

85% occupancy of brain dopamine D_2-receptors. The receptor occupancy lasted for several hours, despite a substantial fall in plasma concentration. It has been established that the relationship between free drug concentrations in the brain and receptor occupancy is curvilinear (Fig. 3.15), and with the doses administered of these antipsychotics, the concentrations remained sufficient to achieve near maximal receptor occupancy for a long period.

Subsequent studies have used PET to develop drugs and establish appropriate doses for further study, such as with tolcapone, the selective monoamine oxidase type B (MAO-B) inhibitor, for the treatment of parkinsonism (Bench *et al*, 1991). In addition, this study was able to validate platelet MAO-B measurement as a marker for central MAO-B inhibition. In the past few years PET has been increasingly used to provide valuable qualitative and quantitative data on new drugs being developed, which have been targeted at a wide range of receptors in the CNS, including NMDA, 5-HT$_{1A}$ and NK$_1$.

Drug development

It takes as many as 10 years and the expenditure of hundreds of millions of pounds to develop new medicines. The common goal of all the parties concerned with this process (i.e. the pharmaceutical industry, the government-appointed regulators, medical practitioners and the patients themselves) is to make available safe and effective treatments as economically and swiftly as possible.

Pre-clinical research and development

The first step in the discovery of a new medicine is the decision by a pharmaceutical company to begin research into a particular disease, and to identify a biological or chemical lead worthy of investigation. Such a decision is based upon a number of factors, including the medical need, the technical feasibility and likelihood of successfully identifying a suitable candidate for development, and the existence (or current development) of competing products. Essentially these factors relate to the costs likely to be incurred relative to the probability of success and the likely return on the investment.

Drug development is a multi-disciplinary endeavour, involving chemists, biochemists, pharmacologists, pharmacokineticists, toxicologists and pharmacists, as well as medical specialists in the disease area being studied. Technological advances have resulted in this research becoming more automated, with combinatorial chemistry machinery synthesising large numbers of molecules to be processed by high-throughput *in vitro* screens that identify chemicals that meet the predetermined biological targets. These biological targets should establish the potential of the molecule to show efficacy in humans.

The elucidation of the human genome has opened up a new and exciting area of research that is likely to have a substantial impact on new medicines. We are beginning to learn that some diseases that were thought to have one common underlying cause in fact have multiple genetic predisposing factors, and some diseases that were thought to have multiple causes have only a single genetic component. This will generate new areas of research and the development of, initially, proteins targeted at overcoming the gene defect.

Once a chemical candidate drug has been identified, toxicology studies in animals are required. The main objective of the toxicology studies is to identify adverse effects of the drug and to establish what doses/concentrations of the drug produce these effects. Studies of toxicology in animals cannot predict with absolute certainty the effects in humans. Some potentially successful drugs will unnecessarily fail and sometimes drugs with human toxicity are undetected (i.e. there are false negatives and false positives). The science of toxicology continues to improve, for instance with the increasing use of *in vitro* human cells and tissue cultures, to minimise such occurrences. Nevertheless, tests of safety and efficacy *have* to be performed in people.

Phase I clinical studies

Following the successful completion of animal toxicology studies, studies in humans can begin. Clinical drug development is divided into four distinct phases: phases I, II and III take place before market approval is obtained, and phase IV continues the evaluation of new medicines after marketing.

Phase I studies are carried out in specialist clinical units, within premises belonging either to a pharmaceutical company or to a company devoted to the conduct of clinical studies (known as a contract research organisation; CRO). The aim of phase I studies is to establish the doses to be investigated for potential efficacy in patients with the target disease. Phase I studies generally involve just tens of subjects.

The emphasis of these first (phase I) studies in humans is the early detection of any potentially harmful effects. This demands close 24-hour medical observation. The initial dose will be very small, typically one-hundredth of the dose per kilogram of body weight that produced the first detectable effects in the most sensitive animal species in the toxicology studies. Thorough physical examinations, measurements of vital functions and laboratory tests of renal, hepatic and haemopoetic function are conducted before subjects are entered into a study and at regular intervals during the study.

It is normally preferable for healthy volunteers take part in phase I studies rather than people with the relevant disease. This is because they are a more homogeneous population and they will not be receiving any other medication which could produce interactions or confounding adverse events; in addition, any adverse events are generally easier to detect and manage in healthy volunteers. Patient volunteers are generally used only in phase I studies with drugs that are expected to have a narrow therapeutic window, as it could be considered unethical to expose healthy volunteers to potentially toxic doses of a drug that can offer them no therapeutic benefit.

Currently, in the UK, regulatory approval is not required for studies in healthy volunteers. All studies in patients require the approval of the Medicines Control Agency at the Department of Health, usually under the CTX (Clinical Trial Certificate Exemption) scheme. All human studies are conducted to Good Clinical Practice (GCP) standards, as defined by the consensus of the regulatory authorities of the USA, Japan and Europe in the International Conference on Harmonisation. In accordance with GCP, all studies are approved by a properly constituted ethics committee and informed consent from the subjects is always obtained.

Women of child-bearing potential are often excluded from phase I studies, as the toxicology studies required to establish that a drug is without effect on a foetus are time consuming and are unlikely to have been completed before the start of phase I. In addition, ethical reasons prevent the inclusion of children in phase I studies. Elderly subjects are also usually excluded, except from trials of drugs targeted at diseases predominantly of the elderly, such as dementia.

Assuming that the initial dose is well tolerated, progressively higher doses are administered until a predefined target plasma drug concentration is achieved, or until a detectable effect is observed – be it clinical, laboratory, therapeutic or adverse. Once the single-dose study has been successfully completed, a multiple-dose study takes place. As in the single-dose study, the results of functional tests and the reports of the subjects themselves are carefully assessed and documented. Similarly, plasma drug concentrations are measured to provide information on steady-state pharmacokinetics.

During phase I studies with potential psychotropic drugs, it is usual to include objective and subjective measurements of the drug's effect on the CNS. The objective measurements are usually psychomotor and electroencephalographic (see 'Behaviour and pharmacodynamics: methods of measuring drug effects on the human CNS', below). With drugs such as hypnotics it is possible to observe potential efficacy during phase I trials. However, with most potential psychotropic drugs – such as antidepressants, neuroleptics and antidementia drugs – the demonstration of potential efficacy must await study in patients with the relevant disease.

Only 10% of drugs that begin to be studied in humans eventually become marketed medicines. The majority of those that fail after initial development do so during phase I studies, and the largest cause of failure in development is unexpected problems encountered with absorption, distribution, metabolism or excretion (Hill, 2001).

Phase II clinical trials

Having established a safe dose range in phase I trials, the assessment of the new drug's efficacy can begin, with phase II trials. The aim of these is to establish the efficacious dosage regimen and the incidence of side-effects in the patient population. In addition, by measuring plasma drug concentrations, important information on the body's handling of the drug can be obtained. Generally, hundreds of patients are studied during phase II.

Open, also known as unblinded, studies (i.e. the pharmaceutical company, clinical investigator and the patient all know the drug and dose being administered) sometimes take place in early patient studies; however, placebo-controlled, double-blind trials are the rule. Depending on the disease and the availability of an existing effective treatment, the initial phase II studies may have the new drug as an 'add-on' therapy. Indeed, such add-on studies may continue through to registration with diseases, such as epilepsy, where it would be unethical to withdraw patients from their existing treatment.

During phase II development, new clinical studies in healthy volunteers usually occur. Such studies are likely to seek to establish the fate of the molecule in the body (through studies using ^{14}C-radiolabelled drug) and to investigate the potential for drug–drug interactions and for drug–disease interactions (e.g. whether or not the drug can be safely administered to patients with renal or hepatic disease). The phase II studies should establish the optimal dose range and frequency of administration for the new drug, and refine the target indication for subsequent phase III trials.

Phase III clinical trials

The aim of phase III trials (which are discussed more fully in Chapter 4) is to establish efficacy in the target population at the recommended dose and to identify any uncommon adverse events. They are generally performed with the dosage regimen that is intended to be recommended for general use. Typically just one or two doses are studied, in thousands of patients. The duration of phase III trials must be sufficient to ensure that safety data are obtained that will enable the drug to be prescribed after registration; for the treatment of chronic diseases this means that studies must include patients who receive the drug for over a year.

A positive control may be included in phase III studies, in addition to a placebo. The inclusion of the current therapeutic 'gold standard' as a positive control provides a means by which the new drug can be measured against existing therapies. A new drug is unlikely to be successfully marketed if it cannot provide comparable efficacy to existing therapy, unless it can be shown to produce fewer side-effects.

Drug registration

A pharmaceutical company is not permitted to market a new drug without first obtaining a licence from the responsible government authority, which in the UK is the Department of Health, acting on the advice of the Committee for the Safety of Medicines, although the central European licensing authorities (the European Agency for the Evaluation of Medicinal Products and the Committee for Proprietary Medicinal Products) have an increasing role in the granting of authorisation across the European Union.

The amount of data that are required to be submitted to the authorities in support of the licence application is immense, and areas covered include the toxicology, clinical pharmacology, pharmaceutical purity and manufacturing processes, and the drug's efficacy and safety in humans.

The recent creation by the UK government of the National Institute for Clinical Excellence (NICE) and similar initiatives in other countries have added the extra regulatory step of having to provide pharmaco-economic data, on the cost-effectiveness of a new treatment to the health care providers, before a new drug is likely to be able to be widely prescribed.

It can take many months or even years to obtain licensing approval and agreement on the data sheet for new drugs. From the time a drug is first chemically synthesised, through pre-clinical research and development, clinical development and licensing discussion, to registration and availability to the prescribing physician, is some 12 years on average.

Development costs and patent life

In view of the long time it takes to develop a new medicine, the risk of potential failure, and the immense costs, the patent life of a drug is an important factor in the calculation of economic viability by a pharmaceutical company. Approximately 100 000 new chemical entities have to be synthesised in order to have one reach the market. The costs of development continue to increase as the regulatory authorities require more information before they will grant a product licence. It now costs several hundreds of millions of pound to develop a new drug. In the UK the patent life for a new chemical entity is 20 years. Given that it takes approximately 12 years to research and develop a new medicine, the innovating company has just 8 years to recoup its investment before generic versions of the drug are marketed. Because the manufacturers of the generic drug do not have to recoup the costs of research and development, they can manufacture the medicine more cheaply.

Phase IV clinical trials

The scientific study of a new drug does not stop once a licence has been obtained and a drug is being marketed. It is common to continue large multi-centre studies, to identify any adverse reactions that were not identified in the earlier studies. Such studies are part of post-marketing surveillance. Also, phase IV trials will further investigate the target patient population, to perhaps extend the target indications beyond those studied during phases II and III.

Behaviour and pharmacodynamics: methods of measuring drug effects on the human CNS

There is often a need, at all stages of psychotropic drug development, for basic information regarding a putative drug's pharmacodynamic profile. This information may help: to find the most appropriate formulation of the product; to assess the most appropriate dose and treatment regimens; to place the pharmacokinetics into a behavioural context; to provide a pharmacodynamic context for observed clinical effects; or to investigate the possible behavioural toxicity of a product in clinical use, when side-effects or the impact of unwanted CNS activity need to be measured to ascertain the drug's potential 'toxicity' on the activities of everyday living, especially those with high intrinsic risks, such as car driving and occupational/industrial tasks.

The problems associated with drug-induced impairment of psychological and cognitive function cannot be ignored. Accidents, both fatal and non-fatal, are the inevitable consequence of the use of medicines which alter human performance (Currie *et al*, 1995). Whereas the measurement of these side-effects is an intrinsic part of any CNS drug development programme, in clinical use such problems can be overcome simply by the use of clinically efficacious drugs with a proven lack of deleterious (behaviourally toxic) effects.

For example, clinically effective benzodiazepine hypnotics – lormetazepam, brotizolam, temazepam and triazolam – have been consistently shown to be free from early-morning hangover effects, as too have the so-called non-benzodiazepine ligands of the GABA–chloride ion receptor complex, namely zolpidem, zopiclone and zaleplon. Broadly speaking, selective serotonin reuptake inhibitors and reversible inhibitors of monoamine oxidase-A, as well as tianeptine, milnacipran and reboxetine, are free from objective impairment on psychometric measures, whereas the tricyclic antidepressants and other drugs, for example mianserin, trazodone and mirtazepine, all cause impairment on similar tests.

The basic model of psychomotor function

Human psychomotor performance and cognitive function are complex phenomena that rely heavily on a number of distinct basic functions and processes. As a person's life experience increases, these basic systems become organised and integrated through the assimilation and accommodation (modification) of information into behavioural responses to environmental demands, which ultimately enable individuals to perform the tasks of everyday living. The information processing model of CNS function (Fig. 3.16) serves to illustrate the way in which sensory information is perceived, processed and passed through a series of transformations which, to a greater or lesser extent, produce a behavioural response (Hindmarch, 1980).

The operational procedures that link received sensations with overt or covert behavioural response are influenced by the personality, needs, motivation, memory and prior learning experiences of the individual subject. The simpler the psychometric test, the less these extraneous and uncontrolled variables are liable to influence scores and assessments.

Tests of psychomotor performance

The successful measurement of the impact of psychotropic drugs on the human CNS depends on the parsimonious use of psychometric tests within a methodologically sound experimental design. Some of these

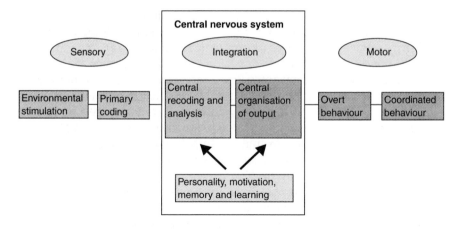

Fig. 3.16 The relationship between the elements comprising the human psychomotor response (adapted from Hindmarch, 1980).

tests require strategy and complex abilities to complete and, as such, do not reflect basic psychological function, as they are, in themselves, too complex for subjects to master without extensive training. Computerised test batteries based on a strategic response or requiring pre-experimental training should be abandoned in favour of simple tests of basic psychological function (including cognitive and psychomotor response) which have been shown to be reliable and valid indicators of the CNS effects of psychotropic drugs.

There are differences between objective psychometric tests and conventional clinical assessments. The former rely on measures of speed of response, number, frequency, rate and so on to measure psychomotor and cognitive function, whereas the latter rely on a subjective impression, which might not always correlate with objective psychometric scores. Patients' subjective reports cannot be regarded as sufficient scientific evidence to support the notion that a particular drug has a specific effect on CNS functioning.

Excluding subjective measures, there are two main approaches to the study of human performance and the effects of psychotropic drugs. A drug can be assessed by means of a battery of tests which are used to build up a profile of effects across the specific psychomotor and cognitive elements. Alternatively, the particular skill of interest, say car driving, can be simulated with as much accuracy as possible. Both approaches have their merits but the majority opinion favours the laboratory-based test battery over direct task simulation. The main reason for this stems from the difficulty of interpreting data derived from simulations. While the visible similarity of a simulation (known as face validity) to a real situation is likely to persuade many that the results are to be trusted, in practice such tests often lack sensitivity in the measurement of performance. The problem is that a task such as car driving comes in a variety of forms, and a simulation can hope to assess only one of these forms. For example, driving an articulated vehicle long distances on a motorway demands different skills to negotiating the evening rush hour after a day at work. Even if it were possible to take account of these differences, uncertainty would remain as to how these effects could be expected to apply to other skills and occupations. However, there is an encouraging link between brake reaction time assessed in a car on the road and laboratory measures of choice reaction time (Ridout & Hindmarch, 2001).

A more coherent picture of the psychomotor effects of psychotropic drugs will emerge if a drug is assessed in terms of a range of basic psychomotor elements common to task and skill groups, rather than if particular skills are tackled individually and directly. A vast array of psychomotor tests have been used to assess the effects of drugs; these often owe more to the ingenuity of their originators than to any serious attempt to produce a reliable and valid psychometric test. It is not possible here to provide an exhaustive list of such tests, but a few of the more common examples are described below under the main groupings, and this should serve as a useful outline (Hindmarch, 1980).

Assessment of sensory function

Stimulus detection, or vigilance tasks, in which a subject is required to respond to predetermined stimuli over an extended period, are good laboratory models of situations that demand alertness to be maintained during boring or repetitive tasks. Sensory recognition or perception has often been examined with simple paper-and-pencil tests, such as digit symbol substitution or letter or digit substitution, and prolonged signal-detection tasks in long-term vigilance situations have also proved useful.

Assessment of CNS arousal

Changes in central arousal are often measured by means of the critical flicker fusion (CFF) threshold. This method exploits the phenomenon that a decrease in arousal of the CNS is accompanied by a fall in the maximum frequency at which the flickering of a light can be perceived.

The electroencephalogram (EEG) is also commonly used to investigate drug-induced changes in central arousal. The EEG measures changes in electrical potential in the cortex by means of electrodes placed on the scalp. By convention, signals obtained from an EEG are classified into four frequency bands: alpha, beta, delta and theta. Changes in the power of these different wavebands provides information on arousal. Although the behavioural correlates with EEG changes are often unclear, sophisticated computer-analysed techniques (pharmaco-EEG) are able to profile drugs into the main psychopharmacological drug classes and thereby assist in establishing the likely therapeutic potential of new agents (Saletu, 1987).

Assessment of motor function

Motor activity and coordination can be classified under four headings – ballistic, gross body balance, fine motor control and motor manipulative activity. Assessment of ballistic activity is often made by measuring the rate of finger tapping, and various stabilometer devices are used to investigate changes in body sway as measurements of balance. Motor control and manipulative skills are modelled by tests such as writing speed and pegboard tasks. More recently, wrist-mounted actigraphs have shown a certain utility in the continuous assessment of overall behavioural activity (Stanley & Hindmarch, 1997).

Assessment of sensorimotor function

Few activities can be classified as being either purely sensory or purely motor – the majority require the coordination of both sensory and motor systems, and a number of tests have been designed to take account of this. Examples of such tests include the Gibson spiral maze test, the pursuit rotor test, card sorting, choice reaction time and the measurement of saccadic eye movement. The last test measures the conjugate shifts of gaze that are produced when a person is instructed to follow a visual target that rapidly moves from one point to another.

Factors affecting psychomotor performance

Whatever tests and test batteries are used to assess psychomotor effects, researchers in this area need to be aware of the extraneous factors that can influence data, and the safeguards that can be taken to overcome or avoid such influences.

The fact that psychomotor performance is greatly modified by age, sex, motivation, socio-cultural factors and personality has long been recognised (Hindmarch, 1980). The motivation generated by the test itself is also important – many psychological tests are regarded by the testees as interesting, and if this motivates the subject to try harder it could mask the effects of a sedative drug.

It is important to use multiple test batteries as, for example, the shorter speed of reaction following dosing with a psychostimulant might, in itself, seem to be the main characteristic of the drug if only reaction time is measured. However, if a battery of tests is used, then it may become evident that the psychostimulant also reduces psychomotor accuracy and impairs logical reasoning skills.

Performance is subject to circadian rhythms, with several peaks and troughs throughout a 24-hour period. Statistics derived from road traffic accidents illustrate this point: the peak period for accidents is between 2 and 6 a.m. and between 2 and 4 p.m. These times correspond with periods of maximum sleepiness and minimum alertness (Moore-Ede, 1993).

In order to combat these pitfalls and others inherent in psychometric studies, proper experimental design and methodology are essential. The number of subjects in a study needs to be sufficiently large to be able to detect subtle or fleeting changes. When studying the effects of psychotropic drugs it is necessary to include both a placebo and an active control (i.e. an established drug with known activity). A crossover design is essential for these studies (i.e. each subject receives all the different treatments, in random order, with a suitable wash-out period between each dose). Subjects need to practise the tests until their performance has reached a plateau, and repeated testing should be performed at the same time of day. The data derived from psychometric studies are improved when a range of doses is studied, preferably covering the therapeutic range, with testing carried out several times after drug administration. Since a very large amount of data can be generated from psychometric studies, it is important to have pre-defined primary end-points and appropriate statistical interpretation of the results. Above all, it is necessary to choose only validated, reliable and sensitive psychometric instruments and to use a protocol that asks a pertinent question.

Implications of performance effects

Tests of psychomotor performance are important in the development of all new psychotropic drugs and drugs that have adverse CNS effects. By way of illustration, two classes of psychotropic agent are discussed below, namely hypnotics and antidepressants.

Hypnotics

The benzodiazepines are widely used as hypnotics in the treatment of sleep disorders, simply because their forebears – the barbiturates and chloral hydrate – were too toxic. As a result much attention has been paid to their psychometric profiles. We have discussed above how the pharmacokinetic properties of benzodiazepines affect their speed of therapeutic onset (see Table 3.1) and duration of effect, and psychomotor testing has shown that for some compounds, such as nitrazepam and flurazepam, there are sedative effects that persist until the morning after administration the previous evening. These findings have important health and safety implications, as increased sleepiness the morning after taking hypnotic therapy is likely to increase the risk of accidents. It is known that, in the UK, approximately a quarter of road traffic accidents can be attributed to daytime sleepiness, and it is unfortunate that accidents caused by sleepiness are inclined to be more serious, with upwards of 80% resulting in fatalities. In addition, residual drowsiness, lethargy and sleepiness during the day disrupt the diurnal balance between sleepiness and wakefulness. Daytime sleepiness can produce sleep-induction problems at night. Paradoxically, treatment with hypnotics that have residual sequelae may result in the very same insomnia that they are designed to overcome. In this context, the differentiation of the potential of hypnotics to produce residual effects through psychometric testing is particularly valuable.

Antidepressants

Tricyclic antidepressants such as amitriptyline, imipramine and desipramine, and atypical drugs such as mianserin, mirtazepine and trazodone are known to affect information processing and cognitive function adversely. The sedation that many antidepressants produce can be a significant problem for out-patients who are trying to carry out everyday tasks; in other words, these drugs can reduce a patient's quality of life. As with hypnotics, such adverse effects can be counter-therapeutic, in that the impairment of quality of life can result in a deepening of the depression that the treatment is trying to alleviate. There are circumstances in which sedating antidepressants are the treatment of choice; however, they must be used with caution in ambulatory patients.

The selective serotonin reuptake inhibitors have, broadly speaking, a favourable profile as regards psychomotor effects and none has serious problems regarding impairment of psychomotor function in clinical use, although the impact on cognitive and psychomotor function following abrupt discontinuation of paroxetine (Hindmarch *et al*, 2000), particularly with respect to the lack of discontinuation effects found with fluoxetine and citalopram, emphasises the importance of objective assessment of CNS activity at all stages of drug development and usage.

Clinical decisions

The problems that are associated with drug-induced impairment of psychomotor function can be overcome through the use of drugs with minimal or no adverse effects.

The importance of developing psychopharmaceuticals with fewer side-effects and greater clinical efficacy is evident. The assumption – so frequently borne out by the results of clinical trials – is that all psychoactive drugs have a similar clinical efficacy. However, a careful assessment of the effects of a particular molecule on psychomotor and cognitive function can not only provide essential data regarding the dose–response pharmacodynamics, but also give vital information regarding the safety of a drug in clinical use.

Ratings of the behavioural toxicity of psychoactive drugs not only inform patients of the potential impact of their prescribed medication on their particular lifestyle, but also give the prescribing physician the means to make an informed decision regarding the most appropriate medication to satisfy the needs of a particular patient.

References

Bench, C. J., Price, G. W., Lammertsma, A. A., *et al* (1991) Measurement of human cerebral monoamine oxidase type B (MAO-B) activity with positron emission tomography (PET): a dose ranging study with the reversible inhibitor Ro 19-6327. *European Journal of Clinical Pharmacology*, **40**, 169–173.

Currie, D. J., Hashemi, K., Fothergill, J., *et al* (1995) The use of antidepressants and benzodiazepines in the perpetrators and victims of accidents. *Occupational Medicine*, **45**, 323–325.

Farde, L., Wiesal, F.-A., Halldin, C., *et al* (1988) Central D_2-dopamine receptor occupancy in schizophrenic patients treated with antipsychotic drugs. *Archives of General Psychiatry*, **45**, 71–76.

Hill, S. A. (2001) Biologically relevant chemistry. *Drug Discovery World*, **2**, 19–25.

Hindmarch, I. (1980) Psychomotor function and psychoactive drugs. *British Journal of Clinical Pharmacology*, **10**, 189–209.

Hindmarch, I., Kimber, S. & Cockle, S. M. (2000) Abrupt and brief discontinuation of antidepressant treatment: effects on cognitive function and psychomotor performance. *International Clinical Psychopharmacology*, **15**, 305–318.

Moore-Ede, M. (1993) *The 24 Hour Society: The Risks, Costs and Challenges of a World That Never Stops*. London: Piatkus.

Ridout, F. & Hindmarch, I. (2001) Effects of mianserin and tianeptine on car driving skills. *Psychopharmacology*, **154**, 356–361.

Saletu, B. (1987) The use of pharmaco-EEG in drug profiling. In *Human Psychopharmacology: Measures and Methods. Vol. 1* (eds I. Hindmarch & P. D. Stonier), pp. 173–201. Chichester: Wiley.

Stanley, N. & Hindmarch, I. (1997) Actigraphy can measure antidepressant-induced daytime sedation in healthy volunteers. *Human Psychopharmacology: Clinical and Experimental*, **12**, 437–443.

Subhan, Z. & Hindmarch, I. (1983) The effects of midazolam in conjunction with alcohol on iconic memory and free recall. *Neuropsychobiology*, **9**, 230–234.

Further reading

Balant, L. P., Benitez, J., Dahl, S. G., *et al* (eds) (1998) *Clinical Pharmacology in Psychiatry: Finding the Right Dose of Psychotropic Drugs*. Luxembourg: European Commision.

Cutler, N. R., Sramek, J. J. & Narang, P. K. (eds) (1994) *Pharmacodynamics and Drug Development: Perspectives in Clinical Pharmacology*. Chichester: Wiley.

Jack, D. B. (1992) *Handbook of Clinical Pharmacokinetics Data*. Basingstoke: Macmillan.

Mann, R. D., Rawlins, M. D. & Auty, R. M. (1993) *A Textbook of Pharmaceutical Medicine*. Carnforth: Parthenon.

O'Grady, J. & Joubert, P. H. (eds) (1997) *Handbook of Phase I and II Clinical Drug Trials*. Boca Raton, FL: CRC Press.

Prien, R. F. & Robinson, D. S. (eds) (1994) *Clinical Evaluation of Psychotropic Drugs: Principles and Guidelines*. New York: Raven Press.

Reid, J. L., Rubin, P. C. & Whiting, B. (1996) *Lecture Notes on Clinical Pharmacology* (5th edn). Oxford: Blackwell.

Ritter, J. M., Lewis, L. D. & Mant, T. G. (1999) *A Textbook of Clinical Pharmacology* (4th edn). London: Arnold.

Rowland, M. & Tozer, T. N. (1995) *Clinical Pharmacokinetics: Concepts and Applications.* Baltimore, MA: Williams and Wilkins.

Spriet, A., Dupin-Spriet, T. & Simon, P. (1994) *Methodology of Clinical Drug Trials* (2nd edn). Basel: Karger.

CHAPTER 4

The clinical principles underlying drug treatment in psychiatric practice

Phil Harrison-Read and Peter Tyrer

Introduction

This chapter addresses some of the general principles surrounding the clinical aspects of pharmacology and therapeutics that are relevant to the treatment of patients with psychiatric disorders. Many of the issues and problems we discuss stem from three important and related facts that are sometimes forgotten in the enthusiasm that greets new drug treatments. First, most 'functional' mental disorders that require drug treatment are recurrent and have a tendency to become chronic. Second, any benefits of drug treatment cannot be viewed in isolation from the setting in which the drug is given. Third, the impairments created by 'illness' are determined as much by personal and social factors as biological ones.

Drug therapy in psychiatry rarely leads to cure, although it may provide suppression or amelioration of symptoms while it is being administered. In such circumstances the personality and persuasion of the doctor is an important aspect of care that has a great deal to do with success. Unfortunately, as Balint (1957) noted many years ago, doctors are often less knowledgeable and aware about prescribing 'themselves' than they are about prescribing drug and other treatments. This comment may arouse some scepticism, but patients, when asked a few questions about their drug treatment over the years, often match 'good drugs' with 'good doctors' – but when 'bad doctors' are identified it is likely to be found that they prescribed the same drugs, although with considerably less benefit.

A great deal also depends on the psychosocial circumstances of treatment. This includes not only the normal environment in which a patient lives but also the physical and social environment in which treatment is given, commonly subsumed under the word 'milieu'. In this context it is worth remembering the alliterative dictum 'milieu matters as much or more than medicine in mending most mental misery'.

The current status and ethics
of drug treatment in psychiatry

Historical background: the drug revolution and its aftermath

The prototypes of most of the psychotherapeutic drugs currently in use were introduced in the late 1940s and 1950s following a remarkable series of adventurous and astute clinical experiments based on 'wrong' hypotheses or accidents (normally translated as serendipity). Nearly all of the original prototypes are still important treatments today. With the possible exception of the selective serotonin reuptake inhibitors (used for the treatment of a wide range of conditions, including affective, obsessive–compulsive and eating disorders), and the rediscovery of the atypical antipsychotic clozapine for treating resistant schizophrenia, no new major advance in psychiatric drug treatment has been planned in the laboratory, despite some promising leads (e.g. the range of serotonin receptor blockers).

One of the first specific psychotherapeutic agents to be used was lithium. Although for a time its long-term safety and therapeutic value were questioned, lithium is probably better known by psychiatrists at present than at any time since its introduction. However, its original application as a specific treatment for acute mania is now less important than its use as a prophylactic agent in affective disorders, where it is currently in competition with carbamazepine and sodium valproate as the main mood stabiliser.

In contrast to the staying power of lithium, the benzodiazepines, at one time popular with prescribers and patients as a universal treatment for anxiety, and widely regarded as exemplars of safety and specificity of action, have now seen a dramatic reversal in their fortunes. Even if this proves to be an overreaction, it reflects a growing (probably healthy) scepticism about the benefits to be expected from psychotropic drugs. It is also fair to say that in the 40 years since benzodiazepines were first introduced in clinical practice, we do not yet have better drugs for the immediate relief of anxiety.

Perhaps the most important prototypal psychotropic drug is chlorpromazine, a phenothiazine with a broad spectrum of actions, which somewhat paradoxically emerged in 1952 as the first specific antipsychotic agent. The impact of its introduction was such that 1952 is often said to mark the date of the so-called 'psychopharmacological revolution', even though new drugs have constantly been introduced over the centuries. After the introduction of chlorpromazine there was a marked increase in the numbers of discharges from mental hospitals and a new wave of therapeutic optimism swept through psychiatry. Although it has been argued that these changes preceded the introduction of chlorpromazine, there is little doubt that this was a major advance. For the first time, a relatively simple drug treatment that could be easily given outside hospital was available to control the symptoms of the most severe and disabling of psychiatric illnesses.

In the 1950s there was a tendency to regard all other new drugs as equally important as chlorpromazine. To some extent this was justified, for example with the introduction of imipramine, the first anti-depressant drug, but in recent years there has been much more concern about the adverse effects of drug treatments as the pendulum of public opinion has gradually swung away from drug treatments and towards psychological treatment and complementary medicines.

The wide spectrum of drug action

Carefully controlled trials carried out in the 1960s (e.g. NIMH-PSC Collaborative Study Group, 1964) confirmed the therapeutic effectiveness of chlorpromazine and related phenothiazine drugs in about 75% of acutely psychotic patients with schizophrenia, compared with only 25% who improved on placebo. These effects were shown to be relatively independent of sedation, since they could not be achieved by treatment with barbiturates or with the sedative but weak antipsychotic pheno-thiazine promazine. Neither did they seem to depend on the production of Parkinsonian-like (extrapyramidal) movement disorders, since another phenothiazine, thioridazine, was as effective an antipsychotic as chlor-promazine but produced fewer extrapyramidal side-effects.

Despite differences in acute and unwanted effects, when used in appropriately matched doses, all 'typical' antipsychotic drugs seem equally effective against the entire spectrum of psychotic symptoms and signs, at least when compared in clinical trials. Thus drugs associated with alerting or sedative effects are equally effective in calming psychotic excitement and in improving mutism and self-neglect in a withdrawn person with schizophrenia. In delusional depression antipsychotic drugs may diminish the psychotic symptoms, while leaving the mood disturbance unchanged. Thus the drugs appear to be selectively anti-psychotic, but not symptom or even syndrome specific, since a drug such as chlorpromazine, in common with many others, seems to have effects on a number of psychiatric syndromes. For example, although chlorpromazine is primarily an antipsychotic, it may also be used as a sedative, a hypnotic or a tranquillising drug for states of excitement due to functional mental disorder or organic brain syndromes. Some of these effects are dose related, and the antipsychotic effects in particular are found only at higher dosage, but the breadth of pharmacological effects is still very pronounced. Thus, although each drug is given a primary label, such as anxiolytic, antidepressant or antipsychotic, most have several therapeutic applications.

There are other reasons – apart from dosage – for the wide spectrum of pharmacological action of many drugs. They include the fact that many drugs are pharmacologically 'dirty', in that they have many different actions irrespective of the ones used for the therapeutic effect under consideration. This issue is mentioned many times in other parts of this book and will not be referred to again. However, there is one general point that ought to be emphasised at this stage. It can be summed up under the heading of teleological error. Teleology is the ascribing of purpose and cause, and a frequent error in psychopharmacology is to assume that because a drug is labelled according to its therapeutic action (e.g. antipsychotic, antidepressant) that it necessarily acts in this way whenever it is found to be therapeutically effective. This was seen in perhaps its most absurd form during the 1960s, after the widespread use of antidepressants to treat anxiety, somatic, hysterical and phobic symptoms (among others) – it was assumed that all such symptoms constituted 'masked' or 'atypical' depression, when the more obvious conclusion, that other symptoms and conditions apart from depression could also be helped by these drugs, was not drawn until much later (Hudson & Pope, 1990; Tyrer, 2001).

The rationale and ethical basis of drug treatment: the medical model of mental illness

The whole notion of using chemicals to alter mental functioning is full of ethical dilemmas. However, many of these problems can be overcome once there is an established rationale for the correct use of drugs. For every medical use of a drug there should be:

(1)   clear indications (normally expressed in diagnostic terms)
(2)   a specified dose range
(3)   a specified duration of treatment.

Even though it is extremely difficult to set these forth exactly (e.g. the indications for antidepressant therapy, the duration of treatment for schizophrenia), the questions always need to be asked and, ideally, the practitioner ought to record at the beginning of treatment what his or her expectations are about each of these three elements. This decision is helped to some extent by the data sheet for each drug, which indicates clearly the best state of knowledge in each of these areas.

If treatment is given within these guidelines it will be approved by the body of opinion in medicine and generally regarded as ethical. Once the practitioner strays from these guidelines (e.g. by giving amphetamines regularly as an antidepressant treatment) the treatment may be not only inappropriate or fundamentally wrong but also unethical, because of the hazards associated with its use.

With these points in mind it is relatively straightforward to prescribe drugs to those who consent to such treatment. It is more difficult to make these decisions when the patient clearly refuses drug treatment. Most of the serious psychiatric disorders are associated with impairment of insight, and refusal to take treatment is extremely common. In most countries of the world treatment cannot be given against a patient's will unless the person is detained in hospital under appropriate legal provision. Even when there is abundant evidence that the patient has responded to drug treatment in the past and relapses only when the drug is stopped, the reintroduction of that drug must be done in the setting of a compulsory admission (although in parts of Australia and the USA compulsory treatment is now given in the community).

Community treatment orders are likely to be introduced into the UK and this is likely to have a significant bearing on drug treatment. It is also fair to add that, in a consumer-driven society, the views of patients are very important, and currently these favour psychological rather than pharmacological treatments, and this is a particular problem in the treatment of schizophrenia (Hale, 1993).

The more 'biological' the symptoms (e.g. impairment of cognitive functions, energy, sleep, appetite, weight, biorhythms and drives), the greater is the expectation that biological treatments such as drugs will ameliorate them or, to put it another way, the more 'ethical' it is to treat them with drugs. On the whole this expectation is justified by empirical research, although symptoms of a mainly psychological or behavioural nature may respond equally well, whether or not biological symptoms coexist. As psychiatrists are frequently put in the position of being encouraged to prescribe more rather than fewer drugs, and newer rather than older drugs, mainly because of the influence of drug marketing procedures, there is an ethical aspect to the treatment of all those conditions in which drugs and non-pharmacological forms of treatment could be equally appropriate. As long as doctors are aware of this tension and tendentiousness, and the tendency for users to prefer non-drug treatments, they should be able to reach a considered, fair and, ultimately ethical, decision about appropriate therapy.

As an alternative to neuropathological concepts, mental or psychological illness can just as easily be conceptualised at the level of a dysfunctional interaction between different aspects of the personality and between the individual and the outside world. An appropriate analogy might be that of a malfunctioning computer program, the cause of which could be either incorrect or inappropriate data input or a fault in the program itself (Harrison-Read, 1984). Such a malfunction might occur despite the fact that the computer's electronics are structurally and functionally sound.

This kind of analogy for psychological illness supports a 're-programming model' of treatment (i.e. some form of psychotherapy,

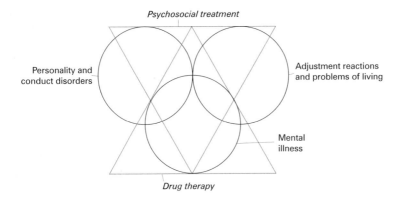

Fig. 4.1 The psychiatric spectrum and the application of drug and psychosocial treatment.

particularly the cognitive–behavioural sort). Drug treatment can then be conceptualised as a physical intervention that indirectly facilitates this process (analogous to switching off parts of the computer while a program is rewritten). Furthermore, 'biological' and 'psychological' mental illness may coexist and be causally related. Using the computer analogy again, repeated program (software) malfunction may eventually lead to a hardware fault such as 'a blown fuse'. Fig. 4.1 illustrates diagrammatically the spectrum of problems and disorders that are the concern of psychiatry, and the relative applications of drug and psychosocial treatments. It argues for combined therapeutic approaches rather than the sterile 'either–or' debate which sometimes divides different schools of psychiatry.

It is likely that for the foreseeable future psychiatric treatment will remain pragmatic, and be based as much on social codes and norms as on scientific and medical foundations.

Evaluation of psychiatric drug treatments in patients (phase III trials)

The earlier stages of evaluating psychiatric drug treatment (phase I and II trials) are discussed in Chapter 3. This chapter is concerned with evaluation of drug treatments at the point at which they are being actively considered for general use in psychiatric disorders.

Open and controlled clinical trials

Open clinical trials involve the administration of a new drug to patients who have the disorder that may become one of the drug's indications, followed by a recording of the effects of administration, with no attempt to control for other factors. These are quite common in preliminary (phase II) drug evaluation but no longer have a place in the formal evaluation of efficacy that is part of phase III studies. The essential feature of the controlled trial is the randomisation of patients to two or more treatment regimens that differ only in the nature of the treatment given. The use of the randomised controlled trial is now commonplace in medicine but there are special features that sometimes make it more difficult to apply in psychiatry (Johnson, 1998).

One of the important tasks of psychiatrists today is to make the best possible choice of drugs for a given patient with information derived not primarily from their own clinical practice but from the 'harder' evidence of controlled clinical trials. This is not easy, because trials are often contradictory and it is far from certain which are the most reliable, but it has been helped by the growth of literature in evidence-based medicine (see below). The psychiatrist can be helped by reading systematic reviews of the subjects concerned, particularly when they employ meta-analysis as a technique for combining the results of several trials (e.g. Cochrane reviews), or by using other methods when there is more limited information available (e.g. Tyrer & Tyrer, 1992).

Some of the essential principles in organising a good clinical trial are described below, and they should always be borne in mind when examining the efficacy of an individual drug.

Selection of patients

Even if considerable sophistication is used in the analysis and interpretation of the results, a poor initial design can invalidate a clinical trial. The selection of patients is the most important issue and the criteria for inclusion and exclusion are critical. The criteria for diagnosis and severity and chronicity of illness must be stated explicitly, and the key variables should be assessed separately using instruments that have accepted validity, sensitivity and reliability.

The aim is to study a relatively homogeneous population that will show a reasonable response to treatment with as little variance in response as possible (high 'signal-to-noise ratio' or large 'effect size', effect size being the mean response divided by its standard deviation). To meet this aim, it is usually necessary to exclude patients with very mild or very severe forms of the disorder under consideration, because they represent the extremes of the population with the disorder and tend to show a relatively small specific response to treatment.

However, imposing excessively strict entry criteria may adversely affect the ability to generalise the results of the trial, and may make it difficult to recruit an adequate number of subjects to the study. The patients entered into the trial may then not be sufficiently representative of the type of patient likely to be considered for treatment in everyday practice, so reducing the practical validity of a trial.

There are several other reasons why the results of a published trial may not be easily generalised to daily practice. The conditions of a research study may result in unusually high levels of patient cooperation and compliance with the treatment, in comparison with ordinary practice. On the other hand, if there are too many non-compliers or non-completers in the trial, this will also affect the extent to which the results of the patients who do conform to the study design can be generalised. These effects are removed by using what is commonly called 'an intention to treat' model, whereby all patients initially randomised are included in the analysis no matter what happens to them subsequently (Johnson, 1998).

Most of the special conditions inherent in controlled clinical trials tend to give an over-optimistic estimate of the practical value of a treatment in ordinary clinical practice. On the other hand, such conditions might also inflate the 'placebo response' and so under-estimate the specific benefit due to the treatment. Of course, if a placebo control group were not included in the trial design, it would not be possible to make any judgement about this at all.

Despite these reasons for caution, overgeneralisation from the results of published trials is common. If the treatment is shown to be effective and useful in a narrowly defined group of patients using narrowly defined outcome criteria and a specified range of doses and duration of treatment, it cannot be assumed that this will be the case in, for example, an older, less ill, more chronic or less cooperative group of patients.

Explanatory versus pragmatic trials

In designing clinical trials, there is a potential conflict between the aim of trying to discover the answer to specific scientific questions about a drug's therapeutic activity (explanatory trials) and attempts to evaluate benefits and problems with the treatment in routine clinical practice (pragmatic trials) (Johnson, 1998). The answer to 'scientific questions' demands rigidly controlled conditions, but these may have less relevance to the conditions of everyday practice. Most designers of clinical trials would like to think that their results are generalisable to general clinical practice, but this is rarely wholly true.

With regard to subject selection, a suggested coping strategy (Kraemer, 1981) that takes all these factors into consideration would be to set rather liberal entry criteria, which would exclude from the trial only the following: those subjects who would not usually be considered for treatment, for legal, ethical or clinical reasons; those who have, *a priori*, little capacity for change (e.g. the very mildly or very severely affected); and those who are unlikely to comply with the requirements of the study protocol. If one wishes to isolate a particular subgroup for *post hoc* (retrospective) analysis, for example to see whether patients with particular symptoms did better than those without, under these liberal criteria, one may easily do so, whereas if more strict entry criteria have been enforced, *post hoc* options are minimised.

Randomisation

Subjects are randomly assigned to study groups in order to ensure that there is no systematic bias in deciding which patients get what treatment. However, because of chance bias, relevant characteristics of the patients in each treatment group must always be stated, to allow a check of any serious imbalances between groups. If there is a patient characteristic that is almost certain to affect the outcome of the trial (e.g the severity of illness), treatment groups can be stratified for this characteristic, so that there are equal proportions in each group.

Measurements: reliability, validity and sensitivity

Measurements used to assess treatment effects must be demonstrably *reliable*, as indicated by test–retest or inter-rater correlations of 0.6 or more (Kraemer, 1981). This usually requires careful standardisation of test conditions, and the use of both highly trained observers and rating scales with precise definitions and 'anchor points'. One way of compensating for the unavoidable use of measures of low reliability is to have very large samples. A better way is to combine the results of several tests or ratings that independently measure various aspects of the same element.

Deciding on the *validity* of measures is a highly complex issue. Clinical trials that use measures that are not generally accepted as valid are suspect. Perhaps the most common reasons for measures being considered invalid are their insensitivity to change in the severity of the condition under study, and their unsuitability for repeated use.

The *sensitivity* of measurements also needs to be considered as a separate issue. A common reason for loss of sensitivity is the arbitrary compression of quantitative measures on a continuous dimension. For example, scores on a rating scale are sometimes used to assign patients to discontinuous categories such as 'no improvement', 'slight improvement' and 'marked improvement'. This may appear to be helpful in deciding on the clinical relevance of a change in rating scores, but unless the steps are independently validated by comparison with a global rating instrument designed for the purpose, this may obscure rather than illuminate, while sacrificing sensitivity and power (see Appendix).

Control groups, experimental design and sample size

In order to assess a drug's merits and demerits, it must be compared with another therapy, either a standard treatment or a placebo. Placebo-controlled trials are essential early in a drug's development in order to

> **Box 4.1** Conditions usually showing marked non-drug-specific
> (placebo) response and/or sustained spontaneous recovery
>
> * Anxiety disorders
> * Adjustment disorders
> * Dissociative and conversion states (hysterical reactions)
> * Reactive mood disorders
> * Drug-induced psychoses
> * Major depressive episodes (placebo responses may occur early in
>   treatment but are often not sustained)
> * Hypomanic and manic episodes

establish that it does have some useful specific efficacy in the condition under study. The use of a placebo is particularly important when the disorder to be treated shows a marked tendency to spontaneous resolution or to respond to non-drug-specific (psychological) aspects of treatment (see Boxes 4.1 and 4.2).

The use of placebos may, however, be considered unethical if the condition under study is highly distressing or dangerous, or if the benefits of existing drug treatments are believed to be substantial. The fact that few, if any, drug treatments for psychiatric disorders have more than about 30% efficacy (that is, measurable benefit over non-specific supportive treatment) does not seem to carry as much ethical weight as it should under these circumstances.

Various strategies have been devised to overcome these objections to placebo-controlled trials (Prien, 1988), but by and large these are unsatisfactory. Even if a formal placebo-controlled design is considered unethical or not feasible, it may be possible to observe all patients for an initial 'run in' period, preferably while taking placebo on a single-blind basis. Any short-term responders can then be excluded from further study so as not to add unnecessary 'noise' to the comparison between a standard and a test treatment. Although it makes good sense to use subjects as their own control, for example by using 'crossover'

> **Box 4.2** Conditions usually showing low placebo response
>
> * Chronic depressive disorders (e.g. dysthymic disorder)
> * Chronic schizophrenia (residual symptoms)
> * Obsessive–compulsive disorder
> * Chronic (generalised) anxiety disorder
>
> Short-term spontaneous fluctuations are common, but sustained spontaneous improvement is less likely

designs, with periods on placebo compared against periods on active treatment, this approach is compromised if there is a significant 'order' effect with treatment – that is, the second treatment is initiated at a different level of pathology from the first (Armitage, 1975), as usually applies (Tyrer *et al*, 1987).

Perhaps the least controversial compromise is to conduct a placebo-controlled study of the new treatment but with the option of 'rescue' treatment if the patient's clinical condition is deemed to warrant additional intervention. The extent to which rescue treatments are used can then be taken as an independent measure of the effectiveness of the trial drug versus placebo. However, there is the risk of adding a further confounding variable if there is an interaction (positive or negative) between the rescue medication and the drug(s) under investigation. Also, this approach is feasible only when rescue treatment has a rapid onset and time-limited beneficial effect. It would therefore lend itself reasonably well to trials of treatments for acute psychosis, but would be less suitable for depressive illness, where rapid treatment effects cannot be expected with rescue drugs.

None the less, this approach has been employed successfully in severe affective disorders, including depression, and most notably by the Northwick Park group (Johnstone *et al*, 1988), who used chlor-promazine as the rescue treatment for acute psychotic distress, and electroconvulsive therapy for worsening depression, in a comparison of lithium, pimozide and placebo for the treatment of affective and non-affective functional psychoses.

At some stage, preferably after placebo-controlled studies have demonstrated superiority of the new drug, it must be compared against existing treatments in order to assess whether there are any advantages of the new over the old. The manufacturers of new drugs are under-standably reluctant to expose their protégés to really stringent com-parisons with the best drugs already available. Where claims are made that a particular drug has special advantages in the treatment of particular conditions, it is common to cite trials in which the drug has been compared with a secondary competitor, and rare to have evidence of comparisons with primary competitors used at optimal doses.

However, there are reasons other than promotional bias that make this kind of comparison difficult and unpopular. If a new drug is tested against a standard treatment, an outcome of 'no difference' may not tell us whether both are equally effective or equally ineffective. For example, with conditions that show substantial spontaneous recovery over a short time, even an effective standard drug may have little or no additional specific activity. The new treatment is unlikely to be any different but it would be quite wrong to conclude that it was 'as good as' the standard. A similar argument applies to situations where the standard treatment is unusually ineffective, such as tricyclic antidepressants in the

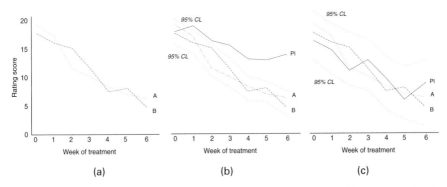

Fig. 4.2 Hypothetical treatment–response curves for groups of subjects treated with drug A or drug B or placebo (Pl). (a) A claim for drug A being 'as good as' drug B would only be valid if: (b) both drugs were effective compared with placebo, and the confidence limits for the mean response effectively ruled out a clinically important difference being missed; otherwise (c) there might be no evidence for a specific effect with either drug treatment, and a substantial difference between them cannot be ruled out, as illustrated by widely spaced confidence limits.

treatment of severe or delusional depression. In view of these consider-ations, any comparision between two or more drugs that are both believed to be active under the conditions of testing needs to be backed up by a placebo comparison as well (see Fig. 4.2).

The other important difficulty in comparing a new with a standard drug concerns the fact that if a real difference exists between the effects of the two drugs, this difference is likely to be much smaller and therefore harder to detect than the difference between either drug and a placebo. In practice this means that in order for a study to have the statistical power to detect a small but clinically important difference between two treatments, a very large number of subjects is required. Put another way, if there is a tiny but real difference between the treatments, this will not be detected if the sample is small (termed a 'type II error', i.e. there is a false negative result).

As a rule of thumb, 10 to 20 subjects per group may provide enough statistical power in a comparison between an active drug such as an antidepressant and a placebo, whereas five or ten times that number may be needed in order not to miss a much smaller but clinically important difference between two active drugs. In order to study sufficient numbers of subjects over a reasonable period of time, there is usually no alternative but to resort to a multi-centre collaborative trial, although this entails a number of major additional problems (see below).

Sequential designs involve an approach in which new subjects are recruited and tested on one of two treatments under comparison until it can be established that there is either a significant difference or no difference within the limits of certain probability assumptions. This avoids the problem of estimating the sample size before doing the trial. However, it requires that the outcome for a pair of subjects allocated to each treatment is known before a new pair of subjects is recruited. Obviously, this is not applicable to the testing of psychotropic drugs with delayed long-term effects or which lead to other changes that are relatively persistent (these are 'carry-over effects', which also invalidate crossover trials to some extent).

There are many small and otherwise inadequate trials that yield negative findings. However, it is difficult to be sure of the number of these studies in comparison with the published ones because most of them are not published. Studies reporting encouraging and positive findings may more easily get into print, despite methodological short-comings, and receive undeserved attention. The results of even a well-designed and conducted trial need to be regarded as highly provisional if the sample size is small, and especially if the results are negative.

Outcome criteria and analysis of results

It is always preferable to measure a patient's response to a drug as a change from the pre-treatment situation. The timing of outcome assessments is also crucial in the detection of treatment effects. Even though so-called delayed therapeutic effects, such as antidepressant and antipsychotic responses, actually begin within the first few days of treatment, sufficient time must be allowed for the drugs under test to reach their maximum effect. This usually but not always takes longer than the time for a placebo response to occur. Placebo responses are typically seen early in treatment, peak after about a week, but then wane as suggestion and wishful thinking evaporate (Quitkin et al, 1984). These considerations caution against assessing outcome too early (unless of course one wishes to measure the placebo effect). Unfortunately, more patients are likely to drop out of longer-term than shorter-term trials, for one reason or another, and large numbers of drop-outs will complicate the analysis of overall outcome.

Even more crucially, the condition under treatment may eventually get better without active treatment (perhaps owing to a combination of spontaneous recovery and remission due to non-drug-specific treatment – see Fig. 4.3). As a result, the difference between the recovery curves of an active and an inactive treatment will shrink as both curves tend to converge exponentially towards an asymptote (Fig. 4.4a).

There are various methods of allowing these masked tendencies of drug effects to be excluded when analysing results (Quitkin et al, 1984). However, these should be anticipated and set in motion before the trial is begun. If an analysis plan is not made in advance, the criticism that a post hoc analysis has been carried out because it happened to suit the data is much more difficult to refute.

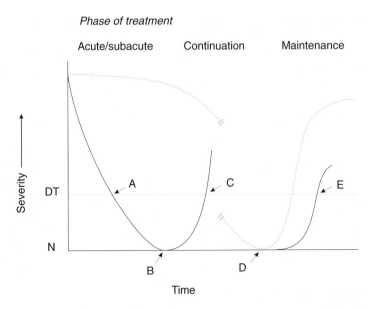

Fig. 4.3 Relationship between phase of treatment, overt symptoms (—) and covert pathogenic processes (---) . DT, diagnostic threshold; N, normality; A response; B, remission; C, relapse; D recovery; E, recurrence. Adapted from Kupfer (1991).

If the trial design allows for repeated measures of response over time, a satisfying theoretical solution to the problem of incomplete data due to drop-outs and convergence of recovery curves towards a common asymptote is provided by using the slope of response on time as a weighted average of observations to characterise each patient's response (Kraemer, 1981; Priest, 1989). Since the recovery curves usually have an exponential form, linear slopes can easily be calculated by converting the time base to a logarithmic scale (Fig. 4.4b). Although this strategy is rarely used, it is simple and effective, and is probably more valid and meaningful than analysis of variance with repeated measures over time (Kraemer, 1981). There are also techniques for replacing missing data in a series and these deserve wider investigation.

A related statistical complication concerns the risk of inflating type I error (false positive results) by making multiple comparisons between treatment groups. If 20 independent comparisons are made, using, say, a t-test with the accepted risk of false positives set at 5% or less ($P < 0.05$), at least one statistically significant difference may arise by chance, even when no such difference exists in reality. It is usual under these circumstances to adjust (reduce) the P value accepted as significant in order to reduce the possibility of false positives or type I errors. Type I errors are unlikely if there are consistent findings among truly independent measures of the same underlying construct, and if the outcomes for analysis were set in advance of trial completion.

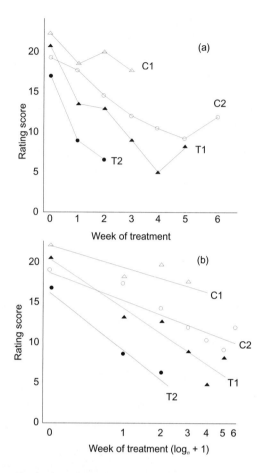

Fig. 4.4 (a) Hypothetical treatment–response curves for two subjects on control treatment (C1, C2) and two subjects on test treatment (T1, T2). Outcome measures, such as final score on a rating scale and change in score from baseline (week 0), are heavily influenced by the period available for assessment and especially by early termination of the trial. (b) Log transformation ($\log_n + 1$) of the x axis (time) results in approximate straight-line plots, the slopes of which provide measures of the amount of improvement on treatment that are relatively independent of the period available for assessment.

Long-term efficacy and prophylaxis

Most psychiatric disorders treated with drugs are recurrent conditions (e.g. affective disorders) or chronic disorders upon which exacerbations or relapses are superimposed (e.g. schizophrenia, obsessive–compulsive disorder). Relapse can be defined as a return of symptoms of severity equal to or greater than the original illness after a period of remission but before full recovery has occurred (Kupfer, 1991). In chronic disorders, such as most cases of schizophrenia, remission is all that can be expected, but in affective disorders remission of symptoms with treatment is followed, after on average 4–6 months, by recovery of the underlying disorder. The period of treatment between remission and recovery is called the 'continuation phase' (Fig. 4.3). Reappearance of illness after full recovery is best called a 'recurrence' rather than 'relapse', and prevention of recurrence is achieved by maintenance therapy or prophylaxis.

Clinical trials investigating the long-term efficacy of drug treatment for relapsing and recurrent conditions can therefore be divided into continuation trials and maintenance trials. In conditions such as major depression, a symptom-free period of at least 4 months is required before a maintenance trial can begin. For chronic conditions such as schizophrenia, long-term drug trials are all in effect continuation (or discontinuation) studies.

Apart from the long-term costs and commitment required for the investigations, continuation and maintenance trials are very difficult to carry out, for the following reasons:

(1) Patients in remission who feel well are often not highly motivated to stay in treatment, and are even less keen to enter or remain in a long-term clinical trial. The refusal rates and drop-out rates are therefore high, and the patient sample is commonly unrepresentative of the target population.

(2) Although there may be benefit from continuation and maintenance treatment with established drugs in conditions such as affective disorders and schizophrenia, the overall balance of risks and benefit is usually unclear. For many investigators this element of doubt justifies carrying out placebo-controlled studies, but as there are no rescue treatments apart from prompt treatment of relapses or recurrences, others feel that long-term placebo-controlled trials are unethical.

(3) Placebo-controlled comparisons of long-term prophylactic treatment requires that the index episode is successfully treated first. This means that patients to be tested on long-term placebo will need to be taken off active treatment, and other patients may need to change treatment too. Unless these changes are made gradually, they may adversely affect the course of the illness and so confound the investigation of the protective effects of long-term therapy (Kupfer, 1991).

(4) It is difficult to decide what are appropriate doses for long-term studies. The understandable desire to reduce the risk of unpleasant or dangerous side-effects has probably led in the past to suboptimal doses being used in maintenance treatment trials, at least with respect to antidepressants and lithium (Kupfer, 1991). With schizophrenia, where traditionally the continuation treatment

has been with doses equivalent to those used for acute treatment, the opposite is true, in that there has been little research into the lower dose limits of long-term antipsychotic treatment.

(5)   There are serious problems in defining and measuring the end-points of continuation or maintenance treatment. Relapses can be defined in terms of a return to drug treatment or the exceeding of a predetermined cut-off on a symptom rating. With drug treatment, the former criterion may overestimate relapse and the latter underestimate it. For example, previous experience of effective drug therapy may encourage patients to return to treatment at the slightest hint of problems which would be too mild to constitute a relapse by other criteria. If the incipient relapse is thereby avoided, symptoms may never deteriorate sufficiently to reach the symptom threshold for relapse. However, if symptoms do deteriorate further despite early treatment, this may reflect a particularly severe relapse. Similarly, if survival time after some form of psychotherapy is being investigated as well, 'subclinical' signs of relapse may encourage the patient to engage in self-help techniques learnt from previous therapy, and if this is not successful, to return to formal treatment only as a last resort (Clark, 1990). In view of these problems, relapse should probably be gauged by agreement on two or more criteria.

Adverse effects

Adverse effects should always be recorded in controlled trials, but wherever possible this should be done in a way that prevents the investigator from finding out enough information to 'break the code' (i.e. identifying the nature of the drug through its particular unwanted effects). This topic is often not addressed in clinical trials, but safeguards can be introduced (e.g. the patient completes a self-rating checklist of adverse effects without the assessor seeing the answers). The detection of rare but potentially serious adverse reactions is usually outside the scope of controlled clinical trials owing to the limitations of sample size. However, provided different controlled studies use similar reporting methods, pooled data may provide an accurate estimate of the incidence of rare adverse drug reactions.

Collaborative multi-centre trials and meta-analysis

When planning a clinical trial it is necessary to estimate the sample size needed, based on power calculations using the expected or hoped for difference between treatments and an estimate of its variance (see Appendix). This may lead to the conclusion that recruitment of a worthwhile sample of patients may be too difficult or will take too long. In this event it may be decided to pool the resources of several centres or sites in order to obtain a reasonable sample size. Differences between the sites in the experience and training of investigators, the study milieu and the sociodemographic attributes of the patients may all be unavoidable and have a profound effect on the outcome. If the results from the different centres are pooled without making allowance for these differences, treatment effects may be obscured or obliterated rather than enhanced (Kraemer & Pruyn, 1990).

None the less, if sufficient time and trouble are taken, it is possible to carry out complex and high-quality multi-centre clinical trials, as exemplified by a National Institute of Mental Health Collaborative Study (Elkin *et al*, 1989), in which the effects of imipramine, two forms of focused psychotherapy, and placebo were compared over a 16-week period in a total of 204 non-bipolar, non-psychotic out-patients with major depression in three centres (Washington, Pittsburgh and Oklahoma). This multi-centre trial is not only unusual in its scope and size, but also in having published its research protocol before the trial was finished. Despite this, the study design met with severe criticism from some experts after the publication of the first results (Klein, 1990), perhaps because some of the findings were neither predicted nor desired.

Since multi-centre studies of this size and quality allow examination of the effects of between-site differences in outcome, important conclusions regarding the generalisability of results can be drawn. If the outcome of a trial is going to influence major policy decisions, at a national or international level, it is obviously important that the results are generalisable to this extent. If results are available from several trials that have addressed more or less the same treatment issues in more or less the same way, the results can be combined using meta-analysis.

Meta-analysis includes a group of techniques for objectively and systematically pooling the results of controlled trials that have investigated similar hypotheses concerning the efficacy of particular treatments. It is a useful technique when trying to reach a conclusion from the results of smaller trials that all differ somewhat in outcome and other respects (e.g. slightly different types of patient or treatment variables). What is important is that all the trials should satisfy minimum standards regarding the homogeneity of their study populations, random allocation of patients, blind assessment, measurements and outcome criteria (Johnson, 1998).

The basic procedure is to calculate a summary outcome statistic for each trial (e.g. effect size of treatments) and then pool these across trials (Kraemer & Pruyn, 1990). Meta-analysis is not to be regarded as a method for homogenising poor results (although if the studies are all poor this will indeed be the result), but rather as a fine filter which clarifies a therapeutic question when there are often conflicting findings (Kraemer & Pruyn, 1990). Good examples are provided by the Quality Assurance Project reports (1983, 1984) on the management of depressive disorders and schizophrenia.

Marketing

Marketing, literally meaning the production of goods for sale, now incorporates the much more contentious issue of promotion. As only about 1 in 3500 potential drugs gets as far as a controlled clinical trial, and only 1 in 20 of these will actually be prescribed, it is easy to see that there is a tremendous amount invested in the launch of each new drug. It is therefore a perfectly reasonable position for a company to encourage as many practitioners as possible to prescribe the new drug in order to recoup research and development costs, never mind make a profit for the company.

Marketing and promotion are respectable activities but doctors have to be aware that they are not agnostic ones; they present products in the most favourable light possible, and this will have the maximum impact if it also appears to be objective. The shiny side of truth always faces the camera. The published word has lost a great deal of its impact in marketing and the pharmaceutical representative is often the key to persuasion, frequently aided by highly polished presentations, with impressive videotapes and slides.

The aim of marketing, to sell the product, and the aim of therapeutics, to find the best remedy, may coincide but do so less often than we would like. In psychopharmacology there are many examples of drugs littering the pages of pharmacopoeias that have no right to be there, some because they are expensive placebos with no significant pharmacological value, and others because they are expensive replicas of early compounds that have proved to be successful but their patents have expired, allowing cheaper 'generic' versions to be manufactured.

Doctors should be vigilant and well informed so that they can detect unnecessary drugs, particularly those that are 'me too' drugs that masquerade as advances and only confuse the practitioner. Many of these drugs are now being removed from clinical practice as a consequence of government bodies such as the Advisory Committee on NHS Drugs. However, it would be better for the profession itself to do the jobs of such committees by no longer prescribing unnecessary drugs and thereby accelerating their demise.

Early and late clinical evaluation, and post-marketing surveillance

Once a drug is accepted as having therapeutic value by clinicians, it will sell itself (although continued advertising will usually increase its share of the market). Clinical experience in practice continues to be the most valuable source of information about a drug, because although it is less economical in terms of time and numbers of patients studied than the controlled clinical trial, it encompasses a broader range, so that unexpected benefits and disadvantages of the drug are detected. Not all these later observations prove to be correct, and many have to be put to the test of further controlled trials, but, on the whole, much more is discovered about a new drug after its introduction to general clinical practice than is known before. There is some advantage in using the diagnostic criteria and rating scales from published studies in routine clinical practice. This may allow better prediction and understanding of treatment effects in the individual patient. An example of a widely used rating instrument that can be applied to all psychiatric patients and to drug-induced changes in their clinical state is the Global Assessment Scale (Endicott *et al*, 1976).

There is a general rule that needs to be borne in mind when assessing the merits of drugs in clinical practice. A compound cannot be regarded as definitely safe or indubitably effective until it has been in use for at least 10 years. The longer a drug is on the market, the less popular it is likely to be, as later discoveries tend to be in the field of unwanted rather than desired effects. If a drug is to satisfy the requirements of marketing, the initial toxicological tests have to be satisfactory and most drugs start their clinical life with a 'good press'. Later, the constant trickle of adverse reports and qualifications about their use bring them down to the level of the drugs that preceded them, or, if the adverse effects are particularly serious, lead to them being withdrawn from clinical use.

Teratogenic adverse effects and those that develop only after chronic use are particularly difficult to detect in early studies, as are the type B (bizarre) effects of drugs (Rawlins, 1981). The type A (augmented) effects are predictable from initial pharmacological testing and are dose dependent, but type B effects are detected only by keen observation and deduction. In the UK, doctors are advised to report all suspected adverse effects on yellow cards to the Committee on Safety of Medicines, and similar systems exist in other countries (see Chapter 15).

In choosing a drug it is therefore important to know what stage it has reached in its life history. If one reads enthusiastic reports of a major advance in treatment and finds that the drug in question has only just been introduced, it is fair to treat the claim with some scepticism. We live in an age in which novelties are mistaken for progress and psychopharmacology has often been the victim. There is another reason for not prematurely abandoning the well-tried and tested drugs. The proper use for each drug requires knowledge not only of its clinical effects and indications, but also of its unwanted effects in acute and chronic dosage, its interactions with other drugs, its full dosage range and its duration of treatment. This information is not obtained overnight and, as a generalisation, older drugs can be prescribed with more confidence than the new, and so inspire greater confidence and compliance in the patients to whom they are prescribed.

However, in recent years there has been increasing pressure on pharmaceutical companies to provide more and more comprehensive information about new drugs at an early stage after their introduction. For this reason newer psychotropic compounds such as the selective serotonin reuptake inhibitors had already been studied extensively in a very large number of patients before they were launched. In many respects, the use of these newer drugs has been tested and validated in a more systematic way than any of the older drugs that they were designed to complement or even replace. Nevertheless, the short-term intensive study of a new drug can never replace the long-term clinical experience with the older compounds, and the intelligent prescriber will judiciously use both old and new.

The aims of drug treatment, the indications for it and the alternatives to it

Aims and stages of treatment

The aims of drug treatment can be summarised as follows:

(1) to reduce distress and disturbed behaviour
(2) to promote remission of symptoms, to improve coping and to reduce associated disturbance in social functioning
(3) to allow recovery from the underlying susceptibility to relapse
(4) to minimise the frequency and severity of recurrences of illness.

These aims roughly coincide with different stages of treatment (i.e. the acute, sub-acute, continuation and maintenance phases). The acute phase of treatment refers to the initial attempts to reduce distress and disturbed behaviour, whereas the sub-acute phase covers the period of treatment necessary to induce remission of symptoms. The continuation phase refers to the treatments aimed at promoting recovery from the underlying neurobiological pathogenic processes and the maintenance phase is aimed at preventing recurrences. The terminology used in these descriptions is summarised in Fig. 4.3.

Acute treatment

Acute treatment is concerned with the rapid relief of symptoms or distress. These psychotropic drug actions can be broadly divided into stimulant and depressant effects on the central nervous system. The acute relief of symptoms is usually pleasant, and there is a danger that it may even lead to euphoria. Drugs that are effective quickly and that lead to a feeling of well-being lend themselves all too readily to misuse. Thus, inappropriate or excessive reliance by the prescriber or patient on the short-term relief provided by anxiolytic drugs may be at the expense of interference with coping behaviour in the face of long-term stress or personal difficulties. This may lead initially to psychological and then later to physical dependence, followed by a cascade of further problems.

Sub-acute drug actions on psychiatric syndromes

Two main features characterise these types of drug effects:

(1) They are gradual or delayed and may take several weeks to develop fully.
(2) Their effects are relatively specific and cannot be replicated in normal subjects or volunteers.

Although clinical improvement appears to lag several weeks behind the direct pharmacological actions of many drugs (e.g. antidepressive and antipsychotic agents), this time delay is a relative matter, since some improvement in symptoms may often be detected very early on in treatment, and may be used to predict which patients will eventually respond best (e.g. Katz et al, 1987).

This has an important implication. In the absence of any detectable early improvement in clinical state, or if there is an actual worsening, such as dysphoric reactions to antipsychotics (Van Putten & May, 1978), it is unlikely that the eventual outcome will be favourable. From this it follows that dogged perseverance with a drug treatment that has shown no early benefit at all is probably a waste of time. (Treatment of very chronic cases that have proved resistant to other treatments may be an exception.)

Sub-acute drug actions tend to affect all aspects of a particular mental state syndrome, regardless of the underlying diagnosis. Thus, neuroleptics exert therapeutic effects across the full range of 'positive' psychotic symptoms (hallucinations, delusions, thought disorder, catatonic behaviour, etc.), regardless of diagnostic labels (schizo-phrenia, paranoid states, delusional depression, mania, etc.). The same can probably be said regarding the mood-normalising properties of lithium (see Johnstone et al, 1988). Despite this apparent lack of specificity, sub-acute drug actions can still be of diagnostic help in a few situations:

(1) treatment with antidepressive drugs to distinguish the reversible dementia (usually inaccurately termed pseudo-dementia) of severe depressive illness in the elderly from the irreversible cognitive impairment of Alzheimer's disease or multi-infarct dementia
(2) the administration of antipsychotic drugs to patients with both psychotic and depressive features may resolve the psychosis but not the depressive syndrome in a case of primary depressive illness, whereas it will cause remission of both aspects of the syndrome where the underlying process is primarily or mainly schizophrenic

(3) a depressed, paranoid patient may become frankly psychotic during antidepressive drug treatment when the underlying condition is a paranoid disorder (e.g. paranoid schizophrenia or paraphrenia).

Continuation and prophylactic treatment

Once remission of symptoms is achieved, the risk of relapse may be reduced by continuing treatment until the underlying disturbance has resolved. In general, the continuation phase of treatment after recovery should last for several months – setting more precise durations is largely a matter of guesswork.

The aim of maintenance treatment is to prevent a new episode of illness (recurrence) (Kupfer, 1991). Since the risk of recurrence and associated morbidity is high for conditions such as depression, this is a very important treatment goal, often described as tertiary prevention. In chronic conditions such as schizophrenia, where full recovery may not occur, long-term treatment may never strictly qualify as maintenance therapy, but the term prophylaxis may still be used to describe this preventive measure.

As with continuation treatment, drug dosage appears to be very important in determining the success of prophylaxis. For example, imipramine is more successful in preventing the recurrence of unipolar depression when it is given in high dosage (250 mg per day) (Frank *et al*, 1990) than in lower dosage (140 mg per day) (Prien *et al*, 1984). A similar conclusion appears to apply to lithium prophylaxis in bipolar affective disorders, at least with respect to recurrence of mania (Gelenberg *et al*, 1989). However, this has to be balanced against evidence that more patients discontinue or fail to comply with maintenance therapy with drugs in higher dosage, because of problems with unwanted effects. In schizophrenia, the benefits of (standard dose) prophylactic treatment are well established. However, the dangers of tardive dyskinesia and other unwanted effects (most of which are dose related) makes it extremely difficult to decide the optimal dosage for maintenance treatment. There is little doubt in clinical practice that for some patients a lower than average dosage may be sufficient to prevent a relapse, but despite this, in larger groups of subjects the benefit of low-dose antipsychotic regimens is fairly marginal. Most patients relapse more frequently when randomly allocated to low-dose treatment compared with standard treatment and the expected benefits of fewer side-effects and better social functioning are often not achieved (Johnstone *et al*, 1988).

Indications, contraindications and alternatives: which treatment for which patient?

Normal unhappy responses to negative life events, the handicaps induced by certain personality traits and the ordinary vicissitudes of life

---

Box 4.3 Depressive symptoms indicating a favourable response to antidepressive drugs (provided not too severe, and not accompanied by delusions or hallucinations)

- Weight loss*
- Morning worsening of mood*
- Reduced appetite*
- Mid and late insomnia*
- Distinct quality of altered mood
- Anhedonia
- Motor retardation
- Hopelessness
- Motor agitation
- Guilt

These symptoms are all characteristic of melancholia, endogenous or vital depression.

*Reversal of these symptoms may suggest favourable response to monoamine oxidase inhibitors.

---

are not normally regarded as sufficient indication for the prescription of psychotropic drugs by doctors (see above). The dividing line between the presence and the absence of 'illness' is difficult to define, but the presence of 'biological' signs and symptoms often helps to justify the use of drug treatment (see Box 4.3).

Diagnosis, syndromes and symptoms

As indicated above, most longer-term psychotherapeutic drug effects tend not to be diagnosis specific. This fact can be used to undermine categorical diagnosis, but it also has to be recognised that there are examples where treatment of the underlying diagnostic condition is the most effective or only way of improving symptoms associated with a non-specific syndrome. For example, the depressive syndromes commonly associated with borderline personality disorder are not usually helped by conventional antidepressive treatment (e.g. Soloff *et al*, 1986). Most of the evidence suggests that antipsychotic drugs in different dosages are more effective in improving the depressive symptoms in such conditions.

Even at a syndromal level, response to treatment can be an uncertain guide to construct validity of the disorder. Thus, the type 2 (negative or defect) syndrome characteristic of chronic schizophrenia, and often described as being non-responsive to antipsychotics, uses treatment resistance as one of its defining features. However, the similar clinical syndrome consisting of poverty of speech and flattened affect that may be seen in depressive disorders is eminently responsive to antidepressive drug treatment. Even in schizophrenia, a negative syndrome defined in these clinical terms may sometimes show a marked improvement with antipsychotics.

Using biological measures or markers as predictors of drug responsiveness seems attractive in theory but has made little impact, except perhaps to indicate in which direction the dose of a particular drug should be moved in order to achieve a therapeutic response.

Severity, chronicity and organicity

It is a consistent finding that the specific benefit of drug treatments tends to be correlated with the initial severity of the disorder. Mild acute conditions tend to show a marked improvement due to non-specific components of drug treatment, and this can be exploited further by employing formal or informal psychotherapeutic techniques. In mild disorders, the benefit of active drug treatment may be little more than that resulting from 'a good placebo'. This generalisation seems to apply particularly to self-limiting conditions such as mild non-chronic forms of major depression (Fig. 4.5).

By contrast mild chronic conditions (e.g. dysthymic disorder) show a very poor placebo response, and although the response to drug treatment may be quite unimpressive overall, the specific component of the response may be relatively great. Chronicity is not necessarily an indicator of poor response to treatment, since the condition may have

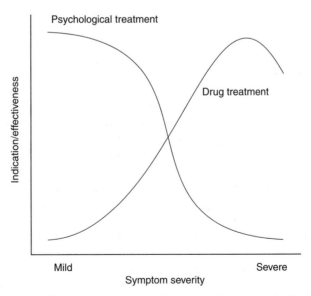

Fig. 4.5 The likely effectiveness of psychological and pharmacological treatments depends upon the initial severity of the mental disorder.

been allowed to become chronic through neglect of treatment, and yet still respond briskly when treatment is at last begun.

Greater illness severity can predict response to drug treatment. Thus, severe forms of depressive illness tend to show a low placebo response and yet respond well to antidepressive drug treatment, whereas mild acute depression (particularly in general practice) shows little specific response to antidepressant drug treatment, or no more than to placebo (Hollyman *et al*, 1988). This may explain in part why certain biological symptoms are also associated with good treatment response (Box 4.3), since they are often associated with the more severe form of depression.

Personality factors: the effects of expectations, attitudes and experience of drug treatment on dependence and compliance

It sometimes surprises psychiatrists that patients are so unwilling to accept medical advice on drug treatment. This problem is certainly not restricted to dealings with patients who are lacking insight and are therefore 'out of touch with reality'. Either patients reject the prescription of a drug, or insist on it when other treatments (e.g. other drugs or psychotherapy) are thought to be more suitable. The causes of this 'non-compliance' are complex, but to some extent reflect two general and recent trends: the first is a growing belief that the consumer should have at least as much say in treatment issues as the prescriber; and the second is that patients increasingly assume that treatments prescribed by psychiatrists, especially drugs, are as likely to do harm as to bring benefit. These general trends, which can be cast epigram-matically as 'the doctor does not necessarily know best', tend to be affected by two other factors: the patient's personality and previous experience of drug treatment.

There are many ways of defining and classifying personality type. When personality traits are extreme and cause problems to the individual or others, they are regarded as disorders. For our present purposes, the four main categories of personality disorders can be used to discuss personality traits as well. Thus, antisocial and dependent personality traits tend to lead to overuse or misuse of certain psycho-tropic drugs, whereas withdrawn and inhibited personality traits tend to result in rejection or intolerance of prescribed medication.

People with an antisocial personality are often impulsive, easily bored and sensation seeking, and may have a propensity to overuse any and all psychotropic drug, 'for kicks'. If such misuse is long term, it may produce secondary effects, such as physical dependence on benzodiazepines or serious mental state changes (e.g. paranoid psy-chosis in amphetamine addicts). People with a dependent personality are timid and anxious, and prone to taking sedative drugs, such as benzodiazepines, long term. Although such people may not take more than the prescribed amount, they are very resistant to any change in or discontinuation of their medication, a tendency that will be exacerbated by their propensity to experience distressing withdrawal effects. For both groups it is wise to avoid psychotropic medication (Tyrer & Murphy, 1992).

Withdrawn (paranoid) and inhibited (obsessional and hypochondriacal) personalities are often very resistant to the idea of drug treatment. Paranoid patients may feel that they are being fobbed off or not taken seriously by the offer of drug treatment. Even worse, the taking of a drug may be experienced as something predominantly intrusive and harmful, especially if administered by injection, although this may also apply to any offer of help that obliges patients to acknowledge and accept their need and vulnerability. People with a withdrawn, hypochondriacal or depressive personality may resist having treatment aimed at reducing or eliminating the very aspect of their life (their problems and complaints) that gives it meaning and permits some contact and communication with other people.

It also has to be borne in mind that many people with a personality disorder have intermittent mental state abnormalities, often of a sufficient severity to qualify as illness, and therefore sometimes requiring treatment. Furthermore, probably a half or more of people with long-term mental illnesses can be regarded as suffering from a personality disorder as well, which has to be taken into account when planning and prescribing treatment. Problems of acceptability and compliance with treatment due to personality factors may be exacerbated by mental state problems such as paranoia and loss of insight.

Unfavourable previous experiences of drug treatment, whether due to adverse effects or failure to perceive benefit, have a major influence on the acceptability of further drug treatment, so this must be taken into consideration by the prescriber. Some of the most subjectively objectionable adverse drug effects (akathisia and dysphoria with neuroleptics, tremulousness and anorgasmia with antidepressants) are the least well understood or appreciated by prescribers. Notwithstanding some ethical and medico-legal obstacles, there is quite a good case for prescribers having to have 'a taste for their own medicine' at some stage in their career in order to improve their appreciation of some of these 'harmless' but highly undesirable drug effects. Personality traits once more may have an important effect in determining the impact of previous experiences of adverse drug effects. Paranoid patients have apparent confirmation of their suspicion that all treatments offered by the doctor are harmful, whereas inhibited, highly controlled patients may experience drug-induced drowsiness as a threat to their ability to stay in control.

Psychotherapy as an adjunct or alternative to sub-acute drug treatments

Although this subject may be considered peripheral to the main point of this chapter it is none the less relevant. Systematic research carried out in the past two decades has shown that various forms of psychological and associated therapies can produce measurable benefits comparable to those of pharmacological treatments. This applies across a range of diagnoses, from depression and anxiety states (Klerman & Schechter, 1982; Clark, 1990) to schizophrenia (Shepherd, 1988). As a generalisation, whereas drugs have most effect in reducing symptoms, psychotherapy has more benefit in improving social maladjustment and interpersonal relationships. Psychological treatments therefore appear to be especially indicated where symptoms are mild but psychosocial impairment is marked (Fig. 4.6), and this has been borne out in several studies (Blackburn *et al*, 1981; Hollyman *et al*, 1988; Elkin *et al*, 1989). The results of the study by Blackburn *et al* (1981) are summarised in Table 4.1; in that study cognitive–behavioural therapy was compared with antidepressant drug therapy and much greater improvement was found in the general practice sample (milder cases of depression) than in the hospital sample (more severe cases) when cognitive–behavioural therapy was used alone.

In most circumstances psychological treatments combine well with pharmacological ones but there are a few exceptions. Perhaps the most

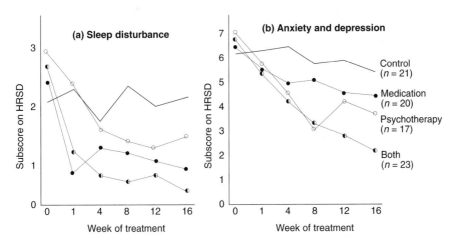

Fig. 4.6 Improvement of somatic (a) and psychological (b) symptoms of depression with psychotherapy, antidepressant medication or combination treatment for relatively chronic patients. The control group received no specific treatment. HRSD, Hamilton Rating Scale for Depression. (Data from DiMascio *et al*, 1979.)

Table 4.1 Comparison of cognitive–behavioural therapy (CBT) and anti-depressive drug therapy (ADT) alone or in combination in mild and severe major depressive illness: percentage reduction in score on the Beck Depression Inventory after 12–20 weeks of treatment

	Milder cases (general practice sample)	More severe cases (hospital sample)
ADT	14	60
CBT	84	48
Both	72	79

Data from Blackburn *et al* (1981).

important is the interaction between benzodiazepines and desensitisation through exposure to feared situations in phobic (avoidant) disorders: if anxiety is banished temporarily but prematurely by drugs, this will preclude the experience of relief of anxiety through desensitisation, and hence prevent long-term resolution of the problem. In mild disorders, psychotherapy alone may be highly effective and drug treatment relatively ineffective, so combining the two types of treatment may confer little additional benefit. In contrast, with severe disorders, drug treatment may be more effective than psychotherapy, but again with no additional benefit from combined treatment. This is exemplified by the study of Blackburn *et al* (1981) (see Table 4.1).

There are, however, several studies that show the benefits of combining psychotherapy with drug treatment. In an early influential study (DiMascio *et al*, 1979) patients with chronic major depression were given brief focused ('interpersonal') psychotherapy, amitriptyline, or both, and compared with an untreated control group. Drug treatment and psychotherapy were both effective in this patient population, and the effects of the two treatments in combination were additive. This additive effect seemed to be due to drug treatment mainly improving vegetative symptoms, such as sleep impairment, while psychotherapy had a greater effect on mood and depressive ideation (Fig. 4.6).

Since benefit from drug treatment does not seem to outlast its administration, there has been much research interest in the possibility that psychotherapy may have protective effects against relapse or recurrence of illness that outlast the period of therapy. The evidence available indicates that this is the case with both cognitive and behaviour therapy (Basoglu & Marks, 1989; Clark, 1990; Durham & Allan, 1993).

Since patients may be able to practise many aspects of psychotherapy on their own, continued treatment can be maintained for long periods, perhaps with occasional refresher courses. In this way, drugs may be seen as only part of an overall treatment strategy for maintenance control of chronic symptoms and prophylaxis against relapses and recurrences of illness.

Evidence-based drug treatment

Over the past 10 years there has been a dramatic growth in evidence-based medicine, a natural development to link practice to research (Geddes *et al*, 2000*a*). Drug treatment has been a beneficiary of this, as most therapeutic drugs are evaluated in randomised controlled trials and there are usually sufficient numbers of these to carry out good meta-analytical studies. Current evidence is constantly being updated and re-evaluated in the context of new studies. It is important to acknowledge both the value and the limitations of evidence-based medicine in determining choice in clinical practice. Evidence reinforces and buttresses practice, it is not a substitute for patient-focused decisions that combine independent evidence of therapeutic value, personal choice and the uniqueness of the individual.

Some examples of the value of an evidence-based approach to clinical practice are summarised below.

(1)   For Alzheimer's disease donepezil, selegeline and *Gingko biloba* may all improve cognitive function more than placebo (Warner & Butler, 2001).

(2)   For depression there is no clear evidence of superior efficacy of any one type of antidepressant drug over psychological therapy (mainly cognitive and interpersonal therapy) for cases of moderate severity, but in severe cases prescription antidepressants are superior to other treatments (Geddes & Butler, 2001).

(3)   For generalised anxiety benzodiazepines are the most rapidly acting treatment, but cognitive therapy, buspirone, imipramine, trazodone, venlafaxine and paroxetine are all effective in the longer term and there is no clear superiority of any one treatment (Gale & Oakley-Browne, 2001).

(4)   For obsessive–compulsive disorder clomipramine has similar efficacy to other (more selective) serotonin reuptake inhibitors, and equivalent efficacy is shown by both cognitive and behaviour therapy (Soomro, 2001).

(5)   For post-traumatic stress disorder there are negative effects from debriefing, and small positive effects from both antidepressants and cognitive–behavioural therapy (Bisson, 2001).

(6)   For schizophrenia the atypical antipsychotics are as effective as older drugs (with fewer adverse effects) and clozapine is more effective than older antipsychotics. There is limited evidence that psychological treatments such as family therapy, compliance therapy and cognitive–behavioural therapy may also have benefits and improve adherence to antipsychotics (McIntosh & Lawrie, 2001).

121

This is all very useful information and helps in particular to specify the value of drug treatments in the context of therapy as a whole. Nevertheless, it really provides a broad-brush background rather than the *pointilism* precision that is necessary for good clinical practice. Because more information is needed by the more expert practitioner, more detailed guidelines have been produced in many areas of psychopharmacology. Thus it is possible to make some comparisons between the efficacy of individual antidepressant drugs (Anderson *et al*, 2000), to judge the importance of dosage in comparing atypical and typical antipsychotic drugs (Geddes *et al*, 2000*b*) and to consider the value of a combination of mood stabilisers compared with monotherapy (Sachs *et al*, 2000). When one strays away from the firmer evidence provided by systematic reviews it is important to realise that the distinction between guidelines and expert opinion (the conventional lowest level of evidence) is sometimes hard to discern and the perceptive reader will sometimes be able to detect conflicts of interest. The cautious practitioner will rarely stray far from current evidence-based practice but will recognise that it is a general guide rather than a definitive rule-book.

Practicalities of treatment

Psychological aspects of treatment: placebo and nocebo effects

At this point we assume that the doctor has decided that drug treatment is necessary for a specific condition and is about to start this treatment. We further assume that a decision has been made regarding which particular drug is to be taken, based on the patient's symptoms, diagnosis and published experience of the treatment of this condition.

Rather than merely writing out the name of the drug on the prescription pad and give it to the patient, it is also crucial to agree on the terms and conditions of the treatment to be undertaken. In other words, a contract is made with the patient, which can be called a therapeutic alliance (a common term in psychotherapy). Just as in any business transaction, the patient must have confidence in the therapist and in the treatment on offer in order to be willing to proceed with it. As any salesperson knows, the first step in winning the trust and cooperation of prospective but apprehensive clients is to bolster their self-esteem and confidence in their decision over whether or not to buy. Patients may have strong misgivings or at least mixed feelings about treatment, and the prescriber must ensure that these do not become strong negative attitudes, while ensuring that appropriate information is given about the likely risks and drawbacks as well as the benefits of medication.

Overcoming ambivalence or negative attitudes to drug treatment, and making the patient feel as much at ease as possible under the circumstances of a distressing condition, constitutes an important part of what is sometimes called a placebo ('I will please'). Conversely, increasing negative attitudes and expectations represents a nocebo ('I will harm') component of treatment, and this can take several forms. Thus unrealistic (and therefore unfulfillable) expections of treatment will inevitably lead to disappointment and disillusionment with the therapist. Suggesting to patients that they need drug treatment because they are too sick to help themselves may foster feelings of helplessness and dependency, which can undermine recovery. A particular form of nocebo effect occurs when patients believe they are being deprived of or withdrawn from a drug that they are convinced will benefit them, even when, at an objective level, no such deprivation or withdrawal has taken place (Tyrer, 1991b). This nocebo effect can produce or amplify adverse responses to treatment withdrawal that is actually taking place, for example in benzodiazepine dependence (Tyrer et al, 1983).

Judging how best to establish a therapeutic alliance and then to enhance the placebo component of treatment requires a careful assessment of the patient, including mental state, personality and past experiences. This may take time and trouble, but unless there is extreme urgency in starting treatment (in which case a placebo response may not be relevant), marking time often pays dividends. Merely paying attention to the factors that constitute a placebo response may be enough to effect a significant improvement in the patient's condition. Unfortunately, such improvement may be short lived, as failure to effect 'a complete cure', and the patient's realisation that their troubles are not all over, may cause the placebo response to switch back into a nocebo reaction.

What may constitute a formula for a good therapeutic alliance and a placebo response in one patient may have the converse effect in another. For example, taking care to probe deeply into the patient's past and present difficulties, and personalising these by minimising the role of an illness process, may make many patients feel that they are being understood and taken seriously, whereas in a severely depressed patient the same approach may cause much distress and increase feelings of guilt and inadequacy. It is necessary to try to predict and understand the patient's reaction and point of view, and as far as possible to share these feelings (empathise), so long as this does not undermine the very basis of drug treatment (e.g. by agreeing with a paranoid patient that all medicine is poison).

The placebo response can be thought of as a positive effect that can be enhanced by appropriate strategies (Perry, 1990). It is often helpful to frame the patient's distress in terms of 'an illness', or 'nervous breakdown', or 'depression in response to adversity', because it confers meaning and importance to the individual even though it may not be satisfactory as a diagnostic description. Just as it can be helpful to demonstrate to the patient that their symptoms and experiences are well understood and not 'freakish', so it can be more reassuring than alarming to specify expected side-effects and their timing in relationship to the benefits of treatment. This helps the patient to have confidence in the prescriber's experience and expertise with the treatment. It may be reinforced by suggesting self-help coping strategies during this period.

As well as advising about the likely delay in recovery, it is a good strategy to inform the patient in advance that the treatment is not the last resort and that if it is ineffective, there are alternatives. For patients who feel threatened by the idea of ingesting a powerful foreign substance, it may be very helpful for the first tablet or injection to be taken in the presence of a doctor, and for the patient's reaction to be monitored over the next few hours. This may be particularly important with antipsychotic drugs, as a small proportion of patients may have a very unpleasant dysphoric reaction after a single dose, which may be associated with later adverse side-effects such as akathisia, dystonia and akinesia. Although little is known about this very important phenomenon (Emerich & Sanberg, 1991), it may be associated with poor treatment response and non-compliance (Van Putten & May, 1978). Similar reactions may occur in a proportion of patients taking tricyclic antidepressants and related drugs. Witnessing the patient going through such a subjective reaction and taking it seriously greatly improves mutual credibility and understanding, and may prevent unnecessary distress and waste of time by persevering doggedly with a treatment that is unacceptable to the patient for very good reasons, even though these may not be well covered in textbooks.

Compliance, side-effects and polypharmacy

Patients in general, and psychiatric patients in particular, are not very good at taking pills. This can be for many reasons. Some of the factors leading to problems with compliance tend to be similar to those that undermine the therapeutic alliance and placebo response. The most important reason is unpleasant side-effects, especially those not adequately understood or taken seriously by the prescriber, such as dysphoric reactions, movement disorders (especially akathisia) and sexual dysfunction. A second factor is failure to convince the patient that treatment is worthwhile or necessary, or that the prescriber has sufficient expertise and experience, or has taken sufficient time and trouble to ensure a good chance of successful outcome. Interestingly, good cooperation may not require that patients agree with the prescriber about the cause of their troubles. Conversely, a patient with 'full insight' may not necessarily be a reliable taker of medication. The ability to convince the patient of the prescriber's concern and goodwill and receptiveness to the patient's point of view, without necessarily sharing it, seem to be the most important considerations.

A long delay before any benefit is felt by the patient will naturally shake confidence in the treatment, especially if side-effects are troublesome at an early stage. In conditions such as depression, an objective improvement may occur before the patient acknowledges feeling any change for the better (Katz *et al*, 1987); it is therefore important to be able to convince patients that progress is being made and that this will soon be felt by them. There is no substitute for frequent and attentive contact with the patient.

A different problem arises during the continuation and maintenance phases of treatment, when the patient may be feeling relatively or completely well. It appears to be a common and not unreasonable assumption that a sense of well-being is incompatible with the need for treatment. Only with careful explanation along the lines of 'treatment is needed for you to stay well' will a reasonable degree of compliance be likely.

Regardless of the phase of treatment, complicated drug regimens hinder compliance. Every effort must be made to keep the number of drugs and the frequency of administration to a minimum. This does not mean that all polypharmacy is inappropriate and there may be several instances in which two or more drugs are given for good pharmacological reasons. In addition to synergistic effects of agents with different pharmacological profiles acting on the same syndrome, it is often valuable to give an additional drug to counteract the adverse effects of the initial drug if it is considered necessary for the first drug to be continued at full dosgae (Table 4.2).

Whenever combinations of drugs are used, there is an increased risk of adverse effects due to drug interactions; these effects may be worse than the original adverse effects for which the additional drug was prescribed (e.g. toxic confusional states resulting from anticholinergic medication given to alleviate antipsychotic-induced parkinsonism).

There is usually much less rationale for giving more than one drug from the same general class, the effects of which are generally additive. Perhaps the most common reason for 'same-class polypharmacy' is the co-administration of an oral and depot antipsychotic. This can often be justified early in treatment, particularly when illnesses are likely to show marked short-term fluctuations, as the oral component of medication facilitates dose adjustment. However, the long-term use of such combinations is almost always a reflection of poor prescribing practice.

Sometimes patients claim that an oral drug, such as chlorpromazine, has special additional properties which cannot be matched by a depot antipsychotic alone, and of course there may be pharmacological grounds to support this argument, because there is considerable patient

125

Table 4.2 Drug treatments for the side-effects of psychotherapeutic medication

Psychotherapeutic medication	Side-effect	Remedial drug
Neuroleptic	Parkinsonism	Anticholinergic (e.g. procyclidine)
	Akathisia	β-blocker (e.g. propranolol)
		Anticholinergic (e.g. procyclidine)
		5-HT$_2$ blocker (e.g. cyproheptadine)
Selective serotonin reuptake inhibitor	Akathisa	As above
	Anorgasmia	5-HT$_2$ blocker (e.g. cyproheptadine)
Tricyclic antidepressant	Erectile impotence	Sildenafil
	Urinary retention	Parasympathomimetic (e.g. bethanecol)
	Excess sweating	α_1-blocker (e.g. terazocin)
Lithium	Tremor	β-blocker (e.g. propranolol)
	Polyuria	Antidiuretic hormone sensitiser (e.g. carbamazepine)
	Hypothyroidism	Thyroxine
Carbamazepine	Leucopenia	Lithium
	Hyponatraemia	Antidiuretic hormone desensitiser (e.g. lithium, demeclocycline)

idiosyncrasy. Taking all these factors into consideration, it is a reasonable rule to confine the treatment of patients to no more than three psychotropic drugs at any one time.

Treatment failure: insufficient treatment or inappropriate selection?

For most drugs it is advisable to start at a low dose and build up gradually to the accepted therapeutic dose range. The rationale for this is that many troublesome side-effects are dose related and most prominent with acute drug treatment, but tend to wane as treatment is continued. For many drugs (e.g. lithium) this caution minimises the risk of overshooting into the toxic range of plasma concentrations.

Drugs that are relatively well tolerated, or that have adverse effects that build up slowly, can usually be given at doses within the therapeutic range from the outset. Examples include the 'second-generation' antidepressants (e.g. selective serotonin reuptake inhibitors) and most antipsychotics. With most drugs and most patients, there are marked individual variations in dose requirements, which can be ascertained only by trial and error. Much of this variation is probably pharmacokinetic in origin, in that there are major variations in the absorption, distribution, metabolism and excretion of different drugs. There can also be important differences between levels of a drug in the blood or plasma and those in the brain, where the drug is exerting its major effect. For this reason there may be a poor relationship between plasma (or blood) level and therapeutic response, even for drugs such as lithium, which is more evenly distributed through the different compartments of the body than other drugs. The early promise of 'therapeutic windows' (i.e. a narrow range of plasma or blood concentrations associated with an optimal therapeutic effect; see Chapter 3) has not been fully realised for most drugs.

What is becoming clear is the notion that, with increasing tissue concentrations, the specific biological effects of particular drugs reach a ceiling associated with a maximal tissue level, so that further increases in drug concentration will have little or no further beneficial response. Patients who fail to respond to drug doses that give maximal tissue concentrations will almost certainly not respond to higher doses that give 'supra-maximal' tissue concentrations, unless another pro-therapeutic drug mechanism comes into play at these higher levels. Thus, patients with a psychosis that proves refractory to drug treatment can be shown on positron emission tomography to be have 'maximal' (greater than 80%) dopaminergic receptor occupancy (Wolkin et al, 1989). Presumably in these patients other factors prevent dopamine blockade from having any important effect in reducing psychotic symptoms.

The implications of all this can be illustrated. With haloperidol, increasing the dose to produce plasma concentrations in excess of 20 ng/ml is unlikely to convert drug non-responsive patients into responsive ones. Unless it can be shown that higher than usual doses are needed to achieve a maximal plasma or tissue concentration of the drug in a particular individual, such higher doses are almost certainly not justified in terms of improved efficacy, and will probably carry greater risk of adverse effects. With imipramine, doses may need to be increased to a level that produces plasma concentrations of imipramine plus its active metabolite desipramine of 225 ng/ml or more, beyond which no further beneficial clinical response is likely in most individuals.

With newer drugs such as the selective serotonin reuptake inhibitors, the situation is more complex, since these drugs have different therapeutic applications, which may depend on their effect on different brain sites and systems. In practice the dose response ceiling appears to be low for conditions such as panic disorder, intermediate for depression, and high for obsessive–compulsive disorder and eating disorders. Pushing doses impatiently beyond their various response ceilings will confer no therapeutic advantage, and of course runs the risk of countertherapeutic actions and other adverse effects.

Doctors often prescribe a drug that appears to be appropriate for a condition but find that no clinical response is achieved. In such refractory patients it is common to go on gradually increasing the dosage, sometimes beyond the agreed maximum dose (which varies from publication to publication but is best identified from the *British National Formulary*). There is considerable controversy over the doses that are clinically acceptable in specialist psychiatric practice. This particularly applies to what is often described as 'megadose' antipsychotic drug therapy, which describes dosages that are sometimes several times greater than the maximum cited in the *British National Formulary*. Because there have been a number of unexplained deaths and other tragedies in patients taking these higher dosages, the prescriber must take extra care and, preferably, ask for a second opinion, if such high doses are to be used in exceptional cases.

Once an adequate dose of a drug has been tried without success for a reasonable period this can be registered as a treatment failure. The next step is usually to try a different drug, although if its basic mechanism of action is similar to that of the first, it may not be any more effective, assuming that the first drug did not fail because of inadequate tissue concentrations of the active agent. However, as has been said, many treatment failures probably do have a pharmocokinetic explanation, although this may be difficult to ascertain in practice. After two trials of separate drugs, it is then usually worth trying an augmentation treatment, i.e. adding a different type of agent to the one that was ineffective alone.

Although the effectiveness of combined treatments may sometimes have a pharmocokinetic explanation, this does not appear to be the case for lithium as an adjunct to antidepressants and antipsychotics in refractory cases of depression and schizophrenia, respectively.

At present, the third stage for treating refractory cases includes electroconvulsive therapy for affective disorders and clozapine for schizophrenia, but the situation is likely to change as more is understood about the biological basis of treatment refractoriness. The fourth stage involves reconsidering the initial diagnostic formulation, and perhaps refocusing on a completely different approach to treatment (e.g. couple therapy for a depressive illness maintained by conflict within the marriage, or 'socio-anthropological treatment' for a culture-bound syndrome previously labelled as schizophrenia). Finally, if all this fails, it will probably be necessary to start all over again from the beginning, on the assumption that treatment responsiveness is likely to change over the time course of the illness.

Treatment discontinuation and withdrawal effects

Planning the discontinuation of treatment should begin from the outset, and patients should be given some idea of the likely duration of treatment even if this is as vague as 'for the foreseeable future' with lithium and neuroleptics, or as definite as '2 weeks or less' with benzodiazepines. Patients with chronic conditions on long-term maintenance treatment may need to be discouraged from thinking about discontinuation, although the patients themselves may be continually pressing for this. In contrast, pressure for the phasing out of 'addictive' drugs such as benzodiazepines may come from the prescriber who perceives a negative risk–benefit balance for the patient with continued treatment.

Under these circumstances, at some stage it is usually worth a planned and controlled attempt at treatment withdrawal, with full awareness of the risks and problems likely to be encountered. The general principle of gradual withdrawal with careful monitoring is recommended in all instances. If the patient is taking drugs that are difficult to withdraw in a gradual manner – either because of their pharmacokinetics (e.g. lorazepam has a short half-life and therefore shows marked changes in plasma levels over the course of a few hours) or because of their limited dose ranges (e.g. loprazolam is marketed only as 1 mg tablets) – it is reasonable to change to a similar drug that has a longer half-life (e.g. diazepam) or a much wider dose range.

Although this policy is now generally accepted as proper practice in the case of drugs such as benzodiazepines, which have established dependence potential, it is important to realise that 'withdrawal syndromes' have been described for almost all the major classes of drugs used in psychiatry. The word 'discontinuation' used before 'effects', 'syndrome' or 'symptoms' (Pecknold *et al*, 1988; Zajecka *et al*, 1997; Michelson *et al*, 2000) is a euphemism for 'withdrawal'.

The syndrome following withdrawal of benzodiazepines represents the best example of this, although it is far from being fully understood. There is a considerable overlap between the symptoms of withdrawal and those of pre-existing anxiety and it is often not possible to distinguish absolutely between the two. However, the presence of more unusual symptoms, such as perceptual disturbance (e.g. hypersensitivity to noise and touch associated with additional symptoms such as tinnitus and itching sensations) and, very rarely, epileptic seizures, emphasises that the condition is not the same as the original. The syndrome becomes marked within 2–3 days after stopping a short-acting benzodiazepine and within 7 days of stopping a long-acting one. Although a withdrawal syndrome is normally self-limiting, there is also evidence that a 'post-withdrawal syndrome' can maintain many of the symptoms for long after the drug has completely left the body (Tyrer, 1991*a*; Higgitt & Fonagy, 1993).

Intepretation of the withdrawal syndrome is also complicated by the 'nocebo effect' referred to earlier. If patients believe that they are likely to get withdrawal symptoms, they may get them even if the drug they are taking does not actually change in dosage. For example, in one double-blind trial of the withdrawal of benzodiazepines from apparently dependent patients, more than 40% of patients experienced 'withdrawal symptoms' when they changed over to the same benzodiazepine as they had been taking previously in exactly the same dose, but in a different-coloured tablet, as they were expecting this to be a lower dose in a withdrawal programme (Tyrer et al, 1983). There is some evidence that this tendency is related to personality status, and that patients with a dependent personality are more likely to experience such symptoms, but this remains a subject for debate.

Withdrawal syndromes in the form of acute psychotic reactions have been described after discontinuation of antipsychotics in schizophrenia (Chouinard & Jones, 1980) and dramatic mood elevation can follow the sudden discontinuation of lithium therapy in patients with bipolar disorder (Mander & Loudon, 1988). The sudden withdrawal of anti-depressants, particularly when they have been taken in high dosage, is associated with a number of new phenomena, including affective change, psychosomatic symptoms, sleep disturbance and movement disorders (Dilsaver & Greden, 1984).

It is important to realise that these withdrawal syndromes vary considerably in their manifestations and, unlike the withdrawal syndromes from addictive drugs, there is often no desire to take the drug again. None the less, these phenomena emphasise the importance of effecting change in neuropharmacology gradually once a positive stable equilibrium has been reached.

Concluding comments

We have moved a long way in understanding the mechanisms and neurochemistry of drug actions in the past 50 years. Nevertheless, our knowledge of psychotropic drugs remains a mixture of anecdotal and scientific evidence, and the anecdotal part still is in the ascendancy. The good clinician has to synthesise the detailed knowledge of a drug's pharmacological and pharmacokinetic actions (see Chapter 3) and to synthesise this with the much less exact science of clinical practice, which extends from the identification of symptoms and diagnostic groups to understanding personal idiosyncrasies and beliefs.

If we sometimes appear sceptical in this account, this is a reaction to the widespread overemphasis of the clinical aspects of pharmacology. Psychopharmacology is blessed by having a much larger research and development budget than other areas of psychiatry (the total exceeds the rest of psychiatry several-fold) but one of the handicaps arising from this imbalance is that there are many more extrapolations or generalisations from research evidence to everyday clinical practice than are sometimes justified. A restatement of our ignorance and confusion about these fundamentals is sometimes necessary to counteract the neat, clean, reductionist explanations of drug effects that are the understandable presentations of pharmaceutical companies, and which sometimes lead all of us in the wrong direction (Shorter & Tyrer, 2003). They are naturally economical with contradiction and profligate with consistency when it comes to promoting their products.

On a positive note, the decision to prescribe a drug for a specific disorder is gradually being made on the basis of more or less objective evidence rather than on the prejudices of the therapist. We have begun to separate the active principles of therapy from the form of its delivery, and the principles outlined here should aid this process. We can look forward to a time when a common body of evidence becomes the basis of treatment in all the mental health disciplines.

Appendix. Power calculations in practice

These notes illustrate the value of making power calculations in designing and evaluating clinical trials. They help to explain why 'quantitative' measures are more likely than 'qualitative' judgements such as 'recovered' versus 'non-recovered' to produce statistically significant differences between treatment groups when using small samples, while pointing out the difference between clinical and statistical significance. Problems with type 1 error (a false conclusion that chance variation is a positive result) and type 2 error (drawing a negative conclusion which is false) are also illustrated, with the help of confidence limit calculations.

You are considering a double-blind comparison of the therapeutic efficacy of 'drug X' compared with the standard treatment, amitriptyline.

You will study patients with DSM–IV major depression, and you expect a 70% 'response rate' in the amitriptyline group, with 'response' defined as a 50% or more reduction in the Hamilton Rating Scale for Depression (HRSD) score at 6 weeks of treatment.

You are hoping that drug X is at least as good as amitriptyline, and preferably a little better. How will you demonstrate this, if it is true, and how many subjects will you need?

First, consider the possibility that the two treatments are indeed of slightly different efficacy. This slight difference may be great enough to be clinically important, and therefore should not be missed.

If the sample size is too small, you will conclude that the 'response rate' on drug X is 'not significantly different from that on amitriptyline', even though there really is a difference (false negative, type 2 error). The solution is to use a big enough sample that a clinically significant difference can be detected if it does in fact exist, while at the same time being able to state that such a difference is real and not due to chance variation (false positive, type 1 error).

Let us assume that you would wish to detect a 20% or greater difference in response rate between the groups:

R_1, response rate on amitriptyline = 70%
R_2, response rate on drug X = 90%

You want to be able to conclude that there was only a 5% probability of detecting such a difference by chance (probability of a type 1 error, $\alpha = 0.05$). Let us also assume that you are prepared to accept a 10% chance of missing this real difference (type 2 error, $\beta = 0.10$), or in other words, that you will be content with a *power* of 0.90 $(1 - \beta)$ to detect this difference. First, an f value must be found from Table 4.A.1 (see Pocock, 1983, p. 125).

The number (n) of subjects required can then be calculated using the equation:

$$ n = \frac{R_1 \times (100 - R_1) + R_2 \times (100 - R_2)}{(R_2 - R_1)^2} \times f(\alpha, \beta) $$

= 80 per group.

Thus a surprisingly large number of subjects are needed (160) considering that a real difference of less than 20% between the treatments would still be missed.

Now suppose in your clinical trial that you decided to use the actual change in HRSD scores as a measure of therapeutic efficacy, what difference in this measure would you consider it necessary to be able to detect, and what would be the required sample size?

We anticipate that amitriptyline will cause a mean fall of 10 points on the HRSD measured after 6 weeks of treatment, and that the standard deviation of this change will be ± 5 points. (We use previously published studies for these figures.)

We then decide that a difference between amitriptyline and drug X groups of 5 points or more in this mean change score (i.e. a mean (s.d.)

Table 4.A.1 f values (for $\alpha = 0.05$ and $\beta = 0.10$, $f(\alpha, \beta) = 10.5$)

		β	
		0.05	0.10
α	0.05	13.0	10.5
	0.01	17.8	14.9

fall in HDRS of 15 (5) points in the drug X group) would be clinically important, and therefore not to be missed, at least with 90% certainty (power). Thus, to calculate the number of subjects needed per group:

Mean (s.d.) change score on drug X, R_X = 15 (5)

Mean (s.d.) change score on amitriptyline, R_A = 10 (5)

$\alpha = 0.05$, $\beta = 0.10$, $f(\alpha,\beta) = 10.5$

R_X minus R_A = 15 − 10 = 5

$$n = \frac{2 \times s.d.^2}{(R_X - R_A)^2} \times f(\alpha,\beta)$$

$\quad$ = $\quad$ (50/25) × 10.5 $\quad$ = $\quad$ 21 per group (see Pocock, 1983, p. 128).

This is a more manageable number of subjects, but we may be unsure whether a 5-point difference in HRSD change scores is as clinically important as a 20% difference in 'response rate', as used in the earlier calculation.

Now, let us assume that we do the trial, but only 20 suitable patients can be found (10 per group). The results are presented in Table 4.A.2.

In terms of the fall in HRSD scores, the results have turned out as predicted, with drug X producing a mean drop in the score of about 5 points more than amitriptyline. However, the 'response rate' is identical in both groups at 7 out of 10, or 70%.

Table 4.A.2 HRSD scores

Amitriptyline				Drug X			
Before	After	R_A	(%)	Before	After	R_X	(%)
20	9	11	(55)[a]	22	5	17	(77)[a]
22	10	12	(54)[a]	23	1	22	(96)[a]
24	10	14	(58)[a]	20	2	18	(90)[a]
30	13	17	(57)[a]	29	5	24	(83)[a]
18	5	13	(72)[a]	17	3	14	(82)[a]
28	12	16	(57)[a]	27	9	18	(67)[a]
21	9	12	(52)[a]	24	8	16	(67)[a]
20	12	8	(40)	19	11	8	(42)
25	21	4	(16)	27	14	13	(48)
18	18	0	(0)	19	10	9	(47)
Mean 22.6	11.9	10.7		22.7	6.8	15.9	
s.d 4.1	4.6	5.3		4.0	4.3	5.1	
s.e.m.		1.68				1.62	

[a]Classed as 'responded'.

Is there a statistically significant difference between the groups in the extent to which the HRSD score falls with treatment?

Let us do a t-test:

$$t = \frac{\text{mean } R_X - \text{mean } R_A}{\sqrt{\text{s.e.m. } R_X^2 + \text{s.e.m. } R_A^2}}$$

$$= \frac{5.2}{\sqrt{1.62^2 + 1.68^2}} = 2.24 \text{ (d.f.} = 18, P < 0.05)$$

As mean R_X is significantly greater than mean R_A, what do we make of the apparently identical 'response rate' in the two groups?

These response rates may not accurately reflect the 'true' response rates, because with such small samples we cannot have much 'confidence' in the measures obtained. What are the 'confidence limits' for the 70% response rates, that is, the limits within which we can be fairly (say 95%) sure that the 'true' response rate falls?

The confidence limits of a percentage depends on its standard error: thus, 95% confidence limit = 2 × standard error of percentage

$$\text{standard error of percentage} = \sqrt{\frac{\% \times (100 - \%)}{n}}$$

(Pocock, 1983, p. 206)

In this case:
$$= \sqrt{\frac{70 \times 30}{10}} = 14.5$$

Thus 95% confidence limits of 70% = ± 2 × 14.5 = ± 29% (i.e. 41% to 99%).

The 'true' response rate with either amitriptyline or drug X might be as high as 99% and as low as 41%, which is compatible with an undetected difference of response rate between the two treatment groups of as much as 2 × 29 = 58%.

Such a large difference between the effects of the two treatments cannot be ruled out by our findings, because the sample size is inadequate. Even if we had not found a statistically significant difference between the groups in the change in HRSD scores, we would have had to conclude from our confidence limits that the identical response rates in the two groups did not prove that the treatments were equally efficacious, but, on the contrary, the true response rates might differ by as much as 58%. In order to avoid this type 2 error, there is no alternative but to use a much larger sample size when using a 'qualitative measure' such as 'responded' versus 'non-responded'. A 'quantitative measure' such as change in actual HRSD score may let us get away with a smaller sample size, but the clinical significance of such results may be harder to evaluate. Nevertheless, by considering both types of measure in our hypothetical drug trial, we can say that:

(1)   the response rate data are compatible with, but do not demon- strate, a difference in efficacy between the two treatments

(2)   this is confirmed by the finding that drug X produces a significantly greater resolution of symptoms than amitriptyline

(3)   drug X is therefore likely to be more efficacious than amitriptyline, but this needs to be confirmed in a clinical trial using a larger sample size (e.g. $n = 160$).

References

Anderson, I., Nutt, D. & Deakin, J. (2000) Evidence-based guidelines for treating depressive disorders with antidepressants: a revision of the 1993 British Association for Psychopharmacology guidelines. *Journal of Psychopharmacology*, **14**, 3–20.

Armitage, P. (1975) *Sequential Medical Trials*. Oxford: Blackwell.

Balint, M. (1957) *The Doctor, the Patient and the Illness*. London: Pitman Medical.

Basoglu, M. & Marks, I. M. (1989) Anxiety, panic and phobic disorders. *Current Opinion in Psychiatry*, **2**, 235–239.

Bisson, J. (2001) Post-traumatic stress disorder. *Clinical Evidence*, **5**, 688–694.

Blackburn, I. M., Bishop. S., Glen, A. I. M., *et al* (1981) The efficacy of cognitive therapy in depression: a treatment trial using cognitive therapy and pharmacotherapy, each alone and in combination. *British Journal of Psychiatry*, **139**, 181–189.

Chouinard, G. & Jones, B. D. (1980) Neuroleptic-induced supersensitivity psychosis: clinical and pharmacological characteristics. *American Journal of Psychiatry*, **137**, 16–21.

Clark, D. M. (1990) Cognitive therapy for depression and anxiety: is it better than drug treatment in the long term? In *Dilemmas and Difficulties in the Management of Psychiatric Patients* (eds K. Hawton & P. Cowen), pp. 55–64. Oxford: Oxford University Press.

Dilsaver, S. C. & Greden, J. F. (1984) Antidepressant withdrawal phenomenon. *Biological Psychiatry*, **19**, 237–256.

DiMascio, A., Weissman, M. M., Prusoff, B. A., *et al* (1979) Differential symptom reduction by drugs and psychotherapy in acute depression. *Archives of General Psychiatry*, **36**, 1450–1456.

Durham, R. C. & Allan, J. (1993) Psychological treatment of generalised anxiety disorder. A review of the clinical significance of results in outcome studies since 1980. *British Journal of Psychiatry*, **163**, 19–26.

Elkin, I., Shea, M. T., Watkins, J. T., *et al* (1989) National Institute of Mental Health treatment of depression collaborative research program. *Archives of General Psychiatry*, **46**, 971–982.

Emerich, D. F. & Sanberg, P. R. (1991) Neuroleptic dysphoria. *Biological Psychiatry*, **29**, 201–203.

Endicott. J., Spitzer, R. C., Fleiss, J. L., *et al* (1976) The Global Assessment Scale. *Archives of General Psychiatry*, **33**, 766–771.

Frank, E., Kupfer, D. J., Perel, J. M., *et al* (1990) Three-year outcomes for maintenance therapies in recurrent depression. *Archives of General Psychiatry*, **47**, 1093–1099.

Gale, C. & Oakley-Browne, M. (2001) Generalised anxiety disorder. *Clinical Evidence*, **5**, 668–678.

Geddes, J. & Butler, R. (2001) Depressive disorders. *Clinical Evidence*, **5**, 652–667.

Geddes, J., Tomlin, A. & Price, J. (2000a) *Practising Evidence-Based Mental Health.* Abingdon: Radcliffe Medical Press.

Geddes, J., Freemantle, N., Harrison, P., *et al* (2000b) Atypical antipsychotics in the treatment of schizophrenia: systematic overview and meta-regression analysis. *BMJ,* **321**, 1371–1376.

Gelenberg, A. J., Kane, J. M., Keller, M. B., *et al* (1989) Comparison of standard and low serum levels of lithium for maintenance treament of bipolar disorder. *New England Journal of Medicine,* **321**, 1489–1493.

Hale, T. (1993) Will the new antipsychotics improve the treatment of schizophrenia? *BMJ,* **307**, 749.

Harrison-Read, P. E. (1984) The use of drugs in psychiatry. In *Aspects of Psychopharmacology* (eds D. J. Sanger & D. E. Blackman), pp. 174–199. London: Methuen.

Higgitt, A. & Fonagy, P. (1993) Benzodiazepine dependence syndromes and syndromes of withdrawal. In *Benzodiazepine Dependence* (ed. C. Hallström), pp. 58–70. Oxford: Oxford University Press.

Hollyman, J. A., Freeling, P., Paykel, E. S., *et al* (1988) Double-blind placebo-controlled trial of amitriptyline among depressed patients in general practice. *Journal of the Royal College of General Practitioners,* **38**, 393–397.

Hudson, J. I. & Pope, H. G. J. (1990) Affective spectrum disorder: does antidepressant response identify a family of disorders with a common pathophysiology? *American Journal of Psychiatry,* **147**, 552–564.

Johnson, D. A. W. (1988) Drug treatment of schizophrenia. In *Schizophrenia: The Major Issues* (eds P. Bebbington & P. McGuffin), pp. 158–171. London: Heinemann.

Johnson, T. (1998) Clinical trials in psychiatry: background and statistical perspective. *Statistical Methods in Medical Research,* **7**, 209–234.

Johnstone, E. C., Crow, T. J., Frith, C. D., *et al* (1988) The Northwick Park 'functional' psychosis study: diagnosis and treatment response. *Lancet,* **ii**, 119–126.

Katz, M. M., Koslow, S. H., Maas, J. W., *et al* (1987) The timing, specificity and clinical prediction of tricyclic drug effects in depression. *Psychological Medicine,* **17**, 297–309.

Klein, D. F. (1990) NIMH collaborative research on treatment of depression. *Archives of General Psychiatry,* **47**, 682–684.

Klerman, G. L. & Schechter, G. (1982) Drugs and psychotherapy. In *Handbook of Affective Disorders* (ed. E. Paykel), pp. 329–337. Edinburgh: Churchill Livingstone.

Kraemer, H. C. (1981) Coping strategies in psychiatric clinical research. *Journal of Consulting and Clinical Psychology,* **49**, 309–319.

Kraemer, H. C. & Pruyn, J. P. (1990) The evaluation of different approaches to randomized clinical trials. *Archives of General Psychiatry,* **47**, 1163–1169.

Kupfer, D. J. (1991) Long term treatment of depression. *Journal of Clinical Psychiatry,* **52** (suppl. 5), 28–34.

Mander, A. J. & Loudon, J. B. (1988) Rapid recurrence of mania following abrupt discontinuation of lithium. *Lancet,* **ii**, 15–17.

McIntosh, A. & Lawrie, S. (2001) Schizophrenia. *Clinical Evidence,* **5**, 695–716.

Michelson, D., Fava, M., Amsterdam, J., *et al* (2000) Interruption of selective serotonin reuptake inhibitor treatment. Double-blind, placebo-controlled trial. *British Journal of Psychiatry,* **176**, 363–368.

NIMH–PSC Collaborative Study Group (1964) Phenothiazine treatment in acute schizophrenia. *Archives of General Psychiatry,* **10**, 246–261.

Pecknold, J. C., Swinson, R. P., Kuch, K., *et al* (1988) Results from a multicenter trial. III. Discontinuation effects. *Archives of General Psychiatry,* **45**, 429–436.

Perry, S. (1990) Combining antidepressants and psychotherapy: rationale and strategies. *Journal of Clinical Psychiatry,* **51** (suppl. 1), 16–20.

Pocock, S. J. (1983) *Clinical Trials: A Practical Approach.* Chichester: Wiley.

Prien, R. F. (1988) Methods and models for placebo use in pharmacotherapeutic trials. *Psychopharmacology Bulletin*, **24**, 4–8.

Prien, R. F., Kupfer, D. J., Mansk, P. A., *et al* (1984) Drug therapy in the prevention of recurrences in unipolar and bipolar affective disorders. Report of the NIMH Collaborative Study Group comparing lithium carbonate, imipramine and a lithium carbonate–imipramine combination. *Archives of General Psychiatry*, **41**, 1096–1104.

Priest, R. G. (1989) Antidepressants of the future. *British Journal of Psychiatry*, **155** (suppl. 6), 7–8.

Quality Assurance Project (1983) A treatment outline for depressive disorders. *Australian and New Zealand Journal of Psychiatry*, **17**, 129–146.

Quality Assurance Project (1984) Treatment outlines for the management of schizophrenia. *Australian and New Zealand Journal of Psychiatry*, **18**, 19–38.

Quitkin, F. M., Fabkin, J. G., Ross, D., *et al* (1984) Identification of true drug response to antidepressants. Use of pattern analysis. *Archives of General Psychiatry*, **41**, 782–786.

Rawlins, M. D. (1981) Clinical pharmacology: adverse reaction to drugs. *BMJ*, **282**, 974–976.

Sachs, G., Printz, D., Kahn, D., *et al* (2000) The Expert Consensus Guideline Series: Medication Treatment of Bipolar Disorder 2000. *Postgraduate Medicine* (special issue 104).

Shepherd, G. (1988) The contribution of psychological intervention to the treatment and management of schizophrenia. In *Schizophrenia: The Major Issues* (eds P. Bebbington & P. McGuffin), pp. 226–243. London: Heinemann.

Shorter, E. & Tyrer, P. (2003) The separation of anxiety and depressive disorders: blind alley in psychopharmacology and the classification of disease. *BMJ*, **327**, 158–160.

Soloff, P. H., George, A., Nathan, R. S., *et al* (1986) Progress in pharmacotherapy of borderline disorders: a double-blind study of amitriptyline, haloperidol and placebo. *Archives of General Psychiatry*, **43**, 691–697.

Soomro, G. M. (2001) Obsessive–compulsive disorder. *Clinical Evidence*, **5**, 679–687.

Tyrer, P. (1991*a*) The benzodiazepine post-withdrawal syndrome. *Stress Medicine*, **7**, 1–2.

Tyrer, P. (1991*b*) The nocebo effect – poorly known but getting stronger. In *Side Effects of Drugs Annual, 15* (eds M. N. G. Dukes & J. K. Aronson), pp. xix–xxv. Amsterdam: Elsevier.

Tyrer, P. (2001) The case for cothymia: mixed anxiety and depression as a single diagnosis. *British Journal of Psychiatry*, **179**, 191–193.

Tyrer, P. & Murphy, S. (1992) The place of benzodiazepines in psychiatric practice. *British Journal of Psychiatry*, **151**, 719–723.

Tyrer, P. & Tyrer, J. (1992) Comparing the quality of data from several clinical trials (Letter). *British Journal of Psychiatry*, **160**, 126.

Tyrer, P., Owen, R. & Dawling, S. (1983) Gradual withdrawal of diazepam after long-term therapy. *Lancet*, i, 1402–1406.

Tyrer, P., Marsden, C. A., Casey, P., *et al* (1987) Clinical efficacy of paroxetine in resistant depression. *Journal of Psychopharmacology*, **1**, 251–257.

Van Putten, T. & May, P. R. (1978) Subjective response as a predictor of outcome in pharmacotherapy. *Archives of General Psychiatry*, **35**, 477–480.

Warner, J. & Butler, R. (2001) Alzheimer's disease. *Clinical Evidence*, **5**, 630–641.

Wolkin, A., Barouch, F., Wolf, A., *et al* (1989) Dopamine blockade and clinical response: evidence for two biological subgroups of schizophrenia. *American Journal of Psychiatry*, **146**, 905–908.

Zajecka, J., Tracy, K. A. & Mitchell, S. (1997) Discontinuation symptoms after treatment with serotonin reuptake inhibitors: a literature review. *Journal of Clinical Psychiatry*, **58**, 291–297.

Further reading

Freeman, C. & Tyrer, P. (eds) (1992) *Research Methods in Psychiatry: A Beginners' Guide* (2nd edn). London: Gaskell.

Hawton, K. & Cowen, P. (eds) (1990) *Dilemmas and Difficulties in the Management of Psychiatric Patients*. Oxford: Oxford University Press.

Lader, M. & Herrington, R. (1990) *Biological Treatments in Psychiatry*. Oxford: Oxford University Press.

Pocock, S. J. (1983) *Clinical Trials: A Practical Approach*. Chichester: Wiley.

Tyrer, P., Harrison-Read, P. & Van Horn, E. (1997) *Drug Treatment in Psychiatry: A Guide for the Community Mental Health Worker*. Oxford: Butterworth/Heinemann.

Part II
Pharmacology of the main psychotropic drug groups

CHAPTER 5

Anxiolytics, sedatives and hypnotics

Stephen J. Cooper

Introduction

Anxiety is one of the most frequent human emotions and is experienced by everyone from time to time. Pathological anxiety is less common and may arise from: general anxiety disorder; one of the many other forms of neurosis; depressive illness; psychotic illness; or from a physical disorder, such as hyperthyroidism. Sleep disturbances are similarly common and have several causes.

While psychopharmacologists may dream of ultimately being able to match specific classes of drugs to specific diagnoses, this is still far from reality for anxiety and sleep disorders. Nevertheless, it is important to remember that where anxiety symptoms arise from a depressive illness, a psychotic illness or a physical disorder, treatment of the primary condition is what may ultimately bring relief from the anxiety symptoms. Furthermore, in endogenous (or melancholic) depression and in other psychoses, antipsychotic drugs are usually most effective for any anxiety symptoms and anxiolytics of the minor tranquilliser type may be of little value.

The principal neurotransmitter systems implicated in anxiety are gamma-aminobutyric acid (GABA), serotonin (5-HT) and noradrenaline (NA). Some authors try to implicate particular systems, or even particular receptor subtypes, in particular clinical syndromes (e.g. Deakin & Graeff, 1991). However, evidence overall is that disturbances of all of these systems can be identified. Whether or not any one of these ultimately turns out to be primarily disturbed in particular types of anxiety, leading to secondary disturbance of the others, remains to be seen.

These points are made in order to avoid any misconceptions that may arise from the fact that many of the drugs described here have very specific pharmacological effects. Although they also have fairly specific effects in relieving anxiety symptoms and causing sedation, this does not necessarily imply that these symptoms are directly mediated by the same specific receptors/transmitters.

Barbiturates

History

Barbiturates were among the first psychotropic drugs to be synthesised for clinical use. The first was diethylbarbituric acid (in 1903) and the second phenobarbital (in 1912), which is still in use for the management of some patients with epilepsy. Barbiturates first began to be supplanted when propanediol derivatives (principally meprobamate) became available (in 1951) but more rapidly fell out of use as hypnotics and anxiolytics when the benzodiazepines were introduced in the 1960s. Benzodiazepines are safer in overdose, less prone to induce tolerance and dependence, and have fewer adverse effects (Box 5.1).

Pharmacology and kinetics

Barbiturates are readily absorbed after oral administration. Those used intravenously for anaesthesia are thiobarbiturates (e.g. thiopental), which are highly protein bound and highly lipid soluble, and so rapidly enter the central nervous system (CNS). Those used orally are oxy-barbiturates (e.g. phenobarbitone, amylobarbitone), which are less protein bound and less lipid soluble. They are distributed and metabolised more slowly and thus have longer durations of action. Elimination half-lives are in the range 30–90 hours. Hepatic metabolism is the principal route of inactivation and this may become more rapid with regular use, because barbiturates induce hepatic microsomal enzymes.

Mechanism of action

Barbiturates depress the activity of neuronal tissues. Their effects generally become more widespread as greater tissue concentrations are reached – they have little selectivity for neurons mediating different functions. Anticonvulsants perhaps demonstrate some selectivity, in that doses producing anticonvulsant effects do not necessarily induce sleep.

Their principal neuropharmacological effect is to enhance the action of GABA at its receptors. Neurophysiological and molecular studies suggest that GABA receptors are coupled to a chloride ionophore in a

---

Box 5.1 Problems with barbiturates

- Impairment of psychomotor function
- Tolerance to their effects
- Cross-tolerance to other drugs
- High potential for physical dependence
- Potent depression of the central nervous system in overdose

---

complex that includes separate binding sites for barbiturates and benzodiazepines. The effect of a barbiturate at this binding site is to modify the structure of the complex to augment the effect of GABA. This enhances the opening of the chloride channel, and so allows increased flux of Cl⁻ into the neuron, resulting in hyperpolarisation. Thus neuronal firing is reduced. (See also 'The $GABA_A$–BDZ receptor complex', below.)

Types and applications

Initially barbiturates were used as hypnotics and anxiolytic sedatives. They are now obsolete for these indications and the only patients continuing to use them as hypnotics are occasional elderly people who started taking them many years ago and who have not been able to stop or transfer to a benzodiazepine. They continue to find occasional use in the management of epilepsy (see Chapter 10), but have been largely replaced by modern anticonvulsants. Intravenous barbiturates are used for the induction of anaesthesia, but again the introduction of more modern agents with less severe 'hangover' effects has tended to supplant them.

Adverse effects and interactions

The main adverse effects are on psychomotor function. Cognitive performance and motor skills are both impaired and this can occur as a hangover effect following a single night-time dose. More chronic cognitive impairments can also occur in children who use barbiturates for the long-term management of epilepsy. Also in children, paradoxical hyperactivity may occur. Other adverse effects are vertigo, nausea, vomiting and diarrhoea.

With chronic use, tolerance develops to their effects. This is partly pharmacokinetic, because barbiturates induce their own metabolism, but also pharmacodynamic, owing to change at the GABA receptor complex. Tolerance is defined as the need to use large doses of a drug in order to achieve similar effects with repeated administration. Cross-tolerance to other general CNS depressants (e.g. benzodiazepines and general anaesthetics) also occurs.

Physical dependence occurs, as evidenced by a wide variety of withdrawal symptoms, similar to those for benzodiazepines (see below), including anxiety, insomnia and epileptic seizures. Dependence is closely linked to tolerance and the severity of withdrawal symptoms generally depends on the degree of tolerance. Tolerance and dependence develop rapidly and easily to barbiturates, which gives them a high potential for misuse.

Barbiturates are extremely dangerous in overdose because of their marked CNS depressant properties. Furthermore, cross-potentiation between the various barbiturates and alcohol leads to exaggeration of the effects of both if they are combined.

Propanediols

The principal drug in this group was meprobamate, first synthesised in 1951. It has a more specific anxiolytic effect than the barbiturates and, while having similar adverse effects, causes less impairment of psychomotor function. However, because of physical dependence and a low margin of safety between therapeutic and lethal doses it was rapidly superseded by the benzodiazpines once they became available. Skin rashes are the other major adverse effect. There is little information regarding its mechanism of action.

The GABA$_A$–BDZ receptor complex

Effects of GABA in the CNS

Benzodiazepines and barbiturates appear to exert their effects through the structure often known as the GABA$_A$–BDZ (benzodiazepine) receptor complex, which controls the opening and closing of a chloride ion channel (Fig. 5.1). Binding of GABA to postsynaptic GABA$_A$ receptors causes opening of chloride channels directly linked to the receptor and thus allows influx of Cl$^-$ ions into the neuron. This makes the inside of the neuron more negatively charged, that is, results in hyperpolarisation. As a result, it becomes more difficult for excitatory influences on the neuron to produce sufficient depolarisation to induce an action potential. Thus, GABA$_A$ receptors have inhibitory effects.

The effects of GABA at GABA$_A$ receptors can be antagonised by bicuculline and picrotoxin (see Fig. 5.1 and Chapter 1). GABA$_B$ receptors are not involved in mediating the effects of benzodiazepines or barbiturates.

There are few 'long' GABAergic pathways in the brain mediating effects in a variety of sites but arising from specific nuclei (as is the case for noradrenaline and serotonin systems). Most GABA-releasing neurons are short inter-neurons. These are widespread and mediate inhibition in many brain areas, including the cerebral cortex, hippocampus, amygdala, brain-stem and cerebral cortex. Inhibition in the brain-stem may modulate the activity of the serotonergic and noradrenergic cell bodies in the raphe and locus coeruleus, respectively. GABA may also influence these systems via presynaptic inhibition at nerve terminals, which reduces the release of neurotransmitter. These systems are of interest because they have been implicated in pharmacological theories of anxiety.

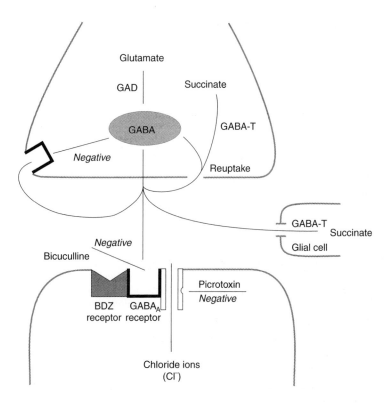

Fig. 5.1 A diagrammatic representation of the pre- and postsynaptic terminals of a synapse that uses gamma-aminobutyric acid (GABA) as a transmitter. Synthesis of GABA from glutamate is catalysed by the enzyme glutamic acid decarboxylase (GAD). Inactivation is by reuptake into neurons or glial cells, followed by metabolism to succinate via the enzyme GABA-transaminase (GABA-T). The postsynaptic receptor complex consists of a $GABA_A$ receptor linked to a chloride ion (Cl^-) channel and a benzodiazepine (BDZ) receptor. Binding of GABA to its receptor opens the Cl^- channel. Bicuculline can block this effect at the $GABA_A$ receptor and picrotoxin can influence it at an independent site on the receptor complex. Binding of a benzodiazepine to the BDZ receptor enhances the effects of GABA by altering the shape of the receptor complex (allosteric modulation).

The $GABA_A$–BDZ receptor complex structure

Binding sites for GABA and benzodiazepines

The receptor complex is made up of five subunits and is embedded in the bimolecular layer that makes up the neuronal membrane. These subunits surround the chloride ion channel. Fig. 5.2 provides a diagrammatic representation of that part of the complex on the outside

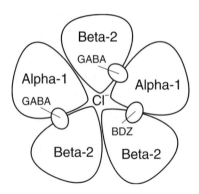

Fig. 5.2 A diagrammatic representation looking down on to that part of the receptor complex that is on the outside of the neuronal membrane. It shows the arrangement of the five subunits (in this case two α-1, two ß-2 and one χ-2) around a chloride ion (Cl⁻) channel. The two GABA binding sites are at the interface between the α-1 and β-2 subunits and the BDZ binding site is at the interface between the α-1 and χ-2 subunits. Opening of the Cl⁻ channel depends on the binding of two molecules of GABA. Binding of a BDZ molecule will increase the degree of opening and amount of time GABA maintains the opening of the ion channel.

of the neuronal membrane and shows where the receptor sites for GABA and benzodiazepines are found. Two GABA molecules are required to increase the conductance of the chloride ion channel (by increasing the length of time for which the channel is open).

Specific binding sites, or receptors, for benzodiazepines were identified in brain tissue in 1978. These are close to, but separate from, the GABA$_A$ receptor (Fig. 5.2). When a benzodiazepine binds to the BDZ receptor it augments the effects of GABA via an allosteric interaction between the BDZ receptor and the GABA$_A$ receptor, that is, it alters the shape of the structure to allow enhanced opening of the ion channel. Thus, benzodiazepines enhance Cl⁻ inflow and the inhibitory effects of GABA. Not all GABA$_A$ receptors are associated with BDZ receptors. Points to note are:

(1) Benzodiazepines have no effect on chloride channels by themselves – removal of GABA by inhibiting its synthesis or blockade of GABA receptors with bicuculline abolishes any effect of a benzodiazepine on chloride channels.
(2) GABA$_A$ and BDZ receptors are separate – benzodiazepines do not bind to GABA$_A$ receptors and neither GABA nor bicuculline will bind to BDZ receptors.
(3) The presence of GABA agonists enhances the binding of benzodiazepines to their receptors and the presence of benzodiazepines enhances the binding of GABA to its receptor.

(4)   BDZ receptors are grouped into two main groups – high affinity and low affinity. Only the high-affinity site is important in the anxiolytic, hypnotic and anticonvulsant effects of benzodiazepines.

(5)   Barbiturates and alcohol also bind to this receptor complex, although at different sites from benzodiazepines. One of the reasons for the lethality of barbiturates in overdose is that while normal pharmacological doses act to enhance the effects of GABA (similarly to benzodiazepines), very high doses can independently cause opening of the chloride ion channel. High doses of benzodiazepines cannot do this.

Structure

The five macromolecular subunits making up the receptor complex come from seven families of subunits – alpha, beta, gamma, delta, epsilon, theta and rho. Each of these families consists of a number of subtypes of units: α – six subtypes; β – three subtypes; γ – three subtypes; ρ – three subtypes; and δ, ε, θ – one subtype each. A receptor complex normally consists of two pairs of subunits from different families, with the fifth subunit coming from one of the other families of subunits. For example, the most commonly found $GABA_A$–BDZ receptor (approximately 50% of the total) consists of two α_1 subunits, two β_2 subunits and one γ_2 subunit.

Clearly, a large number of potential combinations of subunits are theoretically possible. However, studies using genetically modified mice indicate that only some of these combinations are compatible with life. It also seems that to obtain a functional response to a benzodiazepine drug a γ subunit is essential. Those $GABA_A$–BDZ receptor variants that do exist are not equally distributed within the CNS. For example, cholinergic neurons never carry $GABA_A$–BDZ receptors that contain the α_1 subunit. Alternatively, if we consider receptors comprising α_x, $\beta_{2/3}$, and γ_2 subunits, 60% of these will have an α_1 subunit and such receptors are found mainly in the cerebral cortex. On the other hand, 15% will carry the α_3 subunit and most of these are found in the reticular activating system.

Any given drug that binds to $GABA_A$–BDZ receptors will have different effects at different receptor variants (more potent at some, less potent at others) and thus different potency of effects in different brain areas. This creates the potential to develop drugs with effects at specific receptor subtypes, and which may have more specific clinical effects, for example anxiolysis without sedation (Rudolph *et al*, 2001).

Receptor subgroups

Although many variants of the receptor complex may be possible, a simple functional classification is often employed. Thus, of all receptor complexes that have a $GABA_A$ receptor: 10% have no affinity for benzodiazepines; 10% have low affinity for benzodiazepines; and 80% have high affinity for benzodiazepines. These 'high-affinity' sites are then divided according to their affinity for zolpidem: BDZ type 1 receptors (sometimes termed ω_1 receptors) have high affinity for zolpidem and BDZ type 2 receptors (ω_2) low or no affinity for zolpidem.

Benzodiazepine receptor ligands

Agonists, antagonists and inverse agonists

A ligand is a substance that will bind to a particular receptor, or binding site, and generally has a part of its structure complementary to that of the receptor. A particular receptor is usually named according to its principal ligand, which is usually a transmitter substance (e.g. noradrenaline, serotonin) but sometimes it is a drug, as in the case of the BDZ receptor. Subclassification of receptors (e.g. α-adrenergic, β-adrenergic) is usually related to the different physiological effects of the subtypes.

Drugs or ligands binding to most receptors either act to produce the same effect as the transmitter normally active at the receptor or act as straightforward neutral antagonists, blocking the effect of the transmitter but having no effect of their own. However, for BDZ receptors different ligands may have very different physiological effects, even though they bind to the same receptor (Fig. 5.3).

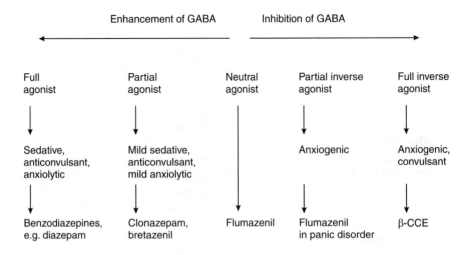

Fig. 5.3 The different effects of various ligands for the benzodiazepine receptor.

Agonists

These have the characteristic effect at the receptor of the normal transmitter substance or drug. In the case of the BDZ receptor, the standard benzodiazepines, such as diazepam, are agonists.

Inverse agonist

These have the opposite effect to the 'agonists': in the case of BDZ receptors 'inverse agonists' are convulsant and anxiogenic. β-CCE (see below) has such effects. While full 'agonists' at the BDZ receptor appear to enhance the binding of GABA to its receptors, there is evidence that 'inverse agonists' inhibit the binding of GABA.

Competitive antagonists

These block the effects of both 'agonists' and 'inverse agonists'. They should have no intrinsic activity of their own and are sometimes termed 'neutral antagonists'. So far no entirely neutral antagonist at the BDZ receptor has been found. Flumazenil acts as a competitive antagonist in many, but not all, situations.

Partial agonist/partial inverse agonist

These compounds occupy the BDZ receptor but have only some of the effects of either full agonists or inverse agonists. By occupying the receptors they are also antagonists towards other benzodiazepines. Flumazenil can act as such a compound. Normally it is a competitive antagonist to standard agonists, such as diazepam, and is therefore useful in treating overdoses. However, in patients with panic disorder it has partial inverse agonist effects and can thus be anxiogenic.

Endogenous ligands

Given that a definite binding site exists in human brain tissue for benzodiazepines, the possibility of one or more endogenous ligands is raised. In 1980 Braestrup and colleagues identified β-CCE (β-carboline-3-carboxylic acid ethylester) in human urine and brain tissue. β-CCE has a high affinity for BDZ receptors, at which it has inverse agonist effects, and little affinity for other receptors, including GABA, noradrenaline and dopamine receptors. Other peptides of similar structure, with similar effects, have been identified as occurring naturally in the mammalian CNS. Indeed, it now seems that β-CCE itself can be derived from these peptides. (In fact, the original identification of β-CCE probably resulted from an artefact of the extraction of one of these peptides from urine samples.)

More recently, evidence for endogenous ligands with agonist effects like benzodiazepines has accumulated. These substances are known as 'endozepines' and have been identified in brain tissue from humans

149

who died before the introduction of benzodiazepines. Increased concentrations of endozepines have been found in the cerebrospinal fluid (CSF) of patients with hepatic encephalopathy. However, they are also found in plants used in the human diet, such as rice and potatoes, and may therefore have dietary origin.

A further substance identified in human brain tissue is the peptide known as diazepam-binding inhibitor (DBI). DBI is present in about half of all GABAergic neurons and when released reduces the efficiency of GABA in opening the chloride ion channels linked to $GABA_A$ receptors. DBI was so named because it was identified and purified through its ability to displace diazepam from its binding sites. The active component is an octadecapeptide sequence known as ODN.

None of these substances is present in large quantities in human tissue and it remains doubtful whether or not they have a physiological role.

Clinical pharmacology of benzodiazepines

History

The benzodiazepines were first identified in 1957 during the systematic screening of a series of compounds for those with muscle-relaxant properties. Randall and his colleagues noted that some of these compounds had a 'taming' effect on test animals at doses less than those producing ataxia or sedation. This suggested a possible role in reducing anxiety. The first benzodiazepine to be tested in patients was chlordiazepoxide, which became available for general use in 1960 and which was followed by diazepam in 1962.

Benzodiazepines rapidly gained popularity in the treatment of anxiety because they were less potent than the barbiturates and meprobamate, and had fewer of the many problems of these drugs (Box 5.1). At the same time, they were more specific for the treatment of anxiety and more pleasant to take than the only other alternatives, the phenothiazine neuroleptics. Nevertheless, it was not until 1965 that barbiturate prescribing began to decline significantly. This was partly because of the degree of dependence of many patients on barbiturates and partly because of caution with new drugs following recognition of the problems caused by thalidomide, a piperidinedione sedative introduced around the same time. At present, 13 benzodiazepines are listed in the *British National Formulary* (seven as anxiolytics and six as hypnotics), as are three non-benzodiazepine hypnotics that also act via the $GABA_A$–BDZ receptor complex.

In the early years of benzodiazepine use physical dependence was not thought to occur with standard therapeutic doses, although it had been described with excessive doses taken over prolonged periods (Hollister *et al*, 1961). In 1973 Covi and colleagues reported evidence of minor withdrawal symptoms after 20 weeks of treatment with chlordiazepoxide, but the complexity of their study protocol slightly obscured the result (Covi *et al*, 1973). However, following the observation of withdrawal symptoms by Petursson & Lader (1981) on discontinuation of treatment in 16 patients, on normal therapeutic doses, it became clear that physical dependence could occur with standard therapy. Since then there has been a reduction in benzodiazepine prescribing and new guidelines for prescribing have been published (see p. 169).

Despite these problems, benzodiazepines remain one of the most effective and safest treatments for anxiety symptoms. Death or serious long-term morbidity from overdose of benzodiazepines alone is rare, and tends to occur only if they are combined with other CNS depressants, such as alcohol. Since their fall from favour and reduced prescribing there has been a fall in the numbers of patients presenting following overdose of benzodiazepines but an almost parallel rise in the numbers presenting with overdose of paracetamol or of non-steriodal anti-inflammatory drugs (NSAIDs) (Hawton & Fagg, 1992). Poisoning with paracetamol and NSAIDs is associated with significantly greater morbidity and mortality.

Pharmacokinetics

In this and the following sections, diazepam will be used as the principal example (Table 5.1).

Bioavailability following oral administration is almost complete and peak plasma concentrations are reached in 30–90 minutes. The presence of food reduces the rate but not the extent of absorption. Absorption following intramuscular administration is erratic and often slower than after oral dosing. This should therefore be avoided unless absolutely necessary.

Diazepam is highly lipid soluble and therefore diffuses rapidly into the CNS. After the peak plasma concentration has been reached there is a phase of falling plasma concentrations as the drug is distributed to

Table 5.1 Pharmacokinetic properties of diazepam

Bioavailability	Almost complete with oral dosing
Peak concentration (single dose)	30–90 minutes
Protein binding	95%
Renal excretion	Negligible for unchanged drug
Metabolism	Phase I to active metabolite, desmethyldiazepam
	Phase II for inactivation of metabolites
Elimination half-life	
young adults	20 hours
elderly	30–100 hours
desmethyldiazepam	30–90 hours

tissues – the distribution phase (see Chapter 3). The pattern of plasma concentrations seen is consistent with a two-compartment model.

Protein binding of diazepam, mainly to albumin, is around 90–95%. High lipid solubility means it is stored in body fat as well as brain tissue. It is found in breast milk and will cross the placenta.

Elimination is largely via hepatic metabolism (see below), with almost negligible renal excretion of unchanged drug. The elimination half-life ($t_{1/2}$) is age dependent: in young adults it is around an average of 20 hours, but over 65 years of age this rises to an average of 40 hours, with a wide range (30–100 hours), indicating a need for care in prescribing to the elderly. It takes approximately five half-lives to wash a drug out of the plasma. Thus for diazepam this may take anywhere from 4 to 10 days, on average.

Newborn infants metabolise benzodiazepines very slowly. Single doses of a benzodiazepine given to a nursing mother may produce quite low concentrations of unbound benzodiazepine in infant plasma. However, chronic dosing of the infant via breast milk, despite the low dose, will result in accumulation in plasma because of the slow metabolism.

Metabolism of benzodiazepines

The major function of drug metabolism is to enhance excretion either into bile or by making compounds more water soluble, thus facilitating renal excretion. For many drugs there are two stages to this process.

Phase I

Functional groups on the drug molecule are altered in some way, for example by hydroxylation, deamination or N-dealkylation. This step often results in the production of an active metabolite. In the case of diazepam, as well as some other benzodiazepines, phase I metabolism produces desmethyldiazepam, an active metabolite with a $t_{1/2}$ much longer than that of diazepam (between 30 and 90 hours in young adults). Drugs that undergo phase I metabolism are subject to the effects of age, liver disease or other enzyme-inducing drugs, which generally have effects on the enzymes mediating this phase.

Phase II

In phase II, drugs or their metabolites undergo processes in which functional groups are added to the molecule, for example by acetylation or conjugation. Conjugations most often involve combining the drug or metabolite molecule with sulphate or glucuronic acid. Conjugation usually inactivates a compound. Thus, this is the final metabolic step for many benzodiazepines, although for some (e.g. lorazepam, temazepam) it is the only step. Drugs only undergoing phase II metabolism do not produce active metabolites.

Physiological and adverse effects

Benzodiazepines act through their effects as agonists at the BDZ receptor. The affinities of different benzodiazepines for their receptor correlate with their anti-anxiety potencies *in vivo*. The inhibitory effects in the brain are responsible for the anti-anxiety, anticonvulsant and sedative/hypnotic effects. Inhibition of afferent pathways in the spinal cord results in relaxation of skeletal muscles. All benzodiazepines exhibit these effects. Which effect is evident is probably a function of the tissue concentration and relative affinity of the drug for the BDZ receptor. At low tissue levels anxiolysis occurs and at high levels sedation will occur for all benzodiazepines. Tolerance develops to many of their effects and this issue is examined in more detail below.

At normal therapeutic doses benzodiazepines have little effect on autonomic, cardiovascular or respiratory function, although they may sometimes (mainly with intravenous use) cause respiratory depression and reduce systolic blood pressure. Benzodiazepines do not cause induction of hepatic microsomal enzymes and standard biochemical indices are not altered during treatment. Leucopenia and eosinophilia are very rare. Neuroendocrine measures are also usually unchanged, although occasionally plasma cortisol levels may decrease.

Chronic, high-dose therapy may interfere with the dexamethasone suppression test. One interpretation of some data from animal studies and a study of prognosis in breast cancer suggested promotion of breast cancer by diazepam. A subsequent large case-control study found no evidence to support this (Kaufman *et al*, 1982).

The principal adverse effects of diazepam are listed in Table 5.2. The most important of these relate to BDZ receptor effects: sedation, amnesia and psychomotor impairment. The sedative, amnestic/psycho-motor and anxiolytic effects of benzodiazepines can be regarded as falling along a continuum of effects which are dependent on the degree of benzodiazepine receptor occupancy. The development of tolerance to these effects would appear to lie along a similar continuum, with the anxiolytic effects being most resistant to the development of tolerance.

Table 5.2 Adverse effects of diazepam

Common	Occasional	Rare
Drowsiness	Dry mouth	Amnesia
Dizziness	Blurred vision	Restlessness
Psychomotor impairment	Gastrointestinal upset	Skin rash
	Ataxia	
	Headache	
	Reduced blood pressure	

However, increasing knowledge of GABA$_A$–BDZ receptor subtypes suggests that these differences may be because different functions involve different subtypes, which have differential susceptibility to different drugs.

Sedation

Sedation is a common effect and occurs with all benzodiazepines, although the extent will depend on the susceptibility of the individual patient. Tolerance to the sedative effects has been shown in many studies and appears to develop over 2–3 weeks of treatment.

Psychomotor impairment

Benzodiazepines have well-known adverse effects on psychomotor performance, which can be shown both in the laboratory setting (using for example reaction time tests or digit symbol substitution) and in real-life tasks. A study of 19 386 drivers involved in first road traffic accidents found an association between the use of benzodiazepines and being involved in an accident; there was in fact a dose–response relationship (Barbone *et al*, 1998). These effects may occur from both daytime use and from hangover effects following the use of benzodiazepine hypnotics. Patients must be warned about impairment of ability to drive, operate machinery or carry out other manual tasks. These impairments arise partly as a result of sedation but also because benzodiazepines affect central processing ability, particularly that concerned with sensory information (Hindmarch, 1980).

The development of tolerance to these impairments, during chronic use of benzodiazepines, has been demonstrated in some studies on some types of test, but findings are not consistent. Results are often difficult to interpret because of failure to examine benzodiazepine plasma concentrations. Steady accumulation of active metabolites may well explain some discrepant findings. It is also important to remember that in highly anxious patients performance is impaired and will improve, in some respects, on treatment with benzodiazepines.

Amnesia

The effects of benzodiazepines on memory were first noted in 1965 and have been reviewed by King (1992). Following benzodiazepine pre-medication, before general anaesthesia, many patients were found to have amnesia for some events that occurred before surgery. Controlled studies of benzodiazepine-induced amnesia indicate that it is for recall and recognition of items presented after receipt of the drug (i.e. it is an anterograde amnesia) – there is no impairment of retention or retrieval of previously stored information (i.e. no retrograde amnesia). Again, sedation plays an important part in this phenomenon and this has been elegantly demonstrated by the ability of flumazenil, a BDZ antagonist, to antagonise equally the amnestic and sedative effects of lorazepam (Preston *et al*, 1989). Not all studies, however, have found a close correlation between sedation and memory impairment, although two factors may make a close relationship difficult to determine. First, effects on memory are likely to last longer than sedation, given that information never learned can never be retrieved. Second, tolerance to the sedating effects may sometimes develop very rapidly, even during the action of a single dose (tachyphylaxis).

Comparison of benzodiazepines

Differences in intrinsic potency are determined by a particular benzodiazepine's ability to bind to the receptor, those drugs with a higher affinity for the receptor being more potent and, thus, in isolated tissue samples, requiring a smaller dose to achieve the same effect (lorazepam > diazepam > oxazepam). While this is one factor that will determine the effects of a drug in the clinical situation, other pharmacokinetic factors are also important.

For single doses of a drug, factors affecting absorption and distribution are relevant. Lipid solubility is the most important of these. A highly lipid-soluble drug, such as diazepam, will be rapidly absorbed and will rapidly reach the brain. However, its high lipid solubility also leads to rapid distribution to other tissues, so plasma concentrations may fall rapidly, resulting in diminished effects. On the other hand, a single dose of lorazepam, of equal potency, which is much less lipid soluble, will take longer to be absorbed and reach the brain but will be more slowly and less extensively distributed to other tissues. Its effects will thus be of slower onset but more sustained.

For chronic dosing, factors relating to metabolism and elimination are more important. Rates of elimination are compared using the elimination half-life ($t_{1/2}$) for each drug. The $t_{1/2}$ is useful in predicting the length of time it will take to reach steady-state concentrations during a schedule of regular chronic dosing (when dosing is once every half-life) and the time to eliminate a drug after stopping regular dosing – approximately $5 \times t_{1/2}$ in both cases. Drugs with a long $t_{1/2}$ will accumulate more slowly and take longer to reach maximum effect (e.g. diazepam). On the other hand, they will have a more sustained effect than a drug with short $t_{1/2}$ (e.g. alprazolam). The $t_{1/2}$ is determined both by volume of distribution (V_d) and clearance (Cl) of a drug:

$$t_{1/2} = \frac{0.693 \times V_d}{Cl}$$

Thus, more lipid-soluble benzodiazepines, with a high V_d, will tend to have a longer $t_{1/2}$. Clearance is determined both by the rate of metabolic inactivation (thus drugs undergoing only phase II metabolism

Table 5.3 Comparison of the pharmacological properties of common anxiolytics and hypnotics

Drug	Absorption	$t_{1/2}$ of drug (h)	Metabolic phases	$t_{1/2}$ of important major metabolites (h)
Diazepam	Rapid	20–100	I + II	30–90
Chlordiazepoxide	Intermediate	5–30	I + II	30–90
Alprazolam	Intermediate	5–15	I + II	Very low concentration
Lorazepam	Intermediate	10–20	II only	None
Nitrazepam	Intermediate	24	I + II	30–90
Flurazepam	Rapid	2	I + II	36–120
Temazepam	Slow	10	II only	None
Zolpidem	Rapid	2	II only	None
Zaleplon	Rapid	1	II only	None
Zopiclone	Rapid	3–4	I + II	3–6

will have greater Cl) and by renal clearance. Table 5.3 shows the elimination half-lives of some common benzodiazepines.

The major metabolic factor is whether or not phase I hepatic metabolism produces active metabolites, which in general have a much longer $t_{1/2}$ than the parent drug. Table 5.3 indicates which undergo phase I metabolism and which only phase II metabolism. While some drugs in these two groups may have a similar $t_{1/2}$, it is clear that, with chronic dosing, the magnitude of effect is going to be greater for those producing active metabolites, which will gradually accumulate. In addition, maximum effects will take longer to achieve, development of tolerance to any effects will be obscured and effects will be slow to wane on cessation of the parent drug (which may protect against withdrawal symptoms).

Reference to particular uses and problems for some specific compounds may help to illustrate these points.

Lorazepam

Its relatively high water solubility makes lorazepam the most suitable benzodiazepine for parentral use. This property also results in low tissue distribution, a more sustained effect of a single dose and hence the drug's utility in the treatment of acute agitation, such as in psychotic illness. On the other hand, its relatively short $t_{1/2}$ may contribute to the difficulty in withdrawal after chronic use.

Alprazolam

The intermediate $t_{1/2}$ of this compound means that fairly regular dosing is necessary (at least three times per day) or else significant dips in plasma concentration will occur through the day.

Flurazepam

The parent drug has a short $t_{1/2}$ (2 hours), but phase I metabolism results in an active metabolite (desalkylflurazepam) with a long $t_{1/2}$ (36–120 hours). This slowly accumulates and may cause pronounced hangover effects.

Triazolam

This has a very short $t_{1/2}$, of between 2 and 5 hours, and no active metabolites. Thus, it should induce sleep and produce few hangover effects the following day.

Clorazepate

This is a pro-drug, being metabolised to desmethyldiazepam, which is what has clinical effects. The onset of these effects is therefore slow but will be prolonged because of the long $t_{1/2}$ of desmethyldiazepam.

Drug interactions

As mentioned above, the most important interaction is with alcohol, which potentiaties the CNS depression, resulting in greater sedation and psychomotor impairment. Fatality from overdose of a benzodiazepine most often occurs if it is combined with alcohol or other CNS depressant. In the case of diazepam this potentiation is also due in part to inhibition of hepatic clearance by alcohol, presumably competing for the same metabolic pathways.

Antacids of the magnesium/aluminium hydroxide type reduce the rate and extent of absorption. Drugs that induce hepatic enzymes, such as barbiturates, phenytoin, carbamazepine and rifampicin, may increase hepatic metabolism and reduce plasma concentrations. Chronic alcohol intake and nicotine (via cigarette smoking) may also increase metabolism. On the other hand, cimetidine and isoniazid may inhibit hepatic enzymes and cause elevated plasma concentrations by reducing metabolism.

Use during pregnancy

Benzodiazepines, like other drugs, are best avoided if possible during pregnancy. There have been reports of cleft lip and cleft palate occurring in association with benzodiazepine use in pregnancy but well-controlled studies are not available. A developmental dysmorphism specific to benzodiazepine use, similar to the foetal alcohol syndrome, was described in seven babies in Sweden (Laegreid et al, 1987). These cases arose from mothers who were taking large daily amounts of benzodiazepines and in three cases other drugs as well. Their alcohol intake was not reported. A subsequent examination of 104 000 pregnancies did not support a close association between benzodiazepines and teratogenic abnormalities (Bergman et al, 1992).

Benzodiazepines taken late in pregnancy or during labour may cause respiratory depression and feeding difficulties in the baby. If the mother has been taking moderate or high doses, then withdrawal symptoms may occur in the infant 2–3 weeks after birth.

Treatment of overdose

Deaths from benzodiazepine overdose alone are rare and patients have survived overdoses of up to 2 g. Management rests largely with gastric lavage (if the overdose is fairly recent) and appropriate supportive therapy. Respiration rate, pulse rate and blood pressure should be monitored. Dialysis is of limited value for most benzodiazepines because they are highly lipid soluble and have a large volume of distribution.

Flumazenil, an antagonist/partial inverse agonist at BDZ receptors, may be useful in reversing sedation following overdose. Side-effects from this may be anxiety, agitation, nausea and occasionally convulsions. The short elimination half-life of flumazenil, of 1–2 hours, means that patients must continue to be monitored until their plasma benzo-diazepine concentrations are likely to be below dangerous levels. Relapse towards coma can occur, necessitating a further dose.

Following recovery, patients should be warned about impairment of ability to drive or carry out other skilled tasks, which may continue for some weeks.

Sleep and hypnotics

Neurophysiology of sleep

Sleep is a recurring state of inactivity that is accompanied by decreased responsiveness to the environment and loss of awareness. It differs from coma by the ease with which a person may be roused to normal awareness and it differs from stupor, in that stupor is a disorder of motor function and not of consciousness.

Neurophysiological studies of sleep began in the 1930s and led to the identification of a number of distinct stages of sleep, which are associated with different physiological states. Many centrally acting drugs have effects on these sleep stages and interest has also focused on possible alteration of these in some psychiatric disorders, particularly depression.

Wakefulness is maintained by the activity of the ascending reticular activating system. However, the onset of sleep is not due to a decrease in activity of this system but to activity arising from other mid-brain centres, particularly the raphe nuclei and locus coeruleus. Before a person falls asleep there is generally a latency period of 10–20 minutes before the four stages of non-rapid eye movement (NREM) sleep begin

(Table 5.4). The development of sleep is marked by increasing amounts of slow-wave activity on the electroencephalogram (EEG). In stage II bursts of higher-frequency (12–14Hz) sleep spindles may be seen but also increasing amounts of the high-voltage, low-frequency complexes, known as K-complexes. Low-frequency activity increases through to stage IV NREM sleep, the first period of which is reached about 30–60 minutes after a person has fallen asleep. After 90 minutes the first period of rapid eye movement (REM) sleep appears and lasts for around 5–10 minutes, before a return to NREM sleep. Through the night, four to six cycles of NREM and REM sleep occur. As the night's sleep progresses, the length of the REM period increases to about 30 minutes and the amount of stage IV sleep in each cycle decreases. After sleep onset most people have a number of brief awakenings. Those reporting insomnia may be more aware of these than normal subjects, who are generally unaware of them.

Table 5.4 gives the overall percentage of total sleep time (TST) spent in each stage for young adults, who generally sleep for around 6½–8 hours a night. Neonates and young children sleep for longer and have a greater percentage of TST as stage IV and REM sleep. With increasing

Table 5.4 The stages of sleep

Stage (% TST)	EEG	Sleep state	Physiological state
I (5%)	Low amplitude, mixed frequency	Drowsy or shallow sleep	Slow, rolling eye movements
II (50%)	As stage I plus sleep spindles and K-complexes	Asleep	No eye movements Decreased muscle tone Decreased HR and RR
III (8%)	Moderate amount of high amplitude, slow frequency (< 2Hz)	Asleep (slow-wave sleep)	As stage II
IV (12%)	Large amount of high-amplitude, low-frequency activity	Asleep (slow-wave sleep)	As stage II
REM (25%)	Low-amplitude, mixed-frequency activity (like stage I)	Dreaming	Bursts of rapid eye movements Loss of muscle tone Increased cerebral blood flow HR, RR, BP very variable

TST, total sleep time; REM, rapid eye movement; BP, blood pressure; HR, heart rate; RR, respiratory rate.

159

age TST decreases and also the amount of stage IV sleep, so that in the elderly less than 5% of TST will be stage IV.

Effects of hypnotics on sleep

The initial effect of a hypnotic is to speed up the induction of sleep and to help maintain sleep. Drugs that are fairly rapidly absorbed will generally be preferable. High lipid solubility may enhance rapidity of action but may also result in extensive tissue distribution, which in turn may rapidly reduce plasma concentrations and result in a longer $t_{1/2}$. The ideal hypnotic should probably have an intermediate $t_{1/2}$ and no active metabolites. This will result in a fairly sustained effect through the night, without risk of a withdrawal effect during the night, but with a low risk of hangover effects the next day. Hypnotics with a long $t_{1/2}$ or that have metabolites with a long $t_{1/2}$ will slowly accumulate in the plasma and tissues. This results in a continuation of their effects through the daytime – the hangover effect.

Barbiturate and benzodiazepine hypnotics suppress both REM and stage IV sleep, although barbiturates do this to a much greater extent. Benzodiazepines mainly suppress REM sleep in the early part of the night. However, with chronic use tolerance develops to this effect, so that after 2 weeks of continuous use the total amount of REM sleep returns towards normal. This tolerance seems to reflect an adaptation and presumed enhancement of the neurochemical/neurophysiological processes driving sleep to cope with the drug effect. On withdrawal of the drug the now enhanced physiological drive to induce REM sleep is unmasked (having previously been inhibited by the drug). Thus a rebound increase above normal amounts of REM sleep occurs (Fig. 5.4). This increase in REM sleep results in increased dreaming, nightmares and nocturnal wakenings. It may take up to 5–6 weeks to see a return to the normal sleep pattern, a phenomenon first noted by Oswald & Priest (1965). This broken sleep pattern on hypnotic withdrawal can be reversed by recommencing the hypnotic and therefore encourages chronic use.

If tolerance develops to one effect of hypnotics, does it also develop to their principal effect of reducing insomnia? Some studies have suggested that this may be the case, but one follow-up of almost 100 patients, using subjective measures, suggested that effectiveness could be maintained for almost 6 months (Oswald *et al*, 1982).

Tolerance, dependence and withdrawal

Tolerance to benzodiazepine effects

The phenomenon of REM sleep rebound described above, following chronic hypnotic use, is one example of the development of tolerance followed by a withdrawal syndrome on cessation of the drug. Interest in

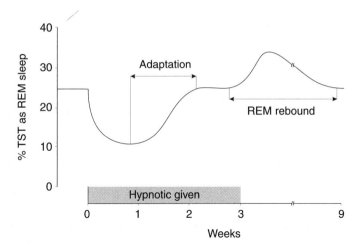

Fig. 5.4 The initial reduction in rapid-eye-movement (REM) sleep as a percentage of total sleep time (TST) following introduction of a benzodiazepine hypnotic. This is maximal around 5 days, after which adaptation or tolerance occurs to this effect. On cessation of the drug a rebound increase in the amount of REM sleep occurs, which may last for up to 6 weeks.

these phenomena has increased greatly since the recognition that a withdrawal syndrome may occur following cessation of benzodiazepines used for anxiolysis at standard doses. As yet, however, our understanding of these phenomena is incomplete. Tolerance to the effects of a drug may be defined as the need to use larger doses to achieve the same effects with repeated administration.

Such phenomena are often more easily studied in laboratory animals, for which conditions can be standardised much better than for humans. The acute sedative effects of benzodiazepines in animals can be measured by decreases in exploratory behaviour and general motor activity. Tolerance develops to these effects and also to the muscle relaxant, ataxic and anticonvulsant properties (File, 1985). Animal models of anxiety have also been used to investigate tolerance to anxiolytic effects. Tolerance has been demonstrated in some of these models and appears to develop more slowly than tolerance to the sedative and anticonvulsant effects.

In human studies, tolerance to the sedative, muscle relaxant and anticonvulsant properties of benzodiazepines has been demonstrated. Tolerance to the sedative effects may begin within a few days and be pronounced by 2–3 weeks. Tolerance to the anticonvulsant effects also occurs rapidly, so that while 'full agonist' benzodiazepines are useful in the acute treatment of epileptic seizures, they are of little benefit in long-term prophylaxis. Acute use of benzodiazepines results in increased fast-wave activity on the EEG, as well as effects on auditory

evoked responses, and tolerance also develops to these neurophysiological effects. Tolerance to their effects on psychomotor performance
may develop (Aranko *et al*, 1983) but is not demonstrated as consistently
as tolerance to the properties described above. Tolerance is usually
demonstrated by repeated testing during chronic dosing. It can also
be demonstrated using a standardised single-dose challenge of, say,
diazepam before and during chronic dosing with another benzodiazepine. These methods were used together by Higgitt *et al* (1988),
who found similar results with both.

Very rapid development of tolerance (tachyphylaxis) may sometimes
occur to a drug effect. This has been demonstrated for the sedative
effects of benzodiazepines in some individuals in whom tolerance to
the physiological effects begins to become evident while plasma
concentrations are still rising after a single dose. If the degree of
physiological effect (e.g. sedation) is plotted against benzodiazepine
plasma concentration following a single dose, the result is a graph
described as a clockwise hysteresis curve (Fig. 5.5).

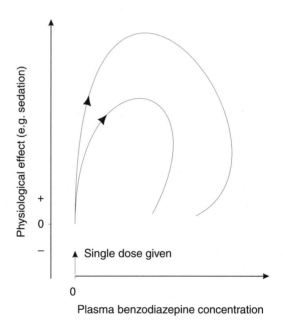

Fig. 5.5 These clockwise hysteresis curves demonstrate the development of tolerance
to the effects of two different doses of a benzodiazepine even as the plasma level
continues to increase following a single dose. Note: these are plots of effect versus
concentration, not time.

Whether or not tolerance develops to the desirable anxiolytic and hypnotic effects of benzodiazepines is less certain. Certainly these effects seem more resistant to tolerance. Some studies report continuing benefits for anxiolysis and hypnotic effects for up to 6 months (Oswald et al, 1982; Rickels et al, 1983). However, others report a group of patients who tend to increase their daily usage over time (Busto et al, 1986) and who presumably have developed tolerance to their initial daily dose. Re-emergence of anxiety symptoms has also been reported during chronic use. While these findings may have alternative explanations, the development of tolerance to the therapeutic effects of benzodiazepines almost certainly occurs in some patients and probably occurs to some degree in many.

Cross-tolerance occurs between benzodiazepines, that is, the tolerance found to the effects of one benzodiazepine during chronic dosing will also be found to the effects of others. There is also cross-tolerance with barbiturates and alcohol, which probably occurs because of the proximity of their sites of action at the $GABA_A$–BDZ receptor complex.

The fact that tolerance develops more readily to some effects than to others (sedation > psychomotor/amnestic effects > anxiolysis) may relate to the different tissue concentrations required to achieve these effects or may be due to the presence of different receptor subtypes. It is still to be determined whether some subtypes may be more prone to the development of tolerance than others. Tolerance to some effects has been suggested to persist for up to 4 months after cessation of the benzodiazepine (Higgitt et al, 1988). This was demonstrated by the use of diazepam challenge following withdrawal. It seems unlikely that this is entirely due to receptor effects and cognitive factors may be important.

Three principal mechanisms may underlie the development of tolerance.

(1) Pharmacokinetic factors may result in induction of metabolism or the production of less active metabolites that compete for the receptor sites. However, these do not appear to be of importance for the benzodiazepines. Enzyme induction is important in the development of tolerance to barbiturates and alcohol but does not appear to occur with normal doses of benzodiazepines.

(2) Pharmacodynamic factors may cause alterations at the receptor sites which affect sensitivity to the drug. This is probably the most important mechanism for the development of tolerance to benzodiazepines. So far there is evidence of two processes through which this may occur: reduction in BDZ receptor number and/or sensitivity with chronic treatment; and uncoupling of the links between the BDZ and the $GABA_A$ receptors.

(3) Cognitive theories suggest that adaptation to the effects of drugs may be seen as the organism learning new responses in order to

restore pre-drug levels of reinforcement. Such mechanisms have not been extensively examined in humans but some recent work suggests that pharmacodynamic factors cannot explain all aspects of tolerance and that cognitive factors may explain many of the remaining aspects (Higgitt *et al*, 1988).

Benzodiazepine dependence and withdrawal

Physiological (or physical) dependence on a drug is generally secondary to the development of tolerance. The adaptive changes that occur during the development of tolerance are left unopposed if the drug is stopped. This then results in a rebound hyperexcitability in the system affected by the drug: a withdrawal syndrome occurs. The withdrawal syndrome can be suppressed by recommencing intake of the drug and hence encourages chronic use and dependence. REM sleep rebound on cessation of hypnotics provides the classic model of benzodiazepine withdrawal.

Withdrawal syndromes often appear only after excessive use of a substance, as with alcohol, and this was thought to be the situation with anxiolytic benzodiazepines. However, in 1981 a withdrawal syndrome following normal therapeutic doses was described (Petursson & Lader, 1981) and has been confirmed by subsequent investigations. The syndrome consists of typical somatic and psychological symptoms of anxiety as well as other symptoms less prominent in anxiety (Table 5.5). Of particular note are symptoms of abnormal sensory perception, such as hyperacusis, paraesthesiae, photophobia and hypersensitivity to touch and pain, and also other somatic symptoms, such as muscle stiffness or twitching. A symptom peculiar to benzodiazepine withdrawal is a sensation of abnormal body sway. More unequivocal symptoms of a physical withdrawal syndrome, such as epileptic seizures, confusional states and hallucinations, may occur but are noted in less than 5% of cases.

Table 5.5 Benzodiazepine withdrawal symptoms

Anxiety symptoms	Disturbance of perception	Severe but rare effects
Anxiety	Hypersensitivity to stimuli	Paranoid psychosis
Dysphoria	Abnormal bodily sensations	Depressive episode
Tremor	Abnormal sense of movement/	Seizures
Muscle pains	body sway	Confusion
Sleep disturbance	Depersonalisation	Hallucinations
Headache	Visual disturbance	
Nausea, anorexia		
Sweating		
Fatigue		

Symptoms of the withdrawal syndrome may be similar to the patient's original anxiety symptoms for which treatment was prescribed. Indeed, its existence was initially controversial, as some believed it was only re-emergence of pre-existing anxiety or some form of rebound anxiety. The occurrence of additional features, as described above, may help in diagnosis, as may continued observation of the patient: a typical withdrawal syndrome will lead to a rebound increase in anxiety above the pre-treatment level with a gradual return towards lower levels over a period of some weeks.

Estimates of the incidence of a withdrawal syndrome following long-term use of benzodiazepines (usually longer than 6 months) vary from 0% to 100%, which reflects different attitudes to the nature of the syndrome. The best estimate is 45% of patients after 6 months (Tyrer *et al*, 1981, 1983). Symptoms usually emerge during the first week of discontinuation, but may also occur following dosage reduction, and persist for 7–10 days. Claims of persistence of symptoms for 6 months or more are likely to be on the basis of re-emergence of anxiety or psychological dependence, rather than any known pharmacological mechanism. That psychological factors are important was demonstrated by Tyrer *et al* (1983), who found that 22% of patients in one study of withdrawal experienced withdrawal symptoms at a stage when their benzodiazepine dose was unchanged, although they thought it had been decreased. The same group also reported that passive and dependent personalities were more likely to develop symptoms (see Chapter 4). Symptoms also appear more commonly following discontinuation of benzodiazepines of short half-life, owing largely to the more rapid fall in plasma concentrations. While most studies have concentrated on long-term users, there is evidence of rebound anxiety and withdrawal symptoms after only 6 weeks of treatment at moderate doses (Power *et al*, 1985).

Management of withdrawal

The majority of patients on long-term benzodiazepines can be withdrawn as out-patients unless there were seizures or psychotic episodes during previous attempts. Those on drugs with a short half-life (e.g. lorazepam) should be changed to one with a long half-life (e.g. diazepam), from which withdrawal syndromes are usually less severe. A process of gradual dose reduction or tapering is preferable to abrupt cessation. Usually 4–16 weeks are required, depending on the initial dose. Dosage should be reduced in steps at either weekly or fortnightly intervals. Suggested steps are either a 25% reduction in daily dose or a reduction in daily dose of 2 mg of diazepam or its equivalent. Regimens should not be rigid and tapering should occur at a rate appropriate to the level of withdrawal symptoms.

A variety of drugs have been tried in attempts to attenuate withdrawal symptoms. Propranolol attenuates some features but does not decrease the frequency of withdrawal symptoms or improve outcome (Tyrer et al, 1981). Initial reports suggested that clonidine reduced withdrawal severity but placebo-controlled trials found no benefit. Similarly buspirone also appears to be ineffective. A recent placebo-controlled trial of carbamazepine found a trend towards reduced severity of symptoms and a significant facilitation of ability to attain complete withdrawal for the carbamazepine-treated group (Schweizer et al, 1991).

Education of the patient and regular psychological support during withdrawal are necessary (Higgitt et al, 1985). Anxiety management training and relaxation therapy are also helpful, probably largely for those patients with chronic anxiety problems. Group therapy seems to have little effect. Some patients may develop a depressive episode during withdrawal and this may require treatment with an antidepressant drug. However, antidepressant drugs do not seem to be useful in assisting withdrawal per se (Tyrer et al, 1996).

Reports of long-term outcome following withdrawal tend to come from specialist centres and may not be applicable to the many patients who discontinue by themselves or with the help of their general practitioner. About 50–60% of those entering a formal withdrawal programme will attain a benzodiazepine-free period of around 3–5 weeks. Follow-up over 3–5 years suggests that around one-third will recommence and continue to take benzodiazepines; another third will recommence for a few weeks but stop again; one-sixth will be on other psychotropic drugs; and only one-sixth are likely not to have required any further psychotropic drugs (Higgitt et al, 1985; Holton & Tyrer, 1990; Rickels et al, 1983). Many patients on follow-up continue to report anxiety symptoms, so the poor outcome probably reflects the chronic nature of the symptoms experienced by many of the patients treated with benzodiazepines.

Use of benzodiazepines

Indications

Anxiety

Anxiety may arise as an acute response to stress in many people. In such instances it is usually short-lived and can be managed by psychological support in primary care. Benzodiazepines are rarely required unless symptoms are severe. Their main use is in the management of patients presenting with the features of generalised anxiety disorder. This tends to be a fluctuating condition, with exacerbations at times of stress and increased life events, and often more chronic, milder symptoms between exacerbations. High levels of somatic and psychic symptoms of anxiety as well as a clearly identified stressor and short duration of symptoms predict a favourable response. Depressive, phobic and hypochondriacal symptoms tend to predict poor response. As with many disorders, chronicity as well as anxious/dependent personality traits are unfavourable factors.

Treatment should be for short periods, ideally less than 4 weeks. The dose should be tailored to the severity of the symptoms and any likely pharmacokinetic variables. It is interesting to note that in some situtations 2 mg diazepam taken three times daily was no more effective than placebo (e.g. Cooper *et al*, 1991). This study compared the effects of a new, potential anxiolytic compound with diazepam and placebo but had used a low dose of diazepam because of concerns about dependence.

Other neuroses

Patients presenting with symptoms of panic or agoraphobia (or both) are often slow to respond to treatment, and so are likely to require several months' treatment. Clearly, this is undesirable, as dependence on a benzodiazepine may develop. Imipramine or a selective serotonin reuptake inhibitor (SSRI) is now often considered the treatment of choice for panic disorder. Alprazolam, a high-potency benzodiazepine, has been put forward as having potent anti-panic effects, but the supporting data have been criticised. Low-potency benzodiazepines, such as diazepam, show benefit for panic patients only at high doses.

The subdivision of anxiety disorders found in DSM–IV and ICD–10 is, to a large extent, due to the emphasis on the symptom of panic and the differential responses of certain symptom groups to particular treatments, both pharmacological and non-pharmacological. Tyrer (1985) has argued that this may be a false division because of flaws in the argument for pharmacological subclassification and lack of stability of many symptoms over time. He favours the use of an overall diagnosis of general neurotic syndrome. This, however, does not negate the findings that certain types of symptoms or symptom clusters may respond well to benzodiazepines and others not.

However, it is also of note that attempts to separate anxiety neurosis from depressive neurosis often fail (Kendell, 1974; Johnstone *et al*, 1980). Furthermore, treatment response does not appear to differ and neurotic symptoms in general seem to respond better to tricyclic antidepressants than to benzodiazepines (Johnstone *et al*, 1980; Tyrer *et al*, 1988). Patients with more clear-cut depressive illness do not benefit from benzodiazepines and those with prominent anxiety symptoms may respond better to a monoamine oxidase inhibitor than to a tricyclic antidepressant (Paykel, 1988).

In the management of simple phobias, benzodiazepines may be a useful short-term adjunct to behaviour therapy. They are of little benefit in the treatment of obsessive–compulsive disorder.

Insomnia

In the management of insomnia, benzodiazepines are best reserved for short-term sleep disturbances, for example during acute stress, after surgery or during recovering from jet-lag. Ideally they should be prescribed only for a few nights.

Patients presenting with chronic insomnia require adequate assessment and diagnosis. If possible, treatment should be of the primary cause (e.g. depressive illness, alcohol dependence, overuse of caffeine or other stimulants) or explanation of the problem (e.g. reduced need for sleep with increasing age). If insomnia is severe or very distressing, a benzodiazepine hypnotic may be tried for a short period, but preferably no longer than 4 weeks.

Alcohol withdrawal

For patients in a state of alcohol withdrawal, benzodiazepines may be prescribed to reduce withdrawal symptoms and to prevent epileptic seizures; those with a long elimination half-life, such as diazepam or chlordiazepoxide, are best. The initial dose should be adequate to abolish most of the symptoms, usually in the region of 20–40 mg per day of diazepam, or its equivalent. This dose should be reduced to zero over 5–10 days, depending on the severity of the alcohol addiction.

Psychosis

In acute psychotic states high-dose treatment, usually with a potent drug such as lorazepam, has been found useful in reducing severe agitation. This should be for only a few days, as tolerance will develop to this effect. However, benzodiazepines are not universally useful for agitation. For example, with 'agitated' depression antipsychotic drugs are preferable. Benzodiazepines should also be avoided in anxious or agitated individuals with personality disorders. Aggressive or suicidal behaviour may be released, in a similar manner to the effects of alcohol.

Guidelines for the use of benzodiazepines

Concern about benzodiazepine dependence grew during the 1980s and prompted the Committee on Safety of Medicines (CSM) and the Royal College of Psychiatrists to publish recommendations on their use. The CSM statement is reproduced in the *British National Formulary*, at the beginning of the section on benzodiazepines, and the College statement was published in the *Psychiatric Bulletin* (Priest & Montgomery, 1988); further guidance was produced by the Royal College of Psychiatrists (1997). These essentially recommend that benzodiazepines should not be used for more than 2–4 weeks at a time and only when symptoms of anxiety or insomnia are severe. When prescribed for insomnia they recommend intermittent rather than continuous use.

Benzodiazepine prescribing patterns

The figures discussed here refer to numbers of prescription items dispensed in England and Wales. In 1960, before benzodiazepines became widely used, around 27 million items were dispensed that could be classified as hypnotics or tranquillisers. Over 15 million of these were barbiturate hypnotics, the remainder other non-benzodiazepine drugs. In 1974 a total of 40 million items of this nature were dispensed, of which 25 million were benzodiazepines and 8 million barbiturates. The peak of benzodiazepine prescribing was reached in 1979, when 31 million prescriptions were dispensed. However, as concern rose about dependence and the overall level of prescribing, there was a steady reduction. In 1985 only 21 million prescriptions were dispensed and in 1990 only 16 million.

The reduction in prescribing is accounted for largely by the fall in prescriptions for benzodiazepine tranquillisers, the numbers of prescriptions for hypnotics remaining fairly constant, at 10–12 million. The figures for hypnotic prescribing suggest there has been increased use of preparations of shorter half-life (such as temazepam) and reduced use of preparations of longer half-life (such as nitrazepam).

Women consume approximately 70% of the benzodiazepines dispensed in the UK, a proportion largely mirrored throughout the world. One study, during the period of peak use, found that during one year 16% of women and 7% of men in one group of general practices were prescribed a benzodiazepine at least once during one year (Skegg *et al*, 1977). Prescribing rises with age, a trend most marked for the hypnotics. Women over the age of 40 years receive around 60% of all benzodiazepines prescribed in the UK. However, for benzodiazepine hypnotics women over 65 years receive about 40% of the UK total and women aged 40–65 years about 25% of the total. The Health and Lifestyle Survey of 1986, in which a representative sample of 9003 UK adults were interviewed, found that, on the day of interview, 4.2% of females and 2.1% of males were currently taking tranquillisers or hypnotics. Of those receiving benzodiazepines in any given year, approximately 25% will have been taking them for one year or more, or, looked at another way, between 1% and 2% of the population may be receiving long-term benzodiazepine treatment.

Studies of long-term users in both the UK and the USA indicate that they have considerable underlying psychological morbidity, with around one-third reaching a criterion for psychiatric 'caseness'. Despite the lack of major antidepressant efficacy for benzodiazepines, depressive disorders appear to dominate these 'cases' (Rodrigo *et al*, 1988). At the same time it should be noted that 30–40% of general practice attenders reach similar criteria for psychiatric 'caseness'. Physical morbidity is even more common, with a third to a half of long-term users having significant physical symptoms or disability. Musculosketetal and cardiovascular disorders seem to predominate. This is perhaps not surprising, as initial use of a benzodiazepine is often in response to insomnia or anxiety in the context of a physical illness.

Predictors of long-term use by patients first prescribed a benzo-diazepine are:

(1) history of previous psychotropic drug use
(2) being female
(3) having significant social problems
(4) length of time on the benzodiazepine (i.e. the greater the duration of treatment, the less likelihood there is of stopping it).

Long-term users themselves generally report the main benefits to be on social functioning, but at the same time would prefer not to have to take any medication.

Alternatives to benzodiazepines

Beta-adrenoceptor antagonists

Clinical trials of propranolol in anxiety followed observations by Turner and colleagues in 1965 on its haemodynamic effects in patients with anxiety associated with thyrotoxicosis. Propranolol has been the principal β-adrenoceptor antagonist tested for efficacy in anxiety, although studies have also been carried out with oxprenolol, atenolol, sotalol and acebutolol.

The first placebo-controlled study in anxiety neurosis used a double-blind, cross-over design with trend analysis (Granville-Grossman & Turner, 1966). Statistically significant benefit for propranolol became evident after 15 patients had completed the pair of treatments. Subsequent similar studies found benefit for practolol versus placebo but no benefit for D-propranolol versus placebo. These results suggested that the benefits arise from peripheral β-adrenoceptor antagonism. (D-propranolol has no effect at β-receptors and practolol does not cross the blood–brain barrier.)

Many, although not all, subsequent clinical trials in anxiety neurosis have demonstrated the effectiveness of β-adrenoceptor antagonists compared with placebo but differ as to whether they are most effective for the 'somatic' or 'psychic' symptoms of anxiety. The fact that they reduce tachycardia and the finding in one study of a relationship between a fall in heart rate and therapeutic response (Hallstrom et al, 1981) suggest that it is their effect on somatic symptoms that is most important. However, if we consider physiological theories of anxiety, such as those of James and Lange or Cannon, then it is clear that physiological and psychic responses are linked (although in different directions in these two theories). Aggravation of physiological symptoms may increase psychic discomfort, and reduction of physiological symptoms may enhance improvement in psychic symptoms. Propranolol is an antagonist at both β_1- and β_2-adrenoceptors. Recent investigations of a specific β_2 antagonist found no advantage for it over placebo in anxiety neurosis, which suggests that the beneficial effects of β-adrenoceptor antagonism are due mainly to β_1 antagonism. This is consistent with the evidence that clinical response does not occur without a drop in heart rate, which is a β_1 effect.

The most clearly demonstrated use for β-adrenoceptor antagonists has been in situational anxiety, for example 'stage-fright' in musicians (James et al, 1977). In such situations both β_1 and β_2 antagonism may be relevant. Studies of panic disorder have found little consistent evidence for benefit from these drugs.

Propranolol has also been found to attenuate the symptoms of withdrawal from benzodiazepines. This interesting finding should lead us to re-examine the data on the efficacy of β-adrenoceptor antagonists in anxiety. A review of 19 published studies in which these drugs appeared to be more effective than placebo in the treatment of anxiety neurosis reveals little data regarding the patients' drug treatment before entry to these clinical trials. Many subjects appear to have been previously treated with a benzodiazepine and to have been withdrawn before the start of the study, but in only one study is it clear that there was a drug-free period of more than 2 weeks. Four studies used a crossover design that included a period on diazepam. Previous studies may therefore, in part, have been assessing the effects of β-adrenoceptor antagonists on benzodiazepine withdrawal as well as anxiety neurosis.

Propranolol is usually begun as a single 20 mg dose, to ensure that the patient does not have undue cardiovascular sensitivity to it. After this, doses in the region of 40–160 mg per day are usually required, dose titration depending on clinical response. Above 160 mg per day little additional β-adrenoceptor blockade can generally be obtained. A common practice is often to use a slow-release preparation that needs to be taken only once per day. If used for an elderly patient, then care is required, as the principal route of excretion is renal.

Side-effects include hypotension, feelings of lethargy, impaired concentration and sleep disturbance. Occasionally nightmares and depression of mood have been recorded. The use of less lipid-soluble compounds, such as atenolol, may help to minimise such central effects. If the patient has asthma or cardiac failure, these drugs are best avoided.

Buspirone

Buspirone is an azaspirodecanedione which acts principally as a partial agonist at 5-HT$_{1A}$ receptors. It does not have affinity for BDZ receptors and does not appear to exert any direct effects on GABA activity. The initial effect of buspirone is to reduce serotonin release because of its agonist effect at the cell body 5-HT$_{1A}$ receptors in the raphe. This effect is partly counterbalanced in the short term by agonism at the post-synaptic 5-HT$_{1A}$ receptors. However, treatment over 2 weeks results in a return to the normal level of serotonin release, which, combined with the postsynaptic agonism, may be responsible for the anxiolytic effect.

Buspirone is also an antagonist at presynaptic dopamine receptors but does not antagonise postsynaptic dopamine receptors. Nevertheless, it can cause increased prolactin secretion and other effects similar to those caused by postsynaptic dopamine receptor antagonism. However, these effects could also be due to direct or secondary consequences of its 5-HT$_{1A}$ agonist property. It does not have direct effects on either α- or β-adrenoceptors.

Buspirone is rapidly absorbed from the gut, reaching peak plasma concentrations within 1 hour. It undergoes fairly extensive 'first-pass' metabolism (see Chapter 3). Plasma concentrations are higher if it is taken with food. One of the principal metabolites, 1-pyramidinyl-piperazine (1-PP), is active and is an α_2-adrenoceptor antagonist. It may contribute to the effects of buspirone. The elimination half-life is short, around 3 hours, so dosing should be three times daily to maintain reasonable plasma concentrations. A slow-release form has an elimination half-life of 9 hours. The starting dose is usually 5 mg two or three times daily; this may be increased initially up to 30 mg per day, in divided doses. If therapeutic benefit is still not apparent, then doses may be increased to 45 mg per day.

The principal adverse effects are nausea, gastrointestinal upset, headache and sometimes dizziness. In contrast to the benzodiazepines, buspirone produces little or no sedation, does not interact with alcohol at therapeutic doses and does not appear to have significant adverse effects on pyschomotor performance or memory. Evidence to date suggests that pharmacological dependence does not occur. Buspirone should not be prescribed in combination with monoamine oxidase inhibitors, because a hypertensive crisis could occur. No significant clinical interactions with tricyclic antidepressants or antipsychotics have been reported. However, buspirone does have pro-convulsant effects and this may indicate a need for care in its use with other psychotropic drugs; it is of course also a contraindication to its use for patients with epilepsy.

The anxiolytic effect of buspirone has a slow onset and may take 3 weeks or more to develop. Some reports suggest it may be less effective than diazepam, but this may in part be a reflection of the slower onset of effect and in part be linked with the evidence that patients previously treated with benzodiazepines seem to respond less well to buspirone. Clinical trials suggest its effectiveness for generalised anxiety disorder.

There is no consistent evidence for benefits with other forms of anxiety disorder.

The delay in onset of action may limit its usefulness for patients with severe, acute anxiety, which often follows stress, who may need short-term, rapid relief. On the other hand, for patients with more chronic anxiety it may provide another approach to treatment.

Zolpidem and zaleplon

Zolpidem is an imidazopyridine and zaleplon a pyrazolopyrimidine. These compounds are not benzodiazepines but they act at the BDZ type 1 receptor. Indeed, they have high affinity for receptors containing α-1 subunits but little or no affinity for other types of $GABA_A$–BDZ receptor. They have quite potent hypnotic effects, similar to those of benzodiazepine hypnotics, but they appear to produce less psychomotor impairment and have relatively weak anxiolytic effects. There seems to be a very low risk of tolerance and dependence with these compounds.

Both are rapidly absorbed. The elimination half-life of zolpidem is 2 hours and the main adverse effects are headache, nausea, dizziness and occasionally diplopia. The usual dose is 5–10 mg. The elimination half-life of zaleplon is 1 hour and thus it can be used to assist return to sleep, after waking during the night, with reduced risk of hangover effects the next day. The main adverse effect reported is headache but dizziness may also occur. The usual dose is 5–10 mg.

Zopiclone

Zopiclone is a cyclopyrrolone compound. Although it is not a benzo-diazepine, it does bind to the $GABA_A$–BDZ receptor complex, but at a different site from the benzodiazepines. It is rapidly absorbed and the elimination half-life is 3–4 hours. The usual dose is 3.75–7.5 mg. Adverse effects include headache, nausea and dizziness. Psychomotor impairment may occur, although to a lesser degree than with benzo-diazepines. However, in a study of road traffic accidents there was evidence of a relationship with use of zopiclone (Barbone *et al*, 1998).

Unfortunately, tolerance to its effects does occur. Rebound insomnia has been noted in healthy volunteers on withdrawal after 3 weeks of continuous use. There are also case reports that suggest that dependence may occur.

Antidepressant drugs

The pharmacology of these drugs is covered in detail in Chapter 6. They are quite often used in the management of anxiety disorders as well as depressive disorders. Although many diagnostic systems separate anxiety states from neurotic depression, not all studies are able to

Table 5.6 Licensed indications for the use of selective serotonin reuptake inhibitors (SSRIs) in anxiety

SSRI	GAD	OCD	PD	SP	PTSD	Mixed
Citalopram			X			
Fluoxetine		X				X
Fluvoxamine		X				
Paroxetine	X	X	X	X	X	X
Sertraline		X			X (F)	X

(F), females only; GAD, generalised anxiety disorder; OCD, obsessive–compulsive disorder; PD, panic disorder; SP, social phobia; PTSD, post-traumatic stress disorder; mixed, mixed anxiety/depression.

separate them and many patients are not able to discriminate anxiety from depression (as discussed under 'Use of benzodiazepines', above). Two large clinical trials have compared the effects of diazepam, a tricyclic antidepressant and placebo in a group of patients, some of whom suffered from neurotic depression and some of whom had anxiety disorders (Johnstone *et al*, 1980; Tyrer *et al*, 1988). While both studies found both drugs to be beneficial, overall the results demonstrated a slightly greater benefit from the antidepressant than from diazepam, including superiority of the antidepressant for symptoms of anxiety. Using current ICD–10 definitions, these patients would probably have been considered to be suffering from generalised anxiety disorder (GAD), mixed anxiety–depression and mild depressive disorder.

Clomipramine has been shown to be effective in obsessive–compulsive disorder and clomipramine and imipramine have been found beneficial in panic disorder. Venlafaxine has demonstrated effectiveness for generalised anxiety disorder and mixed anxiety–depressive disorder.

The SSRIs have been extensively studied and found effective for a variety of anxiety disorders. Their efficacy probably relates to their effects on the serotonin system. Table 5.6 shows the indications for which product licences exist in the UK (as of December 2001). It should be remembered that during the first 2 weeks of treatment of panic disorder with an SSRI the panic symptoms may worsen and patients should be warned of this. Many now regard the SSRIs as the treatment of first choice for generalised anxiety disorder, post-traumatic stress disorder and social phobia.

Other approaches

Antipsychotic drugs

Low-dose antipsychotic drugs, particularly thioridazine and chlorpromazine, have been widely used in the management of anxiety. There is not a good evidence base for this, as most clinical trials have been too small or have lacked a placebo control. These drugs are considered to be effective for psychomotor agitation in association with severe depressive disorder. It is important to remember that their long-term use may lead to the development of tardive dyskinesia and that thioridazine now carries restrictions to its use.

New GABA$_A$–BDZ complex ligands

The traditional benzodiazepines are all full agonists at the BDZ receptor. Partial agonists at this receptor are less potent in their induction of sedation, interaction with alcohol and liability to induce physical dependence. Clonazepam is one such drug. Its efficacy as an anticonvulsant is lower than that of diazepam but tolerance to the anticonvulsant effect is much less likely to occur. Although it is not useful as an anxiolytic or hypnotic, these differences help to illustrate the points made earlier about the possibility of developing new drugs that have more selective effects. There is evidence that drugs targeting GABA$_A$–BDZ receptor complexes containing the α_2-subunit, but not those with the α_1-subunit, may have anxiolytic effects but reduced sedative effects. A number of more selective compounds are at various stages of drug development.

Kava kava

Kava kava comes from the root of a plant grown on some Pacific islands. It has been used there for many generations as an anxiolytic and is now in clinical trials. Recently, however, a small number of patients in these studies have developed liver toxicity and caution is now recommended in its use.

Cholecystokinin (CCK) and other peptides

Infusion of CCK$_4$, an agonist at CCK$_B$ receptors, induces panic and CCK$_B$ receptor antagonists have been found to be anxiolytic in some animal models of anxiety. However, CCK antagonists have not proved efficacious in clinical trials, and bioavailability with oral dosing is a problem that may limit their use.

Corticotrophin-releasing factor (CRF) can be anxiogenic, and CRF$_1$ antagonists are being tested for anxiolytic activity. Neurokinin (substance P) can be anxiogenic in laboratory animals and an antagonist has shown anxiolytic activity in some animal models of anxiety.

Acknowledgements

I would like to acknowledge the help of Dr P. Leech, Department of Health, London, who provided some of the statistics on prescribing.

References

Aranko, K., Mattila, M. J. & Seppala, T. (1983) Development of tolerance and cross-tolerance to the psychomotor actions of lorazepam and diazepam in man. *British Journal of Clinical Pharmacology*, **15**, 545–552.

Barbone, F., McMahon, A. D., Davey, P. G., *et al* (1998) Association of road-traffic accidents with benzodiazepine use. *Lancet*, **352**, 1331–1336.

Bergman, U., Rosa, F. W., Baum, C., *et al* (1992) Effects of exposure to benzodiazepine during fetal life. *Lancet*, **ii**, 694–696.

Busto, U., Sellers, E. M., Naranjo, C. A., *et al* (1986) Withdrawal reaction after long term therapeutic use of benzodiazepines. *New England Journal of Medicine*, **315**, 854–859.

Cooper, S. J., Gilliland, A., Kelly, C. B., *et al* (1991) A comparison of a β_2-adrenoceptor antagonist (ICI 118,551), diazepam and placebo in the treatment of acute anxiety. *Journal of Psychopharmacology*, **5**, 155–159.

Covi, L., Lipman, R. S., Pattison, J. H., *et al* (1973) Length of treatment with anxiolytic sedatives and response to their sudden withdrawal. *Acta Psychiatrica Scandinavica*, **49**, 51–64.

Deakin, J. F. W. & Graeff, F. G. (1991) 5-HT and mechanisms of defence. *Journal of Psychopharmacology*, **5**, 305–315.

File, S. E. (1985) Tolerance to the behavioural actions of benzodiazepines. *Neuroscience and Behavioural Reviews*, **9**, 113–121.

Granville-Grossman, K. L. & Turner, P. (1966) The effects of propranolol on anxiety. *Lancet*, **i**, 788–790.

Hallstrom, C., Treasaden, I., Edwards, J. G., *et al* (1981) Diazepam, propranolol and their combination in the management of chronic anxiety. *British Journal of Psychiatry*, **139**, 417–421.

Hawton, K. & Fagg, J. (1992) Trends in deliberate self-poisoning and self-injury in Oxford, 1976–90. *BMJ*, **304**, 1409–1411.

Higgitt, A., Lader, M. H. & Fonaghy, P. (1985) Clinical management of benzodiazepine dependence. *BMJ*, **291**, 688–690.

Higgitt, A., Fonaghy, P. & Lader, M. H. (1988) The natural history of tolerance to the benzodiazepines. *Psychological Medicine* (monograph suppl. 13), 1–55.

Hindmarch, I. (1980) Psychomotor function and psychoactive drugs. *British Journal of Clinical Pharmacology*, **10**, 189–210.

Hollister, L. E., Motzenbecker, F. P. & Degan, R. O. (1961) Withdrawal reactions from chlordiazepoxide ('Librium'). *Psychopharmacologia*, **2**, 63–68.

Holton, A. & Tyrer, P. (1990) Five year outcome in patients withdrawn from long term treatment with diazepam. *BMJ*, **300**, 1241–1242.

James, I. M., Pearson, R. M., Griffith, D. N. W., *et al* (1977) Effect of oxprenolol on stage-fright in musicians. *Lancet*, **ii**, 952–954.

Johnstone, E. C., Owens, D. G. C., Frith, C. D., *et al* (1980) Neurotic illness and its response to anxiolytic and antidepressant treatment. *Psychological Medicine*, **10**, 321–328.

Kaufman, D. W., Shapiro, S., Slone, D., *et al* (1982) Diazepam and the risk of breast cancer. *Lancet*, **i**, 537–539.

Kendell, R. E. (1974) The stability of psychiatric diagnosis. *British Journal of Psychiatry*, **124**, 352–356.

King, D. J. (1992) Benzodiazepines, amnesia and sedation: theoretical and clinical issues and controversies. *Human Psychopharmacology*, **7**, 79–87.

Laegreid, L., Olegard, R., Wahlstrom, J., *et al* (1987) Abnormalities in children exposed to benzodiazepines in utero. *Lancet*, **i**, 108–109.

Oswald, I. & Priest, R. G. (1965) Five weeks to escape the sleeping pill habit. *BMJ*, **ii**, 1093–1095.

Laegreid, L., French, C., Adam, K., *et al* (1982) Benzodiazepine hypnotics remain effective for 24 weeks. *BMJ*, **i**, 860–863.

Paykel, E. S. (1988) Antidepressants: their efficacy and place in therapy. *Journal of Psychopharmacology*, **2**, 105–118.

Petursson, H. & Lader, M. H. (1981) Withdrawal from long term benzodiazepine treatment. *BMJ*, **283**, 643–645.

Power, K. G., Jerrom, D. W. A., Simpson, R. J., *et al* (1985) Controlled study of withdrawal symptoms and rebound anxiety after six week course of diazepam for generalised anxiety. *BMJ*, **290**, 1246–1248.

Preston, G. G., Ward, C. E., Broks, P., *et al* (1989) Effects of lorazapam on memory, attention and sedation in man: antagonism by Ro 15-1788. *Psychopharmacology*, **97**, 222–227.

Priest, R. G. & Montgomery, S. A. (1988) Benzodiazepines and dependence: a College statement. *Psychiatric Bulletin*, **12**, 107–108.

Rickels, K., Case, W. G., Downing, R. W., *et al* (1983) Long-term diazepam therapy and clinical outcome. *JAMA*, **250**, 767–771.

Rodrigo, E. K., King, M. B. & Williams, P. (1988) Health of long term benzodiazepine users. *BMJ*, **296**, 603–606.

Royal College of Psychiatrists (1997) *Benzodiazepines: Risks, Benefits or Dependence. A Re-evaluation* (Council Report, CR 59). London: Royal College of Psychiatrists.

Rudolph, U., Crestani, F. & Möher, H. (2001) GABA$_A$ receptor subtypes: dissecting their pharmacological functions. *Trends in Pharmacological Sciences*, **22**, 188–194.

Schweizer, E., Rickels, K., Case, W. G., *et al* (1991) Carbamazepine treatment in patients discontinuing longterm benzodiazepine therapy. *Archives of General Psychiatry*, **48**, 448–452.

Skegg, D. C. G., Doll, R. & Perry, J. (1977) Use of medicines in general practice. *BMJ*, **i**, 1561–1563.

Tyrer, P. (1985) Neurosis divisible? *Lancet*, **i**, 685–688.

Tyrer, P., Owen, R. & Dawling, S. (1983) Gradual withdrawal of diazepam after long-term therapy. *Lancet*, **i**, 1402–1406.

Tyrer, P., Rutherford, D. & Huggett, T. (1981) Benzodiazepine withdrawal symptoms and propranolol. *Lancet*, **i**, 520–522.

Tyrer, P., Seivewright, N., Murphy, S., *et al* (1988) The Nottingham study of neurotic disorder: comparison of drug and psychological treatments. *Lancet*, **ii**, 235–240.

Tyrer, P., Ferguson, B., Hallstrom, C., *et al* (1996) A controlled trial of dothiepin and placebo in treating benzodiazepine withdrawal symptoms. *British Journal of Psychiatry*, **168**, 457–461.

Further reading

Higgitt, A., Fonaghy, P. & Lader, M. H. (1988) The natural history of tolerance to the benzodiazepines. *Psychological Medicine* (monograph suppl. 13), 1–55.

King, D. J. (1992) Benzodiazepines, amnesia and sedation: theoretical and clinical issues and controversies. *Human Psychopharmacology*, **7**, 79–87.

Tyrer, P. J. (1984) Benzodiazepines on trial. *BMJ*, **288**, 1101–1102.

CHAPTER 6

Affective disorders:
1. Antidepressants

Elemer Szabadi and Christopher M. Bradshaw

Definitions

Antidepressant drugs were originally defined as drugs that alleviate pathological depression. The two prototype drugs were iproniazid, an inhibitor of the enzyme monoamine oxidase (MAO), and imipramine, a drug of a chlorpromazine-like tricyclic structure. Soon after the discovery of these two classical antidepressant drugs in the 1950s, amphetamine was included as another class of antidepressant drug, mainly on the basis of clinical practice (i.e. it was prescribed by clinicians to depressed patients), although it was subsequently removed from the list.

The meaning of the term 'antidepressant' has, however, become ambiguous. The original definition suggests that a drug cannot be called an antidepressant until its clinical usefulness has been demonstrated, and yet pharmaceutical companies sometimes claim to have developed a new antidepressant even before it has been administered to a single patient. These claims are based on the effectiveness of the new drug in laboratory models of antidepressant drug action. These models were first developed as screening tests to detect the potential antidepressant effects of new compounds, and are based on the known pharmacological actions of the classical ('prototype') antidepressants. This approach has resulted in the development of a large number of 'antidepressant' drugs that belong to the two major classes of antidepressant, namely the monoamine oxidase inhibitors (MAOIs) and the tricyclic antidepressants (TCAs). More recently drugs not belonging to either of these two classes have been developed (i.e. drugs that do not inhibit MAO and that do not have a tricyclic structure) that are effective both in the animal models and in patients with depression. Although the animal models predictive of antidepressant drug action have proved to be successful in the development of new antidepressant drugs, it should be noted that the reversal of a deficit in an animal model by an antidepressant drug does not necessarily mean that the deficit is a valid model of human depression. Therefore, clinical effectiveness is still the *sine qua non* of the definition of a drug as an antidepressant.

Although all antidepressant drugs, by definition, are effective in relieving morbid depression, this does not mean that these drugs do not have other actions. Indeed, the effectiveness of these drugs in the treatment of anxiety disorders (e.g. panic disorder, obsessive–compulsive disorder, phobic disorders) is increasingly recognised. Furthermore, some of these drugs can be used in the treatment of 'non-affective' symptoms, examples being the use of imipramine in nocturnal enuresis and the use of serotonin uptake inhibitors in bulimia.

Classification of antidepressants

The antidepressant drugs constitute a structurally and pharmacologically heterogeneous group of compounds that share the property of being effective in treating pathological depression. No consistent classificatory system has been developed based upon the mode of action of these drugs. The two main classes of drug were the MAOIs and the TCAs, one group being defined by its major biochemical action, and the other by its superficial chemical structure. With the development of newer drugs, it became obvious that not every compound could be accommodated under these two headings. Therefore a third category was added, termed 'novel', 'new-generation', 'second-generation' or 'atypical' antidepressants. Finally, with the development of compounds that selectively and potently inhibit the uptake of either 5-HT (serotonin) or noradrenaline into brain tissue, the separate groups of the selective serotonin (re)uptake inhibitors (SSRIs) and noradrenaline (re)uptake inhibitors (NARIs) were established.

Historical classification

This classification distinguishes between the original (classical) and later developed (novel, second-generation) antidepressants. This distinction is rather arbitrary; the cut-off point seems to be around 1980. In this respect, lofepramine and amoxapine are new-generation TCAs. The use of the terms 'typical' and 'atypical' is also rather misleading: although it may be justified to label the early antidepressants 'typical', the new antidepressants are not all 'atypical' (e.g. lofepramine is very similar to the classical TCAs).

Structural classification

There have been several attempts to classify antidepressant drugs by molecular structure, either according to the number of rings in the molecule or according to the presence or absence of atoms other than carbon in the rings (Richelson, 1984). On the basis of the number of rings one can distinguish the following:

(1)   monocyclic compounds (e.g. fluvoxamine, bupropion)
(2)   bicyclic compounds (e.g. fluoxetine, viloxazine)
(3)   tricyclic compounds (e.g. imipramine, amitriptyline, dothiepin, amoxapine)
(4)   tetracyclic compounds (e.g. maprotiline, mianserin, trazodone).

The tricyclic antidepressants can be further classified according to the final amino group in the side chain:

(1)   imipramine and amitriptyline are *tertiary amines*
(2)   their demethylated derivatives (desipramine and nortriptyline) are *secondary amines*.

On the basis of the presence or absence of atoms other than carbon in the ring, one can distinguish the following:

(1)   *heterocyclic* compounds (e.g. imipramine, desipramine);
(2)   *homocyclic* compounds (e.g. amitriptyline, nortriptyline).

The structural classification of antidepressants has not proved particularly valuable, with the possible exception of the distinction between tertiary and secondary amine TCAs: the tertiary amines are more active inhibitors of serotonin uptake than noradrenaline uptake, whereas the reverse order of potency applies to the secondary amines.

Pharmacological classification

The pharmacological classification of currently available antidepressant drugs is shown in Fig. 6.1. This approach to classification assumes that the most relevant pharmacological effect of the antidepressants can be identified. Although this has considerable attraction, it should be borne in mind that the common mode of action of antidepressants is still controversial.

According to the classic monoamine theory of affective disorders (see below), all antidepressant drugs act by increasing the concentrations of either or both of the monoamines noradrenaline and serotonin at the appropriate central synapses, and thus rectify a biochemical deficit (i.e. lack of sufficient monoamine transmitter) that is assumed to underlie depression. Thus, the MAOIs are assumed to increase monoamine levels by inhibiting the catabolic enzyme MAO, whereas monoamine uptake inhibitors may achieve this by blocking the reuptake of the released monoamine transmitters into presynaptic nerve terminals. The great achievement of the classic monoamine theory is that it could identify a pharmacological effect of the TCAs (i.e. uptake blockade) that could be reconciled with the striking single biochemical effect of the MAOIs.

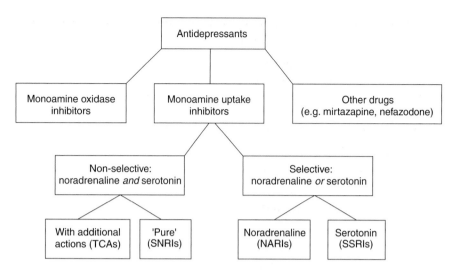

Fig. 6.1 Pharmacological classification of antidepressants.

The monoamine uptake inhibitors can be divided into two major classes: the non-selective group inhibits the uptake of both noradrenaline and serotonin, whereas the selective group affect the uptake of either noradrenaline (the NARIs) or serotonin (the SSRIs). Drugs in the non-selective group may be relatively 'pure', and inhibit the reuptake of noradrenaline and serotonin without any other significant pharmacological action, in which case they are termed serotonin/noradrenaline reuptake inhibitors (SNRIs), or they may have some additional effects, as in the case of the TCAs. The classical TCAs, in addition to the blockade of monoamine uptake, also block a number of neuroreceptors (α_1-adrenoceptors, 5-HT$_2$ receptors, H$_1$ histamine receptors, muscarinic cholinoceptors), which can result in undesirable side-effects.

Some antidepressants do not fit into either the selective or non-selective group (e.g. nefazodone, mirtazapine and buspirone); these are best labelled 'other antidepressant drugs'. It should be noted that some of these drugs may also enhance central monoaminergic transmission by increasing neurotransmitter release (e.g. mirtazapine) or by blocking monoamine uptake (e.g. nefazodone), in addition to modifying the effects of the released transmitter on postsynaptic receptors (see below).

Clinical classification

Attempts have been made to classify the antidepressants according to some aspect of clinical action. Thus, it is customary to distinguish between sedative (amitriptyline, trazodone, maprotiline) and non-sedative (desipramine, amoxapine, fluoxetine) antidepressants, or between 'strongly anticholinergic' (amitriptyline, imipramine) and 'weakly anticholinergic' (desipramine, fluoxetine, trazodone) drugs (Bernstein, 1988).

Pharmacokinetic properties can also be the basis for classification. Thus, on the basis of their elimination half-lives, antidepressants have been divided into four groups (see Richelson, 1984):

(1)   short half-life (3–5 hours) (trazodone, viloxazine)
(2)   intermediate half-life (8–15 hours) (amoxapine, mianserin)
(3)   long half-life (20–24 hours) (dothiepin, clomipramine)
(4)   very long half-life (40–60 hours) (maprotiline, fluoxetine).

Monoamine oxidase inhibitors

As their name implies, these compounds are defined by their ability to inhibit the oxidative deamination of endogenous and exogenous monoamines by the enzymes collectively known as monoamine oxidase.

Chemistry

The structures of a selection of MAOIs are shown in Fig. 6.2.

The prototypical MAOIs – phenelzine, tranylcypromine and iso-carboxazid – bear a close structural resemblance to sympathomimetic amines, a resemblance that is reflected in their pharmacological actions (see below). Phenelzine is a hydrazine derivative of the endogenous trace amine phenylethylamine; tranylcypromine is a close structural relative of amphetamine; and isocarboxazid is a hydrazide derivative, but it is probably its hydrazine metabolite that possesses the MAO-inhibiting property.

Some structural similarity to sympathomimetic amines is also apparent in the case MAOIs with preferential effects on the A and B forms of MAO, clorgyline and selegiline (also known as deprenyl), respectively. However, the more recently developed reversible MAOIs, brofaromine, moclobemide and caroxazone, have more complex structures.

Cellular and receptor pharmacology

It is now well established that MAO exists in two forms, MAO-A and MAO-B, which occur in different proportions in different tissues. The endogenous catecholamines noradrenaline and dopamine, and the indirectly acting sympathomimetic amine tyramine, are substrates for both forms. At low concentrations, serotonin is preferentially metabolised by MAO-A, and phenylethylamine by MAO-B; however, at higher concentrations serotonin and phenylethylamine can serve as substrates for both forms of the enzyme, and in this case apparent selectivity may depend to a large extent on the relative preponderance of the two forms of the enzyme in different tissues.

Irreversible

Non-selective MAOIs

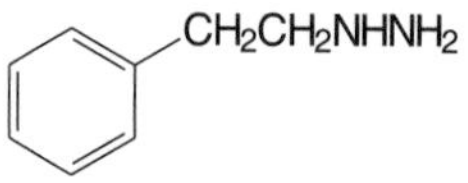

Phenelzine 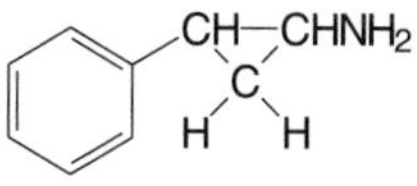   Tranylcypromine 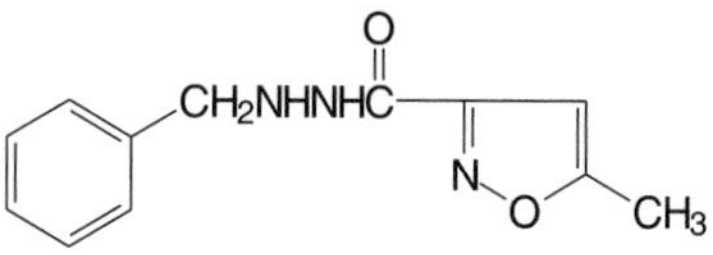   Isocarboxazid

MAO-A selective

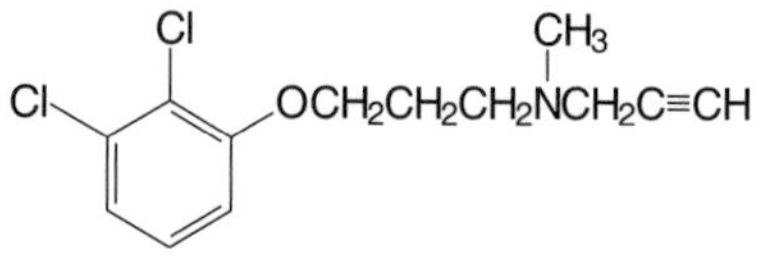

MAO-B selective

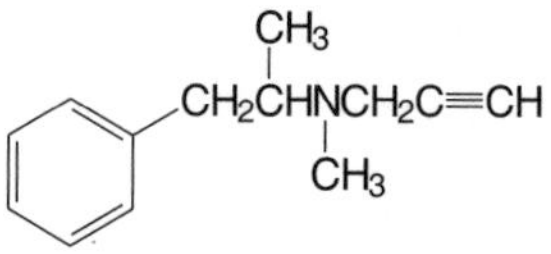

Clorgyline   Selegiline

Reversible

MAO-A selective

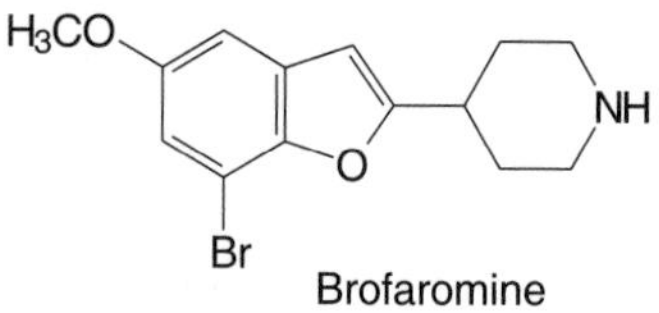

Brofaromine 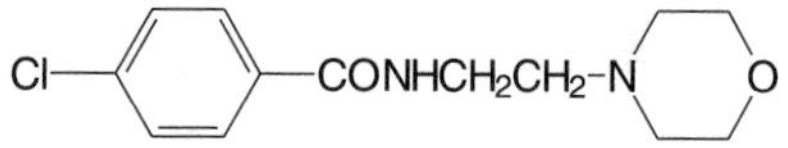   Moclobemide

MAO-B selective

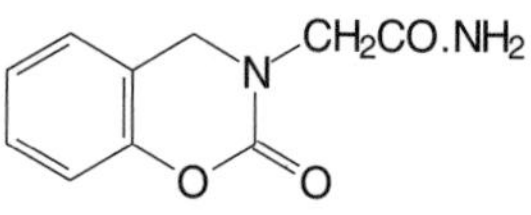

Caroxazone

Fig. 6.2 Chemical structures of some monoamine oxidase inhibitors.

MAO-A is the predominant form in the intestinal mucosa, whereas MAO-B alone is found in platelets; both forms occur in the brain and liver. In the brain, MAO-A is mainly found intraneuronally and MAO-B extraneuronally (the presence of MAO-B in serotonergic neurons of the raphe nuclei is an exception to this generalisation). The deamination of noradrenaline and serotonin in the brain is accomplished mainly by MAO-A; however, the destruction of dopamine in the corpus striatum is largely effected by MAO-B, perhaps reflecting the very high concentration of dopamine in this structure, which may allow a greater proportion of amine metabolism to occur extraneuronally than is the case in other brain structures.

The first generation of MAOIs consists of drugs with irreversible effects on MAO: they permanently inactivate the enzyme, and recovery of MAO activity can be achieved only by synthesis of new MAO molecules. The irreversible MAOIs can be either selective for MAO-A (e.g. clorgyline) or MAO-B (selegiline), or non-selective by inhibiting both MAO-A and MAO-B (e.g. phenelzine, tranylcypromine and isocarboxazid). However, a new class of reversible MAOIs has been developed, which may interact competitively and reversibly with MAO. Moclobemide and brofaromine are reversible inhibitors of MAO-A (RIMAs); caroxazone is selective for MAO-B. Moclobemide is available for clinical use as an antidepressant.

Inhibition of MAO is not the only action exhibited by MAOIs. Some hydrazine MAOIs (e.g. phenelzine) are able to release catecholamines from nerve terminals (an 'amphetamine-like' effect), which may contribute to the 'alerting' effects of these drugs. Others, for example the RIMA brofaromine, block serotonin uptake. Nevertheless, most of the known pharmacological effects of MAOIs are attributable to the direct or indirect results of MAO inhibition.

Acute effects

The acute neurochemical effects of the MAOIs consist of an increase in the concentration of noradrenaline, dopamine and serotonin in the brain, presumably reflecting the protection of intra- and extraneuronal monoamines from degradation by MAO. It is assumed that the functional consequence of this is facilitation of monoaminergic synaptic transmission. However, despite this immediate effect of the MAOIs on monoaminergic function, the therapeutic effect of the MAOIs, like that of the TCAs, tends to develop gradually, over 2 or more weeks of continuous treatment. This finding has led to a search for longer-term adaptive changes produced by MAOIs.

Chronic effects

Prolonged treatment with non-selective MAOIs and selective MAO-A-Is (but not selective MAO-B-Is) is known to result in reduced numbers ('down-regulation') of 5-HT_2 and 5-HT_{1A} receptors in the brain. However, electrophysiological studies have shown that the responses of postsynaptic neurons to stimulation of the serotonergic pathways remain enhanced even in the face of reduced receptor numbers. According to one explanation of these findings (Blier *et al*, 1991), MAO inhibition initially produces an enhanced feedback inhibition of serotonergic neurons. Later, as the somatodendritic (5-HT_{1A}) auto-receptors become desensitised, serotonergic neuronal activity returns to normal: however, the increased availability of intraneuronal serotonin for synaptic release continues to produce increased post-synaptic effects, overriding any attenuating effect of postsynaptic receptor down-regulation.

Chronic treatment with MAOIs also results in down-regulation of central β-adrenoceptors. Here again, however, the net effect on synaptic function may be facilitation rather than suppression, probably due to an increased availability of releasable noradrenaline, resulting from MAO inhibition. For example, melatonin release mediated by β-adrenoceptors is enhanced during chronic as well as acute treatment with MAO-A-Is (see Glue *et al*, 1993).

Interaction with tyramine

Tyramine is a 'pressor amine' which, like adrenaline, noradrenaline and phenylephrine, has the propensity to increase blood pressure on intravenous infusion. It is an indirectly acting sympathomimetic amine: it mimics the effect of sympathetic nerve stimulation on blood pressure by causing the release of noradrenaline, rather than by direct stimulation of postsynaptic adrenoceptors.

The ability of MAOIs to prevent the destruction of tyramine is the basis of the most serious side-effect of these drugs. Tyramine is found in a number of foods and beverages, most notably mature cheeses (hence the 'cheese reaction' seen with MAOIs – see below). Under normal circumstances ingested tyramine is metabolised by MAO-A, mainly in the intestinal mucosa and to a lesser degree in the liver. During treatment with an MAOI, significant quantities of tyramine may enter the circulation and precipitate a sudden release of catechol-amines from stores that are overladen as a result of inhibition of intraneuronal MAO; catastrophic hypertensive crises may ensue. Selective MAO-B-Is do not provoke the cheese reaction, but this is of small comfort to the psychiatrist, because these drugs are ineffective as antidepressants. RIMAs have been shown to be much less liable to provoke the cheese reaction than conventional MAO-A-Is; this is believed to reflect the competitive nature of the inhibition of MAO-A produced by RIMAs, which allows high concentrations of the substrate (tyramine) to overcome the enzyme inhibition (see Tipton & Anderson, 1991).

Organ and systems pharmacology

Many of the peripheral actions of MAOIs are explicable in terms of their effects on the functioning of the sympathetic nervous system; these include tachycardia, hypertension and urinary hesitancy. Xerostomia may result from an enhanced inhibitory noradrenergic influence on the salivatory nuclei of the brain-stem; this is termed the 'clonidine-like' effect (for details see Szabadi & Tavernor, 1999). Orthostatic hypotension is a common side-effect of MAOIs (see below); its cause is uncertain, but it has been suggested that it reflects potentiation of inhibitory dopaminergic transmission in autonomic ganglia.

The MAOIs have a variety of effects on neuroendocrine function, most of which emerge only during chronic treatment and are thought to reflect receptor adaptation processes. (The increased production of melatonin has already been mentioned.) In animals, prolactin secretion elicited by $5-HT_{1A}$ and $5-HT_{1B}$ receptor agonists is reduced during treatment with non-selective MAOIs, presumably reflecting the down-regulation of these receptors. However, studies of patients with depression have shown that the increased secretion of prolactin in response to L-tryptophan challenge is enhanced during treatment with MAOIs, perhaps reflecting the greater availability of serotonin produced from the precursor.

Behavioural pharmacology

A great deal of research effort has been invested in the search for behavioural tests that are sensitive to acute and chronic treatment with antidepressants. Such tests are of considerable value to the pharmaceutical industry, which needs to screen large numbers of compounds for potential antidepressant activity. Since it is generally regarded as an essential feature of such tests that they are sensitive to all known antidepressant drugs, it is not surprising that the profile of the behavioural effects of MAOIs turns out to be very similar to those of antidepressants belonging to other pharmacological families (Willner, 1990; Danysz et al, 1991).

Like TCAs, MAOIs reverse the syndrome induced by the monoamine-depleting agents reserpine and tetrabenazine, which consists of ptosis, hypothermia and catalepsy. They also potentiate the locomotor stimulant effect of amphetamine; this effect is partly centrally mediated, and partly due to interference with the hepatic metabolism of amphetamine.

Operant behaviour maintained under temporal differentiation schedules ('differential reinforcement of low response rates', DRL-72s) is suppressed by MAOIs and other antidepressants, with a concomitant rise in obtained reinforcement frequency; this test is said to be insensitive to drugs without antidepressant efficacy, although there has been some dissent.

Several tests involving stress have been proposed as quasi-veridical animal models of human depressive states, for example the impairment of operant response acquisition consequent upon repeated exposure to unavoidable aversive stimulation ('learned helplessness'), the assumption of immobility after prolonged immersion in water or suspension by the tail ('behavioural despair' or 'forced swim' test), and vocalisation induced in young animals by separation from their mothers or cage-mates ('distress vocalisation'); in general, MAOIs and TCAs reverse or attenuate the behavioural impact of these noxious procedures.

An exception to the rule that MAOIs and TCAs exert similar behavioural effects is the 'olfactory bulbectomy model'. Animals whose olfactory bulbs have been ablated display hyperactivity, 'irritability' and reduced sensitivity to punishment in passive avoidance paradigms. Although these effects are reliably reversed by most other anti-depressants, they are not affected by MAOIs.

A crucial question in trying to relate these behavioural effects to the antidepressant actions of MAOIs is whether the effects are attributable exclusively to MAO-A inhibition. Unfortunately this is not known at present.

Clinical pharmacology

Inhibition of MAO-B activity can be measured directly in platelets, whereas inhibition of MAO-A can only be inferred from reductions in the concentration of the noradrenaline metabolite 3-methoxy-4-hydroxy-phenylglycol (MHPG) in the urine, and dihydroxy-phenylglycol (DHPG) in the plasma. Although there is no direct index of MAO inhibition in the human brain, it has been reported that an 80% inhibition of platelet MAO-B and more than 70% reduction of urinary MHPG is required for the development of an antidepressant effect of non-selective MAOIs (e.g. phenelzine).

The presence of an MAOI in the body can also be detected from the potentiation of the pharmacological effects of tyramine. Thus, it has been shown that the dose of tyramine required to produce a standard pressor effect is greatly reduced by the non-selective MAOIs phenelzine and tranylcypromine, and also by the irreversible (clorgyline) and reversible (brofaromine, moclobemide) selective MAO-A-Is; MAO-B-Is (e.g. selegiline) are much less effective in this respect. Urinary excretion of MHPG declines in parallel with the increase in sensitivity to tyramine. Recovery of normal sensitivity to tyramine and normal urinary levels of MHPG are achieved about 1 week after discontinuing treatment with brofaromine, but is delayed for 4–15 weeks after withdrawal of irreversible MAOIs. Non-selective irreversible MAOIs have also been shown to potentiate the mydriatic response to locally instilled tyramine.

The most prominent behavioural effects of the MAOIs are apparent only in patients suffering from affective disorders. The MAOIs have little effect on the behaviour of euthymic subjects. Tranylcypromine has some amphetamine-like properties (e.g. increase in motor activity and heightened sensitivity to external stimuli). However, there is no tolerance to these effects, and the MAOIs cannot substitute for amphetamine in people addicted to this psychostimulant. The MAOIs have negligible effects on the waking electroencephalogram in healthy volunteers. The non-selective irreversible MAOIs markedly reduce the proportion of sleep spent in the rapid eye movement (REM) phase, resulting in a rebound increase in REM sleep after discontinuation of treatment. Interestingly, this effect is not seen with the reversible MAO-A-I moclobemide.

Pharmacokinetics

The three clinically used irreversible non-selective MAOIs are highly lipid-soluble compounds, and are therefore rapidly absorbed and widely distributed in the body. The peak plasma level after a single oral dose is attained within 2 hours in the case of phenelzine and within 1 hour in the case of tranylcypromine. They are extensively metabolised in the liver; only 1–2% is excreted unchanged in the urine. Phenelzine is believed to exert its pharmacological action via its hydrazine metabolite. Under normal dosage conditions, all the metabolites of tranylcypromine are pharmacologically inactive; however, it has been suggested that in overdose some tranylcypromine may be converted into amphetamine.

The hepatic metabolism of these drugs consists of acetylation, hydroxylation, oxidation and oxidative deamination; the metabolites are excreted in the urine as conjugates of glucuronic acid. The metabolic pathway via acetylation is generally regarded as the primary route of elimination. The effectiveness of this pathway is influenced by the monogenically inherited acetylator status of the individual (fast versus slow acetylators). Approximately half the Caucasian population falls into the 'fast acetylator' category; the ratio of 'fast' to 'slow' is higher in the Oriental population. Acetylator status may have therapeutic implications: slow acetylation may be associated with higher plasma levels of the MAOI, and thus with a quicker antidepressant response but more prominent side-effects. However, the predominant role of acetylation in the metabolic removal of phenelzine has been questioned and the relative importance of oxidation and hydroxylation emphasised (see Mallinger & Smith, 1991).

The RIMAs are also well absorbed and widely distributed in the body. The time to peak plasma concentration after a single oral dose is less than 2 hours for moclobemide and 2–4 hours for brofaromine. Moclobemide undergoes extensive first-pass metabolism in the liver, resulting in an oral bioavailability of about 50%. The elimination of moclobemide is almost entirely via hepatic metabolism; some of the metabolites may possess modest MAO-A-I activity. The elimination half-life of moclobemide is approximately 2 hours, whereas brofaromine is eliminated much more slowly (half-life 12–15 hours).

Therapeutics

The clinical usage of MAOIs has been through three phases:

(1) As the first class of antidepressant drugs developed, they were widely prescribed in the 1950s and 1960s.
(2) Their usage declined in the 1970s and up to the mid-1980s, mainly because of concern about their toxicity and the establishment of TCAs as the drugs of choice.
(3) More recently, there has been a resurgence of interest in them, partly owing to the recognition of their effectiveness in certain types of patients, and partly owing to a more realistic assessment of their risks (see Pare, 1985; Nutt & Glue, 1989).

Three irreversible inhibitors of both MAO-A and MAO-B are available for prescription for the treatment of depression in the UK: phenelzine, isocarboxazid and tranylcypromine, of which phenelzine is the most widely used. It seems to be that the inhibition of MAO-A is essential for the antidepressant efficacy: the selective MAO-B-I selegiline is useful in the treatment of parkinsonism, but is ineffective as an antidepressant. The RIMAs (e.g. moclobemide, brofaromine) are shorter acting and less toxic, and offer a new dimension to the clinical use of MAOIs. Moclobemide is the only RIMA available for clinical use in the UK.

Below, we first review the indications, contraindications, side-effects and interactions of the first-generation, irreversible MAOIs, and then we devote a section to moclobemide, which differs from the irreversible drugs in many important respects.

Indications for irreversible MAOIs

Depression

Irreversible MAOIs are recommended only as a second line of treatment for major depression, that is, they should be prescribed only after a monoamine uptake inhibitor has failed. The reasons for preferring monoamine uptake inhibitors as the first line of treatment are that: there is a much larger database demonstrating their clinical effectiveness, they can be administered without dietary restrictions, and they produce less frequent and less severe side-effects. The irreversible MAOIs are more suitable for treating patients with moderate rather than severe depression. Also, these drugs are generally more effective than TCAs if generalised anxiety is present. Thus, the irreversible MAOIs have been recommended for the treatment of patients with mild/moderate depression, who also show anxiety and who do not respond to TCAs.

Irreversible MAOIs have a reputation for being effective in 'atypical' depression (Pare, 1985); their effectiveness, however, depends on how 'atypical' depression is defined: if it is defined as depression with anxiety, then the irreversible MAOIs certainly have proven effectiveness; however, if the definition of 'atypical' depression also includes personality disorder or hypochondriasis, the effectiveness of the irreversible MAOIs becomes much more marginal.

Anxiety states

These drugs have an anti-anxiety effect that seems to be independent of their antidepressant efficacy. They are best suited for the treatment of patients suffering from chronic anxiety with phobic features or panic attacks; there is much less evidence for their effectiveness in uncomplicated generalised anxiety. Irreversible MAOIs may be more effective than imipramine if phobia, hypochondriacal and hysterical symptoms are present in addition to anxiety.

Phobic states

There is evidence for the effectiveness of irreversible MAOIs in the treatment of agoraphobia and social phobias; however, they are ineffective in the treatment of simple phobias.

Obsessive–compulsive disorder (OCD)

There are isolated case reports showing the effectiveness of irreversible MAOIs in OCD. They have been recommended in chronic, treatment-resistant cases, especially when anxiety and phobic symptoms are also present.

Other uses

Like TCAs, irreversible MAOIs have been recommended for the treatment of chronic pain (especially when features of depression are also present) and bulimia nervosa (especially with anxiety).

Contraindications and precautions of irreversible MAOIs

Cerebrovascular and cardiovascular disease

The risk of a sympathomimetic (hypertensive) crisis (see below) renders these drugs hazardous in patients suffering from these conditions.

Phaeochromocytoma

A phaeochromocytoma that secretes large quantities of catecholamines would augment a sympathomimetic crisis resulting from dietary indiscretion or a drug interaction (see below).

Liver disease and blood dyscrasias

As the irreversible MAOIs can, albeit rarely, lead to hepatocellular jaundice and bone marrow suppression, these drugs should be avoided in patients with liver disease or haemopoetic disorder.

Epilepsy

As the irreversible MAOIs have a slight epileptogenic effect, they should be avoided in patients suffering from epilepsy.

Age

Irreversible MAOIs are not recommended for children. Like all other centrally acting drugs, the irreversible MAOIs cross the placental barrier and pass into the foetus. Although there is no clear evidence for teratogenecity, they should be avoided in pregnant women. As they are excreted in low concentrations in the breast milk, breast-feeding is not recommended to women taking irreversible MAOIs.

Elderly patients are more sensitive to the side-effects and so for them a more gradual build-up of the dosage and a lower final dosage should be applied.

Side-effects and toxicity of irreversible MAOIs

Central nervous system

Daytime drowsiness and insomnia at night are frequent complications. Infrequently psychotic reactions or the precipitation of a manic psychosis can occur.

Autonomic nervous system

The effects of the irreversible MAOIs on the autonomic nervous system are complex: although a sympathomimetic effect predominates, there is also evidence for a sympatholytic effect. The sympathomimetic effect is due to the enhancement of the physiological effects of noradrenaline and adrenaline, resulting from the inhibition of their degradation by MAO, whereas the sympatholytic effect is due partly to sympathetic ganglion blockade (possibly due to potentiation of the inhibitory action of dopamine), and partly to adrenergic neuron blockade (caused by the synthesis of pharmacologically inactive false transmitters in the peripheral nerve endings).

The *sympathomimetic effect* can lead to cardiac arrhythmia and an enhancement of physiological finger tremor, and also to mild

191

'anticholinergic' side-effects in organs that receive a dual noradrenergic/ cholinergic innervation. These 'anticholinergic' side-effects include mydriasis and blurred vision, dry mouth, constipation and urinary hesitancy. It should be noted that most irreversible MAOIs have little affinity for muscarinic cholinoceptors, and thus these 'anticholinergic' side-effects are likely to reflect sympathetic potentiation rather than muscarinic receptor blockade ('pseudo-anticholinergic effects').

The sympathomimetic effects of the irreversible MAOIs are dramatically increased in a *sympathomimetic crisis* ('cheese reaction') evoked by indirectly acting sympathomimetic amines ingested either in food-stuffs (e.g. tyramine) or as drugs (e.g. phenylpropanolamine). The crisis consists of increased sweating and cardiovascular symptoms (tachycardia, increased cardiac output leading to an increase in blood pressure, vasoconstriction leading to pallor and hypertension). If extreme hypertension causes cerebral haemorrhage, death can result. The syndrome therefore requires urgent treatment: the hypertension can be treated by an intravenously injected α_1-adrenoceptor antagonist (e.g. phentolamine, chlorpromazine), and the tachycardia by a β-adrenoceptor antagonist (e.g. propranolol). Foodstuffs containing tyramine in high concentrations (e.g. mature cheese, Marmite and pickled herrings) should be avoided, and the patient should be given a card listing all the dangerous foodstuffs.

The paradoxical orthostatic hypotension (a sympatholytic effect – see above) is one of the most common side-effects of irreversible MAOIs, and in some patients it can be very troublesome. Patients started on an irreversible MAOI often complain of light-headedness and dizziness, and fainting can also occur. It is important to build up the dosage gradually over several weeks. Usually some tolerance develops to this side-effect.

Peripheral nerves

Peripheral neuropathy is a rare complication of treatment with irreversible MAOIs.

Liver

Hepatocellular jaundice is a rare but severe complication of treatment with irreversible MAOIs that restricted the use of these drugs for several years. However, it is now recognised that many of the early cases reported were probably associated with viral hepatitis, and that the risk of this complication is very small.

Bone marrow

Bone marrow suppression is a severe but very rare complication. Regular blood counts are advised in all patients taking irreversible MAOIs.

Skin

Rashes as allergic reactions can occur.

Drug interactions of irreversible MAOIs

Tyramine-containing foodstuffs

Such foods can lead to a sympathomimetic crisis in patients taking irreversible MAOIs (see above).

Sympathomimetic amines

Indirectly acting sympathomimetic amines that are used as nasal decongestants, bronchodilators and appetite suppressants (e.g. phenyl-propanolamine, fenfluramine, phentermine), and also L-dopa can lead to a sympathomimetic crisis in conjunction with irreversible MAOIs (see above). The patient should be warned to avoid 'over-the-counter' cough mixtures that may contain some of these amines.

TCAs

These drugs would be expected to reduce the risk of a sympatho-mimetic crisis resulting from the co-administration of indirectly acting sympathomimetic amines and irreversible MAOIs, since they block the uptake of these amines into the sympathetic nerve terminal, without which the amines cannot exert their pharmacological actions (see Pare, 1985). However, there is evidence that the combination of TCAs and irreversible MAOIs can lead to a severe toxic reaction, characterised by hypertension. It has been suggested that an interaction at central serotonin synapses may underlie this syndrome (the 'serotonin syndrome' – for details see 'Drug interactions', pp. 223–224).

SSRIs

The co-administration of MAOIs with SSRIs can produce a sudden dangerous increase in the brain concentration of serotonin, which in turn can result in a severe toxic reaction (the 'serotonin syndrome'). It is therefore absolutely contraindicated, and a sufficiently long time interval (up to 5 weeks) should be allowed between the discontinuation of an SSRI and the introduction of treatment with an MAOI.

Opiates

Irreversible MAOIs potentiate the pharmacological actions of opiates. This is mainly due to a pharmacokinetic interaction between the two classes of drug (the irreversible MAOIs inhibit the liver enzymes responsible for the metabolism of opiates); however, the possibility of a pharmacodynamic interaction cannot be excluded. The co-administration of irreversible MAOIs and opiates can lead to a severe toxic syndrome characterised by excitement, muscular rigidity, hyperpyrexia, flushing, sweating, hypotension, respiratory depression and finally coma. Therefore opiates should be administered with great caution to patients taking irreversible MAOIs (dosage at 5–10% of the usual level has been recommended). MAOIs should be withdrawn 2 weeks before elective surgery.

Pethidine is absolutely contraindicated in patients taking MAOIs, owing to the rapidity of development and severity of the toxic syndrome following the intramuscular injection of pethidine in patients treated with an irreversible MAOI. The severity of the toxic interaction between MAOIs and pethidine suggests that this reaction may not be due to inhibition of pethidine metabolism alone (Dollery, 1999).

Moclobemide

Moclobemide is a reversible inhibitor of MAO-A and thus has somewhat less potential for evoking hypertensive episodes following ingestion of indirectly acting amines such as tyramine. Owing to its reduced toxicity compared with the classical, irreversible MAOIs, moclobemide can be used as a first-line treatment in depression. Another specific indication for moclobemide is social phobia. There is less information available about the usefulness of this drug for other indications, such as anxiety states in general, or obsessive–compulsive disorder.

Moclobemide has generally been well tolerated in controlled clinical trials; it causes less dry mouth and sedation than the TCAs, and less nausea than the SSRIs. In contrast to the irreversible non-selective MAOIs, which can cause a burdensome orthostatic hypotension, moclobemide can lead to hypertension in some patients. More severe hypertensive reactions can be provoked by the ingestion of tyramine-containing foodstuffs by patients taking moclobemide (the 'cheese reaction'), although the likelihood and severity of such a reaction is much less than with the irreversible MAOIs.

Moclobemide can evoke symptoms of anxiety and agitation in some patients, and therefore it should be avoided in patients with agitated depression. It is non-sedative, and therefore is unlikely to interfere with psychomotor skills such as driving a motor vehicle.

Like the irreversible MAOIs, moclobemide can evoke a severe 'serotonin syndrome', especially when co-administered with SSRIs or TCAs. These drug combinations, therefore, are absolutely contraindicated. Other potentially dangerous drug interactions are the same as with the irreversible MAOIs; that is, both directly acting (e.g. phenylephrine) and indirectly acting (e.g. tyramine, ephedrine) sympathomimetic amines, opiates and serotonergic drugs (e.g. clomipramine) can have deleterious interactions with RIMAs. Moclobemide may also impede the elimination of ibuprofen, and therefore the dosage of ibuprofen may have to be adjusted for patients who are taking both drugs.

Monoamine uptake inhibitors

Drugs in this class have the property of inhibiting the uptake of noradrenaline and/or serotonin into brain tissue; some of these drugs may also inhibit the uptake of dopamine.

Specific uptake is the active (energy-, temperature- and sodium-dependent) accumulation of monoamines into the appropriate nerve endings (e.g. noradrenaline is accumulated by noradrenergic nerve terminals in both the periphery and the CNS); non-specific uptake is the accumulation of the amines by non-neural tissues (e.g. glial cells). The term 'monoamine uptake inhibitors' refers to the inhibition of specific uptake only. Active specific uptake is one of the most important ways by which the released monoamine neurotransmitter is eliminated: when this process is inhibited, the monoamine may remain in the synaptic cleft for a longer time and in a higher concentration than is normally the case, which results in *potentiation* of the pharmacological effects of the released neurotransmitter.

The term 'reuptake' refers to the uptake of the endogenously released transmitter, whereas 'uptake' is a more general term that incorporates the active accumulation of both endogenously released and exogenously administered monoamine transmitters.

Reuptake is an energy-requiring, sodium- and temperature-dependent process, which is carried out by neurotransmitter-specific 'transporters'. The reuptake process is usually studied by measuring the uptake of a radioactively labelled transmitter molecule into tissue samples rich in the relevant presynaptic terminals. Thus, the uptake of noradrenaline can be studied in peripheral tissues that receive a dense sympathetic innervation (e.g. spleen, heart), whereas the uptake of serotonin is often studied in blood platelets, which possess an active serotonin-accumulating mechanism. The uptake of the same neurotransmitters can also be studied in brain tissue samples, using brain slices or synaptosome preparations, consisting of 'pinched-off' nerve endings.

Specific transporter molecules are responsible for the transfer of noradrenaline and serotonin from the extracellular space into noradrenergic and serotonergic neurons. Initially, the noradrenaline transporter was identified as a high-affinity binding site for the tricyclic antidepressant desipramine in brain membrane preparations, and the serotonin transporter as a high-affinity binding site for the tricyclic antidepressant imipramine in brain membrane preparations and blood platelets. This discovery created the possibility of studying the uptake-inhibiting property of antidepressants by examining their ability to displace radioactively labelled desipramine and imipramine from their binding sites in membrane preparations (Langer *et al*, 1984). With the advent of molecular biological techniques, it has become possible to define the molecular structures of the noradrenaline and serotonin transporters and to clone them in cell lines transfected with cDNAs for the respective transporters. The ability of a number of antidepressants to inhibit the binding of noradrenaline and serotonin to these cloned transporters has been studied: the results of these binding studies show good agreement with the effects of the same antidepressants on the uptake of radioactively labelled noradrenaline and serotonin in brain slices and synaptosomes (Lesch & Bengel, 1995).

It is usual to distinguish between non-selective and selective monoamine uptake inhibitors (Fig. 6.1): the non-selective drugs block the uptake of both noradrenaline and serotonin, whereas the selective drugs affect the uptake of only one of these monoamines. *Selectivity* is different from *potency*: a drug may be highly selective and not very potent, or the reverse (see Fig. 6.3). Thus, desipramine, one of the most potent inhibitors of noradrenaline uptake, is classified as non-selective since it also affects serotonin uptake to an appreciable extent. It should be noted that selectivity is always relative, and it is rather arbitrary at what ratio of affinities for the transport processes of noradrenaline and serotonin we start calling a drug selective rather than non-selective. Furthermore, in the distinction between selective and non-selective drugs only the uptake of noradrenaline and serotonin is taken into account, although some of the drugs may also inhibit dopamine uptake.

Non-selective monoamine uptake inhibitors, selective noradrenaline uptake inhibitors and selective serotonin uptake inhibitors are discussed separately below. Drugs that do not fit into these categories are then considered, before a discussion of the general properties of antidepressants.

Non-selective monoamine uptake inhibitors with additional actions (TCAs)

Chemistry

All the drugs in this class have three-ringed structures. The prototypical drug is imipramine, and all the TCAs are analogues of this drug. The structures of a selection of TCAs are shown in Fig. 6.4. These drugs are generally classified according to the substitution of the terminal amino group of the side-chain – thus imipramine, amitriptyline, trimipramine, lofepramine, dothiepin and doxepin are tertiary amines, and desipramine, nortriptyline and amoxapine are secondary amines.

On the basis of the three-ringed nucleus, imipramine, its N-demethylated metabolite desipramine, trimipramine, lofepramine and nortriptyline are *dibenzazepines*, amitriptyline and its metabolite nortriptyline are *dibenzocycloheptadienes*, doxepin is a *dibenzoxapine*,

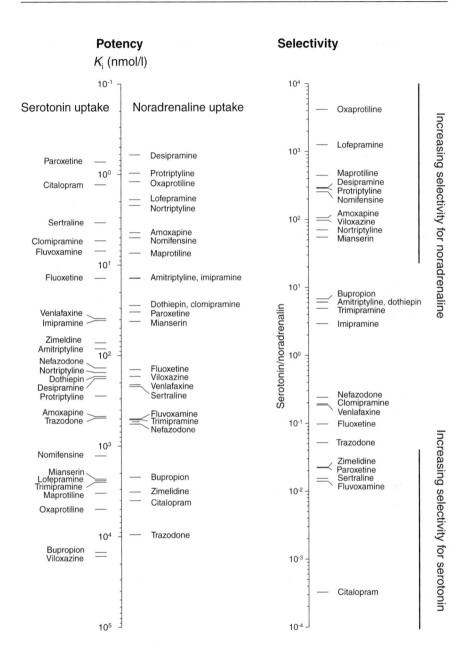

Fig. 6.3 Potencies and selectivities of monoamine uptake inhibitors. K_i is the concentration (nM) of antidepressant required to produce 50% inhibition of monoamine uptake. (Note that high K_i values indicate low potency.) Data from Richelson & Pfenning (1984) and Bolden-Watson & Richelson (1993).

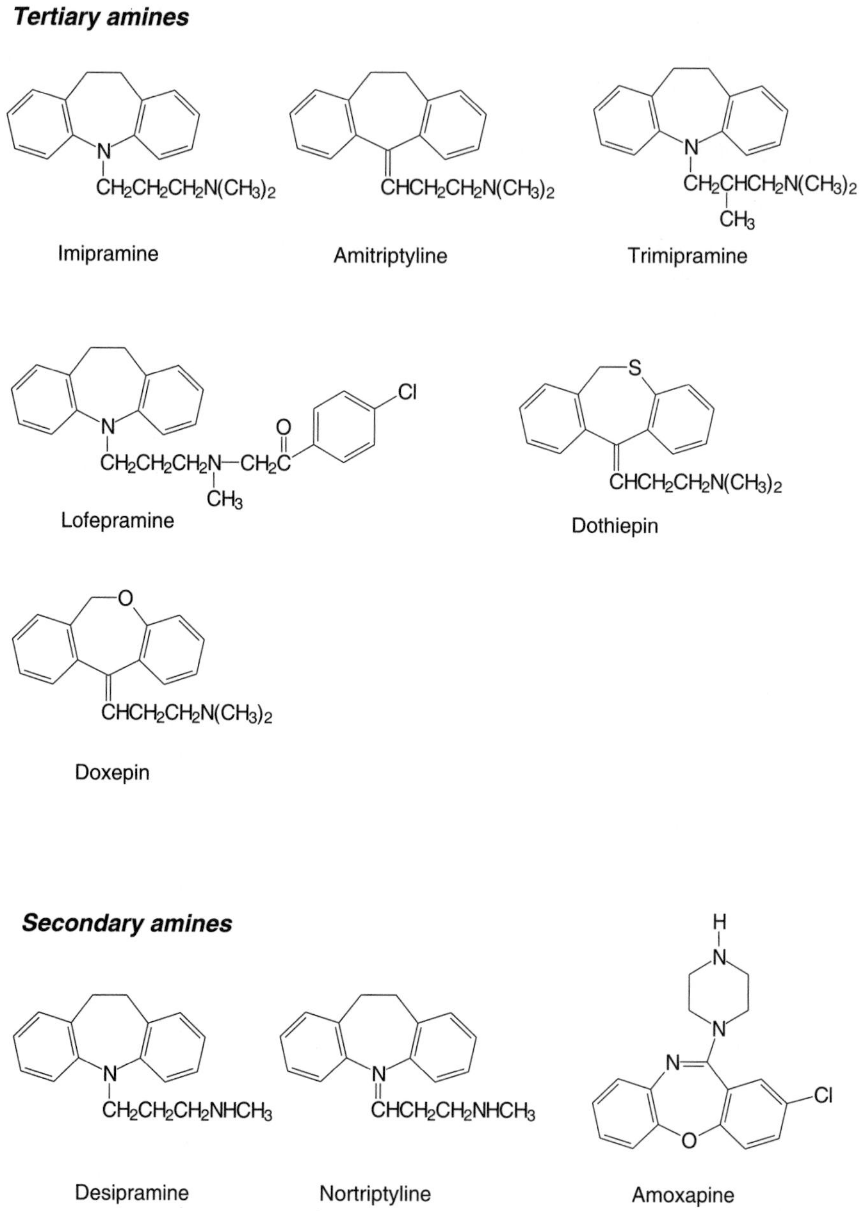

Tertiary amines

Imipramine

Amitriptyline

Trimipramine

Lofepramine

Dothiepin

Doxepin

Secondary amines

Desipramine

Nortriptyline

Amoxapine

Fig. 6.4 Chemical structures of some non-selective monoamine uptake inhibitors (TCAs).

dothiepin a *dibenzothiepin*, and amoxapine a *dibenzoxazepine*. There does not appear to be any systematic relationship between these structural features and the pharmacological profiles of these drugs.

Cellular and receptor pharmacology

Acute effects

Reuptake into nerve terminals is an important mechanism of the inactivation of the monoamine transmitters – noradrenaline, serotonin and dopamine. TCAs have the ability to inhibit the uptake of noradrenaline and serotonin into nerve terminals. As intimated above, the uptake-inhibiting antidepressants differ in their selectivities for the noradrenaline and serotonin uptake mechanisms (see Fig. 6.3). Although all TCAs discussed in this section have a propensity to block the uptake of both monoamines to some degree, desipramine shows considerable selectivity for noradrenaline and clomipramine for serotonin uptake.

Uptake blockade can be demonstrated in various peripheral tissues, in blood cells and in brain. TCAs bind to membrane fragments prepared from these tissues, and it is generally accepted that these 'antidepressant receptors' represent the amine transporter complex; imipramine is generally used to label the serotonin transporter, and desipramine to label the noradrenaline transporter. The immediate consequence of uptake blockade is potentiation of the postsynaptic effects of the transmitter amine. This can be detected using a variety of peripheral preparations, for example the response of the nictitating membrane of the cat to efferent nerve stimulation. Since exogenously applied amines may also be taken up into aminergic nerve terminals, their effects may also be potentiated by the TCAs. Tyramine is an exception to this rule, because its effects are mediated principally by entry into nerve terminals via the uptake 'pump' and release of endogenous noradrenaline; by denying tyramine access to the nerve terminal, uptake-blocking antidepressants generally attenuate the effects of this amine.

The TCAs have a number of other acute pharmacological actions in addition to inhibition of noradrenaline and serotonin uptake. Most of these drugs possess some antimuscarinic activity, amitriptyline being especially potent, and desipramine relatively weak, in this respect; the antimuscarinic action is the basis of many of the peripheral side-effects of these drugs. Blockade of α_1-adrenoceptors and H_1 histamine receptors may underlie the sedative effect produced by some antidepressants; doxepine, trimipramine and amitriptyline have the highest affinities among drugs in this class for both these receptors. The TCAs have little affinity for α_2-adrenoceptors. Most of the drugs in this group also have rather low affinities for dopamine receptors; however, amoxapine is an exception: its D_2 dopamine receptor blocking action is thought to be

199

responsible both for its 'neuroleptic' properties and for its liability to produce extrapyramidal side-effects.

Chronic effects

In contrast to the immediate onset of uptake blockade, the clinical response to the TCAs is typically delayed for 2 or more weeks after the start of treatment. It is generally agreed that pharmacokinetic factors alone cannot account for this delayed onset of action. This has led to an increasing interest in the longer-term changes seen during chronic treatment with these drugs. One such effect is a reduction of the number of central β_1-adrenoceptors ('down-regulation'), associated with diminished activity of β_1-adrenoceptor-coupled adenylyl cyclase. Initially, it was thought that this constituted an adaptation to the enhanced availability of noradrenaline resulting from noradrenaline uptake blockade. However, this was rendered unlikely by the finding that antidepressants with little or no noradrenaline uptake blocking action can down-regulate β_1-adrenoceptors. Subsequently, it was found that destruction of the serotonin-containing pathways prevented β_1-adrenoceptor down-regulation, which suggested that down-regulation may be mediated by altered activity in serotonergic neurons innervating the noradrenergic nuclei of the lower brain-stem. Unfortunately, the picture is now complicated by the finding that antidepressants may alter the proportions of high- and low-affinity β_1-adrenoceptors, even after destruction of the serotonergic pathways. The mechanism of β_1-adrenoceptor down-regulation therefore remains uncertain (see Cowen, 1990; Caldecott-Hazard et al, 1991; Pryor & Sulser, 1991).

Prolonged treatment with TCAs also results in reduced numbers of α_2-adrenoceptors in the brain. The α_2-adrenoceptors located on mono-aminergic nerve terminals play an important inhibitory role in the regulation of transmitter release; thus down-regulation of α_2-adreno-ceptors may facilitate synaptic transmission.

Similarly, 5-HT$_2$ receptors are down-regulated during chronic treat-ment with TCAs, and this is accompanied by suppression of behavioural responses believed to be mediated by these receptors. Changes in the number of 5-HT$_{1A}$ receptors are more controversial. Although many studies have reported no such change, there is evidence for reduced numbers of the subpopulation of 5-HT$_{1A}$ receptors located on serotonergic nerve terminals that are believed to inhibit transmitter release (see Blier et al, 1991).

Although interest has mainly been focused on noradrenergic and serotonergic receptors, it is known that long-term treatment with uptake-blocking TCAs can result in adaptive changes in other receptor systems, including reductions in the number of D_1 dopamine receptors, increases in gamma-aminobutyric acid (GABA)-B receptors, and various species of neuropeptide receptor (see Caldecott-Hazard et al, 1991).

Organ and systems pharmacology

Tricyclic antidepressants have a variety of effects on autonomically innervated tissues. These are attributable to:

(1)   inhibition of noradrenaline uptake, resulting in enhanced noradrenergic neurotransmission (*sympathomimetic effect*)

(2)   muscarinic cholinoceptor blockade, resulting in reduced cholinergic neurotransmission (*anticholinergic effect*)

(3) α_1-adrenoceptor blockade, resulting in suppression of noradrenergic neurotransmission (*sympatholytic effect*).

The blockade of muscarinic cholinoceptors by TCAs leads to both a parasympatholytic effect and a sympatholytic effect (with respect to the eccrine sweat glands, which receive a cholinergic sympathetic innervation).

The observed net effect of an antidepressant depends on the relative importance of these mechanisms for physiological function, and on the relative propensity of the drug to influence the individual mechanisms.

The anticholinergic effects of these drugs include reduced glandular secretion, mydriasis, reduced bowel motility, tachycardia, urinary hesitancy and erectile dysfunction; the sympathomimetic effects include tachycardia and mydriasis; and the sympatholytic effects include hypotension, miosis and ejaculatory incompetence. In the case of tissues that receive a dual sympathetic–parasympathetic innervation, prediction of the net effect of an antidepressant can be quite complicated. For example, the anticholinergic action of these drugs may result in mydriasis; however, desipramine, a weak anticholinergic, is more likely to produce mydriasis than the powerful anticholinergic amitriptyline. The likely reason for this paradoxical observation is that although both drugs also have noradrenaline uptake blocking (mydriatic) action, only amitriptyline has significant adrenolytic (miotic) action (Szabadi & Bradshaw, 1986).

Tricyclic antidepressants have direct effects on the heart, mainly due to the blockade of sodium channels, which leads to membrane stabilisation. This results in reduced myocardial contractility and impaired intracardiac conduction, which in turn may lead to arrhythmias (Baldessarini, 2001).

The neuroendocrine effects of TCAs are in many ways similar to those of the MAOIs. As is the case with MAO-A-Is, chronic treatment with TCAs results in elevated concentrations of melatonin in the plasma; this may reflect enhanced stimulation of postsynaptic β_1-adrenoceptors as a result of potentiated central noradrenergic neurotransmission.

The secretion of growth hormone elicited by the α_2-adrenoceptor agonist clonidine is enhanced following acute treatment with TCAs but attenuated following prolonged treatment. The acute effect may reflect potentiated noradrenergic neurotransmission due to uptake blockade, and the chronic effect the more slowly developing down-regulation of α_2-adrenoceptors.

Acute treatment with the serotonin precursor tryptophan provokes the secretion of *prolactin*, probably via stimulation of 5-HT$_{1A}$ receptors. This response can be potentiated by TCAs, which is consistent with electrophysiological and behavioural evidence for facilitation by these drugs of functions that are mediated by the 5-HT$_{1A}$ receptor.

Treatment with serotonin precursors or with m-chlorophenyl piperazine (mCPP) stimulates adrenocorticotrophic hormone secretion, with a consequent increase in plasma cortisol levels; this response is believed to be mediated by 5-HT$_{2C}$ receptors. The response has been found to be attenuated by uptake-blocking antidepressants, a finding that has been cited in support of the notion that antidepressants alter the functional balance between 5-HT$_{1A}$ and 5-HT$_2$ receptors (see 'Common mode of action of antidepressants', pp. 233–236).

Behavioural pharmacology

As discussed earlier, TCAs share many of the behavioural effects of MAOIs; these effects will not be reiterated here. However, unlike the MAOIs, TCAs reverse the behavioural deficits seen in animals whose olfactory bulbs have been ablated.

Of potential relevance for the mode of action of TCAs are the effects of these drugs on unconditioned behaviours believed to be mediated by different subtypes of 5-HT receptor (see Cowen, 1990). Chronic treatment with TCAs is associated with a reduction of the serotonin-induced head-twitch response in rodents, an effect that parallels the down-regulation of 5-HT$_2$ receptors. The effects of chronic treatment with antidepressants on functions believed to be mediated by 5-HT$_{1A}$ receptors are more complex. These drugs attenuate the hypothermic response evoked by the 5-HT$_{1A}$ receptor agonist 8-hydroxy-2-(di-*n*-propylamino)tetralin (8-OH-DPAT), and suppress the behavioural syndrome produced by this compound ('forepaw treading' and hind-limb abduction). The former effect is believed to reflect desensitisation of inhibitory autoreceptors on serotonergic neurons, and the latter desensitisation of a subpopulation of postsynaptic 5-HT$_{1A}$ receptors. The theoretical implications of these complex findings are discussed below.

Clinical pharmacology

The most prominent, and probably most therapeutically relevant, effect of the TCAs is the blockade of the uptake of noradrenaline and/or serotonin. Although uptake blockade cannot be measured directly in the brain in humans, it can be detected in the periphery. Thus, the presence of TCAs in the plasma can be detected by direct measurement of the inhibition of the uptake of radioactively labelled serotonin into blood platelets. The pharmacodynamic indices of the inhibition of noradrenaline uptake are potentiation of the effects of noradrenaline and inhibition of the effects of the indirectly acting sympathomimetic amine tryamine. Thus, it has been reported that TCAs potentiate noradrenaline-induced pupil dilatation and rise in blood pressure, but antagonise tyramine-induced mydriasis and pressor response (see Szabadi & Bradshaw, 1986). The other peripheral pharmacological effects of the TCAs can also be detected by appropriate pharmacological tests: the blockade of α_1-adrenoceptors can be revealed as the antagonism of methoxamine- or phenylephrine-evoked mydriasis and phenylephrine-evoked sweat gland activation, whereas the blockade of muscarinic cholinoceptors can be demonstrated as the antagonism of pilocarpine-evoked miosis and carbachol-evoked activation of sweat glands (Szabadi & Bradshaw, 1986).

Acute administration of single doses of TCAs to euthymic volunteers does not cause any 'activation' or elevation of mood: most of these drugs cause sedation and dysphoria. TCAs impair psychomotor performance and lower critical flicker fusion frequency, a psychophysiological index of CNS arousal (Hindmarch et al, 1992). The effects on the autonomic nervous system are also apparent in healthy volunteers. Pupil size will reflect the interaction between the pupil dilatatory (noradrenaline uptake blockade, muscarinic cholinoceptor blockade) and constrictor (α_1-adrenoceptor blockade, sedation) effects of the antidepressants. Accommodation is impaired, as evidenced by the elongation of the visual near point, and salivation is decreased; there can also be an increase in heart rate and a postural drop in blood pressure. The TCAs have profound effects on sleep: they decrease the number of awakenings, increase stage IV sleep, increase the latency to the onset of REM sleep, and decrease the total time spent in REM sleep. The effects of the TCAs on sleep architecture, together with their propensity to produce daytime sedation (Reite, 1998), are likely to reflect the blockade of central H_1 histamine receptors, α_1-adrenoceptors and muscarinic cholinoceptors by these drugs, which in turn would lead to a reduction in the effectiveness of the histaminergic, noradrenergic and cholinergic wakefulness-promoting pathways (Saper et al, 2001).

The full human pharmacological profile of these drugs, however, becomes apparent only in patients with clinical depression, when their therapeutic (antidepressant and anti-anxiety) effects can be observed. It usually takes 2–3 weeks before the antidepressant effect becomes obvious; the anti-anxiety effect may appear after a few days. All the core symptoms of the depressive syndrome (low mood, low self-esteem, feelings of guilt, suicidal ideation, insomnia, poor appetite, retardation) are affected. All the pharmacological effects detectable in healthy subjects (see above) are also observable in depressed patients; some of the autonomic effects (e.g. decrease in salivation) may be accentuated in depression owing to the effect of illness itself on autonomic functions. The cardiac effects of these drugs (i.e. impairment of conduction and contractility) are more pronounced in patients in the course of prolonged treatment than in healthy volunteers following acute dosing.

Pharmacokinetics

All TCAs are lipid soluble and therefore are almost completely absorbed from the gut and rapidly and widely distributed in body tissues. They readily cross lipid barriers such as the placenta and the blood–brain barrier. TCAs with anticholinergic properties (e.g. imipramine, amitriptyline) reduce gastric emptying and intestinal peristalsis, and thus can delay their own absorption.

With most of these drugs, peak plasma levels are achieved 2–6 hours after a single oral dose (e.g. 3.5 hours for imipramine and 5 hours for desipramine). The TCAs have relatively long plasma half-lives (8–36 hours); this allows once-daily administration. On multiple dosing, steady-state plasma levels are attained within 1–2 weeks. TCAs are extensively bound to plasma proteins (e.g. 75–95% in the case of imipramine). They are all extensively metabolised in the liver. The prototype drug, imipramine, undergoes presystemic metabolism that reduces its bioavailability to approximately 50%. However, the bioavailability of TCAs varies greatly between subjects.

In the case of imipramine, the two most important metabolic routes are demethylation and hydroxylation. The N-demethylated product desipramine (or nor-imipramine) is pharmacologically active. Other TCAs may also have active metabolites (e.g. amitriptyline is converted into nortriptyline, lofepramine into desipramine, and amoxapine into 7-hydroxy- and 8-hydroxyamoxapine; these two metabolites of amoxapine have both antidepressant and neuroleptic properties). A genetic defect can lead to a deficiency of the isoenzyme of microsomal cytochrome P450 IID6 that is responsible for the 2-hydroxylation of TCAs. Subjects suffering from this deficiency show a reduced clearance of imipramine, leading to the prolongation of the elimination half-life and elevation of the steady-state plasma level of the drug. Metabolism via 2-hydroxylation can also be affected by drugs: neuroleptics inhibit and barbiturates and cigarette smoking facilitate this process.

The rate of metabolic degradation of TCAs is reduced in the elderly, leading to higher plasma levels and increased risk of toxicity in this patient group.

The hydroxylated metabolic products are conjugated with glucuronic acid and are excreted via the kidneys.

Attempts have been made to correlate steady-state plasma levels with therapeutic effect. As with bioavailability, there are great (up to 30–50-fold) inter-individual variations in the steady-state plasma concentrations attained on the same oral dosage regimen (Britton *et al*, 1978). In the case of drugs with active metabolites, it is important that the combined concentrations of parent drug and metabolites should be correlated with the therapeutic response. For several TCAs an optimal range of plasma concentration ('therapeutic window') has been proposed; for imipramine, for example, it is 150–250 µg/l (imipramine and desipramine combined).

The assessment of the steady-state plasma level of TCAs has little relevance for everyday clinical practice. However, if a patient fails to respond even to relatively high oral doses of a drug, it may be informative to check whether the plasma concentration falls within the recommended therapeutic window.

Therapeutics

Until recently, TCAs were the most widely used drugs for the treatment of depression; however, SSRIs are taking over their position. Apart from the 'classical' TCAs (imipramine, desipramine, amitriptyline), there is a new generation of TCAs that possess additional pharmacological properties such as lack of a cardiodepressant effect (lofepramine), and neuroleptic-like properties (amoxapine). The most widely prescribed TCAs in the UK are imipramine, amitriptyline, dothiepin and clomipramine.

Indications

Depression

There is now a large body of evidence from well-controlled clinical trials that TCAs are superior to placebo in the treatment of depression. These drugs are recommended for treating patients suffering from moderate or severe depression. A good therapeutic response is expected in patients with endogenous depression characterised by retardation or agitation.

Anxiety states

These drugs are useful in anxiety disorder; indeed, in certain patients they may be more effective than benzodiazepines. However, the relation between their anxiolytic and antidepressant effects remains unclear.

Obsessive–compulsive disorder (OCD)

TCAs have been shown to reduce the severity of OCD symptoms, usually in parallel with changes in anxiety and depression ratings.

Phobic states

TCAs have been used successfully to treat agoraphobia, both alone and in combination with behaviour therapy. It seems that they enhance the effectiveness of exposure treatment.

Briquet's syndrome

This somatisation disorder occurs mainly in women. TCAs have been found beneficial in this condition, possibly because Briquet's syndrome is often accompanied by depression.

Eating disorders

TCAs have been found beneficial both in bulimia nervosa and anorexia nervosa. Their effectiveness in bulimia is probably related to their antidepressant effect: they decrease binge frequency and binge intensity, and lift the accompanying depression.

Hyperactivity and attention deficit in children

Smaller doses of TCAs (e.g. 25–100 mg imipramine daily) have been found beneficial in this condition. Unlike the case with depression, the therapeutic effect is not delayed after initiation of treatment, and so it is thought that it is independent of the antidepressant effect.

Enuresis

Relatively small doses of TCAs (e.g. 50 mg imipramine daily) are useful in this condition. The therapeutic effect has an instantaneous onset; however, tolerance can occur. Apart from childhood enuresis, these drugs can be useful in alleviating incontinence in the elderly. The mechanism is likely to be noradrenaline uptake blockade leading to sympathetic stimulation of the bladder sphincter.

Cataplexy

The effectiveness of TCAs in this condition may be related to their ability to suppress REM sleep.

Chronic pain

The TCAs are used for the treatment of chronic pain; their effectiveness in this condition may be partly related to the alleviation of the accompanying depression.

Contraindications and precautions

Cardiac disease

As the classical TCAs are cardiotoxic, they are contraindicated when cardiac function is compromised by disease. Thus, a history of recent myocardial infarction is an absolute contraindication, since TCAs could produce arrhythmias or heart failure. Bundle branch block is another contraindication, since these drugs can evoke a full atrioventricular blockade.

Epilepsy

As TCAs lower the seizure threshold, they should be used in epileptic patients with caution (e.g. the dosage of the anticonvulsant drug should be increased).

Prostate hypertrophy

These drugs should be avoided in this condition since they can provoke urinary retention.

Mania

TCAs can provoke mania; they should therefore not be given to patients with mania and should be used only with caution for patients with bipolar illness.

Pregnancy

All TCAs pass the placental barrier. Although there is no clear indication of a teratogenic potential, these drugs should be avoided in pregnancy. However, it should be noted that many of the classical TCAs have been used in pregnant women without obvious ill effects.

Age

TCAs are prescribed for children presenting with depression, hyperactivity, enuresis or school phobia. There is a low therapeutic:toxic ratio in children and thus caution is needed in selecting the appropriate dose. Although children metabolise these drugs faster than adults do, they have relatively little body fat that could act as an inactivating reservoir for the drug.

The elderly are especially sensitive to the toxic effects of TCAs. They also have a lower rate of drug metabolism and thus lower doses should be used. Furthermore, concurrent physical disease (prostate hypertrophy, heart disease) often renders the use of TCAs hazardous in these patients.

Side-effects and toxicity

Central nervous system

Drowsiness and impairment of psychomotor performance are frequent complications (Hindmarch et al, 1992). The lowering of the seizure threshold can result in convulsions. Mania can be precipitated in susceptible patients (e.g. those with a history of bipolar affective illness). A toxic confusional state ('atropine psychosis') is a rare complication of treatment with potent anticholinergic TCAs (e.g. amitriptyline); the risk of this reaction is greatly enhanced by the co-administration of another anticholinergic drug (e.g. phenothiazines, anti-Parkinsonian drugs).

Autonomic nervous system

As discussed earlier, TCAs produce a variety of effects on autonomically innervated tissues as a result of their *anticholinergic, sympathomimetic* and *sympatholytic* actions.

Glandular secretions. The anticholinergic effect of TCAs leads to a reduction in glandular secretions. Thus, these drugs all produce xerostomia and xerophthalmia, and reduce gastric secretion. The xerostomia can be very distressing for the patient, especially since it is added to the reduction in salivary secretion that accompanies depressive illness and can promote dental decay (Szabadi & Tavernor, 1999). The reduction in gastric secretion can be beneficial since it can result in the healing of gastric ulcers. The sympathomimetic effects of these drugs can manifest as increased sweating and an increase in physiological finger tremor.

The eye. The anticholinergic effect results in accommodation block, which the patient experiences as blurred vision. The effect on the size of the pupil depends on the relationship between the multiple actions of these drugs, the anticholinergic and sympathomimetic effects leading to mydriasias and the sympatholytic effect resulting in miosis. Thus, the weak anticholinergic drug desipramine causes mydriasis, probably owing to its potent sympathomimetic effect, whereas the potent anticholinergic drug amitriptyline has little effect on pupil size since the mydriasis resulting from the anticholinergic and sympathomimetic effects is counterbalanced by the miosis resulting from the sympatholytic effect. It is often stated that TCAs can precipitate an attack of glaucoma because of their anticholinergic property. However, amitriptyline, which is the most potent anticholinergic of the TCAs, is unlikely to provoke glaucoma since it has little effect on pupil size, whereas desipramine, a drug that has relatively low anticholinergic potency, is likely to carry a higher risk of provoking glaucoma because of its mydriatic effect (see Szabadi & Bradshaw, 1986).

Cardiovascular system. The autonomic control of both the heart and the blood vessels is affected. Many TCAs produce sinus tachycardia, as a result partly of their vagolytic (anticholinergic) effect and partly of their sympathomimetic effect. Postural hypotension is a frequent complication; it is mainly related to the blockade of peripheral α_1-adrenoceptors.

Gastrointestinal system. The anticholinergic effect reduces gastric secretion, and the anticholinergic and sympathomimetic effects reduce propulsive bowel movements. The clinical manifestation of these changes is constipation, and in extreme cases paralytic ileus.

Genito-urinary system. Both bladder functions and sexual functions are affected. Urinary hesitancy and retention may result, from both the anticholinergic and the sympathomimetic effects of these drugs. Erectile impotence can be related to the anticholinergic property of the drugs, whereas ejaculatory incompetence can result from the blockade of α_1-adrenoceptors in the vas deferens and the seminal vesicles.

Cardiovascular system

Tachycardia and orthostatic hypotension are frequent complications of treatment with TCAs; they are related mainly to the effects of these drugs on the autonomic nervous system (see above). In addition, TCAs have a direct effect on cardiac tissue that impairs cardiac conduction and decreases myocardial contractility (see Cassem, 1982).

Liver

Abnormal liver function test results have been reported in some patients treated with TCAs; these probably reflect a hypersensitivity reaction.

Bone marrow

Agranulocytosis is a rare but severe hypersensitivity reaction that occurs mainly in elderly women during the second month of treatment. Regular blood counts are a useful precaution.

Skin

Rashes (urticaria, photosensitivity reactions and cutaneous vasculitis) can occur in susceptible individuals.

Metabolic and endocrine changes

These include weight gain and inappropriate secretion of the anti-diuretic hormone (ADH).

Drug interactions

MAOIs

Co-administration of TCAs and MAOIs can lead to a toxic reaction characterised by hyperthermia, mydriasis, hyperreflexia, convulsions and coma (see under 'Monoamine oxidase inhibitors', above); therefore, this combination should be avoided.

Sympathomimetic amines

TCAs potentiate the pressor effects of directly acting sympathomimetic amines (e.g. adrenaline, noradrenaline) and so may lead to hazardous hypertension. Therefore, the co-administration of these drugs should be avoided (even the small amounts of these amines present in dental anaesthetics can be dangerous).

Methylphenidate

This has a hypertensive interaction with TCAs.

Antihypertensive drugs

The TCAs inhibit the antihypertensive effects of adrenergic neuron blocking agents (e.g. guanethidine), probably by blocking the uptake of these drugs into the sympathetic nerve terminal. The antihypertensive effects of α-methyl-DOPA and clonidine are also inhibited by TCAs; the mechanism of this interaction remains unknown.

Alcohol

Alcohol can produce drowsiness when co-administered with TCAs and can lead to a decrement in psychomotor performance that is greater than that produced by either drug on its own.

Additive interactions

The antimuscarinic properties of anticholinergic drugs (e.g. benztropine, procyclidine) and TCAs, and the membrane-stabilising effects of quinidine-like drugs (e.g. quinidine, disopyramide) and TCAs are additive and, therefore, caution is needed when these drugs are co-administered.

Pharmacokinetic interactions

Both phenothiazine and butyrophenone neuroleptics inhibit the metabolism of TCAs. Barbiturates facilitate the metabolism of TCAs by the liver, probably through the induction of microsomal enzymes, which leads to a fall in the plasma level of the antidepressant. This can result in the loss of the antidepressant effect. Oral contraceptives can reduce the bioavailability and thus the plasma level of TCAs. Cimetidine interferes with the clearance of imipramine and desipramine and can lead to an increase in the plasma concentration of these drugs. Tobacco smoking has been reported to be associated with a reduction in the plasma level of imipramine.

'Pure' non-selective monoamine uptake inhibitors (the SNRIs)

These drugs block the uptake of both noradrenaline and serotonin without other pharmacological actions. In particular, these drugs do not have any appreciable affinity for neuroreceptors, which are believed to play a role in mediating the side-effects of TCAs. Interestingly, the development of these drugs is the result of the recognition that the tricyclic antidepressants are more effective than the SSRIs for the treatment of patients with severe depression (e.g. severe enough to

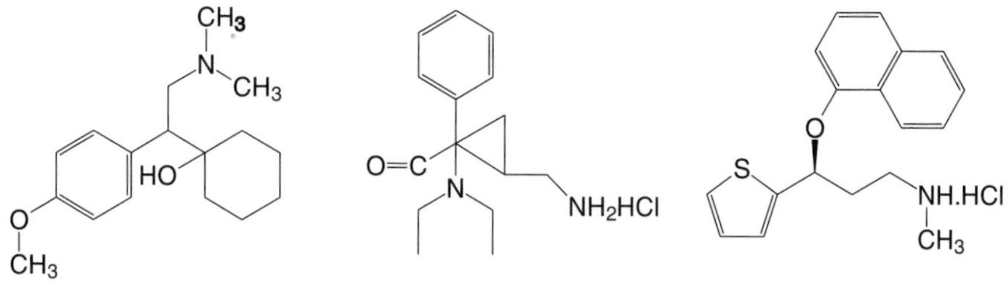

Venlafaxine   Milnacipran   Duloxetine

Fig. 6.5 Chemical structures of some serotonin/noradrenaline reuptake inhibitors (SNRIs).

warrant hospital admission). Therefore, the 'pure' non-selective mono-amine uptake inhibitors were developed as SSRIs with the property of noradrenaline uptake inhibition 'grafted on'. These drugs, usually referred to as 'serotonin/noradrenaline reuptake inhibitors' (SNRIs), include venlafaxine, milnacipran and duloxetine (Fig. 6.5), of which only venlafaxine is available for prescription in the UK.

There is evidence that the action of venlafaxine is dose dependent: at lower doses the drug selectively inhibits the uptake of serotonin, and so acts as an SSRI, whereas at higher doses it inhibits the uptake of both serotonin and noradrenaline. Thus, it has been reported that human volunteers treated with venlafaxine show a reduction of serotonin uptake into blood platelets at all dosage levels, but only at higher doses (e.g. at single doses in excess of 150 mg) is there any indication of the inhibition of noradrenaline uptake (e.g. potentiation of the constriction of the dorsal hand vein evoked by noradrenaline, antagonism of the rise in blood pressure evoked by tyramine) (Abdelmawla *et al*, 1999; Harvey *et al*, 2000). Therefore, it is recommended that treatment should start at a low dose, at which the drug is presumed to act as a pure SSRI, and only when an antidepressant effect is not observable should the dosage be increased in order to 'augment' the effect of the SSRI by recruitment of an additional effect on noradrenaline reuptake.

The side-effects of venlafaxine are the same as those observed with other SSRIs (see below), the most troublesome being nausea. The sleep pattern may also be affected, both insomnia and daytime somnolence having been reported. There are also changes in sleep architecture: while slow wave sleep is unaffected, there is a marked suppression of REM sleep (Reite, 1998). Venlafaxine treatment may be associated with sustained increases in blood pressure, probably reflecting a sympathomimetic effect resulting from noradrenaline uptake inhibition. Venlafaxine can also cause dry mouth: this 'pseudo-anticholinergic' effect is presumably brought about by the inhibition of noradrenaline reuptake at central noradrenergic synapses, leading to the potentiation of the central noradrenergic inhibition of salivary secretion (Szabadi & Tavernor, 1999). Other adverse effects include the precipitation of mania, provocation of seizures, and, in some patients, hyponatraemia. A toxic interaction with MAOIs, leading to a serotonin syndrome, is the most severe drug interaction involving venlafaxine. As venlafaxine has a relatively short half-life (5–7 hours), its abrupt discontination may lead to a 'discontinuation' syndrome (nausea, dizziness, insomnia, headache). Therefore, it is recommended not to discontinue the drug abruptly, but to taper the dosage gradually over several days.

Selective noradrenaline uptake inhibitors (NARIs)

Some antidepressants are potent inhibitors of noradrenaline uptake but have relatively little affinity for the serotonin uptake mechanism. These include oxaprotiline, maprotiline, desipramine, nomifensine, nortriptyline and viloxazine (see Fig. 6.3). Although oxaprotiline and maprotiline are highly selective drugs, desipramine is more potent than either of these. Reboxetine (a more recently developed drug) shows the same potency as desipramine in inhibiting noradrenaline uptake, but a somewhat lower potency than desipramine in inhibiting serotonin uptake (Wong *et al*, 2000).

The chemical structures of some of these drugs are shown in Fig. 6.6. Desipramine and nortriptyline are TCAs (see Fig. 6.4). Oxaprotiline and maprotiline are ethanoanthracene derivatives: the central ring of a tricyclic structure is bridged by an ethylene chain, forming a rigid tetracyclic structure. Nomifensine is a tetrahydroisoquinoline, and viloxazine and reboxetine are morpholines. Thus, the selective noradrenaline uptake inhibitors form a chemically heterogeneous group.

Desipramine and *nortriptyline* share the pharmacological properties of other TCAs; they have a number of effects in addition to noradrenaline uptake blockade (e.g. inhibitory effect on serotonin uptake, blockade of muscarinic cholinoceptors, α_1-adrenoceptors and H_1 histamine receptors). *Nomifensine*, apart from blocking noradrenaline uptake, is a potent inhibitor of dopamine uptake. In fact, radioactively labelled nomifensine can be used experimentally to label the dopamine transporter in brain tissue. As a dopaminergic drug, nomifensine has some behavioural activating ('amphetamine-like') effects. *Viloxazine* is a selective but rather weak inhibitor of noradrenaline uptake. It has only very weak anticholinergic effects.

Desipramine and nortriptyline are considered together with the TCAs. Of the remaining drugs, only maprotiline and reboxetine are clinically important. Viloxazine is available for prescription in the UK but is very rarely used, probably because there is little convincing evidence for its clinical effectiveness. Nomifensine is an effective

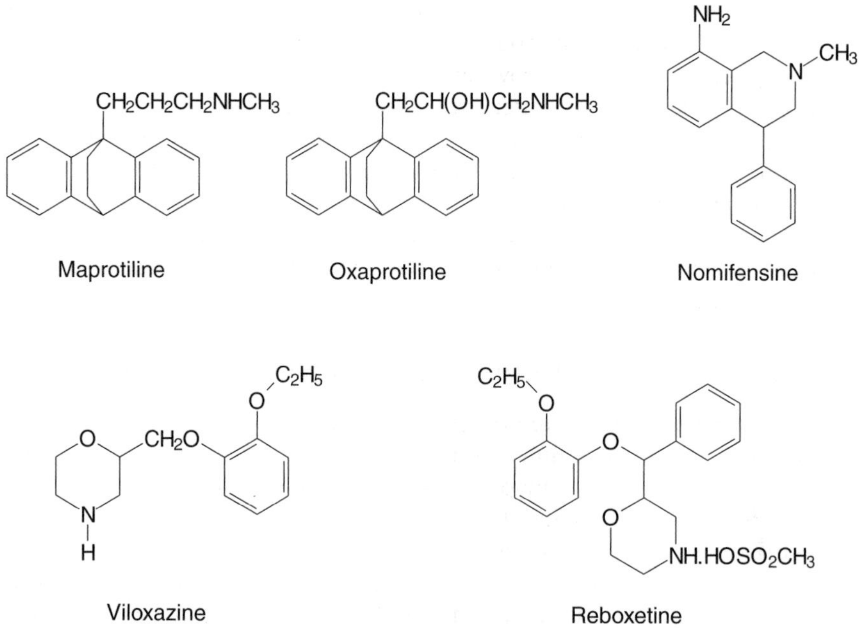

Fig. 6.6 Chemical structures of some selective noradrenaline uptake inhibitors (NARIs).

antidepressant; however, it has been withdrawn due to rare, but severe, idiosyncratic toxic effects (mainly blood dyscrasias).

Maprotiline

Basic pharmacology

Maprotiline and oxaprotiline have very similar pharmacological profiles: they are both potent inhibitors of noradrenaline uptake but have little effect on serotonin uptake. They have relatively low affinities for muscarinic cholinoceptors; for example, maprotiline is 30 times less potent than amitriptyline. They do not block α_1-adrenoceptors. During chronic treatment, like TCAs, they reduce the number of central α_2-adrenoceptors. In behavioural tests of antidepressant activity, oxaprotiline and maprotiline act like TCAs. In general, they are less toxic than the TCAs, and show less toxic effect on the heart.

Clinical pharmacology

Maprotiline has relatively little effect on the autonomic nervous system; there are only weak anticholinergic effects and blood pressure is not affected. It has only weak effects on the heart (impairment of cardiac conduction and some depression of contractility). The waking electroencephalogram (EEG) is only slightly affected: single oral doses may cause an increase in alpha waves, probably reflecting a general relaxant effect; however, there are no EEG changes during chronic treatment. There are changes in the sleep EEG: REM sleep latency decreases and time spent in REM sleep increases. This pattern is opposite to that observed with TCAs.

Maprotiline is slowly, but almost completely, absorbed from the gut; the peak plasma concentration appears 9–16 hours after a single oral dose. It has relatively long elimination half-life (27–58 hours). A high proportion (approximately 88%) of the drug is bound to plasma proteins. The drug readily crosses lipid membranes and is widely distributed in body tissues. It is excreted in breast milk (the milk:blood concentration ratio is 1:5). It is almost fully metabolised in the liver; the two major routes of metabolism are demethylation and hydroxylation. The hydroxylated products are excreted as conjugated glucuronides by the kidneys.

Indications, contraindications and side-effects

Maprotiline is recommended for the treatment of most forms of depression. It is claimed that it produces fewer side-effects and is less toxic in overdose than the conventional TCAs. One single daily dose is appropriate; however, the daily dose should not exceed 150 mg. Above this level the side-effects become troublesome and there is no evidence of an increase in therapeutic effectiveness.

The drug is usually administered on its own; however, the co-administration of a night-time hypnotic is not contraindicated. It is also possible to administer electroconvulsive therapy (ECT) to patients who are being treated with maprotiline.

Contraindications include mania, epilepsy and recent myocardial infarction. The drug should also be avoided in patients suffering from severe liver or kidney disease, since these conditions interfere with removal of the drug and are associated with increased plasma levels.

Although it has only relatively low affinity for muscarinic cholino-ceptors, anticholinergic side-effects can appear at higher dosage levels, and therefore it should not be prescribed to patients suffering from narrow-angle glaucoma or urinary retention. It is generally well tolerated, and there have been very few deaths associated with overdose. Severe idiosyncratic reactions are rare and include agranulocytosis and cholestatic jaundice. Despite the lack of EEG changes, grand mal seizures can occur; drowsiness, nausea and tremor are usually not severe and abate with time.

Autonomic side-effects are sympathomimetic (tachycardia, increased sweating, tremor), sympatholytic (orthostatic hypotension) and anti-cholinergic (dry mouth, constipation, urinary hesitancy). The anti-cholinergic side-effects are more likely to be due to noradrenaline uptake inhibition at central and peripheral noradrenergic synapses than to the blockade of muscarinic cholinoceptors ('pseudo-anticholinergic effects'; for discussion see section on reboxetine, below). The cardio-vascular side-effects are similar to those of TCAs, although they are less pronounced and are reversible. Skin rashes have been reported more frequently than with the classical TCAs.

Although there is no evidence for any teratogenicity, the drug should be avoided in pregnant women. The elderly are more susceptible to some of the side-effects (postural hypotension, urinary hesitancy) and, therefore, lower doses and more gradual build-up to the final dosage is recommended in this patient group.

The most important drug interactions are with directly acting sympathomimetic amines (e.g. adrenaline, noradrenaline), whose pressor effects are potentiated, and with some antihypertensive drugs, whose lowering of blood pressure is attenuated by the co-administration of maprotiline.

Reboxetine

Basic pharmacology

Reboxetine is one of the most potent and selective inhibitors of noradrenaline uptake, and has practically no affinity for neuroreceptors. Reboxetine's high affinity for the noradrenaline transporter and relatively low affinity for the serotonin transporter have been confirmed by direct study of a cell line in tissue culture transfected with the human noradrenaline and serotonin transporters (Wong *et al*, 2000). Reboxetine also shows activity in animal models of antidepressant drug action (see above).

Clinical pharmacology

Reboxetine shows some sympathomimetic activity, as would be expected of a noradrenaline uptake inhibitor, in human subjects: small increases in heart rate and blood pressure have been reported. The drug also increases pupil diameter, which could be related to sympathetic potentiation. However, the increase in pupil diameter may also be due to a 'pseudo-anticholinergic' effect, which may arise from the potentiation of the central noradrenergic inhibition of parasympathetic functions. Such a mechanism may explain some other 'pseudo-anti-cholinergic' effects of the drug, such as attenuation of the pupillary light reflex and reduction in salivary output (which can lead patients to complain of having a dry mouth). The potentiation of the noradrenergic inhibition of the voiding function of the urinary bladder may lead to urinary hesitancy/retention. The potentiation of the noradrenergic inhibition of gut motility may lead to constipation, and the potentiation of the noradrenergic excitatory input to preganglionic sympathetic fibres may increase sweating.

Reboxetine is almost completely absorbed from the gut and it is highly bound to plasma proteins. It shows linear pharmacokinetics: the plasma level directly reflects the administered oral dosage. The drug is eliminated through hepatic metabolism; it has been shown not to affect the metabolism of a large number of other drugs.

Indications, contraindications and side-effects

Reboxetine is indicated for the treatment of all forms of depression. It has been suggested that, because of its noradrenergic 'activating' effect, it may be especially useful for patients who complain of lack of energy and motivation. Reboxetine is recommended for both the acute treatment of depression and the maintenance of clinical improvement in patients who have responded to initial treatment.

Like most novel centrally acting drugs, reboxetine is contraindicated for women who are pregnant or breast-feeding. Adoption of lower doses may be necessary in patients with renal and hepatic failure. Like other antidepressants, reboxetine has the propensity to precipitate mania. Patients suffering from seizure disorders require close monitoring and, if necessary, adjustment of the dosage of the anticonvulsant.

Side-effects include insomnia, dry mouth, increased sweating, urinary hesitancy/retention and tachycardia, consistent with the alerting/sympathetic activating action of the drug (see above). The adverse effect of reboxetine on the urinary bladder, which is due to potentiation of the inhibitory effect of noradrenaline on the detrusor muscle, can be counteracted by co-administration of doxazosin, an α_1-adrenoceptor antagonist which does not pass the blood–brain barrier (Szabadi & Bradshaw, 2000).

As a sympathomimetic drug, reboxetine may enhance the pressor effects of sympathomimetic amines. Co-administration of reboxetine with MAOIs should be avoided owing to the enhanced risk of a 'cheese reaction'.

Selective serotonin uptake inhibitors (SSRIs)

Chemistry

Of the TCAs, clomipramine is a potent inhibitor of serotonin uptake, and it also shows a degree of selectivity for the serotonin uptake mechanism (see Fig. 6.3). However, a number of novel drugs have been developed that are much more selective inhibitors of serotonin uptake than clomipramine. These constitute the group of SSRIs. They include zimeldine, citalopram, fluvoxamine, fluoxetine, paroxetine and sertraline (see Fig. 6.7). It can be seen that they are a chemically heterogeneous group.

Zimeldine was withdrawn following isolated reports of a severe idiosyncratic toxic reaction (Guillain–Barré syndrome). We consider only the other five compounds that are used therapeutically (i.e. citalopram, fluvoxamine, fluoxetine, paroxetine and sertraline). Recently, the pharmacologically active stereo isomer of citalopram (escitalopram) has become available, whose efficacay is approximately twice that of the racemate.

Cellular and receptor pharmacology

The most important common pharmacological feature of these drugs is the selective inhibition of serotonin uptake (see Fig. 6.3); SSRIs have high affinity for the serotonin transporter (radioactively labelled SSRIs can be used to identify it).

Of the six SSRIs shown in Fig. 6.7, citalopram is the most selective and paroxetine is the most potent. The selectivity and potency of the SSRIs for inhibiting serotonin uptake is maintained on repeated administration. These drugs, in contrast to the TCAs, have very little

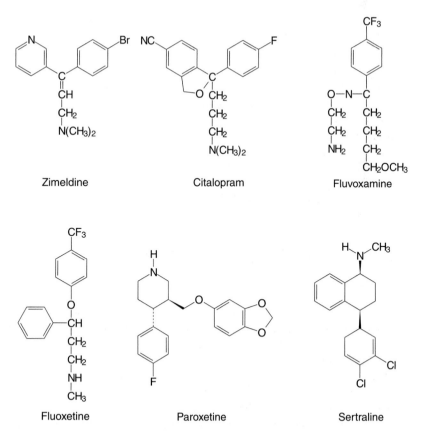

Fig. 6.7 Chemical structures of selective serotonin reuptake inhibitors (SSRIs).

affinity for neurotransmitter receptors, including different subtypes of adrenoceptor, serotonin receptors, muscarinic cholinoceptors and dopamine receptors. On chronic administration, some of the SSRIs (i.e. fluvoxamine, fluoxetine and sertraline), like conventional TCAs, down-regulate central β-adrenoceptors; however, citalopram and paroxetine do not share this effect. Chronic treatment with SSRIs results in complex changes in central 5-HT receptors: 5-HT_{1A} receptors on serotonergic neurons ('autoreceptors') are desensitised, whereas 5-HT_{1A} receptors on postsynaptic cells remain unaffected. Furthermore, like the TCAs, SSRIs down-regulate postsynaptic 5-HT_2 receptors (see Cowen, 1990).

Organ and systems pharmacology

In the brain, the SSRIs may interact with the extrapyramidal dopaminergic system: it has been shown that fluoxetine reduces the turnover of dopamine in the basal ganglia. This interaction may be the basis for the extrapyramidal side-effects observed occasionally in patients treated with the SSRIs. These drugs, like the TCAs and MAOIs, suppress REM sleep in laboratory animals but they do not interact with the autonomic nervous system and have little effect on the cardiovascular system.

Behavioural pharmacology

On their own, the SSRIs have remarkably little effect on unconditioned animal behaviour. However, when they are co-administered with other drugs that increase the availability of serotonin (e.g. the serotonin precursors tryptophan, 5-hydroxytryptophan and tryptamine, or MAOIs), they induce the 'serotonin syndrome'. This is characterised by general locomotor activation and some abnormal movements (e.g. head twitches, 'wet dog shake', reciprocal forepaw treading, etc.). A similar toxic interaction can occur between SSRIs and tryptophan or SSRIs and MAOIs in humans, leading to the human serotonin syndrome. The SSRIs reduce food intake in animals, leading to weight loss.

Like other classes of antidepressant drugs, SSRIs alter performance in the DRL-72s schedule – they reduce the response rate and increase the obtained reinforcement rate. There have also been some reports that SSRIs reduce 'impulsive choice' in animals and promote selection of larger delayed rewards in preference to smaller immediate rewards.

Clinical pharmacology

The presence of SSRIs in the plasma can be detected by inhibition of the uptake of radioactively labelled serotonin into platelets. On acute dosing in human volunteers, SSRIs, unlike TCAs, cause little sedation, and psychomotor performance usually remains unimpaired (Hindmarch *et al*, 1992). The sleep EEG shows suppression of REM sleep. There is little effect on cardiovascular functions, although most SSRIs cause a small drop in heart rate. In general, they do not affect autonomic functions. Fluvoxamine, however, has been shown to be a weak inhibitor of pharmacological responses mediated by cholinoceptors (e.g. carbachol-evoked sweating). The most common effect of acute single doses of SSRIs is nausea.

As with other antidepressants, the full human pharmacological spectrum of the SSRIs can be ascertained only in *patients* suffering from affective disorders. The SSRIs have both antidepressant and anti-anxiety properties. Furthermore, these drugs are effective in alleviating the psychopathological features of OCD: both obsessional thought patterns and compulsive rituals are affected. As with the TCAs, the anti-depressant effect is established gradually, and it may take 2–3 weeks before the effectiveness of an SSRI can be detected.

Pharmacokinetics

The SSRIs are a chemically heterogeneous group with diverse pharmaco-kinetic properties (DeVane, 1992). All SSRIs are rather slowly, but almost completely, absorbed from the gut; the time to peak plasma concentration following a single oral dose varies from 2–8 hours (fluvoxamine) to 6–10 hours (sertraline). They all have rather long elimination half-lives, which allows for once-daily administration of these drugs. Fluvoxamine has the shortest (15 hours) and fluoxetine the longest (84 hours) plasma half-life. It should be noted that norfluoxetine, the active metabolite of fluoxetine, has an elimination half-life of 146 hours.

Because of the slow clearance of fluoxetine and its active metabolite, at least 5 weeks should be allowed before an MAOI is introduced after discontinuation of treatment with fluoxetine (to avoid the danger of the serotonin syndrome – see 'Contraindications and precautions', below).

All these drugs are extensively metabolised in the liver, mainly by hydroxylation to inactive metabolites that are excreted in the urine as conjugates of glucuronic acid. Fluoxetine and sertraline, however, are also metabolised by demethylation, and the demethylated derivatives of both drugs (norfluoxetine and desmethylsertraline) show SSRI activity. These lipid-soluble drugs are widely distributed in tissues and thus show large volumes of distribution.

Fluoxetine displays non-linear elimination kinetics, probably owing to the saturation of liver enzymes: higher doses can result in dispropor-tionately high plasma levels. Moreover, fluoxetine may accumulate during treatment with higher doses over several weeks; this may explain the appearance of some side-effects (e.g. sedation) rather late in the course of treatment with this drug.

All SSRIs bind to plasma proteins, fluoxetine, paroxetine and sertraline to approximately 95% of the saturation level, fluvoxamine to 77%. Thus, fluvoxamine may be safer than the other SSRIs for patients who are being treated with a highly protein-bound drug with a low therapeutic index (e.g. warfarin), since fluvoxamine is less likely to displace the other drug from the protein binding sites.

Indications

Depression

According to clinical trial data, these drugs are probably as effective as the TCAs in treating depression; however, earlier claims that they act faster have not been confirmed. There is no evidence that they are effective in depression that is resistant to treatment with more conventional antidepressants (see Edwards, 1992). In addition to the treatment of acute depressive episodes, SSRIs are suitable for continued treatment in order to prevent relapse.

Anxiety

These drugs have anti-anxiety and antipanic effects, which may be independent of the antidepressive effect.

Obsessive–compulsive disorder

The SSRIs have a unique role in treating OCD: they may reduce both obsessional thinking and compulsive rituals. Their effectiveness in this regard seems to be independent of their antidepressant effect. They are probably more effective than clomipramine, which is regarded as the TCA of choice for OCD.

Eating disorders

There is increasing evidence for the effectiveness of these drugs in bulimia nervosa: they decrease carbohydrate craving and reduce both the frequency and the intensity of binges. As SSRIs have an anorectic effect in animals and can lead to weight loss, they have been tried for the treatment of obesity. There is no convincing evidence for their usefulness in this condition, although, unlike TCAs, they do not lead to weight increase in depressed patients.

Impulse control disorders

Patients suffering from aggressive outbursts and repetitive self-harming behaviours may benefit from these drugs (Kavoussi & Coccaro, 1998). The rationale for this use is supported by some evidence that there is a deficiency of central serotonergic activity in impulse control disorders in general, and in impulsive aggression in particular (Coccaro, 1998).

Neurological disorders

The SSRIs have been tried in a number of neurological conditions; their effectiveness in some of these requires confirmation. There are reports that fluvoxamine can alleviate the psychological symptoms of Gilles de la Tourette's syndrome but not the motor stereotypies. There are reports that some myoclonic syndromes, cataplexy and chronic pain syndromes (e.g. pain associated with diabetic neuropathy) may benefit from the administration of SSRIs.

Other potential indications

The SSRIs may have a role in the treatment of substance misuse: there are reports that they can reduce craving and alcohol intake in alcoholic patients.

Contraindications and precautions

Treatment with MAOIs

This is an absolute contraindication since the combined use of the two classes of drug can evoke a toxic reaction ('serotonin syndrome') that can be fatal. In order to avoid this complication at least a fortnight should be allowed after the discontinuation of treatment with an MAOI before an SSRI is introduced; if an SSRI is replaced by an MAOI, an even longer gap may be required between the two treatments (at least 5 weeks in the case of fluoxetine, as discussed above).

Mania

The SSRIs are contraindicated in mania and should be used cautiously in bipolar illness.

Severe renal failure

Fluoxetine should be avoided in this condition since there can be an accumulation of both the parent drug and its metabolite.

Liver disease

Caution is needed, since liver cirrhosis may increase the elimination half-life of fluoxetine.

Diabetes mellitus

Caution is needed, since fluoxetine can produce both hypoglycaemia (during treatment) and hyperglycaemia (on discontinuation of treatment).

Age

Although these drugs are not recommended for children (ABPI, 1999/2000), their use is increasing for the treatment of OCD in patients under 18 years of age. The SSRIs are not recommended for pregnant and breast-feeding women.

The favourable side-effect profile of these drugs (see below) would indicate that they are especially suitable for the treatment of elderly patients (they cause little sedation and psychomotor impairment, there is no interaction with the autonomic nervous system and little effect on cardiovascular functions). It should be noted, however, that paroxetine is metabolised more slowly by elderly people, whereas age does not seem to influence the pharmacokinetics of fluvoxamine. Fluoxetine has been reported to be poorly tolerated by some elderly patients.

Side-effects and toxicity

Central nervous system

The most severe, but rare, psychiatric adverse effect is the precipitation of mania. More commonly these drugs can induce feelings of anxiety ('nervousness') and insomnia, or, paradoxically, drowsiness and daytime somnolence. This latter complication is especially likely to occur with higher doses of fluoxetine (above 20 mg daily).

There have been reports of increased suicidal ideation in depressed patients treated with fluoxetine; this, however, has not been confirmed and it is likely that the reported increase in suicidal ideation was due to personality factors and other aspects of the psychopathology rather than to the SSRI (see Edwards, 1992). In fact, the SSRIs have been specifically recommended for depressed patients with suicidal tendencies.

In contrast to the TCAs, the SSRIs have little effect on psychomotor functions.

Neurological side-effects include tremor, various extrapyramidal syndromes (akathisia, dystonia, orolingual dyskinesia, worsening of neuroleptic-induced parkinsonism) and convulsive seizures. The precipitation of seizures can be observed with all antidepressants, although it seems to be less likely with SSRIs than with TCAs.

Gastrointestinal system

Anorexia, nausea (and vomiting) and diarrhoea are frequent complaints, with nausea being reported by over 20% of patients in clinical trials with SSRIs (Edwards & Anderson, 1999). Fluvoxamine seems to induce nausea more frequently than fluoxetine, probably because of its faster absorption. The development of nausea can be mitigated by gradual build-up to the final dosage or co-administration of a small dose of a phenothiazine (e.g. 25 mg chlorpromazine three times daily), or both.

Cardiovascular system

These drugs cause a small drop in heart rate; this effect does not seem to have any clinical significance. Otherwise the cardiovascular system is unaffected.

Sexual functions

Delayed ejaculation and anorgasmia (in both men and women) have been reported and can be distressing for some patients. Libido can also be reduced by SSRIs.

Drug interactions

MAOIs

The co-administration of SSRIs and MAOIs results in a toxic reaction (the 'serotonin syndrome'), which is believed to be due to a sudden rise in the concentration of serotonin at the relevant synapses in the brain due to inhibition of the elimination of serotonin by the two classes of drug. The syndrome is reminiscent of the neuroleptic malignant syndrome: initially the patient is restless and agitated and complains of nausea, vomiting or diarrhoea; later, hyperthermia, rigidity, myoclonus or tremor, autonomic instability (tachycardia, hypertension), fluctuating levels of consciousness, and finally convulsions and coma supervene. This is a potentially lethal condition; deaths have been reported when an MAOI was introduced too soon after discontinuing fluoxetine (less than 5 weeks; Edwards, 1992). For treatment, cyproheptadine (a serotonin antagonist), chlorpromazine and dantrolene (a muscle relaxant) have been recommended (Gillman, 1999).

Tryptophan

This precursor of serotonin can result in the 'serotonin syndrome' in the presence of an SSRI (see above).

Lithium

Both pharmacokinetic and pharmacodynamic interactions have been reported. In terms of the former, SSRIs may change the plasma level of lithium – both increases and decreases have been described – and there have been instances of manifest lithium toxicity. Therefore, especially careful and frequent monitoring of lithium plasma levels is required in patients who are on lithium maintenance treatment and in whom an SSRI is introduced. In terms of the latter, lithium may enhance the serotonergic effect of the SSRI and lead to the 'serotonin syndrome'.

Alcohol

Although the SSRIs have little effect on psychomotor performance, they have been shown to potentiate the detrimental effect of alcohol.

Pharmacokinetic interactions

The SSRIs inhibit the metabolism of drugs by oxidative microsomal enzymes in the liver and thus can increase the plasma levels of drugs that are metabolised by these enzymes. Thus, twofold increases in the plasma levels of TCAs have been described in patients also taking an SSRI. Other drugs affected are warfarin, phenytoin, theophylline and propranolol (but not atenolol). As SSRIs bind to plasma proteins, they can displace other drugs from the binding sites and thus increase the free level and potential toxicity of the displaced drug. Fluvoxamine has been reported to reduce the clearance of diazepam and thus prolong its half-life.

Other drugs

This group comprises molecules with antidepressant activities that do not fit readily into the categories of MAOIs or monoamine uptake inhibitors. None of these drugs has any appreciable effect on MAO, and if they have some uptake-inhibiting property it is combined with some complex interactions with neuroreceptors. This group includes mianserin, mirtazapine, trazodone, nefazodone, tryptophan, buspirone, and a mixture of compounds contained in the medicinal plant St John's wort (*Hypericum perforatum*).

The structures of some of these drugs are shown in Fig. 6.8. It is apparent that there is no common structural pattern: mianserin and mirtazapine are tetracyclic compounds, trazodone and nefazodone are triazolopyridine derivatives, tryptophan is an amino acid with an indole nucleus, and buspirone is a member of the azaspirodecanedione family. *Hypericum* contains numerous compounds with biological activity, of which hypericin and pseudohypericin have been most extensively studied; these compounds are naphthodiathrones.

Most of the compounds in this varied group share the propensity to enhance central monoamine transmission, either by blocking mono-amine uptake (mianserin, trazodone and nefazodone) or by increasing monoamine release (mianserin, mirtazapine and tryptophan). There is evidence that *Hypericum* extract acts in the former manner. In addition, these drugs may also interact with neuroceptors in a way that is thought to lead to an antidepressant effect (i.e. either antagonism of 5-HT_2 receptors or stimulation of 5-HT_{1A} receptors, or both: for details, see the section 'Common mode of action of antidepressants', below).

Mianserin

Basic pharmacology

Mianserin has a multiplicity of pharmacological actions. It is about as potent as amitriptyline or clomipramine in inhibiting the uptake of noradrenaline; however, it has little effect on the uptake of serotonin or dopamine (see Fig. 6.3). It has considerable α_2-adrenoceptor blocking property: the blockade of prejunctional release-modulating α_2-adreno-ceptors results in an increased release of noradrenaline. Owing to the

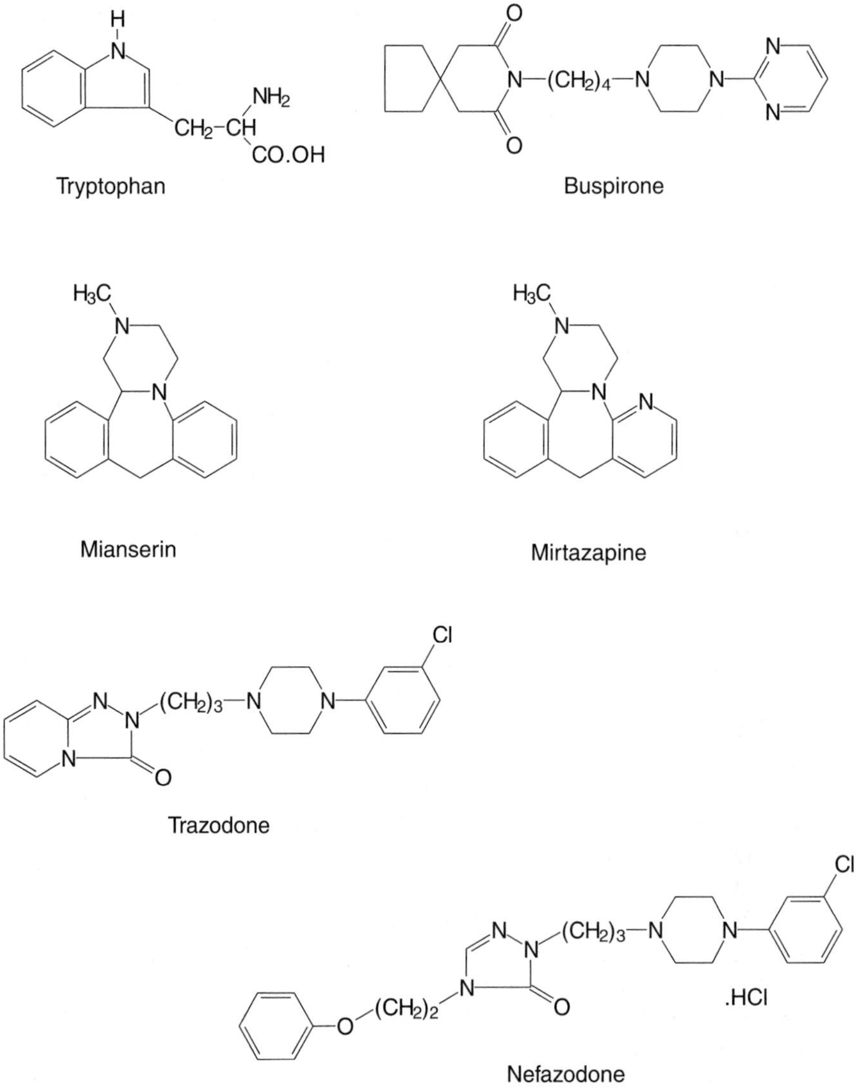

Fig. 6.8 Chemical structures of some antidepressants with multiple actions on central monoaminergic mechanisms ('other drugs').

blockade of α_2-adrenoceptors, mianserin antagonises the pharmacological actions of clonidine, an α_2-adrenoceptor agonist. It also has weak α_1-adrenoceptor antagonist properties. After chronic administration, mianserin down-regulates central β-adrenoceptors: it reduces cyclic AMP production via β-adrenoceptors without changing the number of β-adrenoceptors themselves.

Mianserin antagonises 5-HT$_2$ and 5-HT$_{1C}$ receptors and H$_1$ histamine receptors. It also inhibits the activation of adenylyl cyclase via H$_2$ histamine receptors in the brain. It is only a very weak antagonist at muscarinic cholinoceptors.

Mianserin has at least three pharmacological actions that may be related to its antidepressant efficacy: blockade of noradrenaline uptake, blockade of α_2-adrenoceptors and blockade of 5-HT$_2$ receptors. The blockade of α_2-adrenoceptors results in increased release of noradrenaline, which may correct a functional deficiency in depressed patients: indeed, there is some evidence that selective α_2-adrenoceptor antagonists (e.g. idazoxan) have antidepressant effects (Berlan et al, 1992). Furthermore, it has been suggested that the blockade of central 5-HT$_2$ receptors may also be associated with an antidepressant effect (Charney & Delgado, 1992).

Clinical pharmacology

Mianserin in acute doses has little effect in euthymic subjects. It is mildly sedative, and there are no anticholinergic effects. It reduces both spontaneous and pentagastrin-evoked gastric acid secretion, owing to an interaction with the H$_2$ histamine receptor complex. Although it has weak α_1-adrenoceptor blocking properties, cardiovascular functions remain largely unaffected. As with most other antidepressants, the antidepressant effect develops gradually, over 2–3 weeks of treatment.

Mianserin is rapidly absorbed from the gut, the peak plasma concentration appearing less than 3 hours after a single oral dose. The plasma half-life is 10–20 hours, which allows for once-daily administration. The elimination half-life is longer in the elderly (up to 40 hours). On multiple dosing, a steady-state plasma level is usually attained by the sixth day. The drug undergoes extensive presystemic metabolism in the liver, reducing its bioavailability to 20–30%. The hepatic metabolism involves demethylation, hydroxylation and oxidation; the hydroxylated products are excreted in the urine as conjugates of glucuronic acid. Two of its metabolites (desmethylmianserin and 8-hydroxymianserin) show weak α_2-adrenoceptor blocking properties.

Therapeutics

Mianserin is indicated for the treatment of people with relatively mild depression who can be treated as out-patients. As this drug does not have any anticholinergic or cardiotoxic effects, it is recommended for patients with prostate hypertrophy, glaucoma or cardiovascular disease. Furthermore, as it is relatively safe in overdose, it can be considered for impulsive patients with self-destructive behaviours. Like other antidepressants, mianserin is contraindicated in mania.

A common side-effect is drowsiness, which is most marked during the first few weeks of treatment. Increased appetite and weight gain are also common complications. Idiosyncratic reactions include blood dyscrasias (aplastic anaemia and agranulocytosis), liver necrosis leading to hepatocellular jaundice (especially in the elderly), polyarthropathy and fever. These reactions are unpredictable; monthly blood counts are recommended during the first three months of treatment, when the risk of bone marrow suppression is highest. Bone marrow suppression is a potentially severe complication: 12 deaths were reported in the UK between 1975 and 1985. The drug is not recommended for children and pregnant women; women taking the drug should avoid breast-feeding. Although some elderly patients may benefit from the lack of cardio-vascular and autonomic side-effects, special caution is needed in this patient group because of their lower rate of elimination and the increased risk of bone marrow and liver damage.

The only important drug interaction is enhancement of the sedative effects of alcohol and other CNS-depressant drugs.

Mianserin has recently been withdrawn from the UK market for commerical reasons; it is still available in some other European countries, including Ireland.

Mirtazapine

Basic pharmacology

Mirtazapine is closely related to mianserin (Fig. 6.8). It binds with high affinity to central α_2-adrenoceptors, 5-HT$_2$ and 5-HT$_3$ receptors, and H$_1$ histamine receptors; it has little affinity for α_1-adrenoceptors and muscarinic cholinoceptors. Mirtazapine enhances the release of both noradrenaline and serotonin, and these effects are attributed to the blockade of release-modulating α_2-adrenoceptors by the drug. The following chain of events has been proposed (Stimmel et al, 1997): blockade of release-modulating α_2-adrenoceptors leads to enhanced noradrenaline release; the released noradrenaline stimulates serotonergic neurons via the activation of α_1-adrenoceptors, which in turn results in an enhanced release of serotonin. The final result may be selective stimulation of 5-HT$_{1A}$ receptors, since other subtypes of postsynaptic 5-HT receptor (i.e. 5-HT$_2$ and 5-HT$_3$ receptors) cannot be activated, owing to blockade of these receptors by mirtazapine. It has been suggested that the enhanced noradrenergic effect, together with the selective activation of 5-HT$_{1A}$ receptors, may underlie the antidepressant activity of the drug.

The preserved activity of central α_1-adrenoceptors seems to be crucial for the linkage between the enhancement of noradrenaline and serotonin release, since mirtazapine fails to enhance serotonin release after pre-treatment with the α_1-adrenoceptor antagonist prazosin. Indeed, mianserin, which possesses α_1-adrenoceptor blocking activity, does not enhance the release of serotonin, although, like mirtazapine, it enhances the release of noradrenaline by virtue of its α_2-adrenoceptor blocking activity (de Boer et al, 1996).

Clinical pharmacology

The clinical pharmacological effects of mirtazapine are related to its receptor-blocking profile. On the basis of its ability to block central release-modulating α_2-adrenoceptors, mirtazapine might be expected to have an alerting/activating effect. However, this potential activation is counteracted by sedation produced by the blockade of central H_1 histamine receptors. Indeed, drowsiness/sedation is the most prominent side-effect of mirtazapine. The blockade of some subtypes of 5-HT receptors is likely to be responsible for the lack of some adverse effects that are common with SSRIs: the blockade of 5-HT$_2$ receptors by mirtazapine has been implicated in the lack of agitation, anxiety, insomnia and sexual dysfunction, and the blockade of 5-HT$_3$ receptors may underlie the absence of nausea/vomiting and headache with this serotonergic drug.

Mirtazapine is well absorbed from the gut, and the presence of food in the stomach has little effect on the rate and extent of absorption. The peak plasma level is obtained approximately 2 hours after the administration of a single dose. The drug is metabolised by the microsomal enzymes of the liver, the two metabolites being N-demethyl- and 8-hydroxy-mirtazapine. Mirtazapine has linear pharmacokinetics and a steady-state plasma level is obtained after 5 days. The elimination half-life is around 22 hours, which allows for once-daily administration.

Therapeutics

Mirtazapine is indicated for the treatment of all forms of depression. As with most other antidepressants, it takes 2–4 weeks for the therapeutic effect to develop, although there may be improvement in sleep pattern earlier than that.

The potentially most severe, albeit rare, adverse drug reactions are leucopenia and granulocytopenia, which occasionally can develop into agranulocytosis. Therefore, it is recommended to monitor the blood cell count regularly and to look out for possible signs of throat infection and fever.

As other antidepressants, mirtazapine can precipitate mania.

The most common side-effects are drowsiness and weight gain: the drowsiness is likely to be related to central H_1 histamine receptor blockade. Patients taking the drug should be advised to refrain from driving a motor vehicle or operating machinery.

Trazodone

Basic pharmacology

Trazodone also has more than one pharmacological action. It is a weak inhibitor of serotonin uptake (it has 7% of the potency of clomipramine) and has little affinity for the noradrenaline and dopamine uptake mechanisms (see Fig. 6.3). It antagonises both α_1- and α_2-adreno-ceptors; this can be demonstrated as the reversal of the central cardiovascular effects of the α_2-adrenoceptor agonist clonidine.

In animal behaviour tests it shares some properties with anti-depressant, antipsychotic and anxiolytic drugs. However, unlike the conventional antidepressants it does not potentiate the behavioural effects of L-dopa, and unlike the SSRIs it does not potentiate the behavioural effects of the 5-HT precursor 5-hydroxytryptophan in animals treated with an MAOI. Like the antipsychotics, trazodone reduces conditioned avoidance responses without affecting unconditioned responses, and protects mice from the toxic effects of amphetamine. However, in contrast to the antipsychotics, it does not antagonise amphetamine- and apomorphine-induced stereotypies, and has no cataleptogenic or hypothermic effect.

Trazodone causes sedation and suppresses REM sleep. Its anti-depressant property has been related to the inhibition of serotonin uptake and the release of noradrenaline (via α_2-adrenoceptor blockade).

Clinical pharmacology

Trazodone causes sedation and orthostatic hypotension in healthy subjects, and impairs psychomotor performance. Apart from hypotension, the α_1-adrenoceptor blockade leads to miosis, and can be demonstrated as the antagonism of phenylephrine-evoked sweat gland activation. The priapism observed occasionally in patients treated with trazodone is also likely to reflect α_1-adrenoceptor blockade. There are, however, only very weak anticholinergic effects, and, apart from orthostatic hypotension, there is little effect on the cardiovascular system.

Trazodone is rapidly and completely absorbed; the peak plasma concentration is attained 2 hours after a single dose. It has biphasic elimination kinetics: the half-life of the first phase is 1–4.5 hours and that of the second phase is 7–13 hours. On multiple dosing, the steady-state plasma level is attained within a few days. The plasma protein binding is 80–90%. It is widely distributed in the body; its concen-tration in the brain is higher than in the plasma. It is extensively metabolised in the liver (by hydroxylation, splitting of the piperidine ring, epoxidation followed by hydrolysis). One of its metabolites, mCPP, is a non-selective 5-HT receptor agonist with anxiogenic properties.

Therapeutics

Trazodone is indicated for the treatment of major depression (as defined in DSM–IV) with or without accompanying anxiety; the drug improves depressed mood, insomnia, anxiety and somatic symptoms. As trazo-done has only weak anticholinergic properties, it is recommended for depressed patients who also suffer from glaucoma, prostate hypertrophy or urinary retention. Contraindications include mania. Some people are hypersensitive to trazodone: if signs of drug allergy appear, trazodone should be discontinued immediately, and future prescription of the drug should be avoided.

Side-effects relating to the CNS include drowsiness, impaired memory and incoordination. The autonomic side-effects reflect the blockade of α_1-adrenoceptors: orthostatic hypotension (dizziness, syncope); nasal congestion; priapism; and ejaculatory incompetence.

The injection of an α_1-adrenoceptor agonist (e.g. phenylephrine, ephedrine) into the cavernous bodies may resolve the symptom of acute priapism. Although trazodone shows little cardiotoxicity compared with the conventional TCAs, in some susceptible patients cardiac arrhythmias may occur, including premature ventricular contractions, ventricular couplets, or short bursts (3 or 4 beats) of ventricular tachycardia. Bone marrow suppression is rare and usually mild: low but reversible white cell counts have been reported. Special caution is recommended in patients with a history of heart disease, epilepsy (because of a possible decrease in seizure threshold), and hepatic or renal insufficiency (because impaired elimination will give rise to a risk of toxicity). In light of the risk of priapism, some psychiatrists exclude male patients from treatment with trazodone. The white cell count should always be checked if a patient on trazodone develops fever and sore throat. Trazodone is not used in children, and it is not recommended for pregnant or breast-feeding women. In general, trazodone is better tolerated by the elderly than are the conventional TCAs.

Trazodone may interact with alcohol (enhancement of sedative effect), digoxin and phenytoin (inhibition of metabolism resulting in increased plasma levels and possible toxicity of these drugs). Although there are no data on the possible interaction between trazodone and MAOIs, this combination should be avoided.

Nefazodone

Basic pharmacology

Nefazodone is closely related to trazodone (Fig. 6.8). It is a moderately potent serotonin uptake inhibitor (Fig. 6.3) and has a relatively high affinity for postsynaptic 5-HT$_{2A}$ receptors. It has little or no affinity for muscarinic cholinoceptors, H$_1$ and H$_2$ histamine receptors, or α_1-adrenoceptors.

Nefazodone has some pharmacologically active metabolites. Hydroxy-nefazodone exhibits similar affinities for 5-HT$_2$ receptors and serotonin uptake sites to the parent compound. Another metabolite, mCPP, has multiple actions at 5-HT receptors, the most prominent being an agonistic action at 5-HT$_{2C}$ receptors. Other actions of mCPP include stimulation of 5-HT$_{1A}$ receptors and antagonism of 5-HT$_{2A}$ and 5-HT$_3$ receptors.

Clinical pharmacology

Nefazodone has been shown to inhibit serotonin uptake into blood platelets in human subjects treated with the drug. It causes dose-related increases in serum prolactin and oral temperature in healthy volunteers, reflecting its serotonergic property. In contrast to most other antidepressants, nefazodone does not suppress REM sleep.

Nefazodone is rapidly and completely absorbed after oral administration. It is extensively metabolised in the liver. The elimination half-life is approximately 6 hours. The drug is extensively bound to plasma proteins.

Therapeutics

Nefazodone is indicated for the treatment of all types of depressive illness, including depressive syndromes accompanied by anxiety or sleep disturbance.

On the whole, nefazodone is well tolerated. It shows a lower propensity to cause sexual dysfunction than the SSRIs, probably because of its 5-HT$_2$ receptor blocking activity. As do other antidepressants, nefazodone may precipitate mania.

Special caution is required with patients who suffer from liver failure, since the pharmacokinetics of the drug are very susceptible to alterations in liver function. Caution is also recommended in patients suffering from epilepsy, as the drug may lower the seizure threshold.

Pharmacokinetic interactions may occur with drugs metabolised by the same liver isoenzyme (cytochrome P450 IIIA4). These drugs include the benzodiazepines alprazolam and triazolam, and the antihistamine terfenadine.

Combined administration of nefazodone with other serotonergic drugs (MAOIs, SSRIs) should be avoided, in order to prevent the risk of the serotonin syndrome.

Nefazodone has recently been withdrawn from the European market for commercial reasons; it is available in the USA. In the UK nefazodone is still obtainable off-licence from suppliers in the USA.

Tryptophan

Tryptophan, an amino acid that is a constituent of normal food, is a precursor of serotonin. It is believed that it acts by being converted into serotonin, and thus it has effects that are similar to those of the SSRIs. On its own, it shows low potency as an antidepressant; however, when co-administered with MAOIs or TCAs it may produce an enhanced effect. The combination of an MAOI or a TCA and tryptophan has been recommended for the treatment of resistant (or refractory) depression (see Katona, 1991). However, it has recently been withdrawn owing to reports of a severe toxic reaction (eosinophilia–myalgia syndrome), and is available only on a named-patient basis. It is possible that the toxic reaction was due to some hitherto unidentified contaminant rather than tryptophan itself. The co-administration of tryptophan and SSRIs should be avoided since this combination can provoke the serotonin syndrome.

Buspirone

The anxiolytic drug buspirone, together with its analogues (e.g. gepirone, ipsapirone), also has some antidepressant efficacy. This has been related to an agonistic effect of these drugs at central 5-HT$_{1A}$ receptors (Charney & Delgado, 1992). However, buspirone is rarely prescribed as an antidepressant in the UK.

St John's wort

St John's wort (*Hypericum perforatum*) has been used as a medicinal herb for centuries. In recent years it has become popular as a treatment for depression. In Germany it is available on prescription, and it has become the most widely used antidepressant in that country. In the USA and Australia it is regulated as a dietary supplement, whereas in the UK it is freely available in health food stores and pharmacies without any regulation. In recent years a number of clinical trials and pharmacological studies have been conducted with different extracts of St John's wort. There is still considerable controversy regarding both its pharmacological properties and its clinical effectiveness (Nathan, 2001).

Chemistry

Hypericum contains numerous compounds with biological activity, such as naphthodiathrones (hypericin and pseudohypericin), tanins, pro-anthocyanidins, flavonoids and phloroglucinol derivatives (hyperforin). *Hypericum* extracts have not been standardised and may contain the various constituents in different proportions, which renders the comparison of different studies very difficult.

Basic pharmacology

Early studies indicated that hypericum may act as a reversible MAOI-A. This finding, however, was not confirmed in subsequent studies, and the positive results on MAO in the early studies are generally attributed to impurities in the *Hypericum* extract. There is, however, considerable evidence that hypericum may act as a non-selective monoamine reuptake inhibitor. It has been shown that hypericum non-competitively inhibits the uptake of all three monoamines (noradrenaline, serotonin and dopamine). It is believed that in the *Hypericum* extract, hyperforin is the active principal responsible for monoamine uptake inhibition. After long-term administration, hypericum has been shown to down-regulate α_1-adrenoceptors, an effect shared by many other antidepressants. *Hypericum* extract has also been shown to have activity in a number of animal models capable of predicting antidepressant response.

Clinical pharmacology

There is a paucity of information on the pharmacodynamic actions of hypericum in human subjects. On the other hand, there is considerable information on the pharmacokinetics of the constituents of *Hypericum* extracts. The peak plasma level of the active constituents is obtained approximately 4 hours after administration, and the elimination half-life of hypericin and hyperforin are around 9 hours. Steady-state plasma levels of these constituents are obtained 3–4 days after initiation of repeated dosing. Hypericum interacts with microsomal enzymes of the liver, and this is likely to underlie the observation that the plasma concentrations of a number of drugs (e.g. theophylline, cyclosporin, warfarin, digoxin, the HIV-1 protease inhibitor indinavir, some anaesthetics and oral contraceptives) are reduced in patients taking *Hypericum*. These drug interactions are likely to reflect the inductive effect of hypericum on liver enzymes.

Therapeutics

A number of early clinical trials indicated that *Hypericum* extracts were superior to placebo in the treatment of mild to moderate depression. However, the issue of efficacy remains controversial, and further, larger trials using better standardised extracts are planned, in which St John's wort will be compared both with placebo and established antidepressants.

Hypericum is usually well tolerated. Co-administration with SSRIs should be avoided owing to the risk of the serotonin syndrome, resulting from the additive effects of SSRIs and hypericum on serotonin reuptake. The pharmacokinetic interaction with a large number of drugs (see above) may lead to adverse consequences for patients who are taking those medications for serious, and occasionally life-threatening, conditions. There have been calls to place *Hypericum* extracts under some kind of regulation in the UK. It is important that psychiatrists ask their patients when prescribing antidepressant drugs whether they are also taking any unregulated herbal treatments and to warn them of any risks.

Common mode of action of antidepressants

The discovery that both MAOIs and non-selective TCAs can reverse the behavioural effects of the monoamine-depleting agent reserpine in animals and facilitate recovery from depressive states in humans led to the formulation of the 'classic' monoamine theory of affective disorders. According to this theory, depression results from a deficiency of monoaminergic neurotransmission, occasioned by partial depletion of intraneuronal monoamine stores. MAOIs were deemed to correct this deficiency by limiting the intraneuronal destruction of the monoamine transmitter; TCAs were deemed to do so by blocking monoamine uptake, with a consequent increase in intrasynaptic transmitter concentration. Initially, interest focused on noradrenergic transmission; however, the discovery that some TCAs show relative selectivity for serotonin uptake, coupled with the emergence of evidence for diminished serotonin metabolism in some patients with depression, led first to a shift of emphasis from noradrenergic to serotonergic mechanisms, and later to the proposition that changes in both serotonergic and noradrenergic functions may occur in depression (Prange *et al*, 1974), or that there might be separate noradrenaline-deficiency and serotonin-deficiency depressive syndromes (van Praag, 1978). Unfortunately, the development of highly selective noradrenaline and serotonin uptake inhibitors has failed to generate support for this suggestion, since there is little evidence that depressed patients who fail to respond to 'noradrenergic' treatments benefit from a switch to 'serotonergic' treatments, or vice versa.

A major weakness of the classic monoamine theories is the discrepancy between the rapid appearance of monoaminergic potentiation (typically within minutes or hours of acute treatment with an MAOI or TCA) and the sluggish clinical response to antidepressant treatment. The discovery, in the 1970s, that all known antidepressant treatments produce down-regulation of β-adrenoceptors (reduced numbers of β-adrenoceptor binding sites and diminished activity of β-adrenoceptor-coupled adenylyl cyclase activity) radically altered the theory of antidepressant action. First, the finding that all classes of antidepressants, including some SSRIs, down-regulate β-adrenoceptors shifted the focus of attention back to noradrenergic mechanisms; second, since down-regulation was believed to imply suppression of noradrenergic neurotransmission, the business of antidepressant treatments was now deemed to be the correction of *overactivity* in the noradrenergic pathways.

Unfortunately, there are several problems with β-adrenoceptor down-regulation as a putative common mechanism of action of anti-depressants:

(1)   there may be some exceptions (e.g. trazodone, paroxetine, citalopram) to the generalisation that all antidepressants down-regulate β-adrenoceptors

(2)   some drugs that are effective in producing down-regulation (e.g. clenbuterol, a β-adrenoceptor agonist) have, at best, very modest antidepressant activity

(3) β-adrenoceptor down-regulation is not the only adaptive change produced by antidepressants – as discussed above, down-regulation of α_2-adrenoceptors and 5-HT$_2$ receptors is a common feature of most antidepressants.

In addition, there is the difficult question of the functional consequence of down-regulation. Although logic would seem to dictate that this should be suppression of neurotransmission, there is some evidence that some β-adrenoceptor-mediated functions are enhanced during chronic treatment with TCAs and MAOIs. This has been taken to indicate that down-regulation constitutes an incomplete homeostatic reversal of the increase in noradrenergic function that results from uptake blockade or MAO inhibition.

The observation that destruction of the serotonergic pathways in animals prevents the development of β-adrenoceptor down-regulation again shifted attention back to serotonergic function. Although the interpretation of this observation has been questioned (Pryor & Sulser, 1991), most commentators now agree that the importance of the interaction between different monoamine systems and the functional balance of the various receptor populations was greatly underestimated in earlier theories of antidepressant action.

It is now well recognised that neurotransmitters may act at several subtypes of receptor mediating a variety of physiological effects, so that the functional significance of a change in the number of one receptor subtype is difficult, if not impossible, to predict. Moreover, marked changes in function can occur in the absence of appreciable changes in the numbers of the receptor subtype that mediates that function.

A case in point is the enhancement of serotonin-mediated inhibition of hippocampal neurons seen following chronic treatment with TCAs. At first sight this appears to be paradoxical, since chronic treatment with TCAs does not change the sensitivity of the inhibitory 5-HT$_{1A}$ receptors on hippocampal neurons. However, it has been suggested that the reduced postsynaptic effect may be due to the desensitisation of somatodendritic and terminal 5-HT$_{1A}$ autoreceptors that normally inhibit the activity of serotonin neurons and reduce the release of serotonin from serotonergic nerve terminals (Blier et al, 1991). According to one theory of antidepressant action (see Deakin, 1989), the net increase in postsynaptic 5-HT$_{1A}$ receptor-mediated function, coupled with the decreased 5-HT$_2$ receptor-mediated function, resulting from down-regulation of these receptors is crucial to the antidepressant effect.

It is apparent that no current theory of the mode of action of antidepressant drugs enjoys universal acceptance. Although there is evidence that some drugs with antidepressant efficacy have the ability to increase the availability of noradrenaline and/or serotonin at central synaptic sites – such as MAOIs, monoamine uptake inhibitors and monoamine releasing agents (tryptophan, α_2-adrenoceptor antagonists) – and/or change the balance between 5-HT receptor subtypes (e.g. 5-HT$_2$ receptor antagonists and 5-HT$_{1A}$ receptor agonists), the mechanisms by which these neurochemical changes may lead to the lifting of depressed mood remain elusive.

More recently, theoretical formulations have been developed that take the action of antidepressants beyond the modification of central monoaminergic neurotransmission. Thus, it has been proposed that antidepressants may repair the neuronal damage caused by chronic stress associated with depression (Reid & Stewart, 2001), and thus may protect the hippocampus from atrophy caused by high circulating cortisol levels in depression (Hindmarch, 2001).

Other important common actions of antidepressants of different classes include the rectification of the disordered functioning of the hypothalamic–pituitary–adrenal and hypothalamic–pituitary–thyroid axes, and prevention of the hypersecretion of cytokines, which are the mediators of abnormal immunological responses in depression. Finally, new types of antidepressants, which do not directly interact with monoamine systems, are under investigation, such as antagonists of glucocorticoid receptors, corticotrophin-releasing factor (CRF) receptors and substance P receptors (for review see Hindmarch, 2001).

It is clear that the earlier theories that postulated disturbance of the function of a single neurotransmitter system are simplistic in the light of modern pharmacological knowledge, while the more sophisticated theories are difficult to test. Another major problem is the often poor quality of the clinical evidence on which the theories rely. The sluggish and frequently incomplete clinical response that characterises most current antidepressant treatment regimens, together with the thorny problems of placebo effects, spontaneous remission and the impact of non-pharmacological factors (e.g. life events) on the course of depressive illness, not to mention the considerable controversy that surrounds the diagnosis and classification of affective disorders, make clinical trials of antidepressants difficult to conduct and their results hard to interpret.

General principles of antidepressant treatment

Selection of patients

It is important that antidepressants are reserved for patients suffering from depressive illness of sufficient severity to warrant the prescription of drugs that either have well-documented cardio- and neurotoxicities (e.g. TCAs), or that have been in clinical use for a shorter time than the TCAs and thus may have some rare, hitherto undetected, adverse effects (e.g. SSRIs, SNRIs, NARIs). Although there is general agreement that the antidepressants are effective in alleviating moderate and severe depression, there is little evidence for their effectiveness in minor emotional distress occasioned by adverse life events. Patients presenting with a well-defined depressive syndrome are likely to benefit from an antidepressant irrespective of aetiology (endogenous versus reactive) or previous course (unipolar versus bipolar) of the illness. However, patients with a history of mania are at increased risk of developing a manic episode in the course of treatment with an antidepressant. Antidepressants can be helpful in depression associated with physical or mental illness; however, in these cases it is important to treat not only the depression but also the underlying/accompanying illness (e.g. hypothyroidism, schizophrenia).

Choice of antidepressant

As with any other treatment, the prescriber has to consider the risk:benefit ratio ('therapeutic index') of the individual drugs. The first-generation TCAs have well-documented effectiveness, and none of the newer drugs has been shown to be more effective than the classical TCAs. The major dilemma with the antidepressants is whether to use an old, well-established antidepressant, or to prescribe one of the newer drugs that has a more favourable side-effect profile and is safer in overdose. The advantages of the newer drugs, however, are somewhat mitigated by the possibility that hitherto unidentified rare but severe adverse reactions ('type B side-effects') may emerge in the future, as has been the case with zimeldine, nomifensine and mianserin, whereas the classical TCAs and MAOIs possess mainly dose-related and predictable ('type A') side-effects, whose dangers can be minimised by appropriate monitoring and dosage adjustments. All the same, because of the adverse effects of the TCAs, and the high rate of mortality associated with overdose, the use of the newer drugs, especially of the SSRIs, is increasingly gaining ground, to the extent that most clinicians favour them as drugs of first choice, particularly if patients are living alone, or the medication cannot be supervised, are elderly, have ischaemic heart disease, glaucoma, prostatic problems, or are deemed to be a high suicide risk. Indeed, since the first edition of this book was published (in 1995), the SSRIs have become the first line of treatment for most patients, whereas the TCAs are reserved for patients who fail to respond to an SSRI. However, it should be noted that the picture may be somewhat more complicated when the toxicity in overdose of different classes of antidepressants is compared, since, according to a recent report, the SNRI venlafaxine shows a higher fatal toxity than some of the less toxic TCAs (Buckley & McManus, 2002).

When choosing an antidepressant, it is good practice to aim for monotherapy, that is, to use only one drug at the therapeutically effective dose. The first line of treatment is usually an SSRI. It is advisable to start at a low dose and build up the dosage over 2–3 weeks, while carefully monitoring the patient for both therapeutic response and side-effects. In milder cases of depression, only if a drug has been administered for 6–8 weeks at the recommended dosage without a therapeutic response is it justified to conclude that a particular drug is not suitable for the patient and to consider replacing it with another antidepressant. In the case of severe depression, however, it is hardly justified to wait for 6–8 weeks, and an earlier change in medication, or the introduction of some other form of treatment (e.g. electroconvulsive therapy) may be indicated. If a patient fails to respond to an adequate treatment trial with a second anti-depressant, it is usual to talk about a 'treatment-resistant case'. Such cases constitute a major therapeutic challenge and require special treatment strategies (see below).

An MAOI is usually the second line of treatment, which is introduced if one or more other types of antidepressant have failed. An MAOI may be the first choice in patients who have a history of responding only to this type of drug. The introduction of the RIMAs has increased the scope for this group of drugs; however, the clinical use of moclobemide has not spread to the extent predicted when it was first launched over 5 years ago, probably because of reservations about its efficacy.

There have been attempts to determine which type of drug may be most beneficial for a particular type of patient. Thus, 'sedative' antidepressants (e.g. amitriptyline, mirtazapine) have been recom-mended for patients with agitation and insomnia, and more 'activating' drugs (e.g. desipramine, reboxetine) for patients with psychomotor retardation and lack of energy. However, agitation, insomnia and retardation all improve as the depression lifts, irrespective of the particular antidepressant used. If a patient also has obsessional symptoms, an SSRI may be the antidepressant of choice, and if the depressive syndrome is complicated by delusions, amoxapine, a TCA with antipsychotic properties, could be tried. Delusional depression does not respond well to traditional TCAs, and a combination of a TCA with a phenothiazine antipsychotic has been recommended. In cases of severe delusional depression a course of electroconvulsive therapy may be the best course of action.

Finally, the patient's general medical condition should be taken into account when an antidepressant is being chosen. Thus, a classical TCA would be contraindicated for a patient with a history of cardiac disease or severe epilepsy, and probably should not be chosen for patients with weight problems. Conventional MAOIs should be avoided when orthostatic hypotension and resulting fainting might endanger life (e.g. in patients who operate machinery or work on high buildings).

Duration of treatment

It is customary to distinguish between acute, continuation and prophylactic antidepressant treatments.

Acute treatment

This involves treating a depressive episode until symptoms lift; this may take several weeks or even months. There is a substantial literature showing that there is a high risk of relapse if treatment is discontinued immediately after the patient recovers from a depressive illness.

Continuation treatment

Because of this risk, continuation treatment is recommended for 6–10 months following recovery. At the end of the treatment period the antidepressant is gradually tailed off over several weeks.

Prophylactic treatment

While the justification for continuation of treatment is relatively well established, the issue of prophylactic treatment is more controversial. This involves the patient taking the antidepressant for several years, or even for life, with the objective of preventing relapses. Prophylactic treatment can be considered only for patients who suffer from recurrent unipolar depression, and it is unsuitable for patients who suffer from bipolar affective disorder, for which the prophylactic treatment of choice is lithium. As lithium can also be effective in the prophylaxis of unipolar depression, it can be considered as an alternative to long-term continuation treatment with an antidepressant. It has been pointed out that there may be some advantage in continuing a patient on an antidepressant that has been effective and is well tolerated rather than switching to lithium, whose effectiveness will not have been tested in that particular patient (see Prien, 1992).

Refractory depression

Although depression is usually self-limiting, it may last for several months, and some cases of chronic depression may last for years. If the depressive symptoms do not abate in spite of antidepressant treatment, the label of 'refractory' or '(treatment) resistant' depression is used (see Katona, 1991). There can be numerous causes for resistance to treatment, such as lack of compliance, inadequate dosage or wrong diagnosis (e.g. hysterical dissociation mistaken for depression). Furthermore, a depressive state may be maintained by such factors as physical illness or illness behaviour. It is recommended that at least two different antidepressants in adequate dosages over several weeks, or one antidepressant and electroconvulsive therapy, should have been tried before the depression is declared 'refractory'. At the same time, it is important to search for underlying/maintaining factors. However, if no such factor can be identified, different combination treatments ('augmentation strategies') can be tried.

The combination of some classes of antidepressants is of little practical value: TCAs and MAOIs should not be used together, and the combination of SSRIs and MAOIs is absolutely contraindicated. There are, however, reports of the possible usefulness of TCA/SSRI combinations: this may be related to a pharmacokinetic interaction (i.e. an increase in the plasma level of the TCA). The co-administration of lithium ('lithium augmentation') or thyroid hormones and TCAs or MAOIs has been reported to be effective in some cases of refractory depression. According to some authors, the triple combination of a TCA (or MAOI), lithium and tryptophan may help some patients. These are, however, usually desperate cases of severe, chronic depression in which all available drug treatments should be explored before consideration for psychosurgery (Bridges, 1992).

As a substantial proportion (about 30%) of patients fail to respond to treatment with antidepressants, there is a continuous endeavour to explore the clinical usefulness of novel augmentation strategies. Pindolol is a combined β-adrenoceptor/5-HT$_{1A}$ receptor antagonist, which has a preferential affinity for inhibitory 5-HT$_{1A}$ autoreceptors on serotonergic neurons, and thus it may prevent the 'switching off' of these neurons by excess serotonin made available by an SSRI (Blier & de Montigny, 1997). Indeed, there is clinical evidence that pindolol can be useful in enhancing the efficacy of, or speed up the clinical response to, SSRIs (Perez et al, 2001). More recently, there have been reports of the enhancement of the effectiveness of SSRIs with the co-administration of reboxetine (Lucca et al, 2000) or mianserin (Ferreri et al, 2001).

References

Abdelmawla, A. H., Langley, R. W., Szabadi, E., et al (1999) Comparison of the effects of venlafaxine, desipramine and paroxetine on noradrenaline- and methoxamine-evoked constriction of the dorsal hand vein. British Journal of Clinical Pharmacology, 48, 345–354.

ABPI (1999/2000) Compendium of Data Sheets and Summaries of Product Characteristics. London: Datapharm.

Baldessarini, R. J. (2001) Drugs and the treatment of psychiatric disorders: depression and anxiety disorders. In Goodman & Gilman's The Pharmacological Basis of Therapeutics (10th edn) (eds J. G. Hardman & L. E. Limbird), pp. 447–484. New York: McGraw-Hill.

Berlan, M., Montastruc, J.-L. & Lafontan, M. (1992) Pharmacological prospects for α_2-adrenoceptor antagonist therapy. Trends in Pharmacological Sciences, 13, 277–282.

Bernstein, J. G. (1988) Handbook of Drug Therapy in Psychiatry (2nd edn). London: Mosby.

Blier, P. & de Montigny, C. (1997) Current psychiatric uses of drugs acting on the serotonin system. In Serotonergic Neurons and 5-HT Receptors in the CNS (eds H. G. Baumgarten & M. Göthert), pp. 727–750. Berlin: Springer.

Blier, P., de Montigny, C. & Chaput, Y. (1991) A role for the serotonin system in the mechanism of action of antidepressant treatments: preclinical evidence. *Journal of Clinical Psychiatry*, **51**, 14–20.

Bolden-Watson, C. & Richelson, E. (1993) Blockade by newly-developed antidepressants of biogenic amine uptake into rat brain synaptosomes. *Life Sciences*, **52**, 1023–1029.

Bridges, P. (1992) Resistant depression and psychosurgery. In *Handbook of Affective Disorders* (2nd edn) (ed. E. G. Paykel), pp. 437–452. Edinburgh: Churchill Livingstone.

Britton, D. R., El-Wardany, Z. S., Brown, C. P., *et al* (1978) Clinical pharmacokinetics of selected psychotropic drugs. In *Biology of Mood and Antianxiety Drugs. Handbook of Psychopharmacology, Volume 13* (eds L. L. Iversen, S. D. Iversen & S. H. Snyder), pp. 299–393. New York: Plenum.

Buckley, N. A. & McManus, P. R. (2002) Fatal toxicity of serotoninergic and other antidepressant drugs: analysis of United Kingdom mortality data. *BMJ*, **325**, 1332–1333.

Caldecott-Hazard, S., Morgan, D. G., De Leon-Jones, F., *et al* (1991) Clinical and biochemical aspects of depressive disorder: II. Transmitter/receptor theories. *Synapses*, **9**, 251–301.

Cassem, N. (1982) Cardiovascular effects of antidepressants. *Journal of Clinical Psychiatry*, **43**, 22–28.

Charney, D. S. & Delgado, P. L. (1992) Current concepts of the role of serotonin function in depression and anxiety. In *Serotonin Receptor Subtypes: Pharmacological Significance and Clinical Implications* (eds S. Z. Langer, N. Brunello, G. Racagni, *et al*), pp. 89–104. Basel: Karger.

Coccaro, E. F. (1998) Central neurotransmitter function in human aggression and impulsivity. In *Neurobiology and Clinical Views on Aggression and Impulsivity* (eds. M. Maes & E. F. Coccaro), pp. 143–168. London: John Wiley.

Cowen, P. J. (1990) A role for 5-HT in the action of antidepressant drugs. *Pharmacology and Therapeutics*, **46**, 43–51.

Danysz, W., Archer, T. & Fowler, C. J. (1991) Screening for new antidepressant compounds. In *Behavioural Models in Psychopharmacology: Theoretical, Industrial and Clinical Perspectives* (ed. P. Willner), pp. 126–156. Cambridge: Cambridge University Press.

Deakin, J. F. W. (1989) 5-HT receptor subtypes in depression. In *Behavioural Pharmacology of 5-HT* (eds P. Bevan, A. R. Cools & T. Archer), pp. 179–204. Hillsdale, NJ: Erlbaum.

de Boer, T., Nefkens, F., Van Helvoirt, A., *et al* (1996) Differences in modulation of noradrenergic and serotonergic transmission by the α-2 adrenoceptor antagonists, mirtazapine, mianserin and idazoxan. *Journal of Pharmacology and Experimental Therapeutics*, **277**, 852–860.

DeVane, C. L. (1992) Pharmacokinetics of the selective serotonin re-uptake inhibitors. *Journal of Clinical Psychiatry*, **53**, 13–20.

Dollery, C. (1999) *Therapeutic Drugs* (2nd edn). Edinburgh: Churchill Livingstone.

Edwards, J. G. (1992) Selective serotonin re-uptake inhibitors. *BMJ*, **304**, 1644–1646.

Edwards, J. G. & Anderson, I. (1999) Systematic reviews and guide to selection of selective serotonin reuptake inhibitors. *Drugs*, **57**, 507–533.

Ferreri, M., Lavergne, F., Berlin, I., *et al* (2001) Benefits from mianserin augmentation of fluoxetine in patients with major depression non-responders to fluoxetine alone. *Acta Psychiatrica Scandinavica*, **103**, 66–72.

Gillman, P. K. (1999) The serotonin syndrome and its treatment. *Journal of Psychopharmacology*, **13**, 100–109.

Glue, P., Coupland, N. & Nutt, D. J. (1993) The pharmacological basis for the therapeutic activity of MAOIs. In *Clinical Advances in MAOI Therapies* (ed. S. Kennedy), pp. 1–31. Washington, DC: APA Press.

Harvey, A. T., Rudolph, R. L. & Preskorn, S. H. (2000) Evidence of the dual mechanism of action of venlafaxine. *Archives of General Psychiatry*, **51**, 503–509.

Hindmarch, I. (2001) Expanding the horizons of depression: beyond the monoamine hypothesis. *Human Psychopharmacology – Clinical and Experimental*, **16**, 203–218.

Hindmarch, I., Alford, C., Barwell, F., *et al* (1992) Measuring the side effects of psychotropics: the behavioural toxicity of antidepressants. *Journal of Psychopharmacology*, **6**, 198–203.

Katona, C. L. E. (1991) Refractory depression. In *The Uses of Fluoxetine in Clinical Practice* (ed. H. L. Freeman), pp. 5–13. London: Royal Society of Medicine.

Kavoussi, R. & Coccaro, E. F. (1998) Psychopharmacological treatment of impulsive aggression. In *Neurobiology and Clinical Views on Aggression and Impulsivity* (eds M. Maes & E. F. Coccaro), pp. 191–211. London: John Wiley.

Langer, S. Z., Raisman, R., Sechter, D., *et al* (1984) ^{3}H-imipramine and ^{3}H-desipramine binding sites in depression. In *Frontiers in Biochemical and Pharmacological Research in Depression* (eds E. Usdin, M. Åsberg, L. Bertilsson, *et al*), pp. 113–125. New York: Raven Press.

Lesch, K. P. & Bengel, D. (1995) Neurotransmitter reuptake mechanisms: targets for drugs to study and treat psychiatric, neurological and neurodegenerative disorders. *CNS Drugs*, **4**, 302–322.

Lucca, A., Serretti, A. & Smeraldi, E. (2000) Effect of reboxetine augmentation in SSRI resistant patients. *Human Psychopharmacology – Clinical and Experimental*, **15**, 143–145.

Mallinger, A. G. & Smith, E. (1991) Pharmacokinetics of monoamine oxidase inhibitors. *Psychopharmacology Bulletin*, **27**, 493–502.

Nathan, P. J. (2001) *Hypericum perforatum* (St John's wort): a non-selective reuptake inhibitor? A review of the recent advances in its pharmacology. *Journal of Psychopharmacology*, **15**, 47–54.

Nutt, D. & Glue, P. (1989) Momoamine oxidase inhibitors: rehabilitation from recent research? *British Journal of Psychiatry*, **154**, 287–291.

Pare, C. M. B. (1985) The present status of monoamine oxidase inhibitors. *British Journal of Psychiatry*, **146**, 576–584.

Perez, V., Puigdemont, D., Gilabarte, I., *et al* (2001) Augmentation of fluoxetine's antidepressant action by pindolol. Analysis of clinical, pharmacokinetic, and methodological factors. *Journal of Clinical Psychopharmacology*, **21**, 36–45.

Prange, A. J., Wilson, I. C., Lynn, C. W., *et al* (1974) L-Tryptophan in mania: contribution to a permissive hypothesis of affective disorders. *Archives of General Psychiatry*, **39**, 56–62.

Prien, R. F. (1992) Maintenance treatment. In *Handbook of Affective Disorders* (2nd edn) (ed. E. G. Paykel), pp. 419–436. Edinburgh: Churchill Livingstone.

Pryor, J. C. & Sulser, F. (1991) Evolution of the monoamine hypothesis of depression. In *Biological Aspects of Affective Disorders* (eds R. Horton & C. Katona), pp. 77–94. New York: Academic Press.

Reid, I. C. & Stewart, C. A. (2001) How antidepressants work. New perspectives on the pathophysiology of depressive disorder. *British Journal of Psychiatry*, **178**, 299–303.

Reite, M. (1998) Treatment of insomnia. In *Textbook of Psychopharmacology* (2nd edn) (eds A. F. Schatzberg & C. B. Nemeroff), pp. 997–1014. Washington, DC: APA Press.

Richelson, E. (1984) The newer antidepressants: structures, pharmacokinetics, pharmacodynamics, and proposed mechanisms of action. *Psychopharmacology Bulletin*, **2**, 213–223.

Richelson, E. & Pfenning, M. (1984) Blockade by antidepressants and related compounds of biogenic amine uptake into rat brain synaptosomes: most antidepressants selectively block norepinephrine uptake. *European Journal of Pharmacology*, **104**, 277–286.

Saper, C. B., Chou, T. C. & Scammell, T. E. (2001) The sleep switch: hypothalamic control of sleep and wakefulness. *Trends in Neuroscience*, **24**, 726–731.

Stimmel, G. L., Dopheide, J. A. & Stahl, S. M. (1997) Mirtazapine: an antidepressant with noradrenergic and specific serotonergic effects. *Pharmacotherapy*, **17**, 10–21.

Szabadi, E. & Bradshaw, C. M. (1986) Antidepressant drugs and the autonomic nervous system. In *The Biology of Depression* (ed. J. F. W. Deakin), pp. 190–220. London: Gaskell.

Szabadi, E. & Bradshaw, C. M. (2000) Mechanisms of action of reboxetine. *Reviews in Contemporary Pharmacotherapy*, **5**, 267–282.

Szabadi, E. & Tavernor, S. (1999) Hypo- and hypersalivation induced by psychoactive drugs: incidence, mechanisms and therapeutic implications. *CNS Drugs*, **11**, 449–466.

Tipton, K. F. & Anderson, M. C. (1991) Significance of reversibility as a safety factor of MAO-A inhibitors: preclinical data. In *Biological Psychiatry, Volume 1* (eds G. Racagni, N. Brunello & T. Fukuda), pp. 403–405. Amsterdam: Elsevier.

van Praag, H. M. (1978) Amine hypotheses of affective disorders. In *Biology of Mood and Antianxiety Drugs: Handbook of Psychopharmacology, Volume 13* (eds L. L. Iversen, S. D. Iversen & S. H. Snyder), pp. 187–297. New York: Plenum.

Willner, P. (1990) Animal models of depression: an overview. *Pharmacology and Therapeutics*, **45**, 425–455.

Wong, E. H. F., Sonders, M. S., Amara, S. G., *et al* (2000) Reboxetine: a pharmacologically potent, selective, and specific norephinephrine re-uptake inhibitor. *Biological Psychiatry*, **47**, 818–829.

Further reading

Bloom, F. E. & Kupfer, D. J. (1995) *Psychopharmacology: The Fourth Generation of Progress*. New York: Raven.

Brody, T. M., Larner, J. & Minneman, K. P. (1998) *Human Pharmacology: Molecular to Clinical* (3rd edn). St Louis, MO: Mosby.

Charney, D. S., Nestler, E. J. & Bunney, B. S. (1999) *Neurobiology of Mental Illness*. Oxford: Oxford University Press.

Dollery, C. (1999) *Therapeutic Drugs* (2nd edn). Edinburgh: Churchill Livingstone.

Goodwin, F. K. & Jamison, K. R. (1990) *Manic–Depressive Illness*. New York: Oxford University Press.

Hardman, J. G. & Limbird, L. E. (2001) *Goodman & Gilman's The Pharmacological Basis of Therapeutics* (10th edn). New York: McGraw-Hill.

Leonard, B. E. (1997) *Fundamentals of Psychopharmacology* (2nd edn). Chichester: John Wiley.

Paykel, E. S. (1992) *Handbook of Affective Disorders* (2nd edn). Edinburgh: Churchill Livingstone.

Schatzberg, A. F. & Nemeroff, C. B. (1998) *The American Psychiatric Press Textbook of Psychopharmacology* (2nd edn). Washington, DC: APA Press.

Snyder, S. H. (1996) *Drugs and the Brain*. New York: Scientific American.

Stahl, S. M. (1999) *Psychopharmacology of Antidepressants*. London: Martin Dunitz.

Watson, S. J. (1996) *Biology of Schizophrenia and Affective Disorders*. Washington, DC: APA Press.

CHAPTER 7

Affective disorders:
2. Lithium and anticonvulsants

Rory Shelley

Lithium is an alkali metal usually administered as a salt, such as lithium carbonate, chloride or citrate. It was first isolated from the mineral petalite in 1818 by the Swedish chemist Arfwedson. Its name drives from *lithion*, the Greek word for stone, in order to denote this mineral origin. It exists as two stable isotopes, ^{6}Li and ^{7}Li, of which ^{7}Li is the more common (92.4% of naturally occurring lithium) and less toxic.

By the mid-19th century it was being medically recommended for a variety of maladies, including the dissolving of urinary calculi. Lithium salts were prescribed by Garrod for gout, as they would eliminate uric acid from the body and thus prevent the build-up of urate crystals.

Lithium is found in natural mineral or spa waters, consumption of which had been recommended for mania as far back as the 2nd century AD by Soranus of Ephesus. The concentration of lithium in mineral waters is so low, however, as to require a daily intake of more than several times an individual's own body weight to achieve a therapeutic lithium level.

In the 20th century lithium chloride was used as a substitute for table salt for patients suffering from oedema. By 1949 articles were published in the American medical literature that recognised that lithium could be toxic, sometimes fatally so. It was soon banned by the US Food and Drug Administration.

Around this time an Australian psychiatrist, John Cade, began investigating the biological causes of psychotic illnesses. He injected patients' urine intraperitoneally into guinea pigs and found that urine from patients with mania was more toxic to them than that from patients with depression or schizophrenia. Concluding that this related to urea toxicity enhanced by uric acid, he proceeded to administer lithium to guinea pigs. Surprisingly, they became temporarily lethargic and unresponsive. Having tried lithium on himself first, he conducted an open trial on psychotic patients, and he fortuitously selected a dose equivalent to 600 mg lithium carbonate taken three times a day. His famous 1949 paper reports that manic patients responded (Cade, 1949).

244

This discovery is sometimes cited as an example of serendipity. It could also be argued that, although wrong in his original hypothesis, Cade nevertheless followed a scientific approach to arrive at his clinical finding.

Pharmacokinetics

The pharmacokinetics of lithium are important because it has an unusually narrow therapeutic range. That is, compared with other drugs, there is a narrow gap between the minimum blood level (0.4 mmol/l) required for therapeutic efficacy and the level (1.5 mmol/l) beyond which toxicity may ensue. There is, furthermore, a good correlation between blood levels and both clinical response and side-effects.

Lithium is absorbed fairly rapidly from the upper gastrointestinal tract. A peak serum level is reached 2–3 hours after ingestion. There is a distribution phase over the next 5–7 hours, followed by an elimination phase.

Lithium is not bound to serum proteins, is not metabolised by the liver and is excreted, unchanged, almost solely by the kidney. There is some interpersonal variation in absorption and distribution into other tissue departments from blood, but by 12 hours there are no significant fluctuations in blood levels – hence the value of the 12-hour standardised serum lithium (12h-stSLi) estimation in monitoring patients, as well as in allowing comparisons between different groups of patients in receipt of the drug.

Usually blood is drawn in the morning by venepuncture to monitor the lithium blood level, with the last lithium dose ingested 12 hours previously, the night before. A morning dose is omitted until after the blood test. The half-life of lithium lies between 10 and 24 hours for most patients. Steady-state blood levels are achieved after approximately five half-lives. Therefore, the majority of patients will be in lithium steady-state 5–7 days after starting on lithium (or after either a dosage or tablet change). A blood test before this time will provide a less reliable result.

The rate of absorption of lithium into serum is influenced mainly by how quickly the lithium tablet dissolves. In order to reduce side-effects, attempts have been made to reduce the magnitude of the peak serum lithium level by delaying the rate of release of lithium. This should reduce side-effects associated with a higher serum peak, such as nausea or tremor (see below). On the other hand, if the rate of release is too slow, less lithium will be absorbed. Furthermore, the residual lithium in the gastrointestinal tract will have an irritant effect on colonic mucosa, as well as an osmotic effect, drawing fluid into the tract, thereby causing loose bowel motions or diarrhoea. A slow release of lithium will also be at the expense of reduced bioavailability (Shelley & Silverstone, 1986), although this may be of some benefit if a patient takes an overdose of the drug.

Differences between the rates of release of lithium from different preparations of the drug need to be borne in mind when a patient is switched from one product to another, even from say a 250 mg tablet to a 400 mg tablet of the same brand. It is therefore prudent to monitor lithium levels more closely at such times, although in practice any differences are usually modest. The two most commonly prescribed lithium preparations in the British Isles are Priadel and Camcolit. The pharmacokinetic profiles of the 400 mg formulations of both are similar (Shelley & Silverstone, 1986), as they show an equivalent rate of release.

Finally, whereas most lithium formulations contain the carbonate salt, there are some that contain lithium citrate (e.g. liquid preparations). Equivalence in terms of lithium content will not be comparable between the two salts. For example, 564 mg of lithium citrate contains 6.0 mmol lithium, but 400 mg lithium carbonate contains 10.8 mmol lithium.

Lithium is excreted renally, and passes freely through the glomerular membrane. This is independent of serum concentration: renal lithium clearance is relatively constant for each individual, but is proportional to glomerular filtration. Glomerular filtration is measured by creatinine clearance. If creatinine clearance decreases for any reason, lithium excretion will be reduced and serum lithium levels will rise. Sodium is required for renal lithium excretion. Whenever sodium is depleted, for example because of reduced intake or excess loss, lithium renal clearance is reduced, and serum levels of lithium may become toxic. Furthermore, animal studies show that lithium intoxication can itself impair lithium clearance (Thomsen, 1978).

Mechanism of action

Once absorbed, lithium is widely distributed throughout all body tissues. Its potential to influence physiological functions is enormous, yet its clinical effects are specific. This is the essential challenge underlying any attempt to explain its mechanism of action. The principal theories have centred on:

(1)   electrolytes and ion channels
(2)   neurotransmitters
(3)   second messenger systems.

Electrolytes and ion channels

The physical properties of lithium ions are similar to those of other metallic ions, such as sodium, potassium, calcium and magnesium, all of which have key roles in neuronal cell function. Because of its similarity, lithium can, for example, readily pass through sodium ion channels.

Much clinical research has focused on lithium transport mechanisms, in particular through the membranes of red blood cells (RBCs). The concentration of lithium inside RBCs is less than in plasma. This lithium ratio (of RBC to plasma concentrations) is state independent, and is maintained by mechanisms controlling ion movement in and out of the cell. What happens in the RBC may be a model for neuronal membranes. Compared with normal controls, patients with bipolar disorder have altered Li^+–Na^+ countertransport mechanisms which actively carry the Li^+ ion. This mechanism may be under genetic control, and it has been alleged that this might be associated with a vulnerability to affective disorder (Dorus et al, 1983), although this has not been replicated.

A similar approach using the RBC as a model has investigated the activity of Na^+/K^+–adenosine triphosphatase (ATPase), which is an energy-dependent system and is involved in the sodium pump transportation in membranes. Lithium increases Na^+/K^+–ATPase in patients but not in controls. This may correlate positively with lithium's therapeutic effect. Inhibiting it with an antagonist (such as digoxin) may impair lithium's clinical benefits.

Intracellular concentrations of CA^{2+} and Mg^{2+} ions play a key role in a number of neuronal functions. Lithium may displace or compete with these ions. As a consequence, lithium could, for example, affect Ca^{2+}-dependent activities, including neurotransmitter release or activation of cyclic adenosine monophosphate (cAMP).

Neurotransmitters

It is important to differentiate between the acute and long-term effects of lithium, to appreciate that some non-clinical studies may have used toxic levels of lithium, and to remember that neurotransmitter systems do not function in isolation from each other, as shown in an investigation of lithium effects on both serotoninergic and noradrenergic function (Manji et al, 1991).

Serotonin

Animal studies indicate that short-term lithium treatment increases brain serotonin (5-hydroxytryptamine, 5-HT) turnover. By maintaining an increased turnover, lithium may stabilise mood, as the system is then less open to change. Electrophysiological studies also suggest that lithium may increase the activity of presynaptic serotonergic neurons. Chronic lithium administration may reduce serotonin receptor sites, particularly in the hippocampus.

247

It has proved more difficult to demonstrate lithium-enhanced serotonin neurotransmission in humans. The findings of clinical studies have not been consistent. Many investigations have used neuroendocrine probes of serotonin function. The serum cortisol response to 5-hydroxytryptophan (5-HTP) is enhanced during lithium treatment, as is the prolactin response to tryptophan infusion. Lithium enhances drugs that facilitate the release of serotonin, such as fenfluramine, as measured by an increased prolactin and cortisol response.

Platelet serotonin uptake may be reduced in untreated affective disorder. Long-term lithium treatment may increase serotonin uptake into platelets. Chronic lithium administration reduces serotonin receptor sensitivity. This may be more apparent in the hippocampus, and for $5-HT_2$ than for $5-HT_1$ receptors.

The lithium augmentation of antidepressant efficacy has been explained by proposing that lithium and antidepressants have a synergistic effect of boosting serotonergic function. It was by noting this possibility that de Montigny was prompted to investigate the possible clinical benefits of augmenting antidepressants with lithium (de Montigny *et al*, 1981).

Noradrenaline

Lithium's influence on noradrenergic function has been less considered, although animal studies have shown a number of effects. Initially, lithium may increase noradrenaline uptake into synaptosomes. This, however, returns to normal with continued treatment. As with serotonin, the influences of lithium vary between brain regions.

Clinical studies are limited. They suggest a possible lithium-induced reduction in noradrenaline turnover in affective disorder.

Findings regarding the effects of lithium on adrenergic receptor sensitivity are inconsistent, although it seems unable to prevent down-regulation of β-receptors. In patients with depression, lithium may induce a down-regulation of α-receptors in platelets.

Dopamine

Animal studies show responses to lithium to be specific to different brain regions, with increases or decreases in dopamine or its metabolites. One small clinical investigation indicated that lithium reduces the concentration of dopamine and its metabolites. This may explain its antimanic effect.

Lithium can block the development of the supersensitivity that develops in dopamine receptors after chronic inhibition by neuroleptics such as haloperidol. This led to the unfounded hope that prior treatment with lithium would prevent tardive dyskinesia. It has been suggested, however, that mania may be mediated by overactive dopamine pathways, and thus lithium may work clinically by decreasing this.

Second messenger systems

The molecular mechanisms underlying the therapeutic effect of lithium have focused on those systems involved in signal transduction pathways. Lithium affects both cAMP and phosphoinositol (PI) second messenger systems, and thus attenuates the effects of certain neurotransmitters on their receptors without altering receptor density.

Lithium inhibits noradrenaline-induced cAMP activity, and this varies according to region. By stabilising receptor sensitivity at a given level, it may prevent the fluctuations in neurotransmitter function that underlie bipolar mood swings. Inhibition of cAMP may also explain long-term side-effects such as hypothyroidism and nephrogenic diabetes insipidus, as the release of thyroid hormone and the response of renal cells to vasopressin are energy-dependent processes.

In addition, lithium also affects G proteins, which also transduce signals from receptors to enzymes, generating second messengers, the consequences of which could be similar to the effects of cAMP. These effects are not at therapeutic lithium levels.

The PI second messenger system is stored in a latent form as an inositol lipid in neuronal membranes. When a receptor is stimulated, an inositol lipid gives rise to inositol triphosphate (lns(1,4,5) P3) and diaglycerol (DG). The water-soluble inositol triphosphate diffuses into the cytosol and mobilises intracellular calcium, which in turn activates other molecular events. DG remains within the membrane and triggers the enzyme protein kinase C. Its pathway modulates the activity of adenylate cyclase and may control Ca^{2+} channels. Lithium has the capacity to inhibit both these pathways by limiting the supply of inositol. This in turn leads to receptor desensitisation.

Lithium has no effect on normal mood variations, yet it has specific effects on abnormal mood states. It is hypothesised by Berridge (1989), in what is now called the 'inositol depletion hypothesis', that when neurons are functioning normally, the amount of inositol lipid being used is modest. The consequences of lithium will then be insignificant. With overactive neuronal or synaptic function, however, the demand for inositol will be higher as turnover increases. In these conditions the effects of lithium reducing the inositol supply will become significant.

In patients with manic depressive illness a study using magnetic spectroscopy has demonstrated a lithium-induced reduction in the levels of inositol in the right frontal cortex (Moore et al, 1999). This, however, was before clinical improvement. It has therefore been proposed that inositol reduction sets in train a secondary cascade in the protein kinase C signalling system, thereby producing lithium's therapeutic benefits (Manji & Lenox, 2000). Sodium valproate may have similar effects to lithium on the protein kinase C pathway. Of further interest is the preliminary finding that tamoxifen, which happens also to be a protein kinase C inhibitor, has antimanic effects (Bebchuck *et al*, 2000).

Finally, the mechanism of action of lithium needs to be considered in the light of the body of evidence which indicates that structural changes, such as neuronal cell loss, occur in mood disorder. Lithium has been shown to boost concentrations of proteins in the central nervous system (CNS) which are neuroprotective and neurotropic. It is therefore of some interest that a magnetic resonance study in a small group of patients with bipolar disorder found that chronic lithium usage increased the total volume of grey matter (Moore *et al*, 2000).

In conclusion, when considering the mechanisms of action of lithium, it may be less relevant to focus on specific neurotransmitter systems and more profitable to attend to postsynaptic mechanisms. Lithium affects a number of signal transduction systems common to several different monoamine neurotransmitters. It is thus in a unique position to influence the balance between these neurotransmitter pathways.

Main clinical uses of lithium

Mania

Although lithium is generally recognised to be a safe and effective treatment for mania, and despite many reports to support this view, only a few randomised double-blind placebo-controlled trials (e.g. Maggs, 1963) have tested this. The therapeutic benefits of lithium in mania have, however, been confirmed by trials that have compared lithium with antipsychotic medication, such as chlorpromazine. None the less, approximately 20–40% of patients do not respond to lithium, which may take at least 10 days to be effective. Disturbed or severely excited manic patients are better treated with sedative antipsychotics. Lithium works better in the pure form of mania. Atypical features predict a poorer outcome.

Lithium may be the preferred choice:

(1)   for a cooperative patient with mild mania
(2)   where the patient does not respond to antipsychotics
(3)   where antipsychotics are contraindicated.

Higher serum lithium levels are required for clinical effect in acute mania than for prophylaxis. Stokes *et al* (1976) have shown that the higher the level, the better is the outcome. Others have reported particular patients who were unresponsive at levels up to 1.5 mmol/l but who improved with levels up to 2.0 mmol/l. Such a procedure should be attempted only in hospital, with careful clinical monitoring for early toxicity, frequent serum lithium estimations, and fluid intake adequate to avoid dehydration. Higher doses of lithium may be required to achieve a given serum level in mania than in euthymia. This suggests the body may handle lithium differently in different mood states. It also means that patients stabilised while manic may run the risk of toxicity as their mood returns to normal.

Depression

Acute treatment

Although the first report of lithium's benefits in the treatment of depression was probably in 1894, by Lange (see Johnson, 1984: p. 145), it was some time before it was accepted that this drug with antimanic effect could also be effective in depression. There are sufficient trials now to conclude that lithium is more effective than placebo. Clinical effect may take 3 weeks, and patients with bipolar depression do better than those with unipolar depression. The majority of trials comparing lithium with tricyclic antidepressants tend to show an equivalent response (Watanabe *et al*, 1975; Worrall *et al*, 1979).

Lithium augmentation

De Montigny *et al* (1981) are credited with the first report that adding lithium to the regimen of patients who have failed to respond to tricyclic antidepressants alone leads to clinical improvement. Since then some open and a few double-blind trials have confirmed this, although the time to response is longer (mean of 10 days) than the originally reported 48 hours.

A quantitative analysis of the literature estimated that the odds of remaining ill when lithium is added are reduced by between 56% and 95% (Austin *et al*, 1991). This synergism is found as well with monoamine oxidase inhibitors (MAOIs), and people with depression who do not respond to a tricyclic with lithium may respond to an MAOI with lithium. The mechanism of action is thought to be a combined facilitation of central serotonin neurotransmission. There is animal-based research to support this hypothesis. Investigations of humans, using neuroendocrine probes of serotonergic central activity, lend further support. The correlation, however, between these measures of enhanced serotonin activity and antidepressant outcome is modest (Cowen *et al*, 1991), although lithium's augmentation effects may be mediated through 5-HT$_{1A}$ receptors. A controlled study that showed the combination's benefits in acute depression also demonstrated the need to continue with maintenance therapy for some months (Bauer *et al*, 2000). In combination with nortriptyline, lithium has a marked advantage over either alone in the prevention of relapse in patients with depression who have responded to ECT (Sackheim *et al*, 2001). Lithium augmentation of selective serotonin reuptake inhibitors (SSRIs) could induce a serotonergic syndrome (on which, see Chapter 6).

Recurrent bipolar affective disorder

The principal use of lithium is prophylactically against recurrences of bipolar mood swings. Its benefits for patients, their families and society have been dramatic.

After Schou in the 1950s reported the use of flame photometry for the measurement of lithium concentrations, to avoid toxicity, there was a growing acceptance of the benefits and safety of lithium. This in turn led to the realisation that lithium could reduce the rate of relapse in manic–depressive psychosis. Studies in the 1960s by Hartigan (1963), Baastrup & Schou (1967) and Melia (1967) confirmed this impression. This did not receive universal approval, which prompted Baastrup *et al* (1970) to carry out a double-blind discontinuation study, which confirmed the benefits found in the previous investigations. Studies using different designs, including prospective studies, added further evidence (Angst *et al*, 1970; Coppen *et al*, 1971; Hullin *et al*, 1972; Prien *et al*, 1973).

There are now a satisfactory number of well-designed trials demonstrating the statistically significant superiority of lithium over placebo in the prophylaxis of bipolar disorder. These suggest that 75% of those on placebo will relapse on prospective follow-up compared with 30% on lithium. There are, however, some dissenting reports, for example evidence indicating that hospital admission rates for affective disorders have not been significantly altered by the introduction of lithium (Symonds & Williams, 1981), or that routine clinical results fail to match those from research investigations (Marker & Mander, 1989). Confusion can arise from failing to distinguish between lithium's efficacy (its treatment potential as shown by clinical trials) and lithium's effectiveness (the actual results obtained in normal clinical conditions), which can be influenced by other factors, such as patient compliance (Guscott & Taylor, 1994).

O'Connell *et al* (1991), however, found that the outcome was good for 40% of patients on lithium, fair for 41% and poor for 19%. Whereas not all patients receiving lithium have their disorder completely controlled, the frequency or severity of their relapses will be reduced. A community-based investigation has found reduced admission rates with lithium (McCreadie & Morrison, 1985). Furthermore, the quality of life between episodes is enhanced by a greater sense of mood stability. Both clinically and when reading the literature, it is important to remember that the prophylactic effect of lithium may not become apparent until after at least 6 months of treatment.

The clinical trials demonstrating lithium's benefits prophylactically have been criticised (Moncrieff, 1995), for example on the grounds that lithium discontinuation trials may have overestimated the benenfits because of rebound relapse after withdrawal. These criticisms have been rebutted (Goodwin, 1995; Davis *et al*, 1999) and the issue of rebound has been addressed in a placebo-controlled trial (Bowden *et al*, 2003) in which patients were tapered off lithium before they entered the double-blind phase to avoid relapse due to abrupt discontinuation while on placebo. This 18-month study provides strong evidence for the efficacy of lithium in the prophylaxis of bipolar mood disorder. Finally, a meta-analysis of nine studies, in which a total of 825 patients were randomly allocated to lithium or placebo, found that lithium was superior in preventing relapse in mood disorder overall, especially in bipolar disorder (Burgess *et al*, 2003).

The indications for starting lithium prophylaxis cannot be clearly defined. A general rule of thumb is to consider prophylaxis when a patient has had two distinct manic–depressive episodes lasting at least 1 month within 2 years, or 3 episodes within 5 years. This is based on clinical data that predict that someone relapsing at this rate is likely to continue doing so. In some cases even a single episode of severe mania may justify prophylaxis (Bowden *et al*, 2000*b*) and this would be in keeping with current practice in American psychiatry. Factors such as position of employment (e.g. where the grandiose plans of a company director may bankrupt a business) may strengthen the indication, or it may be weakened (e.g. a concomitant physical illness may act as a relative contraindication).

Serum lithium concentrations correlate positively with prophylactic benefit, although levels do not need to be as high as once thought (Coppen *et al*, 1983), as these had originally been based on experience in mania. Levels around 0.6 mmol/l will be adequate for many. When the 12h-stSLi concentration is increased to 0.7 mmol/l, 50–60% of patients will have a satisfactory outcome, as will 80% at 1.0 mmol/l. It is a matter of clinical judgement as to what level to aim for. If it is too high, the patient may be exposed to unnecessary side-effects and thus will be more likely to drop out. One approach is to aim for a 12h-stSLi of 0.6 mmol/l and adjust it according to outcome or complications.

Treatment should be continued for at least 3 years. A review of the recurrence of mania after lithium discontinuation in patients with bipolar mood disorder found that doing so within 2 years may increase the risk of relapse (Goodwin, 1994).

Predictors of response in bipolar disorder

The most important predictor of response to lithium is patient compliance. Estimates of lithium non-compliance vary from 20% to 50%. Where side-effects occur, reducing serum levels will enhance compliance, as will patient education, self-help groups, involvement of family and cognitive therapy. Practical measures such as frequent lithium estimations, use of pill boxes, and a positive approach to dealing with side-effects are useful adjuncts. Some patients are more likely to be concerned by weight gain, which should be managed quickly and not ignored; others may be more concerned about memory problems and tremor.

Other predictors of a positive lithium response include:

(1) a good previous response
(2) a 'pure' form of bipolar affective illness or endogenous type of depression
(3) a family history of bipolar illness
(4) an episodic sequence of mania followed by depression, rather than depression followed by mania (Faedda et al, 1991).

A poor response is associated with:

(1) rapid cycling
(2) paranoid features
(3) substance misuse
(4) poor social support.

Living with relatives rated as being of high expressed emotion also leads to a poorer response.

Age, marital status, response to the dexamethasone suppression test, and thyroid and renal function do not act as predictors. A variety of personality traits have been investigated, and low neuroticism and high obsessionality may predict a good outcome.

Prophylaxis of unipolar depression

Schou (1989) was moved to speculate on the reasons why 'doubt about the efficacy of prophylactic lithium treatment in unipolar illness seems almost exclusively a U.S. phenomenon'. The US Food and Drug Administration had not as yet sanctioned lithium for this purpose.

A review using meta-analysis of the literature may help resolve this (Souza & Goodwin, 1991). Analysis of the pooled data from eight controlled trials indicated a 'powerful treatment effect' for lithium over placebo. A comparison of lithium against other antidepressant therapy revealed no statistically significant differences; that is, they are of equivalent benefit, although others believe that patients with more severe depression do better on tricyclics. Adding lithium to a tricyclic antidepressant may fail to provide any additional prophylaxis against depression (Johnstone et al, 1990).

Thus, while lithium is the drug of first choice in the prophylaxis of bipolar affective disorder, it is the second choice in unipolar disorder, since the SSRIs are usually as effective and safer (see Chapter 6).

Antidepressants, however, are contraindicated in the maintenance treatment of bipolar disorder because of the risk of precipitating mania or inducing rapid cycling (four or more mood swings per year).

Suicide risk

Long-term lithium maintenance, including for unipolar depression, is associated with a significant reduction in suicide rates, which has not been shown for anticonvulsants generally. This may result from lithium's particular effects on 5-HT$_2$ receptors (Hughes *et al*, 2000).

Other clinical uses of lithium

Puerperal psychosis

Lithium is important in reducing the increased risk of relapse in the post-partum period for women with either affective psychosis or schizoaffective psychosis (Stewart *et al*, 1991).

Schizoaffective psychosis and schizophrenia

Most work in this area has investigated the prophylactic benefits of lithium for schizoaffective psychosis. There are reports that lithium may be as effective in this regard as it is in bipolar affective illness, but also reports of it having little or no effect. This is not surprising in view of the poor validity and reliability of the concept of schizoaffective psychosis. In general, patients with more affective symptoms respond better than patients with more core schizophrenic or unipolar schizo-affective symptoms (Maj, 1988). Similarly, a family history of affective psychosis predicts a response to lithium, whereas schizophrenia in the family tends to predict a lack of response.

The role of lithium in the treatment of 'functional' psychosis was studied by Johnstone *et al* (1988) and it appears that the benefits are confined to elevated mood.

Aggression

Lithium has been shown to be significantly better at suppressing aggression than placebo in a population of young male prisoners who had a history of impulsive aggression (Sheard *et al*, 1976).

Intellectual impairment

As in the intellectually normal population, lithium is useful where recurring mood swings are apparent. Furthermore, it may also reduce the frequency of either self-injurious behaviour or aggression. One report found that 63% of aggressive persons with a learning disability experienced a 30% reduction in this behaviour after taking lithium (Spreat *et al*, 1989).

Alcohol misuse

Lithium may blunt the euphoriant effect of alcohol. Of two early studies indicating lithium had a beneficial effect on the relapse rate in alcoholism, one found that this was apparent where the alcoholism was associated with depression. A subsequent study, however, failed to show that lithium in these patients was superior to a placebo, irrespective of mood (Dorus, 1989).

Eating disorders

A few patients with eating disorders have benefited from lithium in conjunction with behaviour therapy. The evidence is not yet strong enough to make a recommendation, especially in view of the likely hazards.

Lithium for the elderly

Lithium can be effective in the elderly (Shulman *et al*, 1987). Renal function declines with age, and thus lower does of lithium may be required for patients aged over 50 years. Greater care is required with regard to renal, cardiac and thyroid function, as well as to CNS status. Lithium toxicity may occur at the upper level of the normal therapeutic range in the elderly, and lithium–antipsychotic interactions may be more frequent in those over 65. Augmentation of antidepressants is successful in this age group, although one in five patients may have side-effects.

Lithium for children and adolescents

The absence of randomised, double-blind trials combined with the problem of defining criteria for manic–depressive illness in this age group makes it difficult to evaluate lithium's role. However, some investigations have indicated that mood does respond satisfactorily to lithium (Campbell *et al*, 1984). As in adults, it may also benefit hostility and aggressiveness, regardless of the underlying diagnosis.

Children have a higher renal clearance, so may require higher doses of lithium. It is assumed that similar blood levels are necessary, although this is not proven.

Lithium is tolerated well by the young (Lena, 1979). Specific concerns have been raised about adverse effects of lithium on bone development and on growth hormone release; however, these are not significant. The longer-term consequences on renal function need to be monitored clinically, as well as by more extensive follow-up investigations.

Lithium intoxication

Causes

Lithium intoxication is usually inadvertent. During routine treatment, toxicity can be precipitated by dehydration, reduced renal clearance or by drug interactions, such as with thiazide diuretics (see below). Renal lithium elimination will be impaired by medical illness associated with pyrexia or with vomiting or diarrhoea, and by reduced salt intake.

Adequate sodium levels are necessary for lithium excretion. In severe sodium deficiency states, lithium begins to be reabsorbed from distal portions of the tubules. This elevates serum lithium levels, which in turn inhibits sodium reabsorption by inhibiting aldosterone. By exacerbating sodium deficiency, a vicious cycle may thus start. Vomiting and diarrhoea from lithium toxicity can add to this cycle.

Signs

The signs of lithium intoxication (Box 7.1) may appear at serum levels above 1.3 mmol/l, although levels may be deceptively low in the elderly during the evolution of toxicity. Seizures and coma may follow. Death results from either cardiac effects or pulmonary complications caused by severe viscosity of respiratory secretions. After recovery some patients may be left with permanent neurological deficits.

Treatment

Treatment involves supportive measures and anti-epileptics when indicated. Frequent determination of lithium levels, such as every 6–12 hours, is useful to monitor progress, but is no substitute for clinical assessment. Provided renal function is unimpaired, it is usually necessary only to increase fluid intake. Increasing lithium renal

---

Box 7.1 The signs of lithium intoxication

- Vomiting
- Diarrhoea
- Coarse tremor
- Dysarthria
- Ataxia
- Cognitive impairment
- Lassitude
- Restlessness
- Agitation

---

excretion by saline infusion or by osmotic diuresis can be helpful, but not always.

Haemodialysis is the most effective treatment and should be instituted:

(1)   at serum levels above 3 mmol/l
(2)   where indicated by coma or shock
(3)   where conservative measures fail after 24 hours.

Adverse reactions to lithium

The side-effects of lithium are not uncommon, although generally they are tolerated. The prevalence varies from 60% to as high as 90%. There is a general positive correlation between plasma lithium levels and reported subjective side-effects. They tend to be more troublesome with age. Some reports suggest that there may be a sex difference, such as more tremor complained of by men, but overall there are probably no significant sex differences (Vestergaard, 1983; Vestergaard et al, 1988).

Ghodse (1977) reported the following rates for side-effects:

(1)   memory problems (52%)
(2)   thirst (42%)
(3)   polyuria (38%)
(4)   tremor (34%)
(5)   drowsiness (24%)
(6)   weight gain (18%).

Infrequent complaints include metallic taste and altered psychosexual function. Most complaints occur in the first fortnight of treatment.

The type of lithium preparation prescribed may have limited overall consequence for side-effects (Johnstone et al, 1979). Nevertheless, sustained-release formulations may have advantage over standard preparations in reducing specific complaints such as tremor and nausea by lowering peak serum levels. On the other hand, diarrhoea may be less likely with standard-release formulations.

Kidney

Structural changes

Great concern about the potential nephrotoxic effects of lithium developed after the reports by Hestbech et al (1977) that renal biopsy of lithium patients showed structural damage. These included patchy interstitial fibrosis, tubular atrophy and glomerular sclerosis. Although the population biopsied was biased – having been selected by virtue of lithium toxicity, severe polyuria, or reduced kidney function – extensive evaluation of the renal effects of lithium resulted.

Studies of unselected patients on lithium estimate the prevalence of histological abnormalities to be between 10% and 15%. It should be remembered that patients with chronic psychotic illnesses tend to have more degenerative changes in their kidneys and other organs than other people.

Functional changes

Lithium induces polyuria and a compensatory polydipsia due to impaired renal tubular function. This is secondary to inhibition of the kidneys' ability to concentrate urine (by 15–30%) in response to antidiuretic hormone (ADH), resulting in a form of nephrogenic diabetes insipidus. Lithium inhibits the cAMP response to ADH in the cells of the collecting ducts. A degree of polyuria (i.e. up to 3 l urine/24 h) is generally tolerated by patients, but excessive polyuria can lead to dehydration and lithium intoxication.

Coppen et al (1980) found only modest differences in renal tubular function between patients with manic depression on lithium and not on lithium. The possibility of a primary or psychogenic polydipsia should also be borne in mind. Patients may drink excessively for a variety of reasons, including anxiety about lithium intoxication.

Discontinuation of lithium usually but not invariably leads to reversal of polyuria. Treatment with amiloride can counteract the effects of lithium on water transport in the renal collecting ducts.

Changes in glomerular function (GFR), as measured by creatinine clearance, are modest in comparison with those in tubular function. Although GFR may drop below the normal range, this is usually not serious. Few patients experience a decline to below 40 ml/mm, and there is no clear evidence that lithium will lead to severe chronic renal failure. Again, differences between patients with manic depression on lithium and not on lithium are not significant. It is also possible that changes in GFR may be secondary to impairment of tubular function. Acute renal failure may occur occasionally with lithium toxicity.

To minimise renal side-effects, investigators have examined the consequences of different dosage schedules. Multiple daily doses will give a smaller peak and more plateau-like blood levels over 24 hours, whereas once-daily administration will produce high serum peak levels followed by a marked trough.

Paradoxically, experimental work in rats by Plenge et al (1982), backed up by a clinical comparison of these two approaches, suggests that once-daily dosage is safer for the kidney (Schou et al, 1982; Hetmar et al, 1987; Bowen et al, 1991). This finding is explained by reference to the trough in the serum level each day. This allows regeneration for repair in any damaged renal cells, which cannot happen with a more plateau-like serum profile. This may be analogous to the effects of alcohol on the liver, where cirrhosis may be more prevalent with high, but not toxic, constant intake than with intermittent intoxication. The benefits of lithium are diminished, however, when patients are switched to administration every second day.

In summary, most studies have not found a relationship between histological changes and longitudinal reductions in GFR. It is now generally considered that the microscopic structural abnormality and both the tubular and glomerular changes correlate best with a history of lithium toxicity.

Thyroid

Hypothyroidism and non-toxic goitre occur in approximately 3% and 5%, respectively, of patients on lithium. It is more common in women of late middle age. An elevated concentration of thyroid-stimulating hormone (TSH) is often the first sign of reduced thyroid output and so is a good biochemical marker. Thyroid function should be checked every 6–12 months. Minor fluctuations in thyroid function may spontaneously return to normal.

Hypothyroidism may be mistaken clinically for a new depressive episode. With persistent hypothyroidism, replacement thyroxine may be safely prescribed with lithium, and this may be required in 2 per 100 patient-years. Rapid-cycling mood swings may be associated with subclinical hypothyroidism.

There have been case reports of hyperthyroidism in lithium patients. It is unclear whether this is a coincidental finding or whether it is induced by lithium.

Parathyroid

A raised serum parathormone (PTH) level early in treatment may occur because of a failure in the feedback regulation of parathyroid secretion by calcium. This not clinically significant and is not a true hyperparathyroidism. The modest elevation in serum calcium and PTH are usually transient.

Weight gain

Weight gain can occur in a third of patients and is one of the most frequent reasons (along with cognitive changes) for non-compliance. It may be secondary to increased carbohydrate craving, polydipsia-induced increase in calorific drinks, altered glucose metabolism, or hypothyroidism. The strongest correlation is probably between weight gain and polydipsia. Treatment can be successful with appropriate measures, including reduced calorie intake. Caution is necessary that any reducing diet does not result in sodium deficiency. Anticipating this problem can reduce its extent.

Cardiovascular effects

Electrocardiographic monitoring shows that T-wave flattening and inversion occurs in up to 30% of patients. This is benign and reversible. Rare cases of sinus node dysfunction are reported, making the 'sick sinus' syndrome a contraindication for lithium. Syncope should alert to the need for a cardiovascular review. Transient pedal oedema may occur early in treatment. Toxic levels may cause cardiac failure and arrhythmias.

Central nervous system

Fine tremor is the most frequent non-toxic side-effect affecting the CNS. It may be alleviated by β-blockers such as propranolol. Decreased motor coordination and muscle weakness may be missed clinically. Extrapyramidal side-effects are uncommon when lithium is administered on its own, but are frequent when it is combined with antipsychotics. Electroencephalography often records an increased wave amplitude and generalised slowing, although lithium does not exacerbate epilepsy.

The effect of lithium on cognitive function was initially underestimated, perhaps because of confounding variables such as the effects of mood or other medication. Studies of healthy volunteers show small but consistent decreased ability to learn, concentrate and memorise (Judd, 1979).

Skin

A variety of rashes have been noted, of which a maculopapular one is the most common. This is reversible and usually does not reappear on reinstatement of treatment. Flare-up of pre-existing psoriasis is not uncommon. Acneiform eruptions and exfoliative dermatitis occur rarely.

Hair

Hair loss and change in hair texture may be reported, especially in women. If this is associated with hypothyroidism, it may improve with thyroxine.

Blood

Lithium can cause a mild leucocytosis. This has no clinical relevance to lithium patients, but can be of use in medical disorders associated with leucopenia.

Pregnancy

Data from a lithium birth register (Schou & Weinstein, 1980) indicated an excess of congenital malformations (occurring in 11% of births) in children born to mothers taking lithium during pregnancy, especially of the cardiac malformation called Epstein's anomaly (occurring in 8% of births), which involves the tricuspid valve as well as the right atrium and ventricle. Although further register data suggest that the risks may be as low as 0.1% for Epstein's anomaly, this is still 20 times greater than that in the normal population.

A more recent report (Jacobson et al, 1992) on women exposed to lithium in the first trimester concluded that lithium was not a major teratogen. Where possible, however, lithium should be avoided during the first trimester, although the risks to mother and foetus of not taking lithium need to be considered, such as self-destructive or disinhibited behaviours. Relapse rates of approximately 50% over 40 weeks are the same in pregnant as in non-pregnant women (Viguera et al, 2000) and increase where the lithium discontinuation is rapid. Thus, the hazards of lithium discontinuation, especially if it is abrupt, need to be considered in the risk–benefit analysis. The impact of a major relapse on the developing foetus is unknown. If lithium is required, then ultrasound and foetal echocardiography monitoring should be considered.

Lithium can be recommenced later in pregnancy, especially if there are concerns of post-partum relapse.

Foetal goitre has been reported to complicate delivery by pressing on the trachea during birth.

In pregnancy there is a gradual improvement in GFR, which means that lithium dosage will require compensatory increases to maintain a constant blood level. Shortly after delivery, however, GFR rapidly reverts to baseline. Frequent lithium tests are therefore required to avoid toxicity.

Lithium passes readily through the placenta and into breast milk as well. Concentrations in breast milk are 50% of the maternal serum concentration, although infants may have similar blood levels, as their capacity to handle lithium is less. Breast-feeding is therefore relatively contraindicated, although supplementation with bottle-feeding will reduce the infant's exposure.

Anticonvulsants have been regarded as safer in breast-feeding, but, as a recent review points out, there is a paucity of data available, and haematological and hepatic complications may arise in the infants (Chaudron & Jefferson, 2000).

Drug interactions

Diuretics

Thiazide diuretics reduce renal clearance of lithium by as much as 40%, and may therefore cause toxicity. Other types of diuretics have been less well studied, so caution is required with their use. Nevertheless, loop diuretics, such as furosemide, are thought to be without significant effects. Amiloride, a potassium-sparing diuretic, can reduce the polyuria induced by lithium.

Antipsychotics

Great concern resulted from the report by Cohen & Cohen (1974) of irreversible brain damage following the combination of lithium with haloperidol. The original report has been critically analysed. It failed to mention serum lithium levels, and the cases occurred at the same time in the same institution. It is therefore possible that the patients experienced either lithium toxicity or a viral encephalopathy. Although other reports followed of neurotoxicity with lithium and other anti-psychotic combinations, both retrospective and prospective studies of hundreds of patients have failed to confirm a specific lithium–antipsychotic interaction. Lithium, however, may increase intracellular concentrations of haloperidol. The combination does produce worse than expected extrapyramidal side-effects (the 'Methuselah syndrome') and some of the reactions have been likened to the neuroleptic malignant syndrome (see Chapter 9).

One can conclude that the combination of lithium and antipsychotic, a potent regimen in severe mania, is not contraindicated. Caution is required, however; for example, there should be more frequent lithium estimations, use of the lowest doses possible of both drugs, close clinical monitoring to detect significant CNS side-effects, and accurate recording of fluid intake to avoid dehydration. Atypical antipsychotics seem safer in combination with lithium.

Antidepressants

An increase in tremor has been reported with tricyclic antidepressant–lithium combinations.

Anti-inflammatory agents

Non-steroidal anti-inflammatory drugs (NSAIDs) inhibit prostaglandin synthesis. This may result in reduced renal lithium clearance and thus elevate lithium plasma levels (Shelley, 1987), as has been reported for indomethacin, ibuprofen, phenylbutaxone, diclofenac and piroxicam. Aspirin and paracetamol appear to be safe. Sulindac may not be as risk free as was once thought. Patients stabilised on lithium need to be monitored carefully (twice weekly initially) when started on these drugs, especially those who rely on prostaglandins to maintain an optimum renal function, such as the elderly or those with a history of cardiac failure.

263

Cardiovascular drugs

Drugs that reduce renal perfusion may elevate lithium plasma levels. A few cases of lithium neurotoxicity with methyldopa have been reported. Verapamil may cause either neurotoxicity or reduction in lithium levels, and bradycardia has been reported. Digoxin and lithium may produce severe nodal bradycardia. Lithium may decrease the antihypertensive effects of clonidine.

Anticonvulsants

Combinations of carbamazepine and lithium may produce neurotoxic reactions even when both drugs are within their normal therapeutic range. A few cases of neurotoxicity with phenytoin have been reported, with irreversible cerebellar damage. The mechanism is unclear; it could be pharmacological, or perhaps some people with epilepsy may be more vulnerable to lithium toxicity at normal levels. Sodium valproate may reduce lithium concentrations.

Antibiotics

A few case reports suggest that some antibiotics, such as the tetra-cyclines, metronidazole and levofloxacin, may elevate lithium levels, perhaps by a renal interaction.

General anaesthetics

Prolonged apnoea has occasionally occurred when lithium was combined with the muscle relaxants succinylcholine or pancuronium. Cholinergics (neostigmine and pyridostigmine) are antagonised. Lithium discontinuation is therefore advisable when electroconvulsive therapy is used on the patient, both for these reasons and because patients may become confused afterwards.

Lithium therapy in practice

Medical examinations and tests

Once a clinical decision to start lithium has been made, the advantages and disadvantages should be discussed with both patient and relatives. As well as being necessary to obtain consent, this is also an important educational exercise (see also below). A medical history is taken and a note made of any concomitant medication. Following an appropriate medical examination, biochemical screening is required. The following are usually recommended:

(1) thyroid function
(2) urea and electrolytes
(3) urinalysis
(4) creatinine clearance.

These further act as measurements against which future test results can be compared. The practice of measuring urea and electrolytes routinely, without a clinical indication, has limited value. The 24-hour urine volume of the creatinine clearance test should be recorded, as this can be a simple measure of future alterations in renal concentrating capacity, whereas serum creatinine is more an index of glomerular function. Generally, thyroid function, of which TSH is the most sensitive test, should be carried out every 6 months, especially in women who are middle aged or older. Nevertheless, thyroid supplementation is not required unless the T4 level falls or there is clinical evidence of hypothyroidism. A similar frequency is recommended for a serum creatinine test. It is important not merely to ensure that serum creatinine remains within the normal range, but also to detect any pattern of progressive deterioration over time from the baseline. This, or any abnormally high result, alerts the clinician to the need to perform a repeat creatinine clearance test. Additional tests recommended by some include a full blood count and an electrocardiogram in those aged over 50. A baseline body weight and regular repeats are useful.

Dose and serum monitoring

The initial dose will lie within the range 400–600 mg lithium carbonate per day. A 12-hour standard lithium test should be carried out within 5 days and the dose adjusted. Weekly tests are indicated until the required plasma level is established. Steady-state conditions are reached within about a week. There is good correlation between adjustment of dose and the resulting change in plasma levels; for example, doubling the dose will nearly double the plasma concentration. A technique to estimate the dose required has been devised from the result obtained from a 24-hour estimation after a priming dose of 600 mg lithium carbonate (Cooper & Simpson, 1976; Perry et al, 1986). Once the desired level is achieved, levels can be checked less and less frequently; many patients will eventually require checks only every 3–4 months. Regular attendances for venepuncture reinforce the importance to the patient of lithium levels, as well as improving compliance.

Routine checks should encompass a 12-hour standard serum lithium level and a review of side-effects, including an estimate of fluid intake per 24 hours. Indications of increasing polydipsia and polyuria (>3 l urine/24 h) may indicate the need to measure fasting urine osmolarity and for hospital admission for a water-deprivation test if necessary.

A consultation with a nephrologist may be appropriate when an abnormality in renal function is detected.

Education

It is important to educate patient and family about the situations in which more frequent lithium estimations or dose adjustments or discontinuation are required. These include the taking of other medications (e.g. diuretics or NSAIDs), febrile illness, renal or gastro-intestinal symptoms, crash diets, moving to a hot, humid climate or using saunas, taking up vigorous exercise, pregnancy, or the presence of any signs of toxicity. If a patient forgets a dose, the next dose should not be doubled. Lithium should be discontinued 24–48 hours before surgery and recommenced when the patient is able to tolerate oral fluids again. During the procedure adequate hydration should be maintained intravenously.

Education about lithium is essential. This can be done in one-to-one counselling sessions, supplemented by information leaflets such as the fact sheet available from the Royal College of Psychiatrists, or those usefully made available by the pharmaceutical industry. The value of more intensive programmes using video-tape lectures supplemented with follow-up home visits to answer questions has been demonstrated (Peet & Harvey, 1991).

The lithium clinic

In the 1970s and onwards, lithium clinics became an important develop-ment in the care of patients, as well as being a new model of psychiatric service (Fieve, 1975). With a wider range of therapy now available, they are perhaps more appropriately renamed 'mood disorder clinics'. The advantages are that they allow psychiatrists to develop special interests and to keep abreast of an extensive and growing body of literature. They facilitate the setting up of databases and foster research.

Such clinics are usually located in an out-patient setting. Patients preferably attend in the morning, as this allows for 12-hour standard lithium estimations. On arrival, blood is taken for lithium measurement and sent in a batch to a laboratory that is ready to analyse the samples, so that ideally the psychiatrist has the result available when assessing the patient. While waiting to be seen, the patients can complete mood rating scales or questionnaires on side-effects. They can also attend support or education groups.

Discontinuation of lithium

Up to 50% of patients on lithium prophylaxis will discontinue it (McCreadie & Morrison, 1985; Cooper, 1988), with one in four stopping within the first 6 months (Aagaard *et al*, 1988). Long-term follow-up studies indicate that most of these patients will relapse (Abou-Saleh & Coppen, 1986; Page *et al*, 1987). Where patients stabilised on lithium had been randomly assigned to either placebo or lithium, relapse occurred only during placebo treatment (Mander & Louden, 1988). A review of 14 studies of the discontinuation of previously successful lithium treatment for affective disorder revealed that 50% of relapses occurred within 10 weeks of stopping treatment (Suppes *et al*, 1991). Survival analysis estimated that the time to relapse was shorter for mania than for depression: the time to 25% recurrence of mania was 2.7 months, compared with 14 months for a depressive relapse. Overall, there was a 28-fold greater risk of a mood swing after discontinuation compared with during lithium therapy. Discontinuation studies suggest that the peak risk time to relapse is actually within the first 2 days to 2 weeks (Greil & Schmidt, 1988).

Sudden discontinuation of lithium should be avoided. It may be more likely to precipitate a relapse than a gradual phasing out of the drug. Furthermore, there have been case reports of withdrawal symptoms, including irritability, increased anxiety and emotional lability (King & Hullin, 1983).

Following a successful period of treatment the decision whether or not to stop lithium prophylaxis is ultimately the patient's. The role of the psychiatrist is to provide information, advice, counsel, and support for both patient and family.

Pharmacological alternatives to lithium

Most of the alternatives to lithium are anticonvulsants (Post, 1990; Small, 1990).

Carbamazepine

Carbamazepine, which is used in the treatment of temporal lobe epilepsy and trigeminal neuralgia, has a pharmacological structure similar to that of tricyclic antidepressants. Some of the first reports of its use in psychiatry came from Japan, where it was found that it had both antimanic and prophylactic benefit in manic–depressive psychosis. Controlled clinical trials have confirmed this, and it is claimed to be as effective as lithium (Coxhead *et al*, 1992), although the overall data suggest it is not. It may be beneficial where lithium has failed, in particular in rapid-cycling manic depression. The combination of both is clinically potent with refractory affective disorder (Peselow *et al*, 1994), although neurotoxic side-effects may occur in about 10% of cases, even when both are within their normal therapeutic range.

The starting dose is 100–200 mg daily, which can be built up gradually to 1600 mg daily in divided doses. Blood levels need to be monitored. Unlike lithium, there are no guidelines for appropriate blood levels in affective disorder, although it is suggested that therapeutic effect can be achieved at 8–12 µg/ml without toxic side-effects. In contrast to lithium, there is no clear positive correlation between blood levels and either clinical benefit or side-effects (Box 7.2). Carbamazepine is well tolerated, and initial minor side-effects may ameliorate after 2 weeks of treatment.

A full blood count should be carried out before treatment, weekly for the first month, monthly for the subsequent 5 months, and two to four

---

Box 7.2   Side-effects of carbamazepine

Central nervous system
- Dizziness
- Diplopia
- Headache
- Somnolence
- Ataxia
- Blurred vision
- Confusion

Gastrointestinal tract
- Dry mouth
- Nausea
- Constipation/diarrhoea
- Loss of appetite

Metabolic
- Hyponatraemia
- Abnormal liver function tests

Cardiovascular system
- Depression of atrioventricular conduction
- Oedema

Skin
- Allergic rash
- Exfoliative dermatitis

Haematology
- Leucopenia
- Thrombocytopenia
- Agranulocytosis
- Aplastic anaemia

Hypersensitivity
- A rare multi-organ disorder

times a year thereafter. Lithium may induce a leucocytosis, but unfortunately prior lithium treatment does not prevent the induction of leucopenia by carbamazepine. Carbamazepine does not have to be automatically discontinued if an asymptomatic or non-progressive leucopenia develops. If it is severe, progressive or produces clinical symptoms such as a sore throat, then carbamazepine should be stopped. Liver function tests should be carried out before treatment and periodically during treatment, as should serum folic acid estimations. Driving a car may be impaired initially. Arterioventricular conduction defects are a contraindication unless a pacemaker is used.

Carbamazepine may induce its own metabolism, and so blood levels may drop. Likewise, it may reduce blood levels of other drugs, including antipsychotics.

Because of its structural similarity to tricyclics, carbamazepine should preferably not be combined with an MAOI. It may reduce the efficacy of the combined oral contraceptive pill.

There appears to be an increase in developmental disorders, such as spina bifida, in children born to mothers on carbamazepine for the treatment of epilepsy. The influence of anti-epileptics on coagulation and also on folic acid levels need to be borne in mind during pregnancy. Injections of vitamin K are therefore recommended in the last few weeks of pregnancy, as well as for the infant. Carbamazepine is present in breast milk, but not in amounts sufficient to make it an automatic contraindication, provided the infant is closely monitored.

Unlike lithium, carbamazepine does not appear to cause weight gain, hypothyroidism or diabetes insipidus. It may therefore be an alternative where these are a concern. The transfer from lithium to carbamazepine should be done gradually, as rapid discontinuation of lithium may provoke a rebound emergence of symptoms.

Its mechanism of action, as with that of other anti-epileptics used for affective disorder, is uncertain. The effects on neurotransmitters are not similar to those of lithium. It is thought that carbamazepine may stabilise synaptic transmission by dampening the influx of sodium ions into neurons via sodium channels. Presynaptically it blocks the reuptake of both dopamine and noradrenaline and enhances the release of dopamine. How this explains its therapeutic effects is unclear. One interesting theory postulated by Post et al (1982) is that it works by the prevention of electrophysiological 'kindling' in the brain.

Sodium valproate

This drug, whose use is increasing in mood disorder, was first reported in France in the 1960s. There are a few controlled trials of its usefulness in mania, some of which are double blind and placebo controlled (Pope et al, 1991). Its prophylactic effectiveness has been recently shown in a randomised placebo-controlled trial in America, where the Divalproex formulation is used (Bowden *et al*, 2000*a*). As with carbamazepine, lithium-refractory patients and those with mixed or dysphoric mania may benefit from valproate (McElroy *et al*, 1992).

The initial dose is 300–400 mg/day, in divided doses. This is increased gradually under monitoring until therapeutic blood levels are achieved. Peak doses range from 750 to 3000 mg/day, with blood levels in the range 50–100 µg/ml. No correlation between therapeutic efficacy and blood levels has been found.

Valproate, as does carbamazepine, reduces the activity of gamma-aminobutyric acid (GABA) in the CNS. It has therefore been suggested that mania may result from a GABA-ergic overactivity. The side-effects of valproate are listed in Box 7.3.

Lamotrigine

This established anticonvulsant, whose psychiatric use is on the increase, had been noted to enhance the mood of patients with epilepsy. Clinical studies suggest a role in the prophylaxis in mood disorder, especially treatment-resistant or rapid-cycling bipolar disorder (Calabrese *et al*, 2000) or treatment-resistant depression. Lamotrigine is superior to placebo in preventing a depressive relapse in patients with bipolar disorder (Bowden *et al*, 2003) and as such may have an advantage over other mood stabilisers. The dose range is 100–200 mg/day; a starting dose of 25 mg/day should be gradually increased every 1–2 weeks. Common side-effects include rash (especially with high starting doses or if combined with valproate) and headache. It lacks direct effects on CNS kindling, but it may prove relevant that it can be neuroprotective.

Box 7.3 Side-effects of valproate

Common
• Tremor
• Weight gain
• Ankle swelling
• Hair thinning
• Cognitive dysfunction

Less common
• Hepatotoxicity
• Thrombocytopenia

Metabolic abnormality
• Hyperammonaemia/glycinaemia
• Encephalopathy
• Toxicity (1–2%)

Clonazepam

This is a benzodiazepine used in the treatment of epilepsy. It has been advocated in the treatment of mania, especially to control acute manic symptoms. There appear to be no controlled trials of its efficacy in prophylaxis.

Gabapentin

Gabapentin is an anti-epileptic drug that is used as adjunctive therapy in some types of refractory cases and it has a clinical role in neuropathic pain. An open-label study suggested that it has antimanic properties (Cabras *et al*, 1999) but a placebo-controlled trial as adjunctive therapy failed to show any efficacy (Pande *et al*, 2000), as did one in refractory mood disorder (Frye *et al*, 2000). It may prove more effective in anxiety disorders.

Topiramate

In common with other anticonvulsants, topiramate has been assessed in open-label clinical trials in a variety of bipolar mood states, in doses of 100–300 mg daily. It may have a role in resistant cases as monotherapy or in combination with other mood stabilisers, but placebo-controlled double-blind trials are required. Side-effects include cognitive and other CNS complications. Paraesthesia and visual problems have been reported. Unlike other mood stabilisers, it is associated with weight loss in up to 50% of cases and this is greater the more overweight the patient is. Arising from this it has been tried in bulimia nervosa with reported improvement in satiety.

Verapamil

Preliminary reports suggest that this calcium-channel blocker may have antimanic benefits (Dubovsky *et al*, 1986). Theoretically it may work, as Ca^{2+} influx is required for neurotransmitter release, but passage through the blood–brain barrier has not been confirmed at therapeutic levels. It is claimed to be effective in both lithium-responsive and non-responsive mania. The dose lies within the range 240–480 mg/day in divided doses. Initial monitoring of the cardiovascular system, including electro-cardiography, is recommended. It may cause neurotoxicity if combined with lithium.

Clonidine

Clonidine is an α_2-adrenoreceptor agonist. By simulating these pre-synaptic receptors it has an inhibitory effect on CNS noradrenergic activity. It has been reported to have a variety of therapeutic benefits, including alleviation of opiate withdrawal symptoms. A small percentage of patients with mania may respond to it, although smaller than with lithium or verapamil.

Other metallic ions

Vanadium

It has been hypothesised that mood change may result from abnormal activity of the enzyme Na-ATPase. Vanadium may be an endogenous inhibitor of this enzyme. Therefore reducing the concentration of vanadium could be therapeutic in manic depression. This has reportedly been achieved by using ascorbic acid or EDTA (ethylene diamine tetra acetic acid) (Naylor et al, 1984), but remains unconfirmed.

Rubidium

Rubidium is a monovalent cation similar to lithium and potassium, but it has many differences from lithium. Although it may have antidepressant benefits it may also prolong mania or facilitate experimentally induced aggression. Unlike lithium, it increases central noradrenergic activity when given chronically to rats, and in vitro it increases cAMP formation (Mork & Geisler, 1991), whereas lithium inhibits its accumulation.

Summary

Attitudes to the role of anticonvulsants in bipolar disorder differ in the UK and Ireland from those in North America, where they are increasingly being recommended as first-line treatments. The current European view is that anticonvulsants are not a proven alternative to lithium but have a clear therapeutic role where lithium is either insufficiently effective or not tolerated. Their combination with lithium may often be appropriate and they are also worth consideration in mixed affective states or rapid-cycling mood disorder. A further transatlantic difference is in the management of acute mania, where antipsychotics are routinely used in the UK but in North America mood stabilisers are used on their own and antipsychotics are added only if psychotic phenomena are present.

References

Aagaard, J., Vestergaard, P. & Maarhjergk, K. (1988) Adherence to lithium prophylaxis. *Pharmacopsychiatry*, **21**, 166–170.

Abou-Saleh, M. T. & Coppen, A. (1986) Who responds to prophylactic lithium? *Journal of Affective Disorders*, **10**, 115–125.

Angst, J., Weis, P., Grof, P., et al (1970) Lithium prophylaxis in recurrent affective disorders. *British Journal of Psychiatry*, **116**, 604–614.

Austin, M.-P., Souza, F. G. M. & Goodwin, G. M. (1991) Lithium augmentation in antidepressant-resistant patients. A quantitative analysis. *British Journal of Psychiatry*, **159**, 510–514.

Baastrup, P. C. & Schou, M. (1967) Lithium as a prophylactic agent: its effect against recurrent depression and manic–depressive psychosis. *Archives of General Psychiatry*, **16**, 162–172.

Baastrup, P. C., Poulsen, J. C., Schou, M., *et al* (1970) Prophylactic lithium: double blind discontinuation in manic-depressive and recurrent-depressive disorders. *Lancet*, **2**, 326–330.

Bauer, M., Bschor, T, Kunz, D., *et al* (2000) Double-blind placebo-controlled trial of the use of lithium to augment antidepressant medication in continuation treatment of unipolar major depression. *American Journal of Psychiatry*, **157**, 1429–1435.

Bebchuck, J. M., Arfken, C. L., Dolan-Manji, S., *et al* (2000) A preliminary investigation of a protein kinase inhibitor in the treament of acute mania. *Archives of General Psychiatry*, **57**, 95–96.

Berridge, M. J. (1989) Inositol triphosphate, calcium, lithium, and cell signaling. *Journal of the American Medical Association*, **262**, 1834–1841.

Bowden, C. L., Calabrese, J. R., McElroy, S. L., *et al* (2000a) A randomized, placebo-controlled 12-month trial of divalproex and lithium in treatment of outpatients with bipoar I disorder. *Archives of General Psychiatry*, **57**, 481–489.

Bowden, C. L., Lecrubier, Y., Bauer, M., *et al* (2000b) Maintenance therapies for classic and other forms of bipolar disorder. *Journal of Affective Disorders*, **58**, S57–S67.

Bowden, C. L., Calabrese, J. R., Sachs, S., *et al* (2003) A placebo-controlled 18-month trial of lamotrigine and lithium maintenance treatment in recently manic or hypomanic patients with bipolar I disorder. *Archives of General Psychiatry*, **60**, 392–400.

Bowen, R. C., Grof, P. & Grof, E. (1991) Less frequent lithium administration and lower urine volume. *American Journal of Psychiatry*, **148**, 189–192.

Burgess, S., Geddes, J., Hawton, E., *et al* (2003) Lithium for the maintenance treatment of mood disorders (Cochrane Review). *The Cochrane Library*, Issue 3 2003. Available at http://www.update-software.com/abstracts/ab003013.htm.

Cabras, P. L., Hardoy, J., Hardoy, M. C., *et al* (1999) Clinical experience with gabapentin in patients with bipolar or schizoaffective disorder: results of an open-label study. *Journal of Clinical Psychiatry*, **60**, 245–248.

Cade, H. F. H. (1949) Lithium salts in the treatment of psychotic excitement. *Medical Journal of Australia*, **36**, 249–352.

Calabrese, J. R., Suppes, T., Bowden, C. L., *et al* (2000) A double-blind, placebo-controlled, prophylaxis study of lamotrigine in rapid-cycling bipolar disorder. *Journal of Clinical Psychiatry*, **61**, 841–850.

Campbell, M., Perry, R. & Green, W. H. (1984) Use of lithium in children and adolescents. *Psychosomatics*, **25**, 95–106.

Chaudron, L. H. & Jefferson, J. L. (2000) Mood stabilizers during breast feeding: a review. *Journal of Clinical Psychiatry*, **61**, 79–90.

Cohen, W. J. & Cohen, N. H. (1974) Lithium carbonate, haloperidol, and irreversible brain damage. *Journal of the American Medical Association*, **230**, 1283–1287.

Cooper, A. J. (1988) Guide to the long-term drug treatment of major affective disorder: a review. *Psychiatric Journal of the University of Ottawa*, **13**, 144–148.

Cooper, T. B. & Simpson, C. M. (1976) The 24-hour serum lithium level as a prognosticator of dosage requirements: a 2-year follow-up study. *American Journal of Psychiatry*, **133**, 440–443.

Coppen, A., Noguera, R., Bailey, J., *et al* (1971) Prophylactic lithium in affective disorders. *Lancet*, **ii**, 275–279.

Coppen, A., Bishop, M. E., Bailey, J. E., *et al* (1980) Renal function in lithium and non-lithium treated patients with affective disorders. *Acta Psychiatrica Scandinavica*, **62**, 343–355.

Coppen, A., Abou-Saleh, M., Milin, P., *et al* (1983) Decreasing lithium dosage reduces morbidity and side-effects during prophylaxis. *Journal of Affective Disorders*, **5**, 353–362.

Cowen, P. J., McCance, S. L., Ware, C. J., *et al* (1991) Lithium in tricyclic-resistant depression. Correlation of increased brain 5-HT function with clinical outcome. *British Journal of Psychiatry*, **159**, 341–346.

Coxhead, N., Silverstone, T. & Cookson, J. (1992) Carbamazepine versus lithium in the prophylaxis of bipolar affective disorder. *Acta Psychiatrica Scandinavica*, **85**, 114–118.

Davis, J. M., Janicak, P. G. & Hogan, D. M. (1999) Mood stabilizers in the prevention of recurrent affective disorders: a meta-analysis. *Acta Psychiatrica Scandinavica*, **100**, 406–417.

De Montigny, C., Grunberg, F., Mayer, A., *et al* (1981) Lithium induces rapid relief of depression in tricyclic antidepressant drug non-responders. *British Journal of Psychiatry*, **138**, 252–256.

Dorus, E., Cox, N. J., Gibbons, R. D., *et al* (1983) Lithium ion transport and affective disorders within families of bipolar patients: identification of a major gene locus. *Archives of General Psychiatry*, **40**, 545–552.

Dorus, W. (1989) Lithium treatment of depressed and nondepressed alcoholics. *Journal of the American Medical Association*, **262**, 1646–1652.

Dubovsky, S. L., Franks, R. D., Allen, S., *et al* (1986) Calcium antagonists in mania: a double-blind study of verapamil. *Psychiatric Research*, **18**, 309–310.

Faedda, C. L., Baldessarini, R. J., Tohen, M., *et al* (1991) Episode sequence in bipolar disorder and response to lithium treatment. *American Journal of Psychiatry*, **148**, 1237–1239.

Fieve, R. R. (1975) The lithium clinic: a new model for the delivery of psychiatric services. *American Journal of Psychiatry*, **132**, 1018–1022.

Frye, M. A., Ketter, T. A., Kimbrell, T. A., *et al* (2000) A placebo-controlled study of lamotrigine and gabapentin in refratory mood disorders. *Journal of Clinical Psychopharmacology*, **20**, 607–614.

Ghodse, K. (1977) Lithium salts: therapeutic and unwanted effects. *British Journal of Hospital Medicine*, **18**, 578–583.

Goodwin, G. M. (1994) Recurrence of mania after lithium withdrawal. Implications for the use of lithium in the treatment of bipolar affective disorder. *British Journal of Psychiatry*, **164**, 149–152.

Goodwin, G. M. (1995) Lithium revisited: a reply (commentary). *British Journal of Psychiatry*, **167**, 573–574.

Greil, W. & Schmidt, S. (1988) Lithium withdrawal reactions. In *Lithium: Inorganic Pharmacology and Psychiatric Use* (ed. N. Birch), pp. 149–153. Oxford: IRL Press.

Guscott, R. & Taylor, L. (1994) Lithium prophylaxis in recurrent affective illness. Efficacy, effectiveness and efficiency. *British Journal of Psychiatry*, **164**, 741–746.

Hartigan, G. P. (1963) The use of lithium salts in affective disorders. *British Journal of Psychiatry*, **109**, 810–814.

Hestbech, J., Hansen, H. E., Amdisen, A., *et al* (1977) Chronic renal lesions following long-term treatment with lithium. *Kidney International*, **12**, 205–213.

Hetmar, O., Brun, C., Clemmensen, L., *et al* (1987) Lithium: long-term effects on the kidney, 2: structural changes. *Journal of Psychiatric Research*, **21**, 279–288.

Hughes, J. H., Dunne, F. & Young, A. H. (2000) Effects of acute tryptophan depletion on mood and suicidal ideation in bipolar patients symptomatically stable on lithium. *British Journal of Psychiatry*, **177**, 447–451.

Hullin, R. P., McDonald, R. & Allsopp, M. N. E. (1972) Prophylactic lithium in recurrent disorders. *Lancet*, **i**, 1044–1046.

Jacobson, S. N., Jones, K., Johnson, K., *et al* (1992) Prospective multicentre study of pregnancy after lithium exposure during first trimester. *Lancet*, **339**, 530–533.

Johnson, F. N. (1984) *The History of Lithium Therapy*. London: Macmillan.

Johnstone, B. B., Dick, E. G., Naylor, G. J., *et al* (1979) Lithium side-effects in a routine lithium clinic. *British Journal of Psychiatry*, **134**, 482–487.

Johnstone, E. C., Crow, T. J., Frith, C. D., *et al* (1988) The Northwick Park functional psychosis study: diagnosis and treatment response. *Lancet*, *ii*, 119–125.

Johnstone, E. C., Owens, D. G. C., Lambert, M. T., *et al* (1990) Combination antidepressant and lithium maintenance medication in unipolar and bipolar depressed subjects. *Journal of Affective Disorders*, **20**, 225–233.

Judd, L. L. (1979) The effect of lithium on mood, cognition, and personality function in normal subjects. *Archives of General Psychiatry*, **36**, 860–865.

King, J. R. & Hullin, R. P. (1983) Withdrawal symptoms from lithium: four case reports and a questionnaire study. *British Journal of Psychiatry*, **143**, 30–35.

Lena, B. (1979) Lithium in childhood and adolescent psychiatry. *Archives of General Psychiatry*, **36**, 854–855.

Maggs, R. (1963) Treatment of manic illness with lithium carbonate. *British Journal of Psychiatry*, **109**, 56–65.

Maj, J. (1988) Lithium prophylaxis of schizoaffective disorders: a prospective study. *Journal of Affective Disorders*, **14**, 129–135.

Mander, A. J. & Louden, J. B. (1988) Rapid recurrence of mania following abrupt discontinuation of lithium. *Lancet*, *ii*, 15–17.

Manji, H. K. & Lenox, R. H. (2000) Signaling: cellular insights into the pathophysiology of bipolar disorder. *Biological Psychiatry*, **48**, 518–530.

Manji, H. K., Hsaio, I. K., Risby, E. D., *et al* (1991) Mechanisms of action of lithium: 1 & 2. *Archives of General Psychiatry*, **48**, 505–524.

Marker, H. R. & Mander, A. J. (1989) Efficacy of lithium prophylaxis in clinical practice. *British Journal of Psychiatry*, **155**, 496–500.

McCreadie, R. C. & Morrison, P. P. (1985) The impact of lithium in south-west Scotland. I. Demographic and clinical findings. *British Journal of Psychiatry*, **146**, 70–74.

McElroy, S. L., Keck, P. E., Pope, H. O., *et al* (1992) Valproate in the treatment of bipolar disorder: literature review and clinical guidelines. *Journal of Clinical Psychopharmacology*, **12** (suppl.), 42s–52s.

Melia, P. I. (1967) A pilot trial of lithium carbonate in recurrent affective disorders. *Journal of the Irish Medical Association*, **40**, 160–170.

Moncrieff, J. (1995) Lithium revisited. A re-examination of the placebo-controlled trials of lithium prophylaxis in manic–depressive disorder. *British Journal of Psychiatry*, **167**, 569–573.

Moore, G. J., Bebchuck, J. M., Parrish, J. K., *et al* (1999) Temporal dissociation between lithium-induced changes in frontal lobe *myo*-inositol and clinical response in manic–depressive illness. *American Journal of Psychiatry*, **156**, 1902–1908.

Moore, G. J., Bebchuck, J. M., Wilds, I. B., *et al* (2000) Lithium-induced increase in human brain grey matter. *Lancet*, **356**, 1241–1242.

Mork, A. & Geisler, A. (1991) The influence of lithium and rubidium on cyclic AMP formation *in vitro* and *ex vivo*. In *Biological Psychiatry, Vol. 1* (eds I. C. Racagni, *et al*), pp. 200–201. Amsterdam: Elsevier Science.

Naylor, C. I., Smith, A. A. H., Bryce-Smith, D. *et al* (1984) Tissue vanadium levels in manic–depressive psychosis. *Psychological Medicine*, **14**, 767–772.

O'Connell, R. A., Mayo, J. A., Flatow, L., *et al* (1991) Outcome of bipolar disorder on long-term treatment with lithium. *British Journal of Psychiatry*, **159**, 123–129.

Page, C., Benaim, S. & Lappin, F. (1987) A long-term retrospective follow-up study of patients treated with prophylactic lithium carbonate. *British Journal of Psychiatry*, **150**, 175–179.

Pande, A. C., Crockatt, J. G., Janney, C. A., *et al* (2000) Gabapentin in bipolar disorder: a placebo-controlled trial of adjunctive therapy. *Bipolar Disorder*, **2**, 249–255.

Peet, M. & Harvey, N. S. (1991) Lithium maintenance. I. A standard education programme for patients. *British Journal of Psychiatry*, **158**, 197–200.

Perry, P. J., Alexander, B., Prince, R. A., *et al* (1986) The utility of a single-point dosing protocol for predicting steady-state lithium levels. *British Journal of Psychiatry*, **148**, 401–405.

Peselow, E. D., Fieve, R. R., Difiglia,C., *et al* (1994) Lithium prophylaxis of bipolar illness. The value of combination treatment. *British Journal of Psychiatry*, **164**, 208–214.

Plenge, P., Mellerup, E. T. & Bolwig, T. C. (1982) Lithium treatment: does the kidney prefer one daily dose instead of two? *Acta Psychiatrica Scandinavica*, **66**, 121–128.

Pope, H. C., McElroy, S. L., Keck, P. E., *et al* (1991) Valproate in the treatment of acute mania. *Archives of General Psychiatry*, **48**, 62–68.

Post, R. M. (1990) Non-lithium treatment for bipolar disorder. *Journal of Clinical Psychiatry*, **51**, 9–6.

Post, R. M., Uhde, T. W., Putman, F. W., *et al* (1982) Kindling and carbamazepine in affective illness. *Journal of Nervous and Mental Disease*, **170**, 717–731.

Prien, R. P., Caffey, E. M. & Klett, C. J. (1973) Prophylactic efficacy of lithium in manic–depressive illness. *Archives of General Psychiatry*, **28**, 337–341.

Sackheim, H. A., Hasket, R. F., Mulsant, B. H., *et al* (2001) Continuation pharmaco-therapy in the prevention of relapse following electroconvulsive therapy. *Journal of the American Medical Association*, **285**, 1299–1307.

Schou, M. (1989) Lithium prophylaxis: myths and realities. *American Journal of Psychiatry*, **146**, 573–576.

Schou, M., & Weinstein, M. R. (1980) Problems of lithium maintenance treatment during pregnancy, delivery and lactation. *Agressologie*, **21A**, 7–9.

Schou, M., Amdisen, A., Thomsen, K., *et al* (1982) Lithium treatment regimen and renal water handling. *Psychopharmacology*, **77**, 387–390.

Sheard, M. H., Marini, J. L., Bridges, C. I., *et al* (1976) The effect of lithium on impulsive aggressive behaviour in man. *American Journal of Psychiatry*, **133**, 1409–1413.

Shelley, R. K. (1987) Lithium toxicity and mefenamic acid. A possible interaction and the role of prostaglandin inhibition. *British Journal of Psychiatry*, **151**, 847–848.

Shelley, R. K. & Silverstone, T. (1986) Single dose pharmacokinetics of 5 formulations of lithium: a controlled comparison in healthy subjects. *International Clinical Pharmacology*, **1**, 324–331.

Shulman, K. I., Mackenzie, S. & Hardy, B. (1987) The clinical use of lithium carbonate in old age: a review. *Progress in Neuropsychopharmacology and Biological Psychiatry*, **11**, 159–164.

Small, J. C. (1990) Anticonvulsants in affective disorders. *Psychopharmacology Bulletin*, **26**, 25–35.

Souza, F. G. M. & Goodwin, G. M. (1991) Lithium treatment and prophylaxis in unipolar depression: a meta-analysis. *British Journal of Psychiatry*, **158**, 666–675.

Spreat, S., Behar, D., Reneski, B., *et al* (1989) Lithium carbonate for aggression in mentally retarded persons. *Comprehensive Psychiatry*, **30**, 505–511.

Stewart, D. E., Klompenhouwer, J. L., Kendell, R. E., *et al* (1991) Prophylactic lithium in puerperal psychosis. The experience of three centres. *British Journal of Psychiatry*, **158**, 393–397.

Stokes, P. E., Kocsis, J. H. & Arcuni, U. J. (1976) Relationship of lithium chloride dose to treatment response in acute mania. *Archives of General Psychiatry*, **33**, 1080–1084.

Suppes, T., Baldessarini, R. J., Faedda, G. L., *et al* (1991) Risk of recurrence following discontinuation of lithium treatment in bipolar disorder. *Archives of General Psychiatry*, **48**, 1082–1088.

Symonds, R. L. & Williams, P. (1981) Lithium and the changing incidence of mania. *Psychological Medicine*, **11**, 193–196.

Thomsen, K. (1978) Renal handling of lithium at non-toxic and toxic serum lithium levels. *Danish Medical Bulletin*, **25**, 106–115.

Vestergaard, P. (1983) Clinically important side-effects of long-term lithium treatment a review. *Acta Psychiatrica Scandinavica*, **67** (suppl. 305), 11–33.

Vestergaard, P., Poulstrup, I. & Schou, M. (1988) Prospective studies on a lithium cohort. 3: Tremor, weight gain, diarrhea, psychological complaints. *Acta Psychiatrica Scandinavica*, **78**, 434–441.

Viguera, A. C., Nonacs, R., Cohen, L. S., *et al* (2000) Risk of recurrence of bipolar disorder in pregnant and nonpregnant women after discontinuating lithium maintenance. *American Journal of Psychiatry*, **157**, 179–184.

Watanabe, S., Ishino, H. & Ctsuki, S. (1975) Double-blind comparison of lithium carbonate and imipramine in the treatment of depression. *Archives of General Psychiatry*, **32**, 659–668.

Weinstein, M. R. (1980) Problems of lithium maintenance treatment during pregnancy, delivery and lactation. *Agressologie*, **21A**, 7–9.

Worrall, E. P., Moody, J. P., Peet, M., *et al* (1979) Controlled studies of the acute antidepressant effects of lithium. *British Journal of Psychiatry*, **135**, 255–262.

Further reading

Abou-Saleh, M. T. (1992) Lithium. In *Handbook of Affective Disorders* (ed. E. S. Paykel). Edinburgh: Churchill Livingstone.

Birch, N. J. (ed.) (1988) *Lithium: Inorganic Pharmacology and Psychiatric Use*. Oxford: IRL Press.

Johnson, F. N. (ed.) (1980) *Handbook of Lithium Therapy*. Lancaster: MTP Press.

Johnson, F. N. (ed.) (1987) *Depression and Mania: Modern Lithium Therapy*. Oxford: IRL Press.

Journal of Clinical Psychiatry (2000) *Fifty Years of Lithium Use in the Treatment of Bipolar Disorder*. *Journal of Clinical Psychiatry*, **61**, suppl. 9.

Manji, H. K., Bowden, C. L. & Belmaker, R. H. (eds) (2000) *Bipolar Medications: Mechanisms of Action*. Washington, DC: American Psychiatric Press.

Schou, M. (1989) *Lithium Treatment of Manic–Depressive Illness. A Practical Guide* (4th edn). Basel: Karger.

Schou, M. (1997) Forty years of lithium treatment. *Archives of General Psychiatry*, **54**, 9–20.

Watson, W. & Young, A. H. (2001) The place of lithium salts in psychiatric practice. *Current Opinion in Psychiatry*, **14**, 57–63.

CHAPTER 8

Affective disorders: 3. Electroconvulsive therapy

Stephen J. Cooper, Christopher B. Kelly
and Robert J. McClelland

Historical background

The introduction of convulsive therapies into regular use in psychiatric practice should probably be attributed to the Hungarian physician Ladislas Meduna (1896–1964). During investigations into the relationship between epilepsy and schizophrenia he noted two patients with dementia praecox whose acute symptoms were relieved when they developed spontaneous epileptic seizures. Following experiments in animals, he began using camphor (intramuscularly) to induce seizures in patients in 1934. The first patient was a man in a catatonic stupor, in the Budapest–Lipotmezo State Hospital, who recovered after five injections. Meduna then went on to treat more patients with schizophrenia, and found that about half improved. It is worth noting that this therapy was initially introduced for the treatment of schizophrenia rather than depression. Although some of the means used to induce seizures, in the early years, now seem somewhat primitive, it must be remembered that at that time no other useful treatments existed for these conditions.

Camphor was extremely unreliable in its effects and Meduna found pentylenetetrazol, which continued to be used for some years, more reliable. However, all of these substances were irritant, often unreliable in their effects and unpleasant for the patient, as seizures could take some minutes to develop.

In 1938 Cerletti, Bini & Accornero, in Italy, developed an electrical means for induction of seizures. This proved to be more reliable and more acceptable to patients and thus electroconvulsive therapy (ECT) was born.

Initially ECT was also used for the more acutely disturbed schizophrenic patients, but this more readily controlled treatment was soon tried for patients with severe depression and mania, for whom its effectiveness became evident. The introduction of neuroleptic drugs in 1952 supplanted ECT for many cases of schizophrenia and mania. Thus, severe depressive illness became the main indication for its use. It remains useful in patients with schizophrenia and mania who have not responded to pharmacotherapy.

At first ECT was used without an anaesthetic, partly because of the difficulties and risks of the available anaesthetics, and partly because of concerns that anaesthesia might reduce its efficacy. In order to prevent injury to patients during the seizure, it was necessary to have nursing staff restrain their limbs and trunk. Injuries such as fractures of the vertebrae or other bones could still occur, however. Muscle relaxants were introduced to prevent fractures, curare in 1940 and succinylcholine in 1952. As safe, short-acting anaesthetic agents became available they were used to make the procedure less unpleasant for the patients. Thus we arrived at the modern version of modified ECT.

A survey of the use of ECT in England (Department of Health, 1999) found that in a 3-month period 5.8/100 000 of the population received ECT, of whom 68% were female and 41% were aged over 65 years. Only one patient under 16 years received ECT. The number of treatment applications was generally around 5–7 per patient. Between 1985 and 1998 the number of administrations of ECT fell by just over 50%.

There have been criticisms of the use of ECT from within the psychiatric profession as well as from outside it. Until the mid-1970s these may have had some degree of justification, as the evidence for the efficacy of ECT was based largely on professional experience and open clinical studies, but very few well-designed clinical trials. However, subsequently there have been a number of well-conducted clinical trials as well as detailed reviews of practice by professional bodies, both in the British Isles and in the USA (Pippard & Ellam, 1981; Royal College of Psychiatrists, 1995).

Clinical trials

Early studies in depressive illness

Bennett (1938) was among the first to report the efficacy of convulsive therapy for melancholia (in his cases using pentylenetetrazol) but, like many early papers, his was a descriptive report. In 1965 Wechsler and colleagues published a summary of 153 studies of antidepressant treatments published between 1958 and 1963 in British, US and Canadian journals in which ECT was one of the treatments. The mean percentage of patients regarded as improved was 72% for ECT, 65% for tricyclic antidepressants, 50% for monoamine oxidase inhibitors and 23% for placebo. If only studies dealing with depressive illness of recent onset were examined the effectiveness of ECT was more marked, with improvement in 86% compared with 24% for placebo. Studies dealing with 'chronic depression' demonstrated much smaller benefits (ECT

37%; drugs 32%; placebo 21%), although these included patients with schizophrenia and dementia. Many of the studies were uncontrolled, as the use of placebo-controlled trials with random allocation to treatment group was only then beginning to become commonplace.

However, two large controlled trials, one in the USA (Greenblatt *et al*, 1964; n = 281) and one in the UK (Medical Research Council, 1965; n = 259), found very similar results, with 76% and 71% respectively of patients improving with ECT. The main difference was a better placebo response, of around 40–45%, in these controlled studies, although in the US study this was due to a high placebo response in patients with 'psychoneurotic' depression. Even these studies, however, were not double blind, this being a particular ethical problem when an anaesthetic is involved.

Barton (1977) reviewed six studies in which some form of simulated ECT was given and in which the patients and clinical raters were both blind to the treatment used. Overall, outcome was better in patients receiving full ECT, but some of the studies were too small to allow conventional statistical significance to be achieved, and others used an antidepressant as a comparator rather than placebo.

Mortality is another outcome measure of interest in depressive illness. Untreated or inadequately treated illness results in higher death rates from physical disorders as well as from suicide. Slater (1951) carried out a re-analysis of data on death rate from all causes in patients with depression admitted to hospital in Edinburgh in the periods 1900–39 and 1940–48. Those patients treated with ECT had lower mortality and spent less time in hospital than patients admitted before ECT became available or who were not treated with it after its introduction. Similar data from Iowa, for patients with depression admitted between 1959 and 1969, demonstrated lower mortality for those patients receiving ECT or adequate antidepressant drug therapy compared with those given inadequate antidepressant drug therapy or those not treated with ECT or antidepressant drugs (Avery & Winokur, 1976).

Modern clinical trials in depression

Between 1978 and 1985 six randomised controlled trials (RCTs) were published, which each met at least five out of the six following criteria: clear patient selection criteria; random allocation to treatment group; comparison of 'real' versus 'simulated' ECT rather than versus an antidepressant drug; full 'simulated' ECT procedure used, including giving the anaesthetic (but no shock); control of other antidepressant therapy; and use of a standardised symptom rating scale. These studies are summarised in Tables 8.1 and 8.2. Some of these refer to the use of 'MRC criteria' for depression. These were the criteria applied in the

Table 8.1 Methods of important ECT trials

Study	No. of applications	Stimulus	Monitoring	Design
Lambourn & Gill (1978)	6	Brief-pulse; right unilateral	None	Random allocation to equal-sized groups for real or simulated ECT
Freeman et al (1978)	3+ (decided by clinical team)	Sine wave; constant voltage; bilateral	None	Random allocation to equal-sized groups. In simulated ECT groups, only first 2 ECTs simulated, rest real
Johnstone et al (1980)	8	Sine wave; constant voltage; bifrontal	Cuff	Random allocation to real or simulated ECT
West (1981)	6	Square wave; constant voltage; bitemporal	None	Random allocation to real or simulated ECT
Brandon et al (1985)	8	Sine wave; constant voltage; bitemporal	None	Random allocation to real or simulated ECT
Gregory et al (1985)	4+ (decided by clinical team)	Sine wave; constant voltage: (a) right unilateral; (b) bitemporal	Cuff	Random allocation to (a) or (b) or simulated ECT. Analysis only for those receiving at least 6 applications

Medical Research Council study of treatment of depression (Medical Research Council, 1965) and are:

'a persistent alteration of mood, exceeding customary sadness, accompanied by at least one of: self-deprecation with a morbid sense of guilt, sleep disturbance, hypochondriasis, retardation of thought or action'.

Only one of these studies (Lambourn & Gill, 1978) failed to demonstrate a difference between real and simulated ECT. However, their electrical stimulus may well have been too low, given more recent experience (see under 'Stimulus dosage' below), and subsequent work (e.g. Abrams et al, 1983; Gregory et al, 1985) suggests that in many respects unilateral stimuli are also less effective.

The study by Johnstone et al (1980) found only small differences between real and simulated treatment, the main benefit being in speed of response. However, further analysis suggested that it was the presence of delusions that was most likely to predict benefit for real versus simulated ECT in this group (Clinical Research Centre, Division of Psychiatry, 1984). Nevertheless, it would seem that many of these

Table 8.2   Clinical criteria and outcome of important ECT trials

Study	No. of patients (no. completed)	Mean age (years)	Selection criteria	Other treatments	Outcome
Lambourn & Gill (1978)	32 (32)	54	Diagnosis depressive psychosis by clinician	Benzodiazepine hypnotics	No difference between real and and simulated
Freeman *et al* (1978)	40 (38)	51	MRC criteria plus Hamilton score of at least 15	Antidepressants ($n = 18$)	Simulated ECT group required more treatments (7.15 *v.* 6)
Johnstone *et al* (1980)	70 (62)	49	All of MRC, Newcastle and Feighner	Benzodiazepine only	Small, but significant benefit for real ECT
West (1981)	25 (22)	53	Feighner criteria	All given 50 mg amitriptyline at night	Real ECT better. Used self-rating scale
Brandon *et al* (1984)	95 (77)	54	All in-patients referred for ECT	Anxiolytics only	Real ECT better
Gregory *et al* (1985)	69 (60)	Not stated	ICD–9 plus MRC	Benzodiazepine only	Bilateral and unilateral better than simulated. Bilateral gives more rapid response

patients were still quite unwell even at the end of the trial, as their mean score on the Hamilton Rating Scale for Depression was sufficiently high to qualify for entry to many trials of antidepressant treatments. Although the occurrence of a seizure was confirmed by use of the 'cuff technique', the electrode placement was bifrontal rather than bitemporal. Some types of bifrontal placement may be less effective than the standard bifrontotemporal electrode placement (Abrams & Taylor, 1973). Again, given more recent experience in relation to the possible importance of seizure threshold, we cannot exclude inadequacy of the stimulus as a reason for the small effect of ECT.

The other trials demonstrated improvements of around 60–70% with real ECT compared with around 25% for simulated treatment.

Continuing antidepressant therapy complicated two studies. However, in that by Freeman et al (1978) it was more prevalent in the simulated ECT group, who did less well, and in that by West (1981) all patients received what would normally be regarded as a subtherapeutic dose of amitriptyline.

While other criticisms may be levelled at individual details of some studies, it is clear that a number of RCTs arrive at the same conclusion, that for certain types of depressive illness ECT is an effective treatment. Further research is required to determine those factors that give rise to a good response, something that is discussed further under 'Principles of use of ECT' below.

Studies in mania

Now, ECT is not commonly used for mania, but it was before antipsychotic drugs became available. It was regarded as effective, but no entirely adequate controlled clinical trial was ever carried out. A comparison of ECT alone versus chlorpromazine alone in patients with either mania or schizophrenia (Langsley et al, 1959) found similar symptom reduction with these treatments, but those treated with chlorpromazine left hospital sooner.

A retrospective case-control study (McCabe, 1976) compared 28 patients with mania treated with ECT versus 28 not so treated, but matched in other respects, from a cohort of patients admitted to Iowa Psychopathic Hospital between 1935 and 1941. Those treated with ECT left hospital sooner, demonstrated better recovery and had a lower mortality. Interestingly, the number of ECT treatments required was quite high, ranging from 6 to 32, with a mean of 17.

A further retrospective review (Thomas & Reddy, 1982) examined the case notes of patients admitted to Runwell Hospital between 1950 and 1965. Three out of four key features of mania had to be present and patients included had to have had only one form of treatment: ECT or chlorpromazine or lithium. The authors were left with 10 patients in each treatment group, reasonably matched for age and sex, out of an initial 299 who satisfied the diagnostic criteria. There were no significant differences between the treatment groups in terms of either length of stay in hospital or length of time from discharge to readmission, although the trend was for chlorpromazine-treated patients to go home sooner and for ECT-treated patients to have longer remissions.

In one study 34 patients were randomly allocated to treatment with either ECT or lithium carbonate (Small et al, 1988) for up to 8 weeks. The investigators were not completely blind to treatment allocation and some patients also received neuroleptics, although there was no difference in mean daily doses between the treatment groups. Any differences in the effectiveness of the treatments were small but favoured

ECT. During follow-up, when both groups continued on lithium carbonate, there were no differences in clinical symptoms or relapse rates.

Thus, ECT would appear to be an effective treatment for mania but not superior to drug therapy. Its main place is probably in patients who are non-responsive to drugs or very severely ill at the outset, with either risk of exhaustion or manic stupor. In such situations it may also be considered in childhood bipolar disorder (Carr *et al*, 1983).

Studies in schizophrenia

Approximately 10–15% of patients given ECT in the UK have a diagnosis of schizophrenia. The frequency of use of ECT for schizophrenia fell rapidly after the introduction of neuroleptic drugs. Sadly, before this no studies that would conform to modern criteria were carried out to assess its effectiveness. Early descriptive reports, however, provide a fairly consistent view of ECT as effective for symptomatic relief in acutely ill patients, with consequent improvements in social functioning and increased likelihood of discharge from hospital. Patients with a short duration of illness appeared to do best, and chronic, deteriorated patients gained little benefit.

Salzman (1980) provides a review of studies that compared ECT with neuroleptic treatment or the combination of ECT plus neuroleptics with neuroleptic treatment alone. The trend was for a shorter stay in hospital for patients treated with neuroleptic drugs alone versus ECT alone. Relapse rates were fairly similar in a number of these studies, but they were carried out before the introduction of depot neuroleptic drugs. The best study was that of May & Tuma (1965), who examined the acute and long-term effects of five treatments in patients of moderate prognosis: individual psychotherapy, neuroleptic treatment, neuro-leptics plus psychotherapy, ECT and milieu therapy. The neuroleptic treatment groups demonstrated the best acute response (approximately 95% were discharged within 1 year) and ECT was the next best treatment (79% of patients discharged within 1 year). A 3-year follow-up found that the number of days in hospital following initial treatment did not differ between groups treated with drugs or ECT, and this was confirmed in a subsequent 5-year follow-up.

Although most of the studies that have examined the combination of ECT and neuroleptics do not conform to modern standards, the majority suggested a more rapid response than for neuroleptic treatment alone. The best of the older studies (Smith *et al*, 1967) found that 12 applications of ECT, plus chlorpromazine (400 mg per day), produced a faster response than chlorpromazine alone (655 mg per day). Response at 6 months was similar for the two treatments but at 1 year the ECT group had had fewer readmissions.

Janakiramaiah *et al* (1982) compared two dosages of chlorpromazine (300 mg and 500 mg per day) both alone and in combination with (on average) ten ECT treatments. The response rate for ECT plus 300 mg chlorpromazine per day was faster than for 300 mg chlorpromazine per day alone, but similar to the response rate for 500 mg chlorpromazine per day, to which the addition of ECT did not provide further benefit.

Two studies examined the effects of real versus simulated ECT, in addition to antipsychotic drug treatment, in patients who fulfilled the criteria of the Present State Examination for schizophrenia. These studies used full double-blinding and random allocation of patients to treatment group. In the first of these (Taylor & Fleminger, 1980) all ten patients in the real ECT group demonstrated improvement, but only half of the ten in the simulated ECT group did so. The clinical ratings demonstrated significant improvement for both groups at the end of the treatment period, but the group who received real ECT did statistically significantly better. Significant differences emerged specifically for a group of positive psychotic symptoms. The second study (Brandon *et al*, 1985) also demonstrated significantly better improvement with real ECT in schizophrenic symptoms in a study of 19 patients. In both studies the doses of antipsychotic drugs were equalised as far as possible between the treatment groups. However, at follow-up over the following weeks differences between the treatment groups disappeared.

Common clinical wisdom has it that the response to ECT in schizophrenia is largely for depressive symptoms and that such symptoms should be present for the use of ECT to be of value. This idea goes back to studies such as that by Pacella & Barrera (1943), who commented that patients who improved 'almost always had strong affective components of depression, guilt, worthlessness, hopelessness, self-condemnation and suicidal tendencies'. Given the lack of objective diagnostic criteria at that time one wonders if some of their patients suffered from an affective disorder rather than schizophrenia.

Three chart review studies covering, respectively, patients admitted around 1950, 1970 and 1985 were inconclusive. Two found the absence of Schneiderian 'first rank' symptoms to predict better response but also found that patients with such symptoms did better if affective symptoms were also present. The third study did not report any relationship to affective symptoms.

The two clinical trials (Taylor & Fleminger, 1980; Brandon *et al*, 1985) failed to find statistically significantly better improvement in the symptoms of depression in patients with schizophrenia with real ECT (compared with simulated ECT) and this is also true for some of the older studies of inferior design. Brandon *et al* (1985), in particular, reported a proportionately greater improvement in schizophrenic symptoms than in depressive symptoms and this perhaps gives a clue to one of the difficulties in resolving this issue. Many studies have shown that in schizophrenia, the severity of depression correlates with the severity of delusions and hallucinations and that improvement in these positive psychotic symptoms is paralleled by improvement in the depressed mood.

There is no evidence that ECT is of any benefit for chronic patients with predominantly negative symptoms. A clinical trial by Miller *et al* (1953) found no difference between unmodified ECT, anaesthesia and a non-convulsive stimulus under anaesthesia in a group of 30 patients with chronic schizophrenia.

Thus, ECT has a role in the management of schizophrenia. The effect would appear to be primarily on the positive psychotic symptoms; its role in relation to affective symptoms is still unclear. In combination with antipsychotic drug treatment it seems to produce a more rapid response, but the drug-treated patients 'catch up' within a few weeks, which suggests this is therefore not useful as a routine strategy. However, if patients are very severely psychotic or have not responded to drug therapy, then ECT should be considered.

It is a widespread belief that patients with schizophrenia require longer courses of ECT than patients who are affectively ill and indeed the early studies often used 20 or more treatments. However, there is no good evidence on which to base this assertion.

Biochemical effects of electroconvulsive shock in animals

Methods

Much of the research into the biochemical effects of ECT has been carried out in animals rather than in humans. The main advantage of studying electroconvulsive shock (ECS) in animals is the availability of direct access to the brain. However, major drawbacks are: species differences in neurochemistry; lack of equivalence of the electrical stimulus used in most studies to that used in patients; and the fact that one is studying normally functioning animals as against, presumably, pathologically functioning brain systems in humans.

As in humans, a variety of approaches have been used to study the effects of ECS in animals. Methods include: direct assay of the chemical content of brain tissue; measurement of chemically evoked release or reuptake of neurotransmitters; microdialysis, with cannulae *in situ*, allowing direct measurement of regional biochemical changes (Glue *et al*, 1990); and measurement of change in receptor number (B_{max}) and affinity ($1/K_d$) by ligand binding studies. Indirect means involve observation of a number of simple animal behaviours that appear to be mediated by specific neurochemical systems. Quantification of these behaviours (e.g. the degree of hind-limb abduction in the rat mediated by the serotonin system) allows functional estimation of change in activity of these systems.

Dopaminergic effects

Electroconvulsive shock increases the behavioural response to non-specific dopaminergic agonist drugs, such as apomorphine (Green *et al*, 1977). This occurs without evidence of change in dopamine receptor density or affinity (Deakin *et al*, 1981). Depletion of dopamine has been reported in the hypothalamus but not other brain areas. Microdialysis studies have demonstrated increased dopamine concentrations in the striatum after a course of ECS.

Use of specific D_1 and D_2 receptor agonists suggests that D_2 receptor activity is not affected by ECS. Behaviour mediated by D_1 receptors is increased by ECS but this is reversed if the animals are pre-treated with reserpine. However, where pre-treatment with haloperidol (to induce supersensitivity of dopamine receptors) has been used, the effects of concomitant ECS are to attenuate the development of supersensitivity (Lerer *et al*, 1982). This illustrates the difficulties of trying to link different animal paradigms (and even more so of making comparisons with the human situation).

Serotonergic effects

The 1990s saw an explosion of knowledge with regard to serotonin systems and receptor subtypes (Peroutka, 1995). A number of experiments have shown that serotonin-mediated behaviours, induced by non-specific serotonin agonists, are increased following ECS (Grahame-Smith *et al*, 1978). Electrophysiological studies have suggested increased postsynaptic $5-HT_{1A}$ function after a course of ECS, although this has not always been supported by more direct biochemical measures.

Early studies, using non-specific ligands, suggested that serotonin receptor number was unchanged by ECS (Deakin *et al*, 1981). Studies that have employed specific receptor ligands have produced some evidence for differential effects of ECS at different receptor subtypes. Postsynaptic $5-HT_2$ receptors have been shown to increase in number in rat cortex following ECS (one study found this only in male animals), but $5-HT_1$ receptor numbers show no consistent change. ECS does not alter serotonin reuptake or the numbers of imipramine binding sites in animals.

Noradrenergic effects

The most consistent change produced by ECS on the noradrenergic system is a down-regulation (reduction in receptor number and function) of β-adrenoceptors (Deakin *et al*, 1981). This also occurs with most other effective antidepressant treatments. Doubts have been raised about the specificity of some of the receptor ligands used in these studies, such as dihydroalprenolol.

There is no consistent evidence for changes in the numbers of α_1- or α_2-adrenoceptors. Behavioural and hormonal studies in animals suggest possible subsensitivity of α_2-adrenoceptors following ECS. Differences between studies may be due to site-specific effects and differences between pre- and postsynaptic receptors.

In vivo microdialysis studies demonstrate acute release of noradrenaline by ECS. Baseline concentrations of noradrenaline in extracellular fluid from rat frontal cortex are elevated by a course of ECS and the intracellular content of noradrenaline is reduced. This does not occur in other cortical areas (Glue *et al*, 1990).

Effects on GABA and other mechanisms

The basal release of gamma-aminobutyric acid (GABA) in neurons is unchanged after a course of ECS. However, evoked release and synthesis both appear to be reduced (Green & Vincent, 1987). Changes in GABA receptor function appear to be restricted to $GABA_B$ receptors, where increased receptor function and number have been noted, although not in the same brain areas as the metabolic changes in GABA. GABA is an important inhibitory neurotransmitter with anticonvulsant properties and modulatory effects on other monoamine systems.

An awareness that intraneuronal chemistry may also be altered by ECS has stimulated the study of changes in second messenger systems, such as cyclic adenosine monophosphate (cAMP) and inositol phosphate, enzymes (e.g. protein kinase C), intracellular calcium and receptor coupling mechanisms. The most consistent finding following a course of ECS is a reduction in the level of cAMP production induced by stimulation of cortical β-adrenoceptors.

Intrathecal levels of thyrotrophin-releasing hormone (TRH) have been shown to increase with ECS. There is evidence for TRH having antidepressant effects in patients (Marangell *et al*, 1997).

Biochemical effects of ECT in humans

Problems of interpretation

Our understanding of the causes of depression are far from complete, despite a number of biochemical theories having been put forward to explain its origin (see Chapter 6). The most useful have been the catecholamine and indoleamine hypotheses, which developed from observations of the pharmacological effects of antidepressant drugs rather than ECT. However, observations on the effects of ECT should not be ignored, as it is a treatment that is applied only to the brain and whose effects are not complicated by the continuous peripheral effects of drugs. Thus we may learn something about how ECT works, but also something about the causation of the disorders for which we use ECT. Furthermore, ECT is effective in patients with severe psychotic depressive illness, which differentiates it from other antidepressant treatments. The origin of this difference is unclear.

The brain is well protected physically and biochemically by the blood–brain barrier. This excellent protection impedes the investigation of central neurochemical events. Although knowledge of cellular biochemistry is advancing rapidly, current technology allows only limited access to processes at the human cerebral synaptic level and even less to intracellular changes. Thus peripheral sources have been used, such as lumbar cerebrospinal fluid (CSF) or plasma.

Study of receptor function in the central nervous system (CNS) has also been limited and so peripheral tissues carrying the same receptors, such as platelets and white blood cells, have been used. The rationale for this is that these tissues carry the same receptor subtypes and, in some cases, have the same embryonic origin as neuronal tissue. Clearly this approach is limited by the distance from the brain at which measurements are being made.

A further strategy has been to use stimulation tests for hormones whose secretion is under the control of receptors situated in the CNS. Pituitary hormones are controlled by neurotransmission at hypothalamic level and above. It has been suggested that altered hormone concentrations may indicate abnormalities in 'tone' of specific neurotransmitters. However, such is the complexity of the neuromodulation of hormonal release that little useful information is likely to be gained by simple single hormonal measurements – hence the use of drugs with fairly specific effects to stimulate hormone secretion via a particular receptor system. This, however, can be limited by the fact that few drugs have effects on one receptor system only.

Finally, care must always be taken when interpreting biochemical changes and relating them to clinical state. Biochemical alterations may occur that are not of primary clinical importance or are secondary to other changes. The most interesting changes may be those that correlate closely with clinical improvement, as they may provide information on the therapeutic action of ECT.

The biochemical effects of ECT in humans are reviewed below; each neurochemical system is taken in turn. 'Acute changes' refer to those noted within a few minutes or hours of an ECT treatment and are therefore mainly ascertained from blood samples rather than CSF or urine.

Noradrenaline

Acute changes

Plasma noradrenaline concentration rises acutely for up to 5 minutes with each ECT treatment. This occurs with unmodified and modified ECT. This change in plasma noradrenaline is not related to clinical improvement and in some studies is found to attenuate over chronic treatment. There is no acute change in plasma concentration of 3-methoxy-4-hydroxy-phenythyleneglycol (MHPG), the principal central metabolite of noradrenaline.

Changes over the course of treatment

There is evidence of plasma levels of noradrenaline being elevated in depressive illness (Lake *et al*, 1982; Kelly & Cooper, 1998). It is surprising, therefore, that few studies have looked at changes in plasma levels of noradrenaline during a course of ECT, although there are recent reports that it falls over a course of ECT in patients with melancholic or psychotic depressive illness, but not in non-melancholic depression (Cooper *et al*, 1985; Kelly & Cooper, 1997) and this fall may correlate with the clinical improvement. The concentration of MHPG in plasma is not affected by ECT.

Total body turnover of noradrenaline (as measured by the urinary output of noradrenaline plus its metabolites), which is elevated in depressive illness, is reduced by a course of ECT (Linnoila *et al*, 1983). The effect of ECT on CSF noradrenaline has not been studied. A course of ECT has been found to decrease CSF concentrations of MHPG in patients with schizophrenia but not in patients with depressive illness.

The number and function of peripheral lymphocyte β-adrenoceptors have been studied in depressed patients. Generally these receptors are reduced in number (B_{max}) and are less responsive to stimulation with the agonist isoprenaline (measured by production of intracellular cAMP) in patients with depression. A course of ECT does not appear to affect the number of receptors (Cooper *et al*, 1985) but does appear to affect their responsivity, returning β-adrenoceptor function towards normal (Mann *et al*, 1990). Studies of platelet α-adrenoceptors generally do not indicate an effect of ECT on either the number or function of this receptor.

The response of pituitary growth hormone to the α-adrenoceptor agonist clonidine has been found to be blunted in patients with depressive illness. In a small study this appeared to be unchanged by a course of ECT (Slade & Checkley, 1980).

Summary

Overall, there is evidence for elevated peripheral noradrenaline activity in depressive illness which may be associated with peripheral β-adrenoceptor subsensitivity. Both appear to normalise with a course of ECT.

Serotonin

Acute changes

The plasma concentration of the main metabolite of serotonin, 5-hydroxyindoleacetic acid (5-HIAA), is not altered acutely by ECT. There are no data on serotonin itself. The brain availability of tryptophan, the amino acid precursor of serotonin, is not altered.

Changes over the course of treatment

Studies examining changes in serotonin function with a course of ECT have focused on alterations in 5-HIAA. The concentration of 5-HIAA has not consistently been found to change in CSF or plasma with ECT but 24-hour urinary 5-HIAA excretion may fall. The 24-hour urinary serotonin excretion is unaltered by ECT.

The indoleamine theories of depression centre on abnormal serotonin function at the synaptic level and include the possibility of altered serotonin reuptake. Patelets are rich in serotonin, which is captured by similar reuptake mechanisms. Studies suggest that the speed of serotonin uptake into the platelet (V_{max}) may be reduced in patients with depression. ECT normalises this reduction in V_{max}.

A course of ECT is also associated with a rise in platelet 5-HT$_2$ receptor number (Stain-Malmgren et al, 1998) and a reduction in 5-HT$_2$ receptor function, as measured by intracellular calcium response to serotonin (Plein & Berk, 2000).

Prolactin

The most common acute hormonal change associated with ECT is a rise in plasma prolactin concentration. The secretion of prolactin is stimulated by serotonin and inhibited by dopamine inputs. It has been shown that fenfluramine (an agent that specifically releases serotonin from presynaptic stores and blocks its reuptake) causes elevations of prolactin when given orally. The stimulation of prolactin secretion by a standard dose of fenfluramine is enhanced after a course of ECT. This would suggest that ECT enhances serotonergic function at the hypothalamic level and possibly at higher centres. This change does not correlate with clinical improvement in patients with depression (Shapira et al, 1992).

Acute tryptophan depletion after ECT does not appear to cause any transient relapse in patients who have recovered from an episode of depression (Cassidy et al, 1997). Although the mechanism underlying return of symptoms in acute tryptophan depletion has not been fully elucidated, this finding may suggest that ECT does not exert its principal effect via the serotonin system.

Summary

There is some evidence for ECT inducing an increase in serotonin function in humans, but this cannot yet be related to a specific receptor subtype or therapeutic outcome.

Dopamine

Acute changes

There is no information on the immediate effects of a single ECT treatment on concentrations of dopamine. The plasma concentration of its principal metabolite, homovanillic acid (HVA), does not seem to be altered.

Changes over the course of treatment

A number of studies have investigated the effects of ECT on the CSF concentration of HVA. Most have failed to find a change. However, most of these studies compared CSF concentrations before and after a complete course of ECT and did not examine changes during the treatment. Studies of antipsychotic drugs have found that they initially increase dopamine turnover, evidenced by an increase in CSF HVA. Subsequently tolerance develops to this effect (i.e. a reduction back to baseline concentrations of HVA) and the development of tolerance seems to indicate a good clinical response in patients with schizophrenia. It is interesting that one study of the effects of ECT on patients with schizophrenia found that the CSF concentrations of HVA were increased 24 hours after a single ECT treatment but that this change disappeared by the end of the course, in a similar fashion to the changes seen over time with antipsychotic drugs (Cooper *et al*, 1988).

The dopamine agonist apomorphine increases the secretion of growth hormone from the anterior pituitary gland by stimulation of dopamine receptors located in the hypothalamus. The growth hormone response to apomorphine can be used as a measure of dopamine receptor sensitivity. Studies comparing the effects of ECT on the growth hormone response to apomorphine have found either no change or a slight increase after ECT (Christie *et al*, 1982).

The effects of ECT in patients with movement disorders serve only to provide further confusion. There is evidence that ECT may temporarily benefit patients with Parkinson's disease (Douyen *et al*, 1989), possibly through an increase in dopamine receptor sensitivity. However, there is also evidence for both improvement and worsening of tardive dyskinesia following ECT.

Summary

Electroconvulsive therapy appears to affect dopamine systems in humans but the exact nature of this effect is unclear. There is not yet consistent evidence of the increased functioning of dopamine systems demonstrated in many of the animal studies.

Hypothalamic–pituitary–adrenal (HPA) axis

Acute changes

Plasma concentrations of adrenocorticotrophin-releasing hormone (ACTH) are elevated by each ECT treatment, with similar effects throughout the course of treatment. The increase is present by 2 minutes after ECT. Plasma cortisol rises acutely 5–15 minutes after ECT and remains elevated for at least 60 minutes. The rise in plasma cortisol is most pronounced in those patients with non-psychotic depression. None of the above effects appears to be directly related to clinical change. These acute hormonal changes are not shown by patients undergoing cholecystectomy (Whalley et al, 1982), which suggests they are not part of a general stress response. Similar hormonal changes have been found after direct-current cardioversion, which indicates they may be related to high-energy electrical stimulation and not be unique to ECT (Florkowski et al, 1996).

Changes over the course of treatment

Depressive illness is associated with increased release of cortisol and ACTH. The increased cortisol release is most pronounced in the evening and so involves a loss of the normal diurnal variation. Most ECT studies that have examined change in plasma ACTH and cortisol have used single, morning measurements, which have not always shown a change in baseline values after a course of ECT. However, consistent with results from studies of other antidepressant treatments, more intensive studies have shown a decrease in baseline plasma cortisol levels after a course of ECT in patients with severe depression (Christie et al, 1982; Cooper et al, 1985). Patients with higher afternoon plasma cortisol levels after ECT appear to have a greater risk of relapse (Cosgriff et al, 1990).

Corticotrophin-releasing hormone (CRH) is a 41-amino-acid peptide produced in the paraventricular nucleus of the hypothalamus. It controls the release of ACTH at pituitary level. CRH concentrations in the CSF are elevated in depressive illness and have been shown to fall over a course of ECT (Nemeroff et al, 1991).

The dexamethasone suppression test (DST) was initially thought to be a biological diagnostic test for depressive illness. Unfortunately this turned out not to be the case, as abnormal results were also given by patients with several other psychiatric disorders. Despite this, it has been investigated for its predictive value with regard to immediate outcome and relapse after a course of ECT. While the abnormal DST results of some patients will normalise after ECT, as with other antidepressant treatments, the test has no specific predictive ability (Katona *et al*, 1987).

Neurophysins

Neurophysins are carrier peptides, detectable in plasma, which are released mole for mole with secretion of posterior pituitary hormones. However, they have a longer half-life than the associated hormones, which themselves are difficult to measure in plasma, and they give an indication of the amount of the hormone secreted. Oxytocin-associated neurophysin is stimulated by the release of oestrogen and is also named oestrogen-stimulated neurophysin; vasopressin-associated neurophysin is stimulated by nicotine and is also named nicotine-stimulated neurophysin.

Acute changes

Plasma concentrations of oxytocin, vasopressin and their associated neurophysins increase acutely with ECT, reaching a maximum at 2 minutes. There is no change in response between first and last administration of ECT. The increase in oestrogen-stimulated neurophysin following the first ECT treatment correlates with clinical improvement at the end of a course of ECT but not with outcome at 2 months (Scott *et al*, 1991). The reason for the association between oestrogen-stimulated neurophysin secretion and outcome in unclear. It does not appear to be related to the duration of electrical activity during ECT as measured by electroencephalography (EEG). As there is no association between response and baseline or peak oxytocin concentrations following ECT (Smith *et al*, 1994), the significance of the above findings remains uncertain.

Changes over the course of treatment

There is no change from pre-treatment concentrations of oestrogen-stimulated neurophysin, nicotine-stimulated neurophysin or oxytocin with a course of ECT.

Other neurotransmitters, peptides and hormones

A number of other chemical changes have been noted in response to ECT treatment. These are summarised in Tables 8.3 and 8.4 and are briefly outlined below.

Acute changes

Several studies have shown that thyrotrophin-releasing hormone (TRH) is not altered by ECT but that thyroid-stimulating hormone (TSH) rises acutely with ECT. Prolactin rises acutely with each ECT treatment, as it does with spontaneous epileptic seizures. Growth

Table 8.3 Acute hormonal changes with ECT

Hormone	Effect of ECT on concentration
Cortisol	↑
Prolactin	↑
Growth hormone	↑↓
Thyroid-stimulating hormone	↑
Adrenocorticotrophic hormone	↑
Beta-endorphin	↑
Neurophysins	↑
Oxytocin	↑
Vasopressin	↑
Substance P	↑
Insulin	↑

hormone has been found increased, unchanged or decreased after individual ECT treatments. This inconsistency may be related to the post-treatment timing of the measurements, an increase being more likely soon after treatment.

Both CRH and vasopressin, released at the hypothalamic level, induce the release and cleavage of the glycoprotein pro-opiomelano-cortin (POMC). From POMC a family of peptides are produced, which include β-lipotropic hormone, β-endorphin and ACTH. As with ACTH, β-endorphin levels are elevated acutely by ECT.

Of possible medical importance are the rises in serum potassium, insulin and glucose acutely following ECT. It has been suggested that the acute increase in insulin may relate to therapeutic effects, but as yet there is little direct evidence that the above are important to the therapeutic action of ECT.

Attempts have been made to investigate changes in second messenger systems, such as cAMP, in the plasma of patients undergoing ECT. The results are unclear because of the confounding effects of anaesthesia. The relevance to brain activity is questionable.

Table 8.4 Hormonal changes over a course of ECT

Hormone	Effect of ECT on concentration
Cortisol	↓
Prolactin	←→
Growth hormone	←→
Corticotrophin-releasing hormone	↓
Beta-endorphin	↓
Thyroid-stimulating hormone	←→
Thyroxine (FT4)	↓
Neurophysins	←→

Changes over the course of treatment

Baseline TRH and TSH are unaltered by a course of ECT. Likewise, the TSH response to TRH is unaltered. Despite this, free thyroxine (FT4) appears to fall with ECT in a manner unrelated to clinical improvement or plasma albumin or fatty acid concentrations. Prolactin rises with each ECT but the rise is blunted in later treatments. In view of the complexity of release of prolactin it is speculative to apply a neuro-transmitter hypothesis to this change. Pre-treatment concentrations of growth hormone are unaltered by a course of ECT.

Conclusions

It is clear, from the above, that ECT has widespread effects on neurotransmitter and hormonal systems. Many of the changes may be relatively non-specific with regard to treatment response, and reflect only the effects of a generalised seizure. The following are perhaps the most interesting findings in terms of possible explanations of the therapeutic effect of ECT:

(1)   reduction of plasma concentration of noradrenaline
(2)   increase of dopamine function
(3)   increase of serotonin function
(4)   reduction of CRH concentration in CSF.

The relationship between chemical changes and clinical outcome with ECT are summarised in Table 8.5.

Stimulus dosage

Neurophysiological variables

If the principles of psychopharmacology have any relevance for ECT, then at least two groups of questions may reasonably be asked of

Table 8.5   Chemical change in relation to clinical response

Chemical change	Relation to clinical response
Decrease in plasma noradrenaline level (over course)	Some
Increase in oestrogen-stimulated neurophysin level (after first application)	Some
Increase in prolactin level (after first application)	None
Dexamethasone suppression test	None
Increase in cortisol level (after first application)	None
Decrease in cortisol level (over course)	None
Change in prolactin level (over course)	None
Increase in response of prolactin to fenfluramine	None

ECT: questions concerning dosage, in relation to both efficacy and side-effects; and questions concerning kinetics – those variables, related to both the patient and the treatment, that may influence the effectiveness of a given stimulus and account for the great variability in the responses of different patients. Our understanding of these issues has been limited by the difficulty of studying electric currents *in vivo*.

From cellular studies, animal studies and studies of ECT itself, it is clear that small pulsed currents can stimulate neurons, that is, cause an action potential. In intact networks of cells repeated pulsed currents are required to overcome the natural inhibitory systems. There is also evidence that the magnitude of a threshold stimulus, in terms of both amplitude and duration, varies from one cerebral site to another. For example, the parietal region of the cerebral cortex has a much lower threshold for electrically induced convulsion than the frontal region. However, an even greater source of threshold variability resides in the capacitive and resistive properties of the calvarium and scalp. Seizure threshold for ECT is highly variable and a function of factors related to the both stimulus factors (pulse, frequency, duration, train length, electrode position) and the patient (age, gender), as well as others (e.g. medication).

Seizure, stimulus dosage and efficacy

The importance of the induced epileptic seizure in ECT was first demonstrated by the pioneering work of Ottosson (1960). However, the simplicity of this relationship has been challenged by a number of recent studies. One of the most dramatic findings concerned the marked differences in the therapeutic effectiveness of unilateral and bilateral ECT. Sackeim *et al* (1986, 1987*a,b,c*) found that generalised seizures were much more effective clinically when they were produced using near-threshold bilateral stimuli rather than near-threshold unilateral stimuli, even though the seizures were identical in their behavioural and surface-recorded electrophysiological characteristics.

Recent studies have shown that, provided the stimulus intensity is high enough, unilateral and bilateral stimulation are equally effective (McCall *et al*, 2000; Sackeim *et al*, 2000*b*). In these studies stimulus intensity was defined with respect to the stimulus level required to induce a seizure, and they used high suprathreshold stimuli (high-dosage unilateral stimulation = 500% above initial seizure threshold; high-dosage bilateral stimulation = 150% above threshold). This still suggests a close relationship between seizure threshold and efficacy and may indicate that qualitative aspects of the induced seizure are stimulus dependent.

While simple measures of seizure activity, such as fit length, have little relationship to efficacy (Sackeim *et al*, 1987*c*), quantitative EEG studies of the induced seizure have found better therapeutic outcome to be associated with greater EEG power in the low (delta) frequencies, particularly in the prefrontal region. Such seizures were associated with high suprathreshold stimuli.

Another aspect of ECT seizure kinetics, of relevance for efficacy, is the change in seizure threshold across the course of ECT: seizure threshold rises and seizure duration typically shortens, and these changes are correlated with the antidepressant effects of ECT (Sackeim *et al*, 1987*b*; Sackheim, 1999; Chanpattana *et al*, 2000).

While the cognitive side-effects of ECT have been shown to be minimal and short-lived, the evidence suggests that stimulus intensity is an important factor in this process. As with the therapeutic effects, the relationship between stimulus intensity and cognitive impairment may also be mediated by specific seizure characteristics. Recent evidence suggests that these may be different from those associated with therapeutic efficacy (Krystal & Weiner, 1999; Sackeim *et al*, 2000*a*). Of practical significance is the fact that right unilateral ECT at high dosage and of identical efficacy to high-dosage bilateral ECT produces significantly fewer cognitive side-effects (Sackeim *et al*, 2000*a*).

Practical implications for the administration of ECT

The new research evidence has implications not only for the role of ECT in the treatment of depression but also for the practicalities of ECT administration. Seizure threshold (i.e. the stimulus required to induce a seizure) is an important parameter for determining the therapeutic window of ECT but is highly variable. Both the American Psychiatric Association Task Force (1990) and the Royal College of Psychiatrists (1995) recommend one of two methods for estimating the initial stimulus dosage for any given patient. One is a formula based on the effects of factors associated with patient age and gender on threshold stimulus. While this method is widely used (Farah & McCall, 1993), present evidence suggests that it is rather inaccurate and may lead to both under-stimulation and over-stimulation (Gangadhar *et al*, 1998; Mayur *et al*, 1998; Girish *et al*, 2000; Heikman *et al*, 2000; Laidlaw *et al*, 2000; Spicknall *et al*, 2000). The second method is dose titration, and while more time consuming and requiring more training, it is the optimal method for stimulus determination.

The balance of advantages between unilateral and bilateral ECT may be turning again in favour of unilateral stimulation, provided an adequate (high-level) stimulus is used. For unilateral ECT, present evidence suggests this stimulus should be five times that required to achieve seizure threshold, although for patients with a high seizure threshold this dosage may exceed the dynamic range of the stimulus unit. At the present time it may be preferable to reserve right unilateral ECT for those patients in whom even the mild transient cognitive impairments associated with bilateral ECT are clinically unacceptable.

While seizure duration itself may have little relationship to therapeutic efficacy, very short seizures (less than 20 seconds) are likely to be the result of inadequate stimulation and much too close to seizure threshold to produce a therapeutic effect.

It should be noted that factors other than patient variables may influence seizure threshold. Particular attention should be paid to concomitant use of medications with anticonvulsant properties. These include benzodiazepine sedation and propofol as an anaesthetic induction agent (Geretsegger et al, 1998; Martin et al, 1998).

The best guide to the correct number of treatments is a patient's clinical response to the treatment itself. Treatment resistance should not be assumed unless a full course (usually 5–8 treatments) has been administered using adequate suprathreshold stimuli. Individual patients meeting the indications for ECT may require up to 12 treatments to obtain a good clinical response. While the frequency of ECT has little effect on efficacy, frequent ECT stimulation (more than twice a week) results in significantly more cognitive impairment (Shapira et al, 1998).

The therapeutic efficacy of ECT in a given patient can be optimised by careful attention to procedural details. This in turn has implications for training. Within the UK, given that most ECT is administered by non-consultant-grade staff, provision of appropriate training for junior staff is essential to ensure high standards of treatment (Duffett & Lelliott, 1998; Trezise, 1998; Brookes et al, 2000).

Contraindications and morbidity

Contraindications

While there are no absolute contraindications to ECT, it should be avoided within 3 months of a myocardial infarction or a cerebrovascular accident. The treatment itself causes a transient increase in intracranial pressure and should therefore be used with care where this could cause problems. However, it has been used safely and effectively in patients with depression associated with inoperable brain tumours (Greenberg et al, 1988). An acute respiratory tract infection is a contraindication to the anaesthetic.

Particular caution and care are also required if the patient suffers from cardiac arrhythmias, an aneurysm, peptic ulceration, a recent fracture or severe osteoporosis. ECT can be used in pregnancy but thorough muscle relaxation is necessary to protect the foetus.

Common side-effects

Leaving aside memory impairment (on which see below), the most common adverse effect is headache, complained of by up to 30% of

---

Box 8.1 Common, minor side-effects of ECT

The following each affect around 10% of patients who undergo ECT:

- Headache
- Muscular pains
- Confusion
- Palpitations
- Hypotension
- Drowsiness
- Weakness

---

patients and more commonly after bilateral than after unilateral ECT. Muscle aches and pains may occur and usually are due to the muscle relaxant. The common effects, perhaps affecting around 10% of patients each, are listed in Box 8.1.

Major complications

Before the introduction of modified ECT, fractures of the vertebrae or long bones, dislocation of the jaw and fat embolism were a significant risk. However, these are now rare. Some of the major complications are listed in Box 8.2. These are extremely rare and, like the orthopaedic complications, were mainly associated with the use of unmodified ECT. A transient rise in blood pressure does occur with ECT and this is probably responsible for the occasional nasal or subconjunctival haemorrhage or for the rare cerebrovascular accident or bleed from a peptic ulcer. Cardiac complications are rare and are usually associated with pre-existing cardiac disease.

An epileptic seizure following ECT is also rare. A follow-up of 166 patients found late-onset seizures in three cases, at intervals of

---

Box 8.2 Rare, major complications of ECT

The following very rarely affect patients who undergo ECT:

- Myocardial infarction
- Cardiac arrhythmias
- Congestive cardiac failure
- Aspiration pneumonia
- Cerebrovascular accident
- Bleeding from peptic ulcer
- Pulmonary embolism
- Prolonged apnoea

---

4 hours, 2 weeks and 8 years after the ECT. These patients had only one or two seizures and the patient in whom a fit occurred after 8 years had a family history of epilepsy (Blackwood *et al*, 1980). This prevalence rate is within the prevalence rate for epilepsy in the general population. The occurrence of status epilepticus following on from a therapeutic seizure is extremely rare.

Mortality

Surveys of deaths related to ECT generally report figures around the 1 per 22 000 treatments found by Heshe & Roeder (1976) in Denmark. This compares favourably with the reported figure of 1 per 10 000 deaths related to brief anaesthesia for other purposes, where the anaesthesia was held responsible. Death is most likely during or immediately after ECT. The most common cause is probably cardiac arrest due to excessive vagal inhibition, which is best prevented by adequate atropinisation during the induction of anaesthesia.

Effects on memory

Memory impairment associated with ECT appears to relate to the amount of electrical energy given and to the site of electrode placement, rather than to seizure-related variables. It was in order to reduce memory impairment that attempts were made to reduce the stimulus necessary for induction of the seizure, suprathreshold stimuli being more likely to cause cognitive impairment. However, evidence now suggests that minimal electrical stimuli are not clinically as effective as suprathreshold stimuli. Thus, some memory upset may be an inevitable concomitant of effective treatment. Unilateral ECT applied to the non-dominant hemisphere appears to induce less memory impairment than other types of application, but again also appears to be a clinically less effective stimulus.

The situation is complicated by the fact that depressive illness is itself associated with memory impairment. Thus, some aspects of memory may improve as the depression improves, while others are adversely affected by the treatment itself. Most aspects of memory function, if affected by ECT, seem to return to normal over 6 months (Weeks *et al*, 1980; Frith *et al*, 1983).

Four main types of impairment are described:

(1) *Short-term retrograde amnesia.* Many patients have amnesia for events occurring from a few hours to a few days before treatment, and sometimes even for a few weeks. This impairment can be caused both by ECT and by the depressive illness. Other patients have a clear memory right up to the time of treatment.

(2) *Long-term retrograde amnesia.* Some patients complain of loss of discrete memories from the distant past. This is difficult to confirm, but seems more common with bilateral ECT.

(3) *Short-term anterograde amnesia.* This is more common and affects the ability to learn new information. It is more severe with bilateral ECT but resolves rapidly and usually completely by 6 months.

(4) *Permanent anterograde amnesia.* More rarely, some patients complain of persistent memory problems. Lack of pre-treatment information on their memory function makes this difficult to assess. However, there is no definite evidence that ECT causes this.

Structural brain damage

A number of studies have also sought evidence of structural brain damage following ECT. The methods used include computerised tomography, magnetic resonance imaging and examination of serum for brain-specific proteins that might be released if damage occurred. The results of these studies do not suggest that any structural damage occurs with ECT.

One study indeed suggested that ECT induces an increase in protein synthesis (Sermet *et al*, 1998). Studies in laboratory animals suggest that ECS increases the concentration of neuropeptides, such as brain-derived neurotrophic factor (BDNF), which are associated with neuronal sprouting and regrowth (Smith *et al*, 1997). Whether this is of therapeutic importance remains unclear. A course of ECT also increases brain concentrations of choline, as measured by proton magnetic resonance spectroscopy (Ende *et al*, 2000).

Principles of use of electroconvulsive therapy

Patient selection

As discussed above, the principal disorders for which ECT may be indicated are depressive illness, mania and schizophrenia. It is also of value in puerperal psychosis. Depressive symptoms appearing secondary to another primary disorder are best managed by treatment of the primary disorder (e.g. an obsessive–compulsive neurosis or an anxiety disorder). In this instance ECT should be considered only if the depressive symptoms are persistent and doubt arises about the primary diagnosis. The authors of the early clinical studies of ECT are more or less unanimous in the view that it does not benefit patients suffering from psychoneuroses.

Very occasionally ECT has been used in the management of delirium when the underlying cause has been treated but the delirium has failed to respond to standard treatment, such as antipsychotic drugs.

In the treatment of mania, ECT is reserved principally for patients who have not responded to antipsychotic drugs or to a combination of antipsychotic drugs and lithium. Patients with severe mania, and risk of exhaustion, or in a manic stupor, should have ECT as their treatment of first choice.

In the management of schizophrenia, ECT is again reserved principally for patients who have not responded to antipsychotic drugs or who are so disturbed that a more rapid response is required. Although catatonia is often put forward as a specific indication, there is surprisingly little evidence in the literature to support this. However, ECT is useful if a catatonic stupor develops. The role of ECT in treating affective symptoms in schizophrenia is unclear (see above). The evidence suggests that ECT is most effective if used in combination with antipsychotic drugs in schizophrenia.

Predictors of response in depressive illness

In the management of depressive illness, ECT is generally thought to be most useful for patients with a moderate depressive episode with somatic symptoms (termed 'endogenous' or 'melancholic' in older diagnostic systems) or with a severe depressive episode (with or without psychotic symptoms), as well as for patients with bipolar depression. A widely quoted set of symptoms regarded as predictive of response were derived by a group working in Newcastle (Carney et al, 1965). Features predicting good response were: weight loss, pyknic build, early waking, somatic delusions and paranoid delusions. Features weighting against good response were: anxiety, feeling worse in the evening, self-pity, hypochondriasis and hysterical features. However, the prognostic value of some of these features has not been widely replicated.

Mendels (1965) found hysterical features, inadequate personality, neurotic personality traits and the presence of precipitating factors to predict poor response to ECT but did not find evidence for good response in association with variables such as weight loss or early waking. A detailed analysis of predictors of response in the Northwick Park ECT trial (Clinical Research Centre, Division of Psychiatry, 1984) also rejected many of the 'Newcastle' features. However, it did show a relationship between good response and the presence of delusions and psychomotor retardation, although the last feature also predicted good response to simulated ECT. There was also a non-significant trend for patients with fewer life events in the previous 6 months to respond better. The Leicestershire ECT trial (Brandon et al, 1984) also favoured the presence of delusions and retardation as good prognostic factors for ECT.

A few studies have suggested that the presence of psychomotor agitation may predict a good response (Avery & Silverman, 1984), but this feature tends to be found more often in older patients or those with late-onset illness, who tend to have a good response to ECT anyway.

Thus, for depressive illness, although a diagnosis of moderate depressive episode with somatic symptoms, severe depressive episode or psychotic depressive episode may suggest a good response to ECT, the individual features contributing to these diagnoses are not themselves very useful in prognosis, except the presence of delusions and psycho-motor retardation. Although it may be argued that these features are generally predictive of good acute response whatever the treatment, the Northwick Park study showed that, particularly for delusions, these had stronger effects for the group who received real ECT than for the group who had simulated ECT. Indicators of a poor response to ECT seem to be the presence of recent precipitants to the illness and personality factors, the latter also tending to relate to worse long-term outcome for depressive illness in general (Duggan *et al*, 1991).

Prescribing ECT

The decision to give ECT in depression is generally made if treatment with an adequate dose of an antidepressant drug for at least 4–6 weeks has failed. It has been shown in one study that a combination of lithium and tricyclic antidepressant may be as effective as ECT in such cases (Dinan & Barry, 1989), but this has yet to be replicated. Where patients have a history of recurrent depression and a good response to ECT, where there is a high risk of suicide or where a rapid response is necessary for other reasons (e.g. a depressive stupor), then ECT is the treatment of first choice. In patients with psychotic depression, treatment with either a combination of an antidepressant plus an antipsychotic drug or ECT is necessary.

Consent to treatment

Consent to ECT must be in writing and should follow an explanation to the patient of:

(1) the reasons for treatment
(2) the nature and side-effects of treatment
(3) the fact the patient will have a general anaesthetic
(4) the desired outcome
(5) the possible consequence of not having treatment.

The decision to give ECT should be made by the responsible medical officer (RMO), or another senior doctor if the RMO is not available, and this decision should be recorded in the case notes. The consent form should be signed by a doctor as well as the patient and must be retained in the case notes.

In England and Wales, if the patient is detained under the Mental Health Act, then the RMO must certify that the patient is capable of giving informed consent (sections 58[3]a; form 38). In Scotland a similar procedure applies (sections 98[3]a and 98[5]; form 9) and also in Northern Ireland (article 64; form 22).

If a patient refuses consent, a relative cannot give consent on his/her behalf, unless the patient is a minor, in which case parents or guardians must be consulted. If the patient is voluntary (i.e. not detained under the local Mental Health Act), then ECT cannot be given without consent unless it is imperative to give urgent treatment, for example for depressive stupor. In most such cases the common law applies. Following such emergency treatment the patient should be detained under the appropriate sections of the local mental health legislation. Where a patient is incapable of giving properly informed consent, for example an adult with learning disability to a degree rendering him/her incapable of understanding, the common law will again usually apply to the use of urgent treatment, until the patient is detained.

Where a patient is detained but refuses consent, or is unable to give it, then the appropriate sections of the local mental health legislation apply.

England and Wales

The Mental Health Act Commission must be contacted to arrange for an independent psychiatrist, usually from a different hospital, to visit (sections 58[3]b and 58[4] of the Mental Health Act 1983). This doctor may authorise (on form 39) the administration of ECT. If urgent treatment is required, this may be given under the provisions of section 62, followed by immediate notification of the Mental Health Act Commission so that a second opinion may be provided.

Scotland

In most cases the provisions of section 98 in Part X of the Mental Health (Scotland) Act 1984 apply. The Mental Welfare Commission for Scotland must be contacted to arrange for an independent doctor to assess the patient (sections 98[3]b and 98[4]). This doctor may authorise (on form 10) the administration of ECT. If urgent treatment is required, then section 102 applies to detained patients; it requires that the Mental Welfare Commission is notified within 7 days of the treatment being given.

Northern Ireland

Electroconvulsive therapy is included among treatments that require consent or a second opinion under article 64 of the Mental Health (Northern Ireland) Order 1986. Where a patient refuses or is unable to give consent, the Mental Health Commission for Northern Ireland must be contacted and it will arrange for an independent opinion by a psychiatrist appointed under Part IV of the Order, who may authorise ECT (on form 23). If urgent treatment is required, then article 68 applies, which requires immediate notification of the Mental Health Commission by the RMO once treatment has been given.

Republic of Ireland

The Mental Health Act of 1945 did not give guidelines on ECT. However, this is now addressed in the Mental Health Act 2001, Part 4, section 59. This indicates that the consultant psychiatrist responsible for the patient must sign a form to approve the treatment and an independent consultant psychiatrist must also sign a form to authorise the treatment.

Administration of ECT

The Royal College of Psychiatrists' (1995) guidelines provide a detailed description of the facilities and equipment required and procedures to be followed for the administration of ECT. There should be a proper ECT suite, with a waiting area, treatment area and recovery room.

Anaesthesia

The anaesthetic must be administered by a properly qualified anaesthetist with suitable equipment available for monitoring the patient and for resuscitation.

For many years, anaesthesia was induced using methohexitone sodium (Brietal), which gave rapid induction and recovery and produced fewer cardiac abnormalities than other agents. It had little effect on seizure duration. Unfortunately, this drug has ceased to be available because the company that owns the licence for it was unable to find a manufacturer. Were it to become available again, it would be preferred over other induction agents available at the time of writing.

Three other agents are appropriate alternatives: propofol, etomidate and sodium thiopentone. Each has advantages and disadvantages and these have been summarised in a brief statement from the Royal College of Psychiatrists (Freeman, 1999). Propofol is quite widely used but is known to shorten seizure length, although there is no evidence to suggest an effect on overall efficacy of treatment. Etomidate may lengthen seizure duration but can be associated with extraneous muscle movements and, rarely, adrenocortical dysfunction. Sodium thiopentone is associated with a longer recovery time, which may be a particular problem in the elderly.

Muscle relaxation is essential to modify the fit and prevent orthopaedic complications. Suxamethonium chloride at a dose of 30–60 mg is the drug of choice; it is given intravenously after the induction of anaesthesia (from a different syringe but through the same needle as the anaesthetic). It is important to ensure that the period of anaesthesia adequately overlaps the period of muscle relaxation. The use of atropine (usually 0.6 mg) to dry secretions and block the vagus nerve, so limiting bradycardia and hypotension, is not now a universal procedure.

Once anaesthesia has been induced the anaesthetist should adequately oxygenate the patient via a face mask (generally 10–20 inhalations of oxygen). This should prevent cerebral hypoxia during the seizure and has the additional advantage of reducing the seizure threshold. A bite guard must be inserted into the patient's mouth before the electrical stimulus is applied, to prevent damage to the teeth or tongue.

The procedure

The ECT machine should be switched on *before* each treatment session. The instructions for some equipment indicate that a 'warm-up' period of half an hour is necessary. The electrodes should be allowed to soak in a suitable electrolyte solution. The area of the scalp to which they should be applied is 4 cm above the midpoint of a line joining the angle of the orbit to the external auditory meatus (Fig. 8.1(a)). This area should be dry and grease-free. For unilateral ECT the frontotemporal electrode placement is as above, with the second electrode about 9 cm superior and posterior over the parietal region (the 'Lancaster' position; Fig. 8.1(b)).

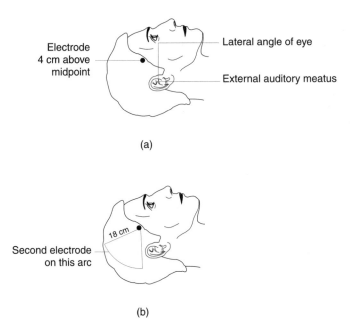

(a)

(b)

Fig. 8.1 The usual electrode positions. (a) The position of the frontotemporal electrode for bilateral ECT. This position also used for one of the electrodes for unilateral ECT. (b) The 'Lancaster' position for the second electrode for unilateral ECT.

The psychiatrist applies the electrodes once the anaesthetist is satisfied with the patient's condition. Firm pressure should be applied throughout the time of passage of the stimulus, which is generally indicated by auditory and/or visual warning signals. The length of the tonic–clonic phase of the seizure should be recorded, as very short seizures are rarely of therapeutic benefit. If no seizure occurs or if there is only a doubtful or very brief seizure (less than 20 seconds) or if a relatively short focal or unilateral seizure occurs, then restimulation should be considered with a more powerful stimulus.

Before restimulating:

(1) the anaesthetist must be satisfied that the patient is still adequately anaesthetised
(2) the patient should be reoxygenated
(3) the psychiatrist should ensure that there is good contact between the electrodes and the scalp.

If there is still no adequate seizure, the patient must be allowed to recover – a third stimulus should not be given.

After treatment the patient should be placed in the 'unconscious position' and should be reoxygenated. Once recovery to the initial level of consciousness has occurred the patient should be taken to a recovery area, where a nurse must monitor the patient until full recovery is achieved.

Course of treatment

Usually between four and eight applications of ECT are required; most patients receive six. There is often some transient indication of improvement within the first three treatments. A few patients can be very slow to respond, but if there has been some sign of response during the first eight treatments, then treatment should be continued at least up to 12 applications before ECT is abandoned.

Treatment is generally given twice per week. There is no evidence that daily ECT induces more rapid improvement but it does cause more severe cognitive impairment.

Failure to have a fit

If seizures do not occur or are very short, even following a second stimulus, then possible reasons for this must be considered. For some patients this is an indication of a high seizure threshold and the solution is the use of a more potent stimulus, by either increasing the electrical energy or altering the frequency of the electrical pulses, depending on which may be altered on the ECT machine available.

Prescription of benzodiazepines may raise seizure threshold. Ideally these should therefore be avoided entirely with patients receiving ECT.

If a benzodiazepine hypnotic is unavoidable, then it should be one with a short elimination half-life and no active metabolites, and it should be omitted on the evenings before ECT treatment sessions.

Antidepressants can also be anticonvulsant for ECT, even though they may be proconvulsant in other situations. One of the authors (SJC) has personally recorded (by EEG) inadequate seizures in patients continued on antidepressants during ECT and noted an increased length of seizure following discontinuation of the antidepressant.

If seizures are very difficult to obtain, some centres have used intravenous caffeine, 5 minutes before treatment, to reduce seizure threshold or prolong seizure time (Shapira *et al*, 1987). It is perhaps ironic to think that 50 years after ECT began to supplant chemically induced seizures that chemical means to augment ECT were again considered.

Transcranial magnetic stimulation

Magnetic stimulation

Transcranial magnetic stimulation (TMS) is a technique for stimulating small areas of cerebral cortex by application of high-intensity magnetic fields of brief duration. The magnetic field is created by rapidly changing an electric current in an insulated coil placed over the scalp. The magnetic field created will induce electric currents in electrical conductors within the field, for example in cortical neurons. The magnetic field strength created is generally around 1 tesla and penetrates the cortex to a depth of approximately 2 cm.

The currents induced in neurons may alter function and result in depolarisation. Motor responses can be developed, for example in the small muscles of the hand, from a coil situated over the vertex.

Repetitive TMS (rTMS) involves the application of trains of magnetic pulses and these can have a variety of physiological effects, which may vary according to the frequency of the rTMS. The use of TMS to stimulate brain function in association with imaging of that function (e.g. by positron emission tomography) is a technique being exploited in the study of brain function (Ebmeier & Lappin, 2001).

Use as a treatment

During the use of rTMS as an investigative technique, some subjects reported changes in affect. This led to its investigation as a treatment for depression and five placebo-controlled trials have now been carried out. These suggest that there may be a useful antidepressant effect. However, as yet there is no clear consensus with regard to mode of stimulation (frequency of pulses, strength of field, length of stimulation) or placement of the coils in order to achieve the best results. Nor is it clear how sustained the effect will be. A meta-analysis of trials has recently been published (McNamara *et al*, 2001). The time for which stimulation is applied is often increased during the course of treatment, from a few minutes to around 15 minutes. The principal adverse effect is headache but occasionally a seizure is induced.

The technique has also been used in schizophrenia and in particular seemed to reduce the severity of auditory hallucinations.

References

Abrams, R. & Taylor, M. A. (1973) Anterior bifrontal ECT: a clinical trial. *British Journal of Psychiatry*, **122**, 587–590.

Abrams, R., Taylor, M. A., Faber, R., *et al* (1983) Bilateral versus unilateral electro-convulsive therapy: efficacy in melancholia. *American Journal of Psychiatry*, **140**, 463–465.

American Psychiatric Association Task Force (1990) *The Practice of Electroconvulsive Therapy: Recommendations for the Treatment, Training and Privileging*. Washington, DC: American Psychiatric Association.

Avery, D. & Silverman, J. (1984) Psychomotor retardation and agitation in depression. *Journal of Affective Disorders*, **7**, 67–76.

Avery, D. & Winokur, G. (1976) Mortality in depressed patients treated with electro-convulsive therapy and antidepressants. *Archives of General Psychiatry*, **33**, 1029–1037.

Barton, J. L. (1977) ECT in depression: the evidence of controlled studies. *Biological Psychiatry*, **12**, 687–695.

Bennet, A. E. (1938) Convulsive (pentamethylenetetrazol) shock therapy in depressive psychoses: a preliminary report of results obtained in 10 cases. *American Journal of Medical Science*, **196**, 420–429.

Blackwood, D. H. R., Cull, R. E., Freeman, C. P. L., *et al* (1980) A study of the incidence of epilepsy following ECT. *Journal of Neurology, Neurosurgery and Psychiatry*, **43**, 1098–1102.

Brandon, S., Cowley, P., McDonald, C., *et al* (1984) Electroconvulsive therapy: results in depressive illness from the Leicestershire trial. *BMJ*, **288**, 22–25.

Brandon, S., Cowley, P., McDonald, C., *et al* (1985) Leicester ECT trial: results in schizophrenia. *British Journal of Psychiatry*, **146**, 177–183.

Brookes, G., Rigby, J. & Barnes, R. (2000) Implementing the Royal College of Psychiatrists' guidelines for the practice of electroconvulsive therapy. *Psychiatric Bulletin*, **24**, 329–330.

Carney, M. W. P., Roth, M. & Garside, R. F. (1965) The diagnosis of depressive syndromes and the prediction of ECT response. *British Journal of Psychiatry*, **111**, 659–674.

Carr, V., Dorrington, C., Schrader, G., *et al* (1983) The use of ECT for mania in childhood bipolar disorder. *British Journal of Psychiatry*, **143**, 411–415.

Cassidy, F., Murry, E., Weiner, R., *et al* (1997) Lack of relapse with tryptophan depletion following successful treatment with ECT. *American Journal of Psychiatry*, **154**, 1151–1152.

Chanpattana, W., Buppanharun, W., Raksakietisak, S., *et al* (2000) Seizure threshold rise during electoconvulsive therapy in schizophrenic patients. *Journal of Psychiatry Research*, **96**, 31–40.

Christie, E. J., Whalley, L. J., Brown, N. S., *et al* (1982) Effect of ECT of the neuroendocrine response to apomorphine in severely depressed patients. *British Journal of Psychiatry*, **140**, 268–273.

Clinical Research Centre, Division of Psychiatry (1984) The Northwick Park ECT trial. Predictors of response to real and simulated ECT. *British Journal of Psychiatry*, **144**, 227–237.

Cooper, S. J., Kelly, J. G. & King, D. J. (1985) Adrenergic receptors in depression. Effects of electroconvulsive therapy. *British Journal of Psychiatry*, **147**, 23–29.

Cooper, S. J., Leahey, W., Green, D. F., *et al* (1988) The effect of electroconvulsive therapy on CSF amine metabolites in schizophrenic patients. *British Journal of Psychiatry*, **152**, 59–63.

Cosgriff, J. P., Abbot, R. M., Oakley-Browne, M. A., *et al* (1990) Cortisol hypersecretion predicts early depressive relapse after recovery with electroconvulsive therapy. *Biological Psychiatry*, **28**, 1007–1010.

Deakin, J. F. W., Owen, F., Cross, A. J., *et al* (1981) Studies of possible mechanism of action of electroconvulsive therapy: effects of repeated electrically induced seizures on rat brain receptors for monoamines and other neurotransmitters. *Psychopharmacology*, **73**, 345–349.

Department of Health (1999). *Electroconvulsive Therapy: Survey Covering the Period From January 1999 to March 1999, England* (Statistical Bulletin, 1999/22). London: HMSO.

Dinan, T. G. & Barry, S. (1989) A comparison of electroconvulsive therapy with a combined lithium and tricyclic combination among depressed tricyclic nonresponders. *Acta Psychiatrica Scandinavica*, **80**, 97–100.

Douyen, R., Serby, M., Klutchko, B., *et al* (1989) ECT and Parkinson's disease revisited: a 'naturalistic' study. *American Journal of Psychiatry*, **146**, 1451–1455.

Duffett, R. & Lelliott, P. (1998) Auditing electroconvulsive therapy. The third cycle. *British Journal of Psychiatry*, **172**, 401–405.

Duggan, C. F., Lee, A. S. & Murray, R. A. (1991) Do difference subtypes of hospitalized depressives have different long-term outcomes? *Archives of General Psychiatry*, **48**, 308–312.

Ebmeier, K. P. & Lappin, J. M. (2001) Electromagnetic stimulation in psychiatry. *Advances in Psychiatric Treatment*, **7**, 181–188.

Ende, G., Braus, D. F., Walter, S., *et al* (2000) The hippocampus in patients treated with electroconvulsive therapy. *Archives of General Psychiatry*, **57**, 937–943.

Farah, A. & McCall, W. V. (1993) Electroconvulsive therapy stimulus dosing: a survey of contemporary practices. *Convulsive Therapy*, **9**, 90–94.

Florkowski, C. M., Crozier, I. G., Nightingale, S., *et al* (1996) Plasma cortisol, PRL, ACTH, AVP and corticotrophin releasing hormone responses to direct current cardioversion and electroconvulsive therapy. *Clinical Endocrinology*, **44**, 163–168.

Freeman, C. (1999) Anaesthesia for electroconvulsive therapy. Statement from the Royal College of Psychiatrists Special Committee for Electroconvulsive Therapy. *Psychiatric Bulletin*, **23**, 740–741.

Freeman, C., Basson, J. V. & Crighton, A. (1978) Double-blind controlled trial of electroconvulsive therapy (ECT) and simulated ECT in depressive illness. *Lancet*, i, 738–740.

Frith, C. D., Stevens, M., Johnstone, E. C., *et al* (1983) Effects of ECT and depression on various aspects of memory. *British Journal of Psychiatry*, **142**, 610–617.

Gangadhar, B. N., Girish, K., Janakiramiah, N., *et al* (1998) Formula method for stimulus setting in bilateral electroconvulsive therapy: relevance of age. *Journal of ECT*, **14**, 259–265.

Geretsegger, C., Rochowanski, E., Kartnig, C., *et al* (1998) Propofol and methohexital as anaesthetic agents for electroconvulsive therapy (ECT): a comparison of seizure-quality measures and vital signs. *Journal of ECT*, **14**, 28–35.

Girish, K., Mayur, P. M., Saravanan, E. S. M., *et al* (2000) Seizure threshold estimation by formula method: a prospective study in unilateral ECT. *Journal of ECT*, **16**, 258–262.

Glue, P., Costello, M. J., Pert, A., *et al* (1990) Regional neurotransmitter responses after acute and chronic electroconvulsive shock. *Psychopharmacology*, **100**, 60–65.

Grahame-Smith, D. G., Green, A. R. & Costain, D. W. (1978) Mechanism of the antidepressant action of elctroconvulsive therapy. *Lancet, i,* 254–256.

Green, A. R. & Vincent, N. D. (1987) The effects of repeated electroconvulsive shock on GABA synthesis and release in regions of rat brain. *British Journal of Pharmacology,* **92,** 19–24.

Green, A. R., Heal, D. J. & Grahame-Smith, D. G. (1977) Further observations on the effects of repeated electroconvulsive shock on the behavioural responses of rats produced by increases in the functional activity of brain 5-hydroxytryptamine and dopamine. *Psychopharmacology,* **52,** 195–200.

Greenberg, L. B., Mofson, R. & Fink, M. (1988) Prospective electroconvulsive therapy in a delusional depressed patient with a frontal meningioma. A case report. *British Journal of Psychiatry,* **153,** 105–107.

Greenblatt, M., Grosser, G. H. & Wechsler, H. (1964) Differential response of hospitalized depressed patients to somatic therapy. *American Journal of Psychiatry,* **120,** 935–943.

Gregory, S., Shawcross, C. R. & Gill, D. (1985) The Nottingham ECT study. A double-blind comparison of bilateral, unilateral and simulated ECT in depressive illness. *British Journal of Psychiatry,* **146,** 520–524.

Heikman, P., Tuunainen, A. & Kuoppasalmi, K. (2000) Value of the initial stimulus dose in right unilateral and bifrontal electroconvulsive therapy. *Psychological Medicine,* **29,** 1417–1423.

Heshe, J. & Roeder, E. (1976) Electroconvulsive therapy in Denmark. *British Journal of Psychiatry,* **128,** 241–245.

Janakiramaiah, N., Channabasavanna, S. M. & Narasimha Murthy, N. S. (1982) ECT/chlorpromazine combination versus chlorpromazine alone in acutely schizophrenic patients. *Acta Psychiatrica Scandinavica,* **66,** 464–470.

Johnstone, E. C., Deakin, J. F. W., Lawler, P., et al (1980) The Northwick Park electroconvulsive therapy trial. *Lancet, ii,* 1317–1320.

Katona, C. L. E., Aldridge, C. R., Roth, M., et al (1987) The dexamethasone suppression test and prediction of outcome in patients receiving ECT. *British Journal of Psychiatry,* **150,** 315–318.

Kelly, C. B. & Cooper, S. J. (1997) Plasma noradrenaline response to electroconvulsive therapy in depressive illness. *British Journal of Psychiatry,* **171,** 182–186.

Kelly, C. B. & Cooper, S. J. (1998) Differences and variability in plasma noradrenaline between depressive and anxiety disorders. *Journal of Psychopharmacology,* **12,** 161–167.

Krystal, A. D. & Weiner, R. D. (1999) EEG correlates of the response to ECT: a possible antidepressant role of brain-derived neurotrophic factor. *Journal of ECT,* **15,** 27–38.

Laidlaw, J., Bentham, P., Khan, G., et al (2000) A comparison of stimulus dosing methods for electroconvulsive therapy. *Psychiatric Bulletin,* **24,** 184–187.

Lake, C. R., Pickar, D., Ziegler, M. G., et al (1982) High plasma norepinephine levels in patients with major affective disorder. *American Journal of Psychiatry,* **139,** 1315–1318.

Lambourn, J. & Gill, D. (1978) A controlled comparison of simulated and real ECT. *British Journal of Psychiatry,* **133,** 514–519.

Langsley, D. G., Enterline, J. D. & Hickerson, G. X. (1959) A comparison of chlorpromazine and EST in treatment of acute schizophrenic and manic reactions. *Archives of Neurology and Psychiatry,* **81,** 384–391.

Lerer, B., Jabotinsky-Rubin, K., Bannet, J., et al (1982) Electroconvulsive shock prevents dopamine receptor supersensitivity. *European Journal of Pharmacology,* **80,** 131–134.

Linnoila, M., Karoum, F., Rosennthal, N., et al (1983) Electro-convulsive treatment and lithium carbonate. Their effects on norepinephine metabolism in patients with primary major depression. *Archives of General Psychiatry,* **40,** 677–680.

Mann, J. J., Mahler, J. C., Wilner, P. J., et al (1990) Normalization of blunted lymphocyte β-adrenergic responsivity in melancholic inpatients by a course of electroconvulsive therapy. *Archives of General Psychiatry,* **47,** 461–466.

Marangell, L. B., George, M. S., Callahan, A. M., *et al* (1997) Effects of intrathecal thyroptopin-releasing hormone (Protirelin) in refractory depressed patients. *Archives of General Psychiatry*, **54**, 214–222.

Martin, B. A., Cooper S. M. & Parikh, S. V. (1998) Propofol anaesthesia, seizure duration and ECT: a case report and literature review. *Journal of ECT*, **14**, 99–108.

May, P. R. A. & Tuma, A. H. (1965) Treatment of schizophrenia. An experimental study of five treatment methods. *British Journal of Psychiatry*, **111**, 503–510.

Mayur, P. M., Subbakrishna, D. K., Gangadhar, B. N., *et al* (1998) Predicting seizure threshold at first ECT: a discriminant analysis study. *Nimhans Journal*, **16**, 193–196.

McCabe, M. S. (1976) ECT in the treatment of mania: a controlled study. *American Journal of Psychiatry*, **133**, 688–691.

McCall, W. W., Reboussin, D. M., Weiner, R. D., *et al* (2000) Titrated moderately suprathreshold vs fixed high-dose right unilateral electroconvulsive therapy – acute antidepressant and cognitive effects. *Archives of General Psychiatry*, **57**, 438–444.

McNamara, B., Ray, J. L., Arthurs, O. J., *et al* (2001) Transcranial magnetic stimulation for depression and other psychiatric disorders. *Psychological Medicine*, **31**, 1141–1146.

Medical Research Council (1965) Clinical trial of the treatment of depressive illness. *BMJ*, i, 881–886.

Mendels, J. (1965) Electroconvulsive therapy and depression. I The prognostic significance of clinical factors. *British Journal of Psychiatry*, **111**, 675–681.

Miller, D. H., Clancy, J. & Cumming, E. (1953) A comparison between unidirectional current nonconvulsive electrical stimulation given with Reiter's machine, standard alternation current electroshock (Cerletti method), and pentothal in chronic schizophrenia. *American Journal of Psychiatry*, **109**, 617–621.

Nemeroff, C. B., Bissette, G., Akil, H., *et al* (1991) Neuropeptide concentrations in the cerebrospinal fluid of depressed patients treated with electroconvulsive therapy. Corticotrophin- releasing factor, beta-endorphin and somatostatin. *British Journal of Psychiatry*, **158**, 59–63.

Ottosson, J. O. (1960) Experimental studies of the mode action of electroconvulsive therapy. *Acta Psychiatrica Neurologica Scandinavica*, **145**, 69–97.

Pacella, B. L. & Barrera, S. E. (1943) Follow-up study of a series of patients treated by electrically induced convulsions and by metrazol convulsions. *American Journal of Psychiatry*, **99**, 513–518.

Peroutka, S. J. (1995) 5-HT receptors: past, present and future. *Trends in Neurosciences*, **18**, 68–69.

Pippard, J. & Ellam, L. (1981) Electroconvulsive treatment in Great Britain. *British Journal of Psychiatry*, **139**, 563–568.

Plein, H. & Berk, M. (2000) Changes in the platelet intracellular calcium response to serotonin in patients with major depression treated with electroconvulsive therapy: state or trait marker status. *International Clinical Psychopharmacology*, **15**, 93–98.

Royal College of Psychiatrists (1995) *The ECT Handbook (Second Report of the Royal College of Psychiatrists Special Committee on ECT)* (Council Report CR59). London: Royal College of Psychiatrists.

Sackeim, H. A. (1999) The anticonvulsant hypothesis of the mechanisms of action of ECT: current status. *Journal of ECT*, **15**, 5–26.

Sackeim, H. A., Decina, P., Prohovnik, I., *et al* (1986) Dosage, seizure threshold and the antidepressant efficacy of electroconvulsive therapy. *Annals of the New York Academy of Sciences*, **462**, 398–410.

Sackeim, H. A., Decina, P., Portroy, S., *et al* (1987*a*) Studies of seizure dosage, seizure threshold and seizure duration. *Biological Psychiatry*, **22**, 249–268.

Sackeim, H. A., Decina, P., Prohovnik, I., *et al* (1987*b*) Seizure threshold in electroconvulsive therapy. *Archives of General Psychiatry*, **44**, 355–359.

Sackeim, H. A., Decina, P., Kanzler, M., *et al* (1987*c*) Effects of electrode placement on the efficacy of titrated low-dose ECT. *American Journal of Psychiatry*, **144**, 1449–1455.

313

Sackeim, H. A., Luber, B., Moeller, J. R., *et al* (2000*a*) Electrophysiological correlates of the adverse cognitive effects of electroconvulsive therapy. *Journal of ECT*, **16**, 110–120.

Sackeim, H. A., Prudic, J., Devanand, D. P., *et al* (2000*b*) A prospective, randomized, double-blind comparison of bilateral and right unilateral electroconvulsive therapy at different stimulus intensities. *Archives of General Psychiatry*, **57**, 425–434.

Salzman, C. (1980) The use of ECT in the treatment of schizophrenia. *American Journal of Psychiatry*, **137**, 1032–1041.

Scott, A. I. F., Shering, P. A., Legros, J. J., *et al* (1991) Improvement in depressive illness is not associated with altered release of neurophysins over a course of ECT. *Psychiatry Research*, **36**, 65–73.

Sermet, E., Gregoire, M., Galy, G., *et al* (1998) Paradoxical metabolic response of the human brain to a single electroconvulsive shock. *Neuroscience Letters*, **254**, 41–44.

Shapira, B., Lerer, B., Gilboa, D., *et al* (1987) Facilitation of ECT by caffeine pretreatment. *American Journal of Psychiatry*, **144**, 1199–1202.

Shapira, B., Lerer, B., Kindler, S., *et al* (1992) Enhanced serotonergic responsivity following electroconvulsive therapy in patients with major depression. *British Journal of Psychiatry*, **160**, 223–229.

Shapira, B., Tubi, N., Drexler, H., *et al* (1998) Cost and benefit in the choice of ECT schedule. Twice versus three times weekly ECT. *British Journal of Psychiatry*, **172**, 44–48.

Slade, A. P. & Checkley, S. A. (1980) A neuroendocrine study of the mechanism of action of ECT. *British Journal of Psychiatry*, **137**, 217–221.

Slater, E. T. O. (1951) Evaluation of electric convulsive therapy as compared with conservative methods of treatment in depressive states. *Journal of Mental Science*, **97**, 567–569.

Small, J. G., Klapper, M. H., Kellams, J. J., *et al* (1988) Electroconvulsive treatment compared with lithium in the management of manic states. *Archives of General Psychiatry*, **45**, 727–732.

Smith, J., Williams, K., Birkett, S., *et al* (1994) Neuroendocrine and clinical effects of electroconvulsive therapy and their relationship to treatment outcome. *Psychological Medicine*, **24**, 547–555.

Smith, K., Surphlis, W. R. P., Gynther, M. D., *et al* (1967) ECT–chlorpromazine and chlorpromazine compared in the treatment of schizophrenia. *Journal of Nervous and Mental Disease*, **144**, 284–290.

Smith, M. A., Zhang, L., Ernest Lyons, W., *et al* (1997) Anterograde transport of endogenous brain derived neurotrophic factor in hippocampal mossy fibres. *Neuroreport*, **8**, 1829–1834.

Spicknall, K., Lisanby, S. H. & Sackeim, H. A. (2000) Determinants of seizure threshold in ECT: benzodiazepine use, anaesthetic dosage and other factors. *Journal of ECT*, **16**, 3–18.

Stain-Malmgren, R., Tham, A. & Aberg-Wistedt, A. (1998) Increased platelet 5-HT$_2$ receptor binding after electroconvulsive therapy in depression. *Journal of ECT*, **14**, 5–24.

Taylor, P. & Fleminger, J. J. (1980) ECT for schizophrenia. *Lancet*, *i*, 1380–1383.

Thomas, J. & Reddy, B. (1982) The treatment of mania: a restrospective evaluation of the effects of ECT, chlorpromazine and lithium. *Journal of Affective Disorders*, **4**, 85–92.

Trezise, K. (1998) Changes in practice of ECT: a follow-on study. *Psychiatric Bulletin*, **22**, 687–690.

Wechsler, H., Grosser, G. H. & Greenblatt, M. (1965) Research evaluating antidepressant medications on hospitalized mental patients: a survery of published reports during a five-year period. *Journal of Nervous Mental Disease*, **141**, 231–239.

Weeks, D., Freeman, C. P. L. & Kendell, R. E. (1980) ECT: III. Enduring cognitive deficits? *British Journal of Psychiatry*, **137**, 26–37.

West, E. D. (1981) Electric convulsion therapy in depression: a double-blind controlled trial. *BMJ*, **282**, 355–357.

Whalley, L. J., Duk, H., Watts, A. G., *et al* (1982) Immediate increases in plasma prolactin and neurophysin but not other hormones after electroconvulsive therapy. *Lancet*, *ii*, 1064–1068.

Further reading

Ebmeier, K. P. & Lappin, J. M. (2001) Electromagnetic stimulation in psychiatry. *Advances in Psychiatric Treatment*, **7**, 181–188.

Fink, M. (1984) Meduna and the origins of convulsive therapy. *American Journal of Psychiatry*, **141**, 1034–1041.

Gleiter, C. H. & Nutt, D. J. (1989) Chronic electroconvulsive shock and neurotransmitter receptors – an update. *Life Sciences*, **44**, 985–1006.

Kendell, R. E. (1981) The present status of electoconvulsive therapy. *British Journal of Psychiatry*, **139**, 265–283.

Royal College of Psychiatrists (1989) *The Practical Administration of Electroconvulsive Therapy (ECT)*. London: Royal College of Psychiatrists.

Sackeim, H. A., Devanand, D. P. & Prudic, J. (1991) Stimulus intensity, seizure threshold, and seizure duration: impact on the efficacy and safety of electroconvulsive therapy. *Psychiatric Clinics of North America*, **14**, 803–941.

CHAPTER 9

Antipsychotic drugs and the treatment of schizophrenia

David J. King and John L. Waddington

Receptor pharmacology: cellular and *in vivo* bases of antipsychotic drug action

Contemporary insights

We have witnessed over the past several years a greater rate of advance in understanding the cellular basis of antipsychotic drug action than occurred over the preceding several decades. This reflects the emergence of deeper insights into brain function furnished by new investigatory tools, including neuroimaging techniques for the direct examination of drug action in living subjects, and the introduction of a still expanding armamentarium of new antipsychotic agents whose actions can be better probed using such technology; this chapter elaborates on recent reviews on these issues (Waddington & Casey, 2000; Waddington *et al*, 2003).

It must be noted that the concept that still underpins much contemporary theorising, namely the dopamine (DA) receptor blockade hypothesis, is now some 40 years old; yet it has been recognised recently as so fundamental an advance as to result in its originator, Arvid Carlsson (Carlsson & Lindqvist, 1963), sharing the 2000 Nobel Prize for Physiology or Medicine. The only cellular property common to *all* known antipsychotic drugs evidencing clinical efficacy in appropriately controlled clinical trials is at least some competitive antagonism of brain DA receptors. Furthermore, recent neuroimaging findings which indicate increased subcortical release of DA in schizophrenia, at least during phases of exacerbation of psychosis (Laruelle & Abi-Dargham, 1999; Abi-Dargham *et al*, 2000), now give this notion pathophysiological relevance.

Origins of the D_2 dopamine receptor blockade hypothesis

Dopamine receptor dichotomy

The relationship of this property to therapeutic efficacy in schizophrenia received strong though indirect support from data that indicated that the *in vitro* affinities of a wide range of antipsychotic drugs for brain DA antagonist binding sites correlate highly with their clinical potencies to control psychotic symptoms (Seeman, 1980). Demonstration that the antipsychotic activity of flupenthixol resides in its α (i.e. *cis*(Z) and DA receptor-blocking) rather than its β (i.e. *trans*(E) and non-DA receptor-blocking) geometric isomer (Johnstone *et al*, 1978) was especially important in this regard.

Conceptually, these now classic notions endure, but have required material modification in their detail as our knowledge base in the neurosciences has expanded. In particular, concepts of DA receptor typology and function have undergone substantial revision. Specifically, it was recognised subsequently that DA receptors exist as two major subtypes, D_1 and D_2 (Kebabian & Calne, 1979). Re-evaluation of the above relationship in terms of this D_1/D_2 schema showed the antipsychotic potencies of antipsychotics to be correlated highly with their affinities for D_2 but not for D_1 receptors. This relationship held not just for rat striatum but also for post-mortem human putamen and, importantly, no differences were apparent between the affinities of such drugs for D_2 receptors in the caudate or putamen (the mesostriatal dopaminergic system, presumed to mediate extrapyramidal side-effects) versus the nucleus accumbens (the mesocorticolimbic system, presumed to mediate antipsychotic efficacy) of human post-mortem brain (Seeman, 1980; Reynolds *et al*, 1982; Seeman & Ulpian, 1983; Richelson & Nelson, 1984; see also Waddington, 1993; Lidsky, 1995). Similarly, selective or preferential D_2 antagonists, such as, respectively, the substituted benzamide sulpiride or the butyrophenone haloperidol, appeared to mimic the essential clinical activity of non-selective antipsychotics, such as the phenothiazines (e.g. fluphenazine) and thioxanthenes (e.g. flupenthixol), which block both D_1 and D_2 receptors (Ehmann *et al*, 1987). On this basis, the primary, even exclusive role in mediating antipsychotic activity was ascribed (Seeman, 1980) to D_2 receptor blockade.

Current concepts of dopamine receptor multiplicity

Gene cloning techniques have indicated that the number of DA receptor subtypes is larger than had been envisaged originally. Until very recently, theory has encompassed six DA receptor protein sequences which, on the basis of structural and pharmacological characteristics, are best subsumed under the umbrella of two *families* of D_1-like (D_1 and D_5) and D_2-like ($D_{2long/short}$, D_3 and D_4) receptors (Waddington, 1993; Missale *et al*, 1998). Within the D_1-like family, the D_1 receptor evidences a general mesostriatal–corticolimbic localisation, whereas its D_5 counterpart evidences primarily a characteristic low-density localisation within particular corticolimbic regions (Waddington *et al*, 1998; Niznik *et al*, 2002). Conversely, within the D_2-like family, the D_2 receptor, having a general mesostriatal–limbic localisation, exists in both 'long' and 'short' isoforms, generated by alternative splicing, and whose functional distinctions are only now being clarified; low-density localisations within distinct corticolimbic regions (Levant, 1997; Tarazi & Baldessarini, 1999) characterise D_3 and D_4 receptors.

Thus, previous studies of the correlation between clinical antipsychotic potencies and affinities for the 'D_2' receptor actually reflect generic affinities for all members of the D_2-like family, because of the inability of the ligands used to distinguish between them. However, subsequent studies using cloned cell lines have indicated that both clinical antipsychotic potencies and the free concentrations of antipsychotics in patient plasma correlate generally with their affinities for the D_2 receptor when expressed independently of its D_3 and D_4 siblings (Seeman, 1992; Waddington, 1993). It has been argued recently that this prepotent binding to D_2 receptors varies also along a dimension additional to conventional affinity, namely 'tightness' relative to that of DA (Seeman & Tallerico, 1998); thus, despite comparable extents of occupancy of the D_2 receptors, those antipsychotics binding more tightly to them may be more likely to induce extrapyramidal symptoms (EPS), while those binding less tightly may be less likely to do so.

Variants of the D_2 receptor blockade hypothesis

Therapeutic potential of selective D_3 antagonists

Much interest in the D_3 receptor as a potentially novel therapeutic target for antipsychotic activity (Sokoloff *et al*, 1992) derives from its high affinity for most antipsychotics and predominantly 'peristriatal' limbic localisation. However, no known antipsychotic shows more than a modest preference for D_3 over D_2 receptors, and clinical antipsychotic potencies appear to correlate less strongly with affinities for the D_3 than for the D_2 receptor (Seeman, 1992; Waddington, 1993). Additionally, it has proved difficult to identify specific functional roles for the D_3 receptor in the absence of antagonists that show material selectivity over its D_2 and D_4 counterparts (Levant, 1997). Furthermore, the most recent preclinical studies with new selective D_3 antagonists (e.g. S33084; Millan *et al*, 2000) do not indicate them to be active in at least traditional models of antipsychotic activity in the manner of D_2 antagonists (selective or non-selective). Only controlled clinical trials with selective D_3 antagonists will ultimately clarify this long-standing conundrum.

Therapeutic potential of selective D_4 antagonists

On the basis of its high affinity for many antipsychotics and its predominantly corticolimbic localisation (Van Tol *et al*, 1991; Tarazi & Baldessarini, 1999), the D_4 receptor has been offered also as a potential novel therapeutic target. However, no known antipsychotics show more than a modest preference for D_4 over D_2 receptors, and clinical antipsychotic potencies appear to correlate less strongly with affinities for the D_4 than for the D_2 receptor (Seeman, 1992; Waddington, 1993). The recent availability of a wide range of selective D_4 agonists and, particularly, of D_4 antagonists for preclinical studies has not indicated activity in at least traditional models of antipsychotic activity (Tarazi & Baldessarini, 1999; Clifford & Waddington, 2000); yet clinical trials with selective D_4 antagonists have proceeded.

In schizophrenia, the D_4 antagonist L 745 870 was initially found to be without either antipsychotic activity or EPS (Kramer *et al*, 1997); indeed, it was associated with some worsening of psychotic symptoms relative to placebo. However, subsequent studies have indicated that L 745 870, and some other such compounds, show partial agonist activity at the D_4 receptor (Gazi *et al*, 1999); hence its capacity to reveal any antipsychotic activity of D_4 antagonists may be compromised. In a subsequent study (Truffinet *et al*, 1999), the mixed D_4/D_5-HT_{2A} antagonist fananserin was also found to be without antipsychotic activity; although it was not associated with exacerbation of psychosis, there appeared to be some worsening of akathisia. Despite these cautionary initial observations, some other selective D_4 antagonists (Tarazi & Baldessarini, 1999; Clifford & Waddington, 2000; Hrib, 2000) continue to attract clinical attention.

Therapeutic potential of selective D_1-like antagonists

Such a considerable body of evidence indicating a primary role for D_2 receptor antagonism in antipsychotic drug action engendered some initial surprise when studies with selective D_1-like antagonists indicated them to be active in essentially all traditional functional models held to predict antipsychotic activity (Waddington, 1993); however, this unexpected profile may have a basis in D_1-like–D_2-like interactions, which play a critical role in regulating the totality of dopaminergic neurotransmission (Waddington *et al*, 1994). Although subsequent clinical trials have indicated that the selective D_1-like antagonists SCH 39166 (de Beaurepaire *et al*, 1995; Den Boer *et al*, 1995; Karlsson *et al*, 1995) and NNC 01-0687 (Karle *et al*, 1995) are without antipsychotic activity, these limited trials have been conducted generally with small numbers of patients, with varying degrees of experimental rigour; unexpectedly, two of these (Den Boer *et al*, 1995; Karle *et al*, 1995) have suggested some amelioration of negative symptoms. Also, no known agent is able to distinguish meaningfully between D_1 and D_5 receptors (Sugamori *et al*, 1998).

It should be noted that cortical D_1-like receptor-mediated processes play an important role in regulating aspects of cognitive function that are known to be impaired in schizophrenia, and that antipsychotics down-regulate D_1 and D_5 receptors in the prefrontal cortex of non-human primates, perhaps via cortical D_2 antagonism (Lidow *et al*, 1998); thus, such findings raise the possibilty of cognitive impairment in schizophrenia being a target for D_1-like receptor-mediated intervention.

PET and SPECT assessment of D_2 receptor blockade in living patients

It must be emphasised that, in the main, the above concepts derive from indirect lines of investigation. One of the major advances of the past decade has been the emergence of functional neuroimaging techniques for the direct visualisation and quantification of drug–receptor interactions in living patients, namely positron emission tomography (PET) and single-photon emission computed tomography (SPECT).

Seminal PET studies by Farde *et al* (1992) confirmed *in vivo* D_2 receptor occupancy as a shared characteristic of all first-generation antipsychotics examined to date, but provided additional insights into how such occupancy relates to clinical effects. They have indicated a general threshold of approximately 65–70% occupancy of available D_2 receptors for therapeutic efficacy over a range of first-generation antipsychotics, with risk for EPS increasing with occupancies above approximately 80%; this suggests a modest 'therapeutic window', over which it could be possible to optimise the risk–benefit ratio of such agents. Using PET and SPECT, increasing D_2 receptor occupancy in patients is correlated with increasing parkinsonism (Heinz *et al*, 1998), reduced handwriting area (Kuenstler *et al*, 1999) and higher levels of prolactin (Schlegel *et al*, 1996; Nordstrom & Farde, 1998). Importantly, PET studies indicate also that patients who are refractory to first-generation agents demonstrate comparable occupancy of D_2 receptors, and that explanations for their non-response should be sought in terms other than inadequate D_2 receptor blockade (Wolkin *et al*, 1989; Coppens *et al*, 1991).

Furthermore, PET data have been instrumental in illuminating the widespread use of inappropriately excessive doses of first-generation antipsychotics. Clinical efficacy at a D_2 receptor occupancy approaching 70% or higher, sometimes with EPS, can often be obtained at 4–6 mg haloperidol (Farde *et al*, 1992) and at 1–5 mg haloperidol in first-episode cases (Kapur *et al*, 2000a); occupancy of D_2 receptors increases in a hyperbolic manner over plasma concentrations of 0.2–2.0 ng/ml haloperidol in patients receiving 1–2.5 mg daily, with an ED_{50} (concentration/dose required for 50% occupancy of available receptors) of 0.4 ng/ml, or 0.7 mg/day (Fitzgerald *et al*, 2000).

This approach has also illuminated aspects of the clinical pharmacology of depot antipsychotics. Thus, regular injection even of a low dose of haloperidol decanoate (30–50 mg/4 weeks) followed by discontinuation is associated with high levels of D_2 occupancy (66–82%) 1 week after injection, falling slowly and persisting (23–34%) 6 months thereafter; thus, commonly used doses of up to 200 mg/4 weeks may be excessive, and likely protect against relapse and influence clinical state and biological measures for prolonged periods after discontinuation (Nyberg *et al*, 1997). Even following discontinuation from regular oral administration at 1.5–15 mg daily, haloperidol can be detected in human brain tissue by high-performance liquid chromatography (HPLC) at concentrations 10–30-fold higher than optimal serum concentrations, with an elimination half-life of 6.8 days (Kornhuber *et al*, 1999).

Although essentially all of the above studies concern striatal D_2 receptors, which are likely mediators of EPS, there is an appreciable body of evidence for the involvement of mesocorticolimbic dopaminergic systems in antipsychotic activity (see 'Dopamine receptor dichotomy', above). Initially, it was not possible to measure receptor occupancies in regions of low receptor density, but advances in PET and SPECT techniques now allow such estimates to be made; a variety of first-generation antipsychotics exert comparable D_2 receptor occupancies in the temporal cortex and thalamus (Farde *et al*, 1997; Bigliani *et al*, 1999).

Actions of first-generation antipsychotics at non-dopaminergic receptors

It is now well established that the shared D_2 antagonist activity of first-generation antipsychotics is manifested on a variable background of affinity for other, non-dopaminergic receptors and additional neuronal processes. Only sulpiride and amisulpride can be said to approach 'selective' affinity for D_2-like ($D_{2/3}$) receptors; haloperidol acts only preferentially thereat, while most phenothiazines and thioxanthenes evidence a yet broader portfolio of receptor affinities, with anti-adrenergic ($\alpha_{1/2}$), antiserotonergic (5-HT_{2A}), antimuscarinic ($M_{1/2}$) and antihistamine (H_1) actions being the most common (Leysen, 2000).

Among these actions, 5-HT_{2A} antagonism has been interpreted as contributing to clinical utility via attenuation of EPS liability and enhancement of antipsychotic efficacy, most controversially in the domain of negative symptoms (Kapur & Remington, 1996; Meltzer, 1999). However, the majority of these actions have been equated with well-recognised side-effect liabilities: $\alpha_{1/2}$ antagonism – cardiovascular effects such as hypotension; H_1 antagonism – sedation; $M_{1/2}$ antagonism is interpreted classically as a 'two-edged sword' which reduces inherent EPS liability but at a cost of increased risk for autonomic side-effects (Kane & Lieberman, 1992).

Indirect examination of these non-dopaminergic actions in relation to clinically manifest side-effects, through correlational analyses similar to those applied to the issue of D_2 affinity versus clinical antipsychotic potency, offers partial support for such notions (Sekine *et al*, 1999). However, unexpected findings have also emerged; thus, the propensity of a wide range of antipsychotics to induce acute dystonic reactions appears correlated also with their affinity for sigma (σ_1 and σ_2) sites (Matsumoto & Pouw, 2000). However, direct examination via PET and SPECT is in its infancy, owing to a paucity of selective ligands and problems relating to the examination of multiple receptors in the same individual. Nevertheless, it should be noted that:

(1) 600 mg chlorpromazine appears to exert almost complete occupancy of cortical 5-HT_{2A} as well as striatal D_2 receptors (Trichard *et al*, 1998)

(2) 100–250 mg/week fluphenazine decanoate, albeit a higher dose than is currently recommended, occupies 89–97% of D_2 receptors and 76–100% of 5-HT_{2A} receptors (Nyberg *et al*, 1998).

Significance of clozapine as the progenitor second-generation antipsychotic

The enigma of the antipsychotic action of clozapine

Clozapine has, over the past decade, materially influenced our perspectives on antipsychotic drug action (Waddington *et al*, 1997). Recent meta-analysis has sustained the superior clinical efficacy and EPS profile of clozapine, although the extent to which this might relate particularly to negative symptoms, manifestation of the deficit syndrome and cognitive impairment, or refractoriness *per se*, and might be reflected in levels of functioning, may have been somewhat overestimated (Keefe *et al*, 1999; Rosenheck *et al*, 1999; Simpson *et al*, 1999; Wahlbeck *et al*, 1999). Its agranulocytosis liability and mandatory blood-count monitoring programme, together with its liability to induce seizures, sedation, hypotension, hypersalivation and weight gain, mean that this important agent is unlikely to attain widespread use as a 'front-line' antipsychotic, although it still appears to be underused for patients who are unresponsive to or intolerant of other agents (Waddington *et al*, 1997; Kane, 1999). Uniquely, however, it indicates that our clinical expectations for new antipsychotics can be heightened (Waddington & O'Callaghan, 1997) and suggests that our pharmacological efforts be directed towards identifying the basis of its advantageous therapeutic profile and resolving the mechanisms of its numerous non-motoric side-effect liabilities so that more utilitarian agents might be identified.

However, clozapine demonstrates an extensive range of actions at multiple levels of neuronal function associated with numerous neuro-transmitter systems (Ashby & Wang, 1996; Waddington *et al*, 1997; Leysen, 2000; Waddington & Casey, 2000). Indeed, in seriously confounding any such goal, the breadth of these actions means that clozapine can be considered either as a rich reservoir for theorising on, or, alternatively, extremely muddy waters in which to fish for, the substrate of a new generation of improved antipsychotic agents.

Dopamine receptor subtypes in relation to clozapine

In the face of modest affinity both for D_2-like ($D_4 > D_2 \approx D_3$) and for D_1-like ($D_1 \approx D_5$) receptors, particular attention has focused on a purported selectivity of clozapine for the D_4 receptor (Van Tol et al, 1991; Seeman, 1992; Leysen, 2000), which might be better described as a limited preference of uncertain functional significance (Waddington et al, 1997; Tarazi & Baldessarini, 1999; Waddington & Casey, 2000). The putative importance of its D_4 antagonist affinity (Seeman, 1992) has recently been downplayed by a major proponent in favour of mechanisms based on the nature of its actions at the D_2 receptor (Seeman & Tallerico, 1998).

More specifically, it has been argued that clozapine has a high dissociation constant with (i.e. binds loosely to and loosely occupies) the D_2 receptor relative to 'tight'-binding first-generation antipsychotics. On this basis, the relationship between affinity for the D_2 receptor and clinical antipsychotic potency appears sustained, in a manner that resolves for clozapine a previously described deviation from this relationship (Seeman et al, 1997; Seeman & Tallerico, 1998); indeed, essentially 'all' aspects of antipsychotic efficacy and EPS liability for clozapine are purported to be explicable in terms of such D_2 receptor-mediated effects (Seeman & Tallerico, 1999).

Non-dopaminergic receptors in relation to clozapine

In vitro, this dibenzodiazepine has a broad and considerably higher antagonist affinity for non-DA than for DA receptor subtypes, particularly α ($\alpha_1 > \alpha_2$), H_1, M ($M_1 > M_2$) and 5-HT (5-HT$_{2A}$ > 5-HT$_{1A[partial\ agonist]}$), together with actions at other levels of synaptic transmission (Waddington et al, 1997; Leysen, 2000). These diverse non-dopaminergic effects of clozapine have engendered many alternative formulations for its clinical profile in terms of antipsychotic efficacy with propensity for numerous adverse effects other than EPS.

A combination of high 5-HT$_{2A}$ with D_2-like antagonism has long been posited to underpin the clinical advantages not only of clozapine but also of other second-generation antipsychotics (Meltzer et al, 1989). This could derive from enhanced release of DA to mitigate EPS due to D_2 blockade in the basal ganglia, and to ameliorate negative symptoms and cognitive dysfunction due to putative dopaminergic deficits in the prefrontal cortex (Meltzer, 1999; but see Carpenter et al, 2000); indeed clozapine, but not haloperidol, has been shown preferentially to augment DA release in the prefrontal cortex relative to the caudate of non-human primates (Youngren et al, 1999). Although this proposition has proved influential and heuristic, some anomalies are evident: the second-generation agent amisulpride is essentially devoid of 5-HT_{2A} antagonism, while the first-generation agent chlorpromazine is a potent antagonist of 5-HT_{2A} as well as D_2-like receptors (Trichard et al, 1998); furthermore, preclinical studies examining the effects of 5-HT_{2A} antagonism on antipsychotic-induced catalepsy are not in overall accordance with such a model (Wadenberg, 1996; Seeman et al, 1997).

One variant posits 5-HT_{1A} partial agonism with D_2-like antagonism (Newman-Tancredi et al, 1996); this may contribute not only to mitigation of EPS (Wadenberg, 1996) but also to enhancement of prefrontal DA release and putative therapeutic effects (Rollema et al, 1997; Prinssen et al, 1999). Another variant posits α_2 antagonism (Blake et al, 1998; Leysen, 2000) also to augment prefrontal DA release and D_2-like antagonist-induced suppression of conditioned avoidance responding, a traditional model of antipsychotic activity (Hertel et al, 1999); indeed, the clinical efficacy of the first-generation antipsychotic fluphenazine can be augmented in the direction of clozapine on co-administration of the α_2 antagonist idazoxan (Litman et al, 1996). In addition to D_2-like antagonism, each of these formulations encompasses an action associated putatively with enhancement of DA release in the prefrontal cortex, in accordance with contemporary perspectives on the pathophysiology of schizophrenia (Waddington & Morgan, 2001). It will be important to clarify whether second-generation antipsychotic activity can be mediated by diverse mechanisms rather than by any generic 'class' action.

Among conceptually novel models at a cellular level, expression of the intermediate–early gene c-fos is induced by numerous physiological and pharmacological stimuli, including antipsychotic drugs, in a manner that might reveal neuroanatomical sites and functional pathways of drug action. As do first-generation antipsychotics, clozapine induces c-fos in the shell region of the nucleus accumbens; however, relative to such agents, which particularly induce c-fos in the striatum as a correlate of EPS liability, clozapine and its desmethyl metabolite induce c-fos preferentially in the thalamic paraventricular nucleus and selectively in the prefrontal cortex (Young et al, 1998), brain regions that are congruent with contemporary formulations of fronto–striato–pallido–thalamo–frontal network dysfunction in schizophrenia (Waddington & Morgan, 2001).

Among conceptually novel models at a behavioural level, some derive from increased understanding of the psychology and pathobiology of this disorder (Higgins, 1998; Ellenbroek & Cools, 2000); these allow us to go beyond more traditional models, whereby attenuation both of hyperactivity induced by DA agonists and of conditioned avoidance responding are held to indicate antipsychotic efficacy, while attenuation of stereotypy induced by DA agonists and induction of catalepsy are held to indicate EPS liability (Kinon & Lieberman, 1996; Arnt & Skarsfeldt, 1998). These newer models include prepulse inhibition of acoustic startle (Swerdlow et al, 1998), phencyclidine-induced social withdrawal (Sams-Dodd, 1999) and neonatal ventral hippocampal lesions (Lipska & Weinberger, 2000). To what extent these new models meaningfully reproduce not only positive but also negative and cognitive aspects of psychopathology, and reflect the therapeutic profile of clozapine and other second-generation antipsychotics, remains to be clarified.

PET and SPECT assessment of clozapine in living patients

Given the importance of understanding the bases of the material advantages and liabilities of clozapine, this agent has attracted considerable attention in PET and SPECT studies. In patients with schizophrenia, initial PET studies indicated that clozapine occupies 20–68% of D_2 receptors at conventional clinical doses, a range materially lower than is encountered with typical doses of its first-generation counterparts (Farde et al, 1992; Nordstrom et al, 1995); using SPECT, the range of D_2 receptor occupancy for clozapine appears wider (Pickar et al, 1996; Kasper et al, 1998). The most recent, systematic PET studies appear to establish that, over a dosage range of 150–600 mg, clozapine occupies 28–65% of D_2 receptors, with doses as high as 850–900 mg occupying only 47–68% thereof, without, therefore, exceeding the 70–80% threshold associated with increased liability for EPS (Kapur et al, 1999).

While these characteristics may explain at least in part its low EPS liability, the challenge is to reconcile the notion of an approximate 70% occupancy threshold for antipsychotic activity using first-generation agents with the at least comparable and apparently greater efficacy of clozapine in the absence of attaining such a threshold. Several factors may be operating. First, there is the concept of clozapine as an agent with 'loose' binding to D_2 receptors and which dissociates more rapidly and can be displaced more readily than is the case for first-generation antipsychotics (Seeman & Tallerico, 1999; see 'Dopamine receptor subtypes in relation to clozapine', above). Second, PET studies indicate that doses of clozapine as low as 150 mg give almost complete saturation of cortical $5-HT_{2A}$ receptors, a figure much higher than for striatal D_2 receptors (Nordstrom et al, 1995; Travis et al, 1998; Kapur et al, 1999), in accordance with an influential model for advantages of second-generation antipsychotics (Meltzer, 1999). Third, clozapine has the highest occupancy of striatal D_1 receptors among all clinically effective antipsychotics (Farde et al, 1992; Nordstrom et al, 1995; see 'Therapeutic potential of selective D_1-like antagonists', above). Finally, there is controversial SPECT evidence that clozapine shows considerably greater occupancy of extrastriatal (temporal cortex) than of striatal D_2 receptors (Pilowsky et al, 1997a), although preliminary PET studies (Farde et al, 1997) suggest otherwise. Further systematic PET and SPECT studies comparing clozapine with first- and subsequent second-generation antipsychotics will be necessary to help resolve the conundrum that is clozapine.

'Atypicality' in relation to mechanisms of second-generation antipsychotics

One level of analysis of 'atypicality' is in mechanistic terms. The diverse pharmacological properties of clozapine reviewed above have prompted exploration as to which combination(s) of these might underpin its advantageous and disadvantageous features, and whether any such combination generalises to some or indeed all second-generation antipsychotics (Kinon & Lieberman, 1996; Arnt & Skarsfeldt, 1998; Meltzer, 1999; Remington & Kapur, 2000; Waddington & Casey, 2000). In overall terms, second-generation agents have generally similar properties in traditional animal models which predict antipsychotic efficacy with low EPS liability (i.e. attenuation of hyperactivity induced by DA agonists and of conditioned avoidance responding vis-à-vis induction of catalepsy), although not all have yet been examined in the newer models of putatively greater homology. However, the appellation 'atypical' may mislead as to any unitary pharmacological basis for their superior profiles; rather, as will be reviewed individually below, they appear mechanistically diverse. Their principal characteristics are summarised in Table 9.1.

Currently available second-generation antipsychotics

Amisulpride

In vitro, this substituted benzamide is a low-affinity, selective antagonist of D_2-like receptors ($D_2 = D_3 \gg D_4$) that has little or no affinity for D_1-like or non-dopaminergic receptors (Coukell et al, 1996; Schoemaker et al, 1997; Waddington et al, 1997).

In patients with schizophrenia, PET studies indicate that lower doses of amisulpride (50–100 mg) occupy only 4–26% of basal ganglia D_2-like receptors, while higher doses (200–800 mg) occupy 38–76% thereof (Martinot et al, 1996). More recently, it has been confirmed that such occupancy of D_2-like receptors by 200–1200 mg amisulpride occurs in the absence of cortical 5-HT_{2A} receptor occupancy (Trichard et al, 1998).

On the basis of preclinical studies using conventional models, it has been argued that lower doses of amisulpride preferentially block presynaptic D_2-like autoreceptors to give a relative enhancement of

Table 9.1 Comparative pharmacology of classical and novel (second-generation) antipsychotics

Receptor profile	c-fos[a]			PCP[b]		PET (SPECT)[c]	
	Nac	Str	Fcx	PPI	SI	D_2 (%)	$5\text{-}HT_2$ (%)
Haloperidol Preferential D_2-like antagonist	++	+++	-	-	-	70–90	0
Amisulpride Selective $D_{2/3}$ antagonist	?	?	?	?	?	36–76	0
Clozapine Multiple antagonist	++	-	++	++	++	20–68	84–100
Olanzapine Multiple antagonist	++	+	+	++	++	43–89	90–100
Quetiapine Multiple antagonist	++	-	++	++	-	22–68	48–70
Risperidone $5\text{-}HT_2/D_2/\alpha_1$ antagonist	++	+	-	++	-	59–89	78–100
Sertindole $5\text{-}HT_2/D_2/\alpha_1$ antagonist	?	?	?	?	+	(50–74)	(90+)
Ziprasidone $5\text{-}HT_2/D_2/\alpha_1$ antagonist + $5\text{-}HT_{1A}$ agonist + NA/5-HT reuptake	?	?	?	?	?	77	95
Zotepine Multiple antagonist + NA reuptake	?	?	?	?	?	(57–61)	?

[a] Induction of c-fos in nucleus accumbens (Nac), dorsolateral striatum (Str) and frontal cortex (Fcx): prominent, + + +; moderate, + +; mild, +; absent, -; unknown, ?

[b] Antagonism of phencyclidine (PCP) effects on prepulse inhibition (PPI) and social isolation (SI): findings indicated as for a.

[c] Occupancy (%) of basal ganglia D_2-like receptors and of cortical $5\text{-}HT_2$ receptors in living patients receiving conventional antipsychotic doses, as estimated by positron emission tomography (PET) or single photon emission computed tomography (SPECT).

From Buckley, N. & Waddington, J. L. (eds) (2000) *Schizophrenia and Mood Disorders: The New Drug Therapies in Clinical Practice*, by permission of Elsevier Science Ltd.

dopaminergic function, which may confer clinical effectiveness against 'negative' symptoms, while higher doses antagonise certain postsynaptic DA receptor-mediated functions, perhaps particularly in corticolimbic regions, to exert antipsychotic efficacy (Coukell *et al*, 1996; Perrault *et al*, 1997); however, this remains to be confirmed clinically, and there are few data on the properties of amisulpride in newer, more homologous models (Depoortere *et al*, 1997; Waddington & Casey, 2000).

Olanzapine

In vitro, this thienobenzodiazepine analogue of clozapine is a broad, high-affinity antagonist of the following receptors: $5\text{-HT}_{2A} = H_1 > M = D_2$-like $(D_2 = D_3 = D_4) = \alpha\ (\alpha_1 > \alpha_2) > D_1$-like (Bymaster *et al*, 1996; Schotte *et al*, 1996; Fulton & Goa, 1997; Waddington *et al*, 1997).

In patients with schizophrenia, PET studies indicate that 5–20 mg doses of olanzapine occupy 43–84% of available D_2 receptors, while higher doses (30–60 mg) occupy 82–89% (apparent ED_{50} 3.2 mg) (Nordstrom *et al*, 1998; Kapur *et al*, 1999); using SPECT, D_2 receptor occupancy with 5–40 mg olanzapine was 36–86% (Tauscher *et al*, 1999; Meisenzahl *et al*, 2000). Over a dosage range of 5–60 mg, olanzapine gives almost complete occupancy of cortical 5-HT_{2A} receptors (Travis *et al*, 1997; Kapur *et al*, 1999). When considered in conjunction with data from controlled clinical trials focusing on efficacy and side-effects, there is thus some consensus of opinion that:

(1) EPS under olanzapine are not absent but mild, even at relatively high levels of D_2 occupancy;
(2) this occurs in association with high M receptor occupancy, which may contribute to mitigation of EPS (Raedler *et al*, 1999, 2000).

However, there is preliminary SPECT evidence that higher D_2 occupancy is associated with greater negative subjective experience (de Haan *et al*, 2000). In relation to the controversy as to whether some second-generation antipsychotics show preferential occupancy of extrastriatal DA receptors, there are preliminary SPECT data that olanzapine occupies a higher percentage of extrastriatal than of striatal D_2 receptors (Bigliani *et al*, 2000).

Olanzapine is active in traditional models of antipsychotic activity in a manner that predicts efficacy with low EPS liability; it has been studied in many of the newer models, in which it has many but not all of the properties of clozapine (Waddington & Casey, 2000).

Quetiapine

In vitro, this dibenzothiazepine analogue of clozapine is a broad, low-affinity antagonist of the following receptors: $H_1 > 5\text{-HT}_{2A} = \alpha_{1/2} > D_2$-like $(D_2 = D_3 > D_4) > D_1$-like $= M$ (Schotte *et al*, 1996; Waddington *et al*, 1997; Gunasekara & Spencer, 1998).

In patients with schizophrenia, initial SPECT studies indicated that quetiapine occupies 0–28% of D_2 receptors 12 hours after receiving a dose of 300–700 mg (Kufferle *et al*, 1997), while PET studies indicated 22–68% occupancy of striatal D_2 receptors and 58–82% occupancy of frontocortical 5-HT$_2$ receptors 2 hours after a dose of 450 mg, although these occupancies fell to 6–54% and 24–64%, respectively, after 12–26 hours (Gefvert *et al*, 1998). The most recent PET studies confirmed that quetiapine manifests transient, 'loose' binding to striatal D_2 receptors, in that occupancy fell from 58–64% at 2–3 hours to 0–20% at 12–24 hours following administration of 400–450 mg; at 12–14 hours after 150–600 mg, D_2 occupancy was 0–27%, while frontocortical 5-HT$_2$ occupancy was 19–94% (Kapur *et al*, 2000*b*); thus, in this regard, it shows some of the properties of clozapine.

Quetiapine is active in traditional models of antipsychotic activity in a manner that predicts efficacy with low EPS liability; it has received less extensive study in newer models, in which it has some but not all of the properties of clozapine (Waddington & Casey, 2000).

Risperidone

In vitro, this benzisoxazole is a high-affinity antagonist of 5-HT$_2$ and a high-affinity antagonist of D_2-like ($D_2 > D_3 = D_4$), α ($\alpha_1 > \alpha_2$) and H$_1$ receptors; an active metabolite, 9-OH-risperidone, shares a generally similar profile and appears to contribute to overall pharmacological activity (Schotte *et al*, 1996; Waddington *et al*, 1997).

In patients with schizophrenia, PET studies indicate that 2–12 mg doses of risperidone occupy 63–89% of D_2 receptors (apparent ED_{50} 0.8 mg) and 72–100% of 5-HT$_2$ receptors, with 3 and 6 mg giving D_2/5-HT$_2$ occupancies of 53–78%/65–100% and 79–85%/86–100%, respectively; at these doses, three of seven and six of seven patients experienced EPS (Kapur *et al*, 1999; Nyberg *et al*, 1999). Using SPECT, 2–10 mg risperidone gave 69–99% occupancy of D_2 receptors (Knable *et al*, 1997), with 5 of 12 patients experiencing EPS unrelated to the extent of D_2 occupancy, while 3–16 mg was associated with substantial occupancy of cortical 5-HT$_2$ receptors (Travis *et al*, 1998).

When considered in conjunction with data from controlled clinical trials focusing on efficacy and side-effects, there is thus some consensus of opinion that:

(1) the overall likelihood of EPS with risperidone is reduced relative to first-generation agents
(2) this may be confined to a low dose range, of 2–6 mg, with higher doses giving a profile that approaches that of a first-generation agent
(3) high levels of 5-HT$_2$ receptor occupancy are unable to prevent the emergence of EPS.

As for olanzapine, there are preliminary SPECT data that higher D_2 occupancy is associated with greater negative subjective experience (de Haan et al, 2000).

Risperidone is active in traditional models of antipsychotic activity in a manner that predicts efficacy with low EPS liability; it has received considerable study in newer models, in which it has some but not all of the properties of clozapine (Waddington & Casey, 2000).

Sertindole

In vitro, this indole derivative is a high-affinity antagonist of the following receptors: $5\text{-HT}_{2A} > \alpha_1 > D_2\text{-like}$ $(D_2 = D_3 = D_4)$ (Sanchez et al, 1991; Dunn & Fitton, 1996; Waddington et al, 1997).

In patients with schizophrenia, initial SPECT studies indicated that 20–24 mg doses of sertindole give 'high' occupancy both of basal ganglia D_2-like receptors and of cortical 5-HT_{2A} receptors (Pilowsky et al, 1997b; Travis et al, 1997). More recently, however, quantitative SPECT studies have indicated that 8–24 mg doses of sertindole occupy 47–74% of basal ganglia D_2-like receptors, and suggest that the earlier, higher estimates might have been influenced by prior treatment with depot antipsychotics (Kasper et al, 1998; Bigliani et al, 2000). Sertindole has yet to receive extensive study using PET. In relation to the controversy as to whether some second-generation antipsychotics may show preferential occupancy of extrastriatal DA receptors, there is preliminary SPECT evidence that sertindole occupies a higher percentage of extrastriatal than of striatal D_2 receptors (Bigliani et al, 2000).

Sertindole is active in traditional models of antipsychotic activity in a manner that predicts efficacy with low EPS liability; regarding new preclinical models, it exerts some reversal of phencyclidine-induced social isolation (Sams-Dodd, 1999), but otherwise it has received less extensive evaluation than has clozapine (Waddington & Casey, 2000).

Prolongation of cardiac QTc interval has engendered the greatest controversy in relation to sertindole (Dunn & Fitton, 1996; Zimbroff et al, 1997; Daniel et al, 1998); indeed, after it became available in Europe it was withdrawn from use owing to regulatory concerns over the clinical significance of such prolongation, particularly liability for potentially fatal ventricular arrhythmias (it was not marketed in the USA). Findings suggest that sertindole may be a pseudo-irreversible α_1 antagonist (a competitive antagonist that can, under certain conditions, act like a non-competitive antagonist) (Ipsen et al, 1997) and a high-affinity antagonist of human cardiac potassium HERG channels (Rampe et al, 1998), and that the latter effect in particular may contribute to prolongation of QTc interval; a similar action at HERG channels appears to characterise pimozide (Kang et al, 2000) (on HERG channels and pimozide, see 'Cardiotoxicity', below). However, while sertindole may prolong QTc interval to a somewhat greater extent than other second-generation antipsychotics, such prolongation does occur with several of these agents; indeed, the first-generation antipsychotic thioridazine has a particular liability in this regard, which appears to exceed that of sertindole (Reilly *et al*, 2000).

In another study, prolongation of QTc interval and dispersion during long-term treatment with first-generation antipsychotics, including thioridazine, did not appear to be associated with ventricular tachy-arrhythmias in patients with schizophrenia in the absence of cardiac disease, although these may occur as a rare side-effect of such antipsychotics, particularly if a patient has additional risk factors (Kitayama *et al*, 1999). Furthermore, drug surveillance data, which are inevitably limited owing to its withdrawal, confirm prolongation of QTc interval by sertindole in the absence of clinical or electro-cardiographic evidence of cardiac arrhythmias or of other clinical evidence of cardiac abnormalities (Pezawas *et al*, 2000). Regulatory authorities appear to have become sensitised to these issues, such that some newer compounds have received increased scrutiny, yet sertindole itself has become the subject of regulatory reappraisal in Europe and the challenges that it presents appear to endure.

Ziprasidone

In vitro, this indole derivative is a high-affinity antagonist at the following receptors: $5\text{-HT}_2 > D_2\text{-like }(D_2 = D_3 > D_4) > \alpha\ (\alpha_1 > \alpha_2) > H_1$. It also exhibits 5-HT_{1A} agonism and inhibits the reuptake of nor-adrenaline and serotonin (Davis & Markham, 1997; Waddington *et al*, 1997; Sprouse *et al*, 1999). It is available in intramuscular as well as oral preparations.

There are as yet no systematic PET or SPECT studies of ziprasidone in patients with schizophrenia. However, in normal subjects PET indicates 77% occupancy of striatal D_2 receptors and 98% occupancy of cortical 5-HT_2 receptors with 20–40 mg doses (Bench *et al*, 1996; Fischman *et al*, 1996).

Ziprasidone is active in traditional models of antipsychotic activity in a manner that predicts efficacy with low EPS liability; particular interest focuses on its 5-HT_{1A} agonist and reuptake-inhibiting actions (Sprouse *et al*, 1999); it has received considerably less study in newer models (Waddington & Casey, 2000).

Zotepine

In vitro, this dibenzothiazepine analogue of clozapine is a broad, high-affinity antagonist of the following receptors: $5\text{-HT}_2 = \alpha_1 = H_1 > D_2\text{-like }(D_2 = D_3 = D_4) > D_1\text{-like}$. It also inhibits reuptake of noradrenaline (Waddington *et al*, 1997; Prakash & Lamb, 1998).

In patients with schizophrenia, preliminary SPECT studies indicate D_2 receptor occupancy of 57–61% with 150–200 mg doses of zotepine (Barnas *et al*, 1997); there are as yet no such studies of 5-HT$_2$ or other receptor occupancies, and zotepine has yet to be evaluated systematically using PET.

In traditional preclinical models, the profile of zotepine is one that would predict antipsychotic efficacy with low EPS liability (Needham *et al*, 1996; Prakash & Lamb, 1998); there are few data on this agent in newer preclinical models (Waddington & Casey, 2000).

Perspective and pharmacogenomics?

Although second-generation antipsychotics represent material progress in the treatment of schizophrenia, it is important that their profiles are not over-interpreted. While several recent reviews and meta-analyses have, in general terms, attested their advantages, at least for those agents available for sufficient time to have generated meaningful bodies of data, they also indicate their limitations (Kasper *et al*, 1999; Leucht *et al*, 1999; Wahlbeck *et al*, 1999; Geddes *et al*, 2000); thus, they are perhaps best conceptualised as more an incremental advance rather than any radical shift in therapeutic armamentarium, and this reinforces the need to continue to search for yet more effective and benign treatments.

One approach to this challenge seeks to improve treatment with second-generation antipsychotics through the pharmacogenetic prediction of optimal responsivity to one of several individual agents in the individual patient. This strategy is now generic to all medical specialties, and continues to be a developing area in clinical psychopharmacology in general and antipsychotic therapy in particular (Arranz *et al*, 2000; and see Chapter 2). More likely to generate fundamental therapeutic advances are ongoing attempts to identify new therapeutic targets in terms of increased understanding of the cellular and molecular pathology of schizophrenia, including avenues such as modifiers of gene expression.

Clinical pharmacology

Historical background and classification

Antipsychotic drugs are effective in the treatment of any type of psychomotor excitement or psychosis, whether on the basis of delirium, mania, psychotic depression or schizophrenia. They can be said to have five clinical properties:

(1) non-specific sedation, which comes on within a matter of hours and is beneficial in anxiety and agitation (tolerance to this effect develops over a matter of days)

(2)   tranquillisation, without impairment of consciousness or cognition, also within hours, which is useful for countering excitation and aggression

(3)   an antipsychotic effect, which takes several days or weeks to develop

(4)   an activating effect which French psychiatrists described as 'disinhibiting', 'releasing' or 'unlocking', which refers to the effect on negative schizophrenic symptoms, and which has the same time course as the antipsychotic effect

(5)   the production of extrapyramidal (or Parkinson-like) symptoms (EPS), which can come on within hours or days or over many weeks (tolerance to these effects develops in most patients after about 6 months).

These drugs frequently cause EPS at doses similar to those required for their antipsychotic effect, and the word 'neuroleptic' (literally 'to grasp the neuron') was first introduced to reflect this. It is now known, however, that these two actions are not invariably linked, and EPS are not necessary for an antipsychotic effect.

Chlorpromazine was the first drug of this class to be shown to have antipsychotic properties. After Laborit, the French surgeon, first observed its tranquillising effect, Delay & Deniker were the first to use it in mental disorders, in 1952. They described a 'neuroleptic syndrome' characterised by psychomotor slowing, emotional quieting and affective indifference. The classic description by Lehmann & Hanrahan (1954) of the effect of chlorpromazine in patients with schizophrenia has never been bettered:

'Although a patient under the influence of chlorpromazine at first glance presents the aspect of a heavily drugged person, one is surprised at the absence of clouding of consciousness. The higher psychic functions are preserved to a remarkable degree and the patients are capable of sustained attention, reflection and concentration ... the drug seems to have little effect on those psychological functions which have their representation in the cortex, but appears to affect selectively those subcortical structures that are concerned with maintaining psychomotor drive and wakefulness.'

Chlorpromazine was nicknamed 'Largactil' because of its large number of (biochemical and physiological) actions, which frustrated early attempts to identify the basis for its antipsychotic effect. It is an aliphatic phenothiazine derivative and it was first noted that a halogen or methoxy group in the ring at the C2 position and a side chain of at least three carbon atoms between two nitrogen atoms was required for a phenothiazine to have antipsychotic properties.

Carlsson & Lindqvist (1963) then demonstrated in animal studies that all clinically effective drugs increase the turnover of catecholamine metabolites, including those of dopamine, and they proposed that the antipsychotic effect was related to monoamine, including dopamine, receptor blockade, which results in increased homovanillic acid (HVA) formation by decreasing negative feedback mechanisms. This was subsequently confirmed for all classes of antipsychotics. The resulting dopamine hypothesis for antipsychotic drug action (which continues to be strengthened by recent studies, as discussed above) should not, however, be confused with its derivative, the dopamine hypothesis of schizophrenia, for which the evidence is still tentative.

Traditionally, antipsychotics were classified according to their chemical class (phenothiazine, butyrophenone, dibenzodiazepine, benzisoxazole, etc.) or chemical potency. The former, however, is not clinically useful and the latter can be misleading, since it is so often confused with efficacy. Furthermore, low-potency drugs (e.g. chlor-promazine, thioridazine, clozapine) have been found to be more hazardous, especially in high doses, probably because of their lack of selectivity, than high-potency drugs (e.g. haloperidol, trifluoperazine or risperidone). Since the reintroduction of clozapine in 1990, a second generation of antipsychotics has been developed which have a reduced tendency to cause EPS and which are commonly called 'atypical' for this reason. There has been some debate as to what constitutes atypicality, or more particularly a 'new atypical', since many of the first-generation drugs could have been hailed as atypical when they were developed. These second-generation drugs can all be said to resemble clozapine in one or more respects but none has proved its equal in the treatment of refractory illness. There is also an implication that 'atypicals' are more effective in treating negative symptoms and cognitive deficits, but a novel effect, as distinct from a reduction in adverse effects, has not been established. Thus 'atypicality' has no pharmacological basis and we prefer to use 'first generation' and 'second generation' to distinguish those newer drugs with less propensity for EPS than their conventional predecessors.

Clinical trials

It is now well established that antipsychotics can curtail all the positive symptoms of an acute schizophrenic episode, and will prevent florid exacerbations of schizophrenia in the majority of chronic patients.

From the 1960s, early trials quickly established that the phenothiazine derivatives were superior to the barbiturates in reducing psychotic symptoms in acute schizophrenia. Although modern diagnostic criteria were not used in these trials, an antipsychotic effect was clearly demonstrated. The first large placebo-controlled trial was carried out under the aegis of the National Institute of Mental Health (1964) in a North American multi-centre study. In that study 463 in-patients with acute schizophrenia were randomly allocated to treatment with chlorpromazine, fluphenazine, thioridazine, or placebo. A flexible dose regimen was used, and for chlorpromazine the mean daily dose was 655 mg. After 6 weeks only 344 patients had completed the study – the majority of drop-outs being on placebo. Less than 40% of the placebo patients had improved substantially, whereas none of the drug-treated patients had deteriorated, 5% were unchanged, 20% had improved minimally, and 75% had improved substantially.

Many hundreds of trials have subsequently explored various aspects of acute and maintenance treatment with different categories of patient and with different antipsychotic drugs.

In an early, influential and very comprehensive study of outcome, May *et al* (1976) followed up 228 first-admission patients with schizophrenia for 5 years after they had received one of the following five types of treatment:

(1)   individual psychotherapy alone
(2)   antipsychotic drugs alone
(3)   psychotherapy plus drugs
(4)   electroconvulsive therapy (ECT)
(5)   milieu therapy alone.

A wide range of psychological, family, social and occupational measures were assayed annually for 5 years, from first admission and first discharge. The principal measure, however, was the number of days spent in hospital during follow-up. Successful treatment leading to discharge was much higher following drug treatment or ECT (95% and 96% of the patients receiving drug alone and drug plus psychotherapy, respectively; 79% of those in the ECT group; 65% of those treated with psychotherapy alone; and 58% of the milieu-treated patients). Furthermore, patients originally treated in hospital with psychotherapy alone stayed significantly longer in hospital over follow-up than those who received ECT, drugs alone, or drugs plus psychotherapy. The findings were similar whether or not the length of the index admission was controlled for. Patients treated with milieu therapy alone had the lowest success rate, but those who were successfully discharged did about as well during follow-up as the patients who received ECT or drugs. This was probably due to an excess of cases with a good prognosis in this group (in spite of the matching of the groups on 74 pre-treatment items of prognostic interest) and is a reminder that not all patients with schizophrenia invariably require maintenance treatment.

The efficacy of maintenance treatment in preventing relapse in outpatients was first shown by Leff & Wing (1971) using oral antipsychotic medication and by Hirsch *et al* (1973) with depot drugs. The Leff & Wing (1971) study highlighted several methodological difficulties inherent in trials of such a heterogeneous condition as schizophrenia. They tried to avoid the problem of selection bias by screening all admissions to the Bethlem Royal and Maudsley Hospitals and using the Present State Examination (PSE) as a diagnostic measure. However, of a total of 116 patients who were discharged after recovering from an acute schizophrenic illness, only 35 entered the trial and, of these, five dropped out within the first few months of the study. Principal reasons for exclusion were: that the clinicians in charge of the patients thought that the patient either did not require maintenance treatment or was too vulnerable to risk entering a placebo-controlled study; and patient non-concordance.

The selected patients were then stabilised on chlorpromazine or trifluoperazine for 6–12 weeks before being randomly assigned to chlorpromazine (100–500 mg daily), trifluoperazine (5–25 mg daily) or placebo for 12 months. The principal outcome measure was 'relapse', which was defined as sufficient concern on the part of the supervising clinician to ensure that the patient was on an active drug. At the end of the trial 80% of the placebo patients had relapsed, as opposed to 35% of those on active medication. A 'relapse rate' (on the basis of a return of schizophrenic symptoms) for 77% of the 81 patients who had been excluded from the trial was estimated by reviewing their case notes, and interviewing their general practitioners and relatives. Their relapse rates ranged from 27.3% (among patients deemed not to have required maintenance medication) to 87.5% (among patients who had not been improved by medication during the index admission). Thus, while the efficacy of maintenance medication in preventing relapse was established in the trial patients, it was concluded that such treatment was likely to be of little value in patients either who had a good prognosis or who were severely ill.

Subsequently, Hirsch *et al* (1973) reported similar findings with depot fluphenazine. In this larger study, 112 patients who had been stabilised on depot fluphenazine for 8 weeks were screened, and 81 entered the trial. They were randomly assigned to active drug or placebo injections and followed up for 9 months. Relapse was again defined as deterioration requiring a review of medication or the need to give active drugs. The two groups were shown to be comparable on a number of clinical and social variables. At the end of the trial there had been seven drop-outs, but the analysis was similar whether they were included or not. Of the placebo patients, 66% had relapsed, compared with 8% of the fluphenazine patients. Of the relapsed patients, 74% also had an increase in PSE-rated symptoms. All the non-relapsed patients were continued on active drug for a further 6 months. After a total of 15 months the relapse rate in actively treated patients had increased to 14–17%, which supported previous impressions that medication delays rather than prevents relapse. Relapse prevention continues to be used as a useful indicator of antipsychotic efficacy in the development of new drugs (King *et al*, 1992).

The prototype 'atypical' is clozapine, with its wide range of central receptor antagonism. This drug was first introduced in Europe in 1975, but after 16 patients in Finland were reported to have developed neutropenia, eight of whom subsequently died as a result, the drug was not licensed in the UK. However, a key study by Kane et al (1988) showed that it was clearly superior to chlorpromazine in 'treatment-resistant' patients and in its effects on negative symptoms. In this important double-blind prospective study, 319 patients with schizophrenia who had failed to respond to at least three different antipsychotics (from at least two different chemical classes) over the preceding 5 years were selected from 16 centres in the USA. The criteria of severity were a total score of at least 48 on the US version of the Brief Psychological Rating Scale (BPRS), a clinical global impression (CGI) score of 4 (moderately ill) and a score of at least 4 (moderate) in two of four key BPRS items: conceptual disorganisation, suspiciousness, hallucinatory behaviour, and unusual thought content. If patients met these criteria, they first entered a single-blind trial with haloperidol (mean dose 61 mg/day) for 6 weeks to ascertain treatment resistance. Patients were excluded if after this haloperidol treatment phase they had improved (20% fall in total BPRS score; and either a total BPRS score of 35 or less or a CGI score of 3 or more, indicating at least mildly ill).

Next, 268 patients entered the randomised double-blind comparison of clozapine (up to 900 mg daily) versus chlorpromazine (up to 1800 mg daily) combined with benztropine (6 mg daily) (in order to maintain blindness, since the chlorpromazine but not the clozapine patients would have been expected to have some EPS), for 6 weeks. The principal findings were that 30% of the clozapine patients responded compared with only 4% of the chlorpromazine patients, and there were similar statistically significant differences between the two groups in the improvements in both positive and negative BPRS symptoms.

Clozapine was granted a limited licence in the UK in 1990. It can be prescribed only for treatment-resistant schizophrenia or patients with schizophrenia who are unable to tolerate conventional antipsychotics, and its dispensing is tightly controlled by the Clozaril Patient Monitoring Service (CPMS), which ensures weekly monitoring of white cell counts. The incidence of agranulocytosis is 1–2%, but since the introduction of the CPMS only two patients have died in the UK as a direct result of this. Clozapine is also commonly associated with sedation, tachycardia, sialorrhoea, lowered seizure threshold, cardio-myopathy (rare) and rebound psychoses on abrupt discontinuation. In spite of this, it is still the preferred drug for treatmen-resistant patients or those who are intolerant of other antipsychotics. About a third of treatment-resistant patients respond within 6 weeks of treatment and a further third will respond within a year.

Future questions for clinical trials in schizophrenia

Each generation of psychiatrists has its own particular aspect of schizophrenia to contend with. For example, it is strange for us now to read that one of the main reasons May *et al* (1976) carried out their study was to test the widely held belief that 'patients who had been initially treated with drugs relapsed more rapidly and spent more time in hospital in the end than non-drug-treated patients' and that 'aborting the schizophrenic process with drugs inhibits long-range potential for growth and adjustment at a higher level of social functioning'. Although this is now no longer an issue, a variety of problems remain. These include, for example:

(1)   Which patients require prolonged maintenance treatment?
(2)   How long should it continue?
(3)   What is the optimum dose of such treatment?
(4)   Do antipsychotics help or exacerbate negative symptoms?
(5)   Does early treatment improve response or prevent the development of negative symptoms?
(6)   What is the best treatment for depression in schizophrenia?
(7)   Can it be distinguished from antipsychotic-induced dysphoria?
(8)   Can antipsychotics improve cognitive deficits?
(9)   How can concordance (adherence, concordance) with medication be improved?

The efficacy of antipsychotics in negative symptoms continues to be controversial and depends to a large extent on whether the trials have identified primary enduring negative symptoms (blunted affect, poverty of speech, avolition and anhedonia) and distinguished them from negative features secondary to positive symptoms (in so far as they cause social withdrawal) or drug-induced sedation, depression or EPS (King, 1998). The second-generation drugs have all been shown to be associated with lower 'secondary' negative symptom scores but for only one of these (amisulpride) has convincing evidence of efficacy in relation to primary negative symptoms in a long (6-month) placebo-controlled trial been published (Loo *et al*, 1997).

The cognitive deficits associated with schizophrenia have been shown to be the best predictor of outcome (Wykes *et al*, 1990; Green, 1996). However, the issue of the efficacy of antipsychotics on these symptoms has not been resolved. Early reviews reported little or no impairment of psychometric test performance (Heaton & Crowley, 1981) or psycho-motor performance (Cassens *et al*, 1990), although memory and fine motor coordination were shown to be impaired (Medalia *et al*, 1988) by antipsychotic drug treatment. There appeared to be no consistent relationship between improvement in psychopathology and cognitive function (King, 1990), which seem, therefore, to be relatively independent aspects of schizophrenia. Recent reviews, however, do suggest that the second-generation drugs are associated with improvements in cognition (King & Green, 1996; Mortimer, 1997; Sharma, 1999; Meltzer & McGurk, 1999). As with negative symptoms, however, it is not yet clear whether this is due to a novel effect or to a reduction in an adverse effect.

There is increasing evidence that the use of antipsychotics in the early stages of schizophrenia can improve outcome by preventing or delaying the onset of negative symptoms and/or cognitive deficits. Crow *et al* (1986) first drew attention to the fact that response to treatment is reduced if there is more than a year's delay in starting treatment in first episodes. Meagher *et al* (2001) have also demonstrated such an effect in chronic patients hospitalised before antipsychotic drugs became available. Although such findings may be confounded by the effects of more insidious onset, negative symptoms and the effect of untreated psychosis on psychosocial networks, the importance of early diagnosis and treatment is increasingly recognised (Loebel *et al*, 1992; McGlashan & Johannessen, 1966) and programmes to ensure these have been established in many centres; one example of such a programme is EPPIC (Early Psychosis Prevention and Intervention Centre) (McGorry *et al*, 1996). Issues such as how early psychosis can be established with confidence and the ethics of placebo-controlled trials in such groups remain.

Compliance, or concordance, with treatment continues to be a major problem in schizophrenia, but some groups have been able to demonstrate that psycho-education programmes can be effective in improving this (Kemp *et al*, 1996).

In the future these questions will increasingly be addressed by systematic reviews of trials, a high standard for which has been set by the Cochrane Schizophrenia Group (see Adams *et al*, 1998).

The ethics of placebo-controlled studies in schizophrenia

Since the basic antipsychotic efficacy of antipsychotics has been established, there can be ethical controversies concerning the use of placebo-controlled studies to answer research questions. From the scientific point of view, there is no doubt that placebo-controlled studies continue to be necessary, for the following reasons:

(1) one cannot presume the efficacy of a standard treatment carried out in different patients at a different time and place by different investigators

(2) only a placebo-controlled study can establish efficacy, because if two active drugs are equivalent, this may mean that:

(a) both are effective
(b) both are ineffective
(c) the study does not have the power to distinguish effective from ineffective treatment (a type 2 error – see Chapter 4).

There is also a humanitarian argument in favour of placebo-controlled studies, which is based on the numbers of patients exposed to potentially inactive treatments. When the placebo response rate is high, as in schizophrenia, where it is about 30%, and the total response is low, perhaps 60%, then to show a statistically significant difference from placebo treatment 60 patients are required per treatment group. In a comparative trial involving two active drugs this figure rises to 500 patients per group. Thus, if the new drug is ineffective, four times as many patients will have been given an inactive drug in a comparative trial compared with a placebo-controlled trial (500 versus 120). It is also clearly unethical to subject patients to trials that are inconclusive or which are not capable of producing statistically significant results.

Placebo-controlled trials can be conducted with patients with schizophrenia in an ethical manner if the following principles are borne in mind:

(1) the patients have given written, informed consent (and since detained patients can give valid consent to ECT they should not automatically be excluded from such studies)
(2) potentially suicidal or dangerous patients are excluded
(3) 'rescue' medication is available where there is deterioration or for use in emergencies
(4) the patient is withdrawn at his/her request or if there is persistent deterioration or signs of relapse.

It is perhaps salutary to recall the words of Claude Bernard in 1865:

'Christian morals forbid only one thing, doing ill to one's neighbour ... so among the experiments that may be tried on man, those that can only harm are forbidden, those that are innocent are permissible, and those that may do good are obligatory.' (Bernard, 1865, p. 102)

Nevertheless, a number of factors have conspired to make such trials all but impossible in the UK at the present time: the majority of patients are cared for in the community or are admitted only for short periods, during which they would be unlikely to fulfil the inclusion criteria; the anxieties of community psychiatric nurses and other carers, who believe a relapse may be prolonged and take many weeks to resolve; and the fear of taking unnecessary risks in a climate of clinical and research governance (and a highly critical public). This has led to more trials being conducted elsewhere, or to the use of sub-therapeutic doses of active drug as a surrogate placebo.

Adverse effects

Adverse drug reactions are traditionally divided into type A (predictable from their known pharmacology and dose dependent) and type B (idiosyncratic and dose independent). Most of these as well as drug interactions are discussed in Chapters 15 and 16 but brief clinical descriptions of the principal ones are given here because of their importance in distinguishing the pharmacological profiles of the classical, first-generation antipsychotics from the newer, second-generation drugs. Nevertheless, as will be seen, apart from propensity to cause movement disorders, there is a great deal of overlap between these two groups of drugs (see Tables 9.2 and 9.3).

The principal pharmacological actions of the classical antipsychotic drugs are listed in Box 9.1 and the consequent clinical problems and adverse effects in Box 9.2. With the exception of reserpine and oxypertine (which act by depleting the storage of catecholamines in synaptic vesicles) the therapeutic and many of the adverse effects of these drugs can be attributed to dopamine receptor antagonism. Blockade of dopamine in the three principal dopamine tracts is presumed to be responsible for their therapeutic (mesolimbic tract), extrapyramidal (nigrostriatal tract) and endocrine (tuberoinfundibular tract) effects.

The endocrine effects are relatively uncommon but can give rise to gynaecomastia, lactorrhoea, amenorrhoea, impotence, false pregnancy tests and weight gain, and are probably largely secondary to elevated plasma prolactin levels, an anterior pituitary hormone whose release is normally inhibited by dopamine, and which may be increased up to threefold in both male and female patients on chlorpromazine or thioridazine.

Table 9.2 'Typical' v. 'atypical' antipsychotics: pharmacology

	Classical (typical)	Second-generation (atypical)
Chemical structure	Various	Various
Site of action	Nigrostriatal and mesolimbic areas	Limbic selectivity (depolarisation block; mRNA; cFOS)
Animal behaviour	Stereotypy hyperactivity	Reduced agonist-induced
	Enhanced latent inhibition	Enhanced latent inhibition
	Enhanced prepulse inhibition	Reduced phencyclidine-induced disruption of prepulse inhibition
Clinical		
Prolactin release	+	±
D_2	+	Low at therapeutic doses (except risperidone)

Table 9.3 'Typical' v. 'atypical' antipsychotics: clinical profiles

	Classical (typical)	Second-generation (atypical)
Sedation	+	±
Extrapyramidal symptoms	+	–
Tardive dyskinesia	+	–
Efficacy in negative symptoms	–	±
Efficacy in depressive symptoms	–	±
Efficacy in cognitive deficit	–	±
Blood dyscrasias	+	+
Increased QTc intervals	+	+
Weight gain	+	+
Hyperlipidaemia	+	+
Diabetes mellitus	+	+

The EPS are more common and can be divided into four types:

(1) parkinsonism
(2) acute dystonias
(3) akathisia
(4) tardive dyskinesia.

The maximum incidence of the first three of these occurs during the first 3 months of treatment and thereafter tolerance develops in most cases and the incidence declines after 6 months. After this time anticholinergic medication can be discontinued; the recurrence rate of EPS

Box 9.1 Pharmacological actions of classical antipsychotic drugs

- Dopamine receptor blockade:
    antipsychotic effect
    extrapyramidal symptoms
    endocrine effects
    anti-emetic effect
- Anticholinergic effects
- α-adrenergic receptor blockade:
    hypotension
- Antihistamine effect
- Allergic reactions
- Other effects on the central nervous system:
    lowered temperature
    lowered convulsive threshold
    increased effect of analgesia, anaesthesia and alcohol

Box 9.2   Clinical problems and adverse effects of classical antipsychotics

- Extrapyramidal side-effects:
  parkinsonism
  acute dystonia
  akathisia
  tardive dyskinesia
- Neuroleptic malignant syndrome:
  severe rigidity
  hyperthermia
  increased serum creatinine phosphokinase (CPK)
  autonomic lability
  clouding of consciousness
- Postural hypotension
- Weight gain
- Water intoxication
- Endocrine changes
- Pigmentation

---

is then only about 10% (Johnson, 1978). Nevertheless, EPS can persist in the elderly, even after discontinuation of the offending antipsychotic drug, for up to 18 months (see Cunningham Owens, 1999).

Tardive dyskinesia is a neurological side-effect that develops after prolonged antipsychotic treatment (often for many years). Although the earliest reported onset is 3–6 months after starting treatment, it does not usually occur until after 2–3 years of continuous medication. Furthermore, in contrast to the other EPS, tolerance does not develop and the symptoms often persist, sometimes irreversibly, particularly in the elderly. The delineation of tardive dyskinesia as an antipsychotic-induced adverse drug reaction has been complicated by the fact that a variety of involuntary movement disorders, particularly orofacial dyskinesias, were described as a feature of dementia praecox from Kraepelin on, long before the antipsychotic era. Senile chorea is also a recognised phenomenon of ageing. Strictly speaking, the term 'tardive dyskinesia' should be used only when antipsychotics are implicated, but the clinical distinction between this and symptoms of the illness is often difficult, if not impossible, and a continuing source of controversy.

Movement disorders – extrapyramidal side-effects

The movement disorders associated with schizophrenia and its treatment have been comprehensively and elegantly reviewed in the monograph by Cunningham Owens (1999). The following brief descriptions are included since they are the single most important adverse effects of the classical, first-generation antipsychotic drugs, and, indeed, the reason for the older appellation 'neuroleptic'. Reduced EPS is the principal distinguishing characteristic of the new second-generation ('atypical') drugs.

Parkinsonism

Symptoms mimicking Parkinson's disease, with akinesia (generalised slowing and loss of movements, particularly the involuntary movements of association and expression), rigidity and tremor, develop gradually after a few weeks and are commoner in older patients, particularly older women. There is usually a satisfactory response to antimuscarinic (anticholinergic) drugs, but these should be used only when indicated and not prophylactically, because they have toxic side-effects themselves (delirium, blurred vision due to paralysis of accommodation and dilated pupils, dry mouth, tachycardia, constipation, paralytic ileus, erectile impotence and urinary retention), and can be fatal in overdose (particularly orphenadrine; Buckley & McManus, 1998). There is also some evidence that they can lower the plasma levels of antipsychotics and possibly reduce their efficacy. They may exacerbate tardive dyskinesia if present, and some have been abused for their euphoriant properties.

Drug-induced parkinsonism can develop quite suddenly at any time during the course of treatment. It can persist for many months, especially in the elderly, even when the offending drug has been withdrawn and anticholinergics added. Indeed, some authorities regard signs of parkinsonism to be iatrogenic in nature if any elderly patient has received an antipsychotic drug, even in small doses, in the previous 18 months (Marsden & Jenner, 1980; Murdoch & Williamson, 1982). Patients with dementia due to diffuse Lewy-body disease (see Chapter 12) are particularly sensitive to antipsychotic-induced EPS. In these circumstances great patience is required because the injudicious use of anticholinergics, particularly in greater than recommended doses, can simply add potentially dangerous toxicity to an already distressing syndrome.

If drug-induced parkinsonism occurs, it should be treated with the careful addition of an anticholinergic drug. The symptoms, unlike acute dystonias (see below), will not remit quickly, and doses beyond those recommended by the manufacturers must not be used in an attempt to speed up the response. Tolerance usually develops to EPS and anti-cholinergics are unnecessary after 6 months in all but about 10% of patients (Johnson, 1978). Dopamine-enhancing drugs such as L-dopa or bromocriptine should not be used because, on the one hand, they cannot be effective in the presence of dopamine antagonism, and, on the other, they can exacerbate psychotic symptoms.

The commonly used anticholinergic drugs are listed in Table 9.4. There are no important differences between them. They all have both central and peripheral antimuscarinic actions, although the peripheral

Table 9.4 The commonly used anticholinergic drugs

Drug	Daily dose	Effects, side-effects and use
Benzhexol	5–15 mg	May cause excitement in high doses in some patients.
Benztropine	1–6 mg	Similar to benzhexol but is excreted more slowly and changes in dose should therefore be carried out very gradually. It has antihistaminic properties and is sedative rather than stimulant. It is also available for intramuscular or intravenous injection in emergencies such as acute dystonias (1–2 mg).
Biperiden	3–12 mg	May also cause drowsiness. It is also available for intramuscular or intravenous injection in emergencies (2–2.5 mg). Transient hypotension may follow parenteral administration.
Orphenadrine	150–400 mg	Tends to have more euphoriant properties than the others and may cause insomnia. It is also a weak antihistamine.
Procyclidine	10–30 mg	Is also available for intramuscular or intravenous injection in emergencies (5–10 mg). Intravenous injection is usually effective within 5 minutes but occasionally it may take up to 30 minutes to act. The duration of the effect is about 4 hours.

actions are less prominent than those of the natural alkaloid atropine; biperiden is also antinicotinic. They may affect performance of skilled tasks, and memory can be impaired, especially in the elderly. They delay gastric emptying and, therefore, the absorption of other drugs, including antipsychotics. Some patients appear to tolerate one better than another. They may be taken before food if dry mouth is troublesome, or after food if gastrointestinal symptoms predominate.

For all the drugs shown in Table 9.4, except benztropine, peak concentrations occur 1–2 hours after an oral dose, and the plasma elimination half-lives are intermediate (10–14 hours). Comparable data are not available for benztropine, but following an oral dose its action is stated to occur in 1–2 hours and to last for 24 hours. Thus, twice-daily dosing is appropriate in most patients. Doses should be started at the lower end of the recommended range and only gradually increased in order to reach an optimal balance between the relief of EPS and the onset of peripheral anticholinergic symptoms, such as blurred vision and dry mouth, and so on.

Acute dystonias and dyskinesias

These are more alarming and dramatic in onset than is parkinsonism, occurring after the first few doses of an antipsychotic drug. They tend to be more common in men and in younger patients. The classic example of acute dystonia is an oculogyric crisis (fixed upward or lateral gaze), but many forms of torsion dystonia and torticollis occur, as well as spasms of the muscles of the lips, tongue, face and throat.

Acute *dyskinesias* (involuntary movements), with grimacing and exaggerated posturing and twisting of the head, neck or jaw, can also occur and must be distinguished from *tardive* dyskinesia by the length of exposure to the antipsychotic drug.

Both these reactions can be quickly and dramatically reversed by the systemic administration of an anticholinergic drug, and thus, like the Parkinsonian reactions, are presumably due to an imbalance between nigrostriatal dopamine and acetylcholine as a result of a drug-induced deficit in dopaminergic function. The pathophysiological mechanisms are reviewed by Marsden & Jenner (1980) and Waddington (1992).

Akathisia

This is probably the most common reaction to antipsychotics and has been reported to occur to some extent in up to 50% of patients. It is characterised by both motor restlessness and subjective agitation, dysphoria or intolerance of inactivity. In mild form there is shifting of the legs or tapping of the feet while sitting, or rocking and shifting of the weight while standing, but in severe forms intensive internal anxiety can be associated with continuous repetitive motor movements or restless pacing.

It is important to consider dysphoria as an early prodrome of akathisia, since many patients do not have a sufficient vocabulary to describe this symptom, which can occur before objective signs of restlessness are present. Furthermore, they may not attribute the effects to their medication, since there can be a delay of 3–4 hours after the last dose. Drug-induced dysphoria and akathisia should be suspected in any patient on antipsychotics who becomes irritable or unsettled and complains of needing to get outside or absconds for no apparent reason. It is important to recognise this possibility, since suicide attempts have been reported in association with these symptoms (Drake & Ehrlich, 1985).

The underlying mechanism is unclear and the response to anticholinergic treatment is variable. Acute forms are related to rapid increases in antipsychotic dose and may respond to anticholinergics. Chronic forms, in which subjective restlessness may be absent and, like tardive dyskinesia (see below), may be exacerbated by antipsychotic withdrawal, respond poorly to anticholinergics but may respond to benzodiazepines. To date, the best-established treatment for either form of akathisia is propranolol, but the response may nevertheless be disappointing. A promising alternative is one of the serotonin antagonists (mianserin, ritanserin or cyproheptadine) (Poyurovsky & Weizman,

2001). For detailed reviews of this syndrome see Barnes (1987) and Adler *et al* (1989).

Akathisia should be distinguished from the idiopathic 'restless legs syndrome' first described by Ekbom (1945), which is not associated with antipsychotics but which, interestingly, often responds to L-dopa.

Tardive dyskinesia

Interest in and concern over this complication of antipsychotic treatment has increased in recent years, both because of its persistence and resistance to treatment and because of its theoretical implications, and there is now a vast literature and a number of excellent reviews on the subject (Crane, 1973; Klawans *et al*, 1980; Kane & Smith, 1982; Barnes, 1987). As a result of the increasing attention given to it, the reported incidence has risen to as much as 56%, but the overall mean, representing the experience of most clinicians, is probably about 15%.

It was first described in the 1960s and the classic clinical picture is of orofacial and buccal–lingual involuntary movements in elderly patients, but choreo-athetoid movements of upper and lower limb girdles can occur, as can a range of tics, abnormal postures and even hemiballismus, grunting vocalisations and disturbances of respiration. It can occur at any age and in non-psychotic patients. Involvement of mouth and face is rare in children, and the more peripheral manifestations usually occur in patients under 50 years of age. It has a higher incidence, greater severity and poorer prognosis with age or organic brain disease, and there is a 2:1 female:male prevalence ratio in patients over 70 years of age.

Neuropharmacologically, tardive dyskinesia is the converse of acute dystonias, since it may be made *worse* by anticholinergic medication, and often appears if antipsychotic drugs are suddenly withdrawn. It has been precipitated by anticholinergic drugs in some cases, but there is no evidence that chronic treatment with combined anticholinergic and antipsychotic drugs is associated with an increased prevalence, and indeed the opposite trend was found in one study. It has therefore been proposed that the aetiological mechanism is dopamine receptor hypersensitivity, induced by prolonged receptor blockade. Consistent with this theory is the fact that an *increase* in antipsychotic medication will produce a temporary remission of symptoms, and the store-depleting antipsychotics (reserpine, tetrabenazine, oxypertine), while causing the other EPS, do *not* produce tardive dyskinesia.

The aetiology has, nevertheless, not been established, and an association with dopamine blockade has not been proven. A number of painstaking clinical studies have failed to establish a link between tardive dyskinesia and amount of antipsychotic drug exposure (Cunningham Owens *et al*, 1982; Waddington & Youssef, 1986; Waddington, 1987). It would therefore appear to be of multifactorial origin, with age, sex and organic brain disease (whether or not associated with psychosis and negative schizophrenic symptoms) as well as antipsychotic drug effects (which may be something other than their dopamine antagonism) all being relevant.

The tardive dyskinesia syndrome continues to present a number of theoretical and clinical puzzles. It can occur concomitantly with any of the other EPS, and it is generally associated with an improvement rather than a deterioration in psychotic symptoms. Thus, the hypothesised receptor hypersensitivity cannot involve all the dopamine receptors or even all the nigrostriatal ones. Clinically it can be difficult to distinguish from drug-induced akathisia, on the one hand, and from a pre-existing stereotyped motor manifestation of the psychosis itself, on the other.

A wide range of medications have been used to treat tardive dyskinesia by attempting to manipulate the levels of dopamine, acetylcholine, gamma-aminobutyric acid (GABA), and other brain neurotransmitters. None of these has proved to be generally successful. The prognosis in patients in whom antipsychotic drugs have been continued or used to suppress the dyskinesias is not as good as in those in whom the drugs have been discontinued. Complete recovery is more likely in young adults and is the rule in children. Accordingly, when tardive dyskinesia has been diagnosed, antipsychotic medication should be reduced gradually and withdrawn if possible. Additional or alternative treatment with a benzodiazepine or a store-depleting antipsychotic (the most effective of which is tetrabenazine) can be tried and anticholinergics should be avoided. Centrally acting cholinergic drugs such as physostigmine can be used experimentally and are associated with temporary improvements, but have no place in routine management.

A number of other 'tardive' syndromes have been described with a similar course and characteristics to tardive dyskinesia, including tardive akathisia, tardive dystonia, tardive Tourette's syndrome, tardive dysmentia, and tardive (or supersensitivity) psychosis.

Neuroleptic malignant syndrome (NMS)

This was first described in France in the early years of the use of phenothiazines, but was forgotten in the UK probably because of its rarity and possibly because it seems to be partially dependent on ambient temperature, and a series of cases during the hot summers of 1983 and 1984 alerted psychiatrists once more to its importance. It is characterised by severe rigidity, hyperpyrexia and highly elevated levels of serum creatinine phosphokinase (CPK). There may also be tachycardia, labile blood pressure and fluctuating levels of consciousness. Levenson (1985) described three major and six minor manifestations of the syndrome, and the reader is referred to this source for detailed case reports.

It may occur with any antipsychotic, but haloperidol and the intramuscular depot drug fluphenazine have been most commonly implicated. Although a report from Israel (Shalev *et al*, 1989) indicated a low mortality in cases associated with haloperidol and thioridazine, the UK Committee on Safety of Medicines' adverse drug reaction database (for the 'yellow card' system) shows that the greatest mortality has been with haloperidol (personal communication).

The aetiology is unknown and both central (hypothalamic temperature regulation) and peripheral (muscular hyperactivity associated with rigidity) mechanisms have been proposed. It is an idiosyncratic (type B) reaction, unrelated to dose or length of drug exposure, and successful re-exposure to antipsychotics without recurrence of NMS has been reported in two-thirds of cases. The duration varies from a few days to 2 weeks. The management is the immediate discontinuation of all antipsychotics and the use of either dantrolene or a dopamine agonist – bromocriptine, L-dopa or apomorphine. Anticholinergics are rarely effective and may exacerbate the fever by reducing sweating. Supportive and symptomatic measures to prevent the most serious complications (rhabdomyolysis with myoglobinaemia and renal failure, which carries a mortality rate of 50%, and dehydration) have reduced the overall mortality rate from 25%, before 1984, to about 10%.

For the immediate control of persistent psychotic symptoms, non-antipsychotic drug management (with benzodiazepines, lithium or ECT) is preferable, but if antipsychotic treatment becomes necessary the use of drugs with minimal potential for EPS (i.e. one of the second-generation drugs) should be tried, with caution.

The extensive literature on this syndrome has been reviewed by Levenson (1985), Pearlman (1986), Kellam (1987) and Dickey (1991).

Other actions on the central nervous system

Further central properties, which have no one simple pharmacological mechanism, are discussed below:

(1) Sedation is a property of most of the classical antipsychotics as well as those second-generation drugs that have a broad-spectrum or multiple-antagonist profile, such as clozapine, olanzapine, quetiapine and zotepine. It is usually attributed to central H_1 antagonism but α_1 antagonism may also be contributory. Although troublesome for some, this is a useful property in actively disturbed or agitated patients. Tolerance generally develops over a few weeks. It should be distinguished from tranquillisation, without impaired consciousness, which persists.

(2) Impairment of the thermoregulatory centre causes a lowering of body temperature (although an increase can also occur, as in the NMS – see above).

(3) A decrease in convulsive threshold can increase the frequency of seizures in epilepsy, as with the tricyclic antidepressants. This is particularly marked with clozapine, where it is dose dependent – a sharp increase in the risk of seizures occurs above 600 mg/day.

(4) The central depressant effects of analgesics, anaesthesia and alcohol are potentiated, which has been exploited in their use as pre-operative medication.

(5) Possible antipsychotic changes in mood (depression) have also been reported. These, like negative symptoms, are controversial, and were based on anecdotal reports after the introduction of high-potency depot drugs. Significant differences in the incidence of depression associated with different antipsychotics have not been found in controlled clinical trials. Depression is a common symptom in schizophrenia, either as a prodrome to more major symptoms or secondary to other symptoms or social circumstances and difficulties in coping. It is also sometimes not easy to distinguish from negative symptoms, or antipsychotic-induced dysphoria with or without akathisia.

Autonomic effects

As with sedation, these adverse reactions are more common with multiple-receptor antagonists.

Anticholinergic effects

The principal anticholinergic effects of antipsychotics are: delirium, blurred vision, dry mouth, tachycardia, constipation, paralytic ileus, erectile impotence and urinary retention. Like the tricyclic antidepressants (Chapter 6), these effects are probably largely responsible for the toxicity of these drugs in overdose. Delirium, although rare, must always be borne in mind when treating elderly patients. It is clearly of central origin and due to blockade of central muscarinic receptors. It is most likely to occur if an antipsychotic is injudiciously combined with both an anticholinergic drug (see 'Parkinsonism', above) and a tricyclic antidepressant, particularly in the elderly. The other symptoms arise because of the peripheral actions of the drugs.

The effects on the eye are particularly complex, as described in Chapter 6. Essentially, the effect on the pupil is the result of the balance between antimuscarinic effects (dilatation of the pupil due to unopposed sympathetic activity) and α-adrenergic antagonism (causing pupillary constriction). Blurred vision, however, is due to paralysis of accommodation.

The cardiac effects are the most serious and toxic of the anticholinergic actions, tachycardia resulting from the unopposed sympathetic action on the heart. The other peripheral effects are predictable from their atropine-like effects on the salivary glands, bowel and bladder, and interference in the balance between adrenergic and cholinergic regulation of the vascular smooth muscle and tissue in the corpora cavernosa (see Chapter 14). Sudden discontinuation of antipsychotics can be associated with cholinergic rebound symptoms, such as vomiting, sweating and bradycardia.

These anticholinergic effects are most marked with thioridazine and clozapine, but there is no simple relationship between this property and chemical structure or subgroup. Since an anticholinergic effect counteracts EPS, the relative proportion of muscarinic and dopamine antagonism can influence the extent to which antipsychotics cause EPS. The anticholinergic effects of antipsychotic drugs, with the exception of thioridazine and clozapine, are generally less than with tricyclic antidepressants, but typical side-effects such as dry mouth and blurred vision are not uncommon and will be increased by the addition of anticholinergic anti-Parkinson medication. Thus, although thioridazine was popular for use with elderly patients because of its low incidence of EPS, it also carried an increased risk of cardiotoxicity (see below) and aggravation of incipient dementia, and has now been withdrawn.

A paradoxical situation arises with clozapine, which can be associated with excessive sialorrhoea, particularly at night. It has been suggested that the mechanism could be a dystonia of the oesophagus leading to failure to swallow saliva, or a partial muscarinic agonist effect. It may be reduced by the addition of small doses of anticholinergic medication. If a traditional anticholinergic is ineffective, hyoscine has been recommended. Most of the second-generation drugs have reduced antimuscarinic effects similar to haloperidol, and olanzapine, which has a relatively low *in vivo* affinity for muscarinic receptors, is reported to produce no changes in heart rate compared with placebo.

α-adrenergic receptor blockade

This is a common property of most first- and second-generation antipsychotics and the reason for gradual dose titration when initiating treatment with clozapine, risperidone, quetiapine and zotepine. It is less marked with amisulpride and haloperidol. It causes orthostatic hypotension and reflex tachycardia, especially with high intramuscular doses (and which are not subject to first-pass metabolism) such as are usually required in psychotic patients, and is particularly dangerous in the elderly. A non-phenothiazine such as haloperidol should therefore be used if intramuscular administration is necessary. Although intravenous administration is possible, and is practised occasionally by anaesthetists, it is a hazardous procedure and should probably be used only in intensive-care units. This α-blocking action is also responsible for the diminished pupil size that is the usual effect of phenothiazine derivatives at therapeutic doses.

Cardiotoxicity

This is similar to the situation with tricyclic antidepressants but it is generally less marked. Like the tricyclics, antipsychotics cause both delayed conduction (with S–T depression and QTc prolongation on electrocardiography, and right bundle branch block) and anticholinergic effects (tachycardia), but the situation is more complex because of their α-receptor-blocking actions.

A sudden cardiac arrhythmia or cardiac arrest is rare, but a high incidence of sudden unexpected deaths has been reported with high doses (greater than 20 mg daily) of pimozide, which is also a potent potassium HERG channel antagonist: the HERG (human 'ether-a-go-go') gene encodes for the delayed rectifier potassium channel (I_{Kr}), which is responsible for ventricular depolarisation. The binding affinity to this I_{Kr} channel appears to determine the potency of QT_c prolongation by different antipsychotics and is particularly marked with thioridazine, sertindole, pimozide, droperidol and haloperidol.

The clinical significance of QTc prolongation is still unclear. Two systematic studies have examined the prevalence of this in patients on antipsychotic medication in comparison with healthy, drug-free controls. QTc prolongation was more likely with very high doses (Warner *et al*, 1996) and with thioridazine and droperidol (Reilly *et al*, 2000). These changes are both age and dose dependent. Nevertheless, concern about this effect and its possible link to sudden death (see below) has led to both thioridazine and droperidol being discontinued and the licence for sertindole being withdrawn.

In addition there appears to be an increased risk of venous thrombo-embolism with these drugs, particularly with chlorpromazine and thioridazine (Zornberg & Jick, 2000). Twelve cases (five fatal) of venous thrombo-embolism have also been reported in association with clozapine (Hägg *et al*, 2000). Furthermore, there appears to be an increased risk of myocarditis (a third of cases proving fatal) and cardiomyopathy associated with clozapine (Kilian *et al*, 1999). There is some recent evidence that both clozapine and thioridazine, but not amisulpride, olanzapine or risperidone, decrease heart rate variability, which further suggests that it is more cardiotoxic than the newer 'atypicals' (Agelink *et al*, 2001; Cohen *et al*, 2001; Silke *et al*, 2002).

Antihistaminic action

Historically, this is one of their oldest known actions because the first-generation antipsychotics were first developed as antihistamines, and this action was thought to account for their anti-emetic properties. However, the anti-emetic effect of phenothiazines is probably due to dopamine blockade at the chemoreceptor trigger zone in the floor of the fourth ventricle, and an anticholinergic action on the emetic centre in the brain-stem.

Weight gain

It has long been recognised that the classical antipsychotics are associated with weight gain. For example, Amidsen (1964) found that 80% of in-patients on chlorpromazine put on weight, a quarter of whom gained more than 25% of their ideal body weight. The new second-generation drugs are also associated with increases in body mass index, with clozapine being particularly culpable, followed by olanzapine (Allison *et al*, 1999). Weight increases of up to 9.1 kg over 1 year with clozapine have been reported. Weight gain is also a recognised problem with risperidone, zotepine and quetiapine. The mechanism is uncertain but 5-HT_{2C} antagonism is a possible factor, since a 5-HT_{2C} receptor gene polymorphism has been reported to be associated with less antipsychotic drug-induced weight gain (Reynolds *et al*, 2002).

As more patients are being treated with second-generation drugs, this is emerging as a greater problem with antipsychotic treatment than EPS. It also has important implications for the general health of patients with schizophrenia because of a strong association with type II diabetes mellitus and an increased risk of hypertension and coronary heart disease.

Hyperglycaemia

Hyperglycaemia has been reported with conventional antipsychotic drugs from time to time since the 1960s but a true drug-induced effect was questionable, particularly since diabetes has a high prevalence in schizophrenia, particularly in untreated patients. Recently, however, there has been an increased number of reports of various degrees of glucose intolerance associated with hyperglycaemia, diabetes mellitus or even diabetic keto-acidosis with the second-generation drugs, particularly clozapine and olanzapine (Mir & Taylor, 2001). Indeed, in a 5-year naturalistic study almost a third of patients taking clozapine were eventually diagnosed with type 2 diabetes. There does not seem to be any direct correlation with weight gain and a concentration-dependent insulin resistance has been proposed for clozapine acting via specific serotonin receptors. Although Mir & Taylor (2001) recommend that all patients starting clozapine or olanzapine should have monthly fasting plasma glucose monitoring for 6 months, this is unlikely to be practicable in most community settings. Nevertheless, constant awareness of the risk of drug-induced diabetes is prudent.

Sexual dysfunction

Current evidence suggests that the first- and second-generation antipsychotics have comparable adverse effects on sexual function

(Barnes & McPhillips, 1999). The complexities of this area include the difficulties in ascertainment, the psychosexual consequences of the problem and the understanding of the pathophysiological mechanisms involved. Muscarinic and α-adrenergic blockade are probably the basis of impaired erectile and ejaculatory function in men, while in women loss of libido, menstrual problems and lactation are thought to be related to elevated prolactin levels. Neither clozapine nor quetiapine elevate serum prolactin levels and, of the second-generation drugs, quetiapine appears to cause fewer sexual side-effects in both sexes. Sertindole (now withdrawn) reduces ejaculatory volume without impairment of libido, erection or orgasm.

Allergic reactions

These can affect a number of systems including:

(1) the liver, causing a cholestatic jaundice
(2) the skin, leading to four types of reaction, namely an urticarial rash (hypersensitivity), contact dermatitis, photosensitivity, and abnormal pigmentation
(3) the eye, which can develop optic neuritis, pigmentary retinopathy (which is dose dependent and occurs notably after high doses of thioridazine) and stellate opacities in the anterior of the lens, the cornea, sclera or conjunctiva
(4) the blood, causing, rarely, an agranulocytosis (an incidence of 1 in 1300 has been reported) or even aplastic anaemia. The risk of agranulocytosis is high with clozapine (1–2%) and remoxipride was withdrawn after eight reports of aplastic anaemia.

The precise mechanisms for these reactions are not known, and both allergic and idiosyncratic reactions may be involved in the adverse effects on the eye and the blood. For a more detailed discussion see Edwards (1986).

Jaundice

Jaundice occurs most commonly with phenothiazines, particularly chlorpromazine, usually during the second to fourth week of treatment. It is an idiosyncratic reaction and therefore not dose dependent. Pruritis is not common but can occur in severe cases. Tests of liver function show a cholestatic picture, with conjugated hyperbilirubinaemia and increased alkaline phosphatase. Serum transaminase may be elevated, in the range 100–200 IU/l, and the white cell count may be normal or slightly elevated, with eosinophilia. The jaundice usually subsides within a few days or weeks but occasionally chronic intrahepatic cholestasis may develop, despite cessation of the offending drug. This may persist for several months, but eventually recovery without cirrhosis is usual. Low doses of a potent, non-phenothiazine should be used if continued antipsychotic treatment is necessary.

Pigmentation

Slate-blue pigmentation in exposed areas was first reported in association with the long-term administration of high doses of phenothiazine medication in 1956. This syndrome has been termed 'oculodermal melanosis'. It has been found in 1–2% of patients but bears no exact relationship to dose, duration of treatment, or presence of tardive dyskinesia. Doses of 125–2900 mg of chlorpromazine equivalents daily (Ban *et al*, 1985) and durations of 2–9 years (Ban & Lehmann, 1965) have been reported in affected patients. Ophthalmological changes are always present (but not vice versa) but visual acuity is unaffected.

Pigmentation occurs most commonly with chlorpromazine but has also been reported with other phenothiazines and non-phenothiazines. Nevertheless, substitution by a non-phenothiazine will usually resolve the disorder (Thompson *et al*, 1988). The nature of the pigment is unknown but the colour may be due to the location of the deposits in the dermis, since a similar slate-blue discoloration also occurs with chloroquine, amiodarone and gold salts.

Rare adverse reactions

Less common adverse effects that have been reported with antipsychotics are: exfoliative dermatitis, systemic lupus erythematosis, elevated serum cholesterol levels, peripheral oedema and fluid retention. Sudden deaths have been reported with all of the antipsychotic drugs from time to time. These fortunately are rare. They are usually unexplained; possible causes that have been suggested are depression of the medullary respiratory centre, a bulbar palsy-like syndrome leading to aspiration or asphyxiation, or a sudden arrhythmia or cardiac arrest. An increased risk of cardiomyopathy has also been reported with clozapine (see above).

Summary

It is now clear that all antipsychotics cause a substantial burden of adverse side-effects and risk of idiosyncratic reactions. Clozapine and the second-generation drugs are a substantial advance, in that they have greatly reduced the risk of EPS, especially dysphoria and tardive dyskinesia. Generally this has made them better tolerated and more acceptable to patients, but weight gain, glucose dysregulation and sexual dysfunction have taken their place as major problems. Furthermore, the clinical significance of prolonged QTc intervals, noted with both groups of antipsychotics, is yet to be fully determined.

Interactions

Drug–drug interactions can be either pharmacodynamic or pharmaco-kinetic in nature. In the latter, the altered response can be related to altered circulating blood levels of the drug(s) involved, while with the former an interaction at the receptor level is implied. They are more frequent in patients with comorbidity and those requiring polypharmacy (e.g. the elderly).

Antipsychotic drugs are generally safe in combination with other drugs. A number of possible interactions can occur, and can lead to either an increase or a decrease in serum antipsychotic levels, but, since there is no good correlation between these serum levels and anti-psychotic response, these are not usually of practical significance. More important are the effects of antipsychotics on the metabolism of other drugs, and the prescriber is advised always to consult Appendix 1 of the most recent edition of the *British National Formulary* before prescribing an antipsychotic in combination with any other drug. The best-known, clinically important interactions are summarised in Chapter 16.

Pharmacodynamic interactions

Effects on the central nervous system

The phenothiazines potentiate the central depressant action of a wide range of drugs, including alcohol, benzodiazepines and antihistamines. They also increase the sedation, analgesia and respiratory depression of opiates. Both the central depressant and hypotensive effects of general anaesthetics are also potentiated.

Although anticholinergics are often used for antipsychotic-induced EPS, additive anticholinergic effects can occur with these drugs or with the concomitant use of tricyclic antidepressants. Possible effects are: confusion, delirium, dry mouth, blurred vision, tachycardia, consti-pation, paralytic ileus, erectile impotence and urinary retention.

Increased EPS and possible neurotoxicity have been described with a number of antipsychotics and lithium (see Chapter 7). Two types of additive interaction may be responsible for this:

(1) the NMS may be exacerbated by a dopamine action of lithium
(2) increased lithium toxicity may occur owing to increased intra-cellular lithium levels.

The phenothiazines, particularly thioridazine, cause marked increases in intracellular lithium and minor increases occur with haloperidol and tricyclic antidepressants. Reports of severe neurotoxicity are rare and have been associated with high serum levels (1.5 mmol/l or above) and high doses of antipsychotics (e.g. haloperidol 40 mg/day or greater) (Baastrup *et al*, 1976). It has been recommended that lithium should not be introduced to a patient who is receiving more than 20 mg/day of haloperidol, and haloperidol should not be given to a patient whose lithium level exceeds 1.0 mmol/l.

Antipsychotics antagonise the dopaminergic effects of anti-Parkinson drugs such as L-dopa and bromocriptine.

Antagonism of anti-epileptic drug effects can occur by lowering the convulsive threshold.

Effects on the cardiovascular system

The quinidine-like action of the phenothiazines can neutralise the inotropic action of digoxin and increase the risk of ventricular arrhythmias with other anti-arrhythmic drugs. The cardiotoxicity of antipsychotics (particularly pimozide, sertindole and thioridazine) is increased by combinations with quinidine-like anti-arrhythmics or the antihistamines astemizole and terfenadine.

The interaction between antipsychotics and antihypertensive drugs can be unpredictable. The phenothiazines, like the tricyclic anti-depressants, also have amine reuptake blocking effects, which can neutralise the effect of drugs blocking adrenergic neurons (guanethidine, debrisoquine and bethanidine), thus leading to an increase in hypertension. On the other hand, an enhanced hypotensive effect may occur with other antihypertensive drugs and severe postural hypotension can occur with angiotensin-converting enzyme (ACE) inhibitors.

Pharmacokinetic interactions

Antacids can reduce the absorption of phenothiazines. Anticholinergics cause delayed gastric emptying and reduced absorption of some antipsychotics, leading to lower serum levels, but the significance of this is controversial.

Enzyme-inducing agents such as the anti-epileptics carbamazepine and phenytoin decrease serum antipsychotic levels.

Enzyme-inhibiting agents such as cimetidine may increase the serum levels of a number of antipsychotics and enhance their adverse effects. The inhibition of a number of cytochrome P450 enzymes by the selective serotonin reuptake inhibitors (SSRIs) has been extensively investigated in recent years (Nemeroff et al, 1996). With the exception of citalopram, the SSRIs inhibit one or more of these enzyme systems. A number of antipsychotics are metabolised by CYP 450 2D6 and consequently their blood levels are elevated by SSRIs. Clozapine is predominantly metabolised by CYP 450 1A2, which is inhibited by fluvoxamine, and this combination can therefore worsen the side-effects of clozapine, especially sedation.

Propranolol increases serum chlorpromazine levels and this was held, by many, to be the explanation for the apparent enhanced antipsychotic response when this β-blocker was used as an adjunctive treatment in schizophrenia.

Pharmacokinetics

Oral preparations

Plasma levels of antipsychotic drugs, as with the tricyclic anti-depressants, show a very wide variation in steady-state levels, differences of up to tenfold being found between individuals on identical doses. The mean plasma elimination half-life is about 16–30 hours for chlorpromazine. It is absorbed erratically and incompletely after oral ingestion, giving rise to five- or tenfold diurnal variations in the plasma level in an individual patient. Chlorpromazine is highly protein bound, is almost entirely metabolised, undergoes extensive first-pass metabolism and gives rise to at least 150 metabolites, several of which are active. Intramuscular doses will thus lead to fourfold or even higher serum levels than the corresponding oral dose. The principal metabolites found in the plasma are chlorpromazine sulphoxide, monodesmethylated chlorpromazine and 7-hydroxy chlorpromazine. After 2 weeks plasma levels tend to fall, which suggests hepatic enzyme induction. About 40% of non-responders are poor absorbers of oral chlorpromazine because of its metabolism to inactive substances in the intestinal wall (active metabolites being formed in the liver). Flupenthixol, but not fluphenazine, has also been shown to cause enzyme induction.

Monitoring of blood levels of the drug has not proved to be of much value in clinical practice since reliable dose–response or even plasma-level–response relationships have not been established. Recently developed PET measures of brain receptor occupancy (discussed above) may be more fruitful but are unlikely to become routinely available. Plasma antipsychotic levels correlate with adverse effects, some electroencephalographic (EEG) changes (increase in delta and theta activity and a decrease in fast beta activity) and increases in prolactin levels, but not with clinical response.

Haloperidol has been widely studied in this respect and a curvilinear dose–response relationship (or 'therapeutic window') has been found by some but not confirmed by others. Unlike chlorpromazine, haloperidol seems to have a relatively steep dose–response curve and little or no further benefit is afforded by doses in excess of 20 mg daily (Bjørndal et al, 1980; Zarifian et al, 1982; Browne et al, 1988; van Putten et al, 1990; McEvoy et al, 1991; Rifkin et al, 1991; Volavka et al, 1992). Indeed, haloperidol has a low therapeutic index, in that the 'neuroleptic threshold' (the dose at which first signs of EPS occur) (3.7 mg daily) appears to be very close to the dose required for an optimum antipsychotic effect in most patients (McEvoy et al, 1991). In another study (van Putten et al, 1990) 35% of patients receiving 20 mg a day discharged themselves against medical advice, probably largely because of akathisia.

Depot preparations

Since patients with schizophrenia lack insight and are frequently paranoid, they are notoriously not concordant with medication regimens. Patients may be non-concordant for a variety of reasons, ranging from impairment of insight, a wish to be independent of medication, adverse drug effects such as akathisia and dysphoria, to poor comprehension and forgetfulness.

Non-concordance for whatever reason is the commonest cause of relapse and has led to the increasing use of depot injections, given at intervals of 2–6 weeks. Even with this route of administration, wide variations in plasma concentrations occur between patients on the same dose, and the variation between patients in the doses used to control symptoms is even greater (e.g. from 12.5 mg fluphenazine decanoate every 6 weeks to 100 mg every 2 weeks). These depot preparations are very slowly and steadily released from an oily depot, taken up into fat stores and hydrolysed by plasma esterases to the parent compound. Thus diffusion from the injection site rather than metabolism is the rate-limiting pharmacokinetic parameter. Since the rate of release from the depot site is slower than the rate of elimination, the pharmacokinetics assume what has been termed a 'flip-flop' model. The 'apparent $t_{1/2}$' of these drugs is not, therefore, a true $t_{1/2}$. For example, the 'apparent $t_{1/2}$' of fluphenazine decanoate is 7–10 days and of flupenthixol decanoate about 50 days, and it can be months before a steady state is reached (Balant-Gorgia & Balant, 1987). By the same token, the drug may be detected in the plasma 9 or even 12 months after the last injection of the depot compound. This has important clinical implications both during the early treatment phase and following the discontinuation of injections, in terms of both therapeutic and adverse effects.

The first second-generation antipsychotic to become available in a depot preparation is risperidone (Risperdal Consta). This is not oil-based but is freshly prepared before each injection from a powder consisting of the drug in biodegradable microtubules.

Therapeutic principles

General guidelines

Dose

The correct dose is the minimum required to control symptoms. Sufficient time (3–4 weeks) should be given for an antipsychotic effect to develop before increasing the dose. A dose above the upper limit stated in the manufacturer's summary of product characteristics (SPC) or the British National Formulary (BNF) is a high dose and should be given only in carefully controlled circumstances (see below).

Polypharmacy

Only one antipsychotic drug should be given at a time (unless an oral preparation is added to a depot drug for an acute exacerbation of symptoms). The administration of two or more antipsychotics to the same patient is illogical, unnecessary and increases adverse rather than therapeutic effects.

Because of the wide range in patients' responses, it is more prudent to adjust the *dose* of one drug according to the patient's requirements and tolerance of the medication, rather than adding an additional antipsychotic.

Combinations of more than one antipsychotic drug are also likely to lead to the inadvertent prescribing of a high dose.

Adjunctive anticholinergics

These should be used sparingly, and never routinely, for the control of EPS (Barnes, 1990). They have, however, been advocated, and could probably be justified prophylactically, in conjunction with high-dose emergency treatments with haloperidol or other high-potency antipsychotics. Anticholinergics are more toxic than antipsychotics and are lethal in overdose. They can be misused for their euphoriant effects. They may precipitate tardive dyskinesia and certainly make it worse. There is some evidence that they reduce both the blood level of antipsychotics and clinical response. Finally, as stated above, tolerance to EPS usually develops and anticholinergics are unnecessary after 6 months in all but about 10% of patients (Johnson, 1978).

Duration of treatment

Treatment may have to continue for an indefinite period, but if a firm diagnosis of schizophrenia is made the initial treatment period should probably be 3–4 years in the first instance. 'Drug holidays' are ineffective and ultimately lead to more rather than less antipsychotic being prescribed (Johnson *et al*, 1983; Jolley *et al*, 1990).

Discontinuation of treatment

Although dependence is not a problem with antipsychotics, abrupt discontinuation should be avoided to prevent a withdrawal dyskinesia or rebound autonomic symptoms. The latter usually take the form of nausea, vomiting and sweating, and are probably due to the release of cholinergic activity following cessation of the anticholinergic effect of the antipsychotic, although supersensitivity of dopamine receptors in the stomach has also been suggested. A rebound psychosis may be precipitated by the abrupt cessation of clozapine, although if there is a warning of possible agranulocytosis there will be no option but to withdraw the drug immediately. Such patients should, therefore, be admitted to hospital if possible.

Depot preparations

Both beneficial and adverse effects of the depot preparations, particularly fluphenazine, may be evident for many months after the last injection. Thus, when these are discontinued many patients will continue to remain well and apparently 'drug free', so that both they and their carers begin to believe that maintenance medication is no longer necessary. However, relapse may occur 9–12 months later and such patients should, therefore, be closely followed up for at least this length of time before a decision is made that maintenance antipsychotic treatment is not required. By the same token, depot-induced EPS can persist for an equally long time in spite of discontinuation of the injections. In such situations patience is necessary, since too vigorous treatment with anticholinergic agents can be both ineffective and hazardous.

Choice of drug

Since the first edition of this book was printed in 1995, many guidelines have been published and readers will now be spoilt for, not to say confused by, choice. They can choose between those published by the Maudsley Hospital (1999) and periodically updated, Frangou & Murray (2000) and Lawrie (1999). These all cover the choice of drug for emergencies, acute episodes, maintenance treatment and treatment resistance, and attempt to base their recommendations on published evidence and meta-analyses. Relevant reviews can also be found in the Cochrane Library.

The principal issue is whether the first-line treatment for first episodes of schizophrenia should be a new second-generation drug (McGrath & Emmerson, 1999; McCreadie, 2000; Taylor, 2000) or a low dose of a conventional (typical) antipsychotic (Frangou & Byrne, 2000; Geddes *et al*, 2000). While there seems little debate about the equivalent efficacy of these options, the question is whether an effective dose of the conventional drugs can be found that does not risk EPS, tardive dyskinesia or hyperprolactinaemia. Many clinicians prefer not to take that risk, as such side-effects could alienate their patients and have negative consequences for the therapeutic alliance, which is essential for successful long-term maintenance treatment.

The National Institute for Clinical Excellence (NICE) (2002) has considered all the issues related to the relative benefits and side-effect profiles of the newer ('atypical') antipsychotic drugs compared with the conventional drugs and has clearly recommended that the oral atypicals amisulpride, olanzapine, quetiapine, risperidone and zotepine should be considered in the choice of first-line treatments for first-episode schizophrenia. They are also recommended for chronic cases in which there is poor tolerance of conventional antipsychotics owing to unacceptable side-effects. The guidance goes on to recommend that clozapine should be introduced 'at the earliest opportunity' for treatment-resistant schizophrenia. This is defined as lack of satisfactory clinical improvement despite the sequential use of the recommended doses for 6–8 weeks of at least two antipsychotics, one (or both) of which should be an atypical. The cost of switching to atypicals was estimated as £70 million per annum, and for the wider use of clozapine in treatment-resistant cases as approximately £41 million per annum. However, since drug costs account for only 5% of the direct costs of schizophrenia they should be set against the estimated total direct treatment costs of £1 billion and indirect costs of £1.7 billion per annum (1990–91). Thus wider use of the new second-generation antipsychotics and clozapine, by improving concordance and response and facilitating the shift from in-patient to residential or community care, could produce substantial savings to the economy as a whole in the long run. While we generally support these NICE guidelines, we believe that a rather longer trial of the new 'atypicals', of say 6–9 months, should be given before clozapine is introduced for treatment-resistant or intolerant patients.

Use of high doses of antipsychotics

Acute, floridly ill and treatment-resistant schizophrenic patients have frequently been given, and seem to tolerate, very high doses of anti-psychotic drugs. However, this raises a number of issues, including:

(1) the relationship between such doses and the incidence of adverse effects
(2) the safety of such doses
(3) the optimum treatment regimen for acutely disturbed patients
(4) whether or not a dose–response or plasma-level–response relationship can be demonstrated for antipsychotics
(5) the efficacy of high or 'mega' doses in treatment-resistant cases.

Adverse effects

In 1971 a side-effect 'breakthrough' phenomenon was proposed, whereby the EPS found at low doses of oral fluphenazine were replaced by mild sedation at high doses (Rifkin et al, 1971), but this was subsequently shown by the same group to have been an erroneous observation (Quitkin et al, 1975). Subsequent studies have confirmed that all adverse effects, including sedation and EPS, are increased on high-dose regimens (Bjørndal et al, 1980; van Putten et al, 1990).

Safety

The risk of sudden death also appears to be increased with high-dose regimens (Flaherty & Lahmeyer, 1978; Ketai et al, 1979; Modestin et al,

1981). Pimozide in doses above 20 mg/day has been reported to be associated with cardiotoxicity and increased risk of sudden death (Committee on Safety of Medicines, 1990).

A widely publicised death of an Afro-Caribbean man in Broadmoor Hospital in 1991 drew attention to the fact that high doses of depot injections combined with intramuscular injections of short-acting phenothiazines can be fatal (Dillner, 1993). Furthermore, a Finnish study of sudden unexplained deaths of patients on normal doses found that most of them were on the low-potency phenothiazine thioridazine (Mehtonen et al, 1991). Hirsch & Barnes (1994) have advised 'that doses of low-potency phenothiazine antipsychotics should be kept at less than 800 mg per day, chlorpromazine equivalents, and high-potency antipsychotics may be more appropriate for high-dose regimes'. In all cases, the use of high doses should not be embarked upon without a careful appraisal of the likely risk:benefit ratio. Such trials should be used only for a defined, limited period.

Increasing concern during the 1990s about sudden unexplained deaths of psychiatric patients taking antipsychotic drugs led to the establishment of the Royal College of Psychiatrists' Working Group on Antipsychotics and Sudden Death. Its report concluded:

'Currently there are insufficient epidemiological data to prove that sudden death is more likely amongst people being treated with antipsychotics than it is among the general population... The possible mechanisms that may underlie such a relationship remain an area for conjecture and hypothesis.' (Royal College of Psychiatrists, 1997)

Nevertheless, it was noted that the risks were increased by high doses, pre-existing cardiac disease and physical restraint (which is associated with high autonomic arousal and elevated levels of circulating catecholamines). It was recommended that benzodiazepines could more safely be used in emergencies (see below).

Treatment of acutely disturbed cases

A rapid antipsychotic (as opposed to sedative) effect is not available, regardless of which drug or dose is used. The objective is therefore rapid tranquillisation rather than rapid 'neuroleptisation'. Although intravenous diazepam can be effective in the management of acute psychotic disturbance (Lerner et al, 1979; Pilowsky et al, 1992), resuscitation equipment should be available in the event of respiratory collapse, and intramuscular diazepam is painful, unreliably absorbed and ineffective. The best and safest choice, therefore, lies between intramuscular haloperidol and a high-potency benzodiazepine, such as lorazepam, alprazolam or clonazepam (Bick & Hannah, 1986; Bodkin, 1990; Pilowsky et al, 1992).

Dose–response relationships

In the 1970s and 1980s numerous pharmacokinetic studies were carried out that sought to establish dose–response or plasma-level–response relationships for a wide range of antipsychotics, but these produced inconclusive results. A linear relationship, a curvilinear ('inverted U') relationship, and no relationship between dose or serum level and response were reported (May & van Putten, 1978; Baldessarini *et al*, 1988; Browne *et al*, 1988). In their review, however, Baldessarini *et al* (1988) pooled the data from a wide range of studies that had used different antipsychotics by converting the doses used to chlorpromazine equivalents. This obscures the possibility that there are different dose–dependent relationships for different antipsychotics. The majority of studies with haloperidol have found that there is no advantage in exceeding standard doses (10–20 mg/day), even in treatment-resistant cases, and that very high doses (100–240 mg/day) are associated with more EPS, sedation and risk of sudden death (Bjørndal *et al*, 1980; Browne *et al*, 1988). (Also see 'Pharmacokinetics', above).

Treatment-resistant cases

Possible reasons for non-response in schizophrenia are either pharmaco-kinetic or pharmacodynamic (inherent insensitivity). The former can occur in about 40% of non-responders – those who are poor absorbers of oral chlorpromazine, owing to its metabolism to inactive metabolites in the intestinal wall (active metabolites are formed in the liver) (Adamson *et al*, 1973). However, further attempts to explain non-response pharmacokinetically have largely been unsuccessful. Although Hollister & Kim (1982) found a better response in treatment-resistant cases with high serum levels of haloperidol, Browne *et al* (1998) were unable to demonstrate any additional therapeutic benefit with doses of haloperidol as high as 160 mg daily in a group of 11 such patients.

In clinical practice, therefore, it would appear that most cases of 'treatment resistance' are due to pharmacodynamic factors. Different pathophysiological mechanisms may also be involved (Abi-Dargham *et al*, 2000). This is consistent with the high D_2 receptor occupancies already noted to occur in such patients (Wolkin *et al*, 1989; Coppens *et al*, 1991).

The only drug with an established superior efficacy in treatment resistance is clozapine (Kane *et al*, 1988). Both dose and duration may be important in determining outcome. Although about a third of such cases show an improvement after 6 weeks, two-thirds will benefit if treatment is continued for 6–10 months (Clozapine Study Group, 1993; King & Mills, 1993). In these trails moderately high doses, in the 400–500 mg/day range, were used. In a first series of 24 treatment-resistant patients, the mean effective daily dose was 488 mg in men and 438 mg in women (Kings & Mills, 1993). Meltzer (1992) recommends a target dose of 450 mg/day given as monotherapy for 6 months. If the response is inadequate after this time, doses up to 900 mg/day (or plasma levels of 360 ng/ml or higher) should be tried. However, the mean dose of clozapine in European clinical trials has been reported to be 310 mg daily, and, after response, the average maintenance dose in the UK is 300 mg/day (Clozapine Study Group, 1993).

Those patients who still fail to respond after an adequate trial of clozapine may benefit from adjunctive amisulpride to augment dopamine $D_{2/3}$ antagonism. Alternatively, lamotrigine, a glutamate release inhibitor, may be effective (Dursun et al, 1999). The proposed mechanism of this is obscure but the complexities of both putative glutamate hypofunction and hyperfunction in schizophrenia have been reviewed by Deakin (2000).

Recommendations

The use of high doses of antipsychotics is being increasingly questioned, on the grounds of both safety and efficacy. In acute psychiatric emergencies, high-potency benzodiazepines, particularly those without active metabolites, such as lorazepam, can be just as effective and are certainly safer.

In treatment resistance, short trials of high doses of conventional antipsychotics may be justified, and seem to be necessary in some individual cases, particularly if clozapine is refused, contraindicated or ineffective. More detailed guidelines have been provided in a consensus statement by the Royal College of Psychiatrists (Thompson, 1994), which will be updated for 2004.

Antipsychotics in pregnancy and lactation

All unnecessary drugs should be avoided in pregnancy and during lactation, but the question of whether antipsychotics should be used in such circumstances will arise if a patient with schizophrenia on maintenance treatment becomes pregnant, pregnancy precipitates a schizophrenic relapse, or in the management of puerperal psychoses. The risks of a psychotic relapse to both the mother and unborn foetus, due to denial or delusional ideas about the pregnancy which can lead to neglect, self-mutilation or suicide, generally outweigh the risks of antipsychotic medication.

There is no good evidence that antipsychotic drugs are teratogenic. Follow-up studies over long periods of the children of mothers who took chlorpromazine have failed to show any adverse effects on development (Loudon, 1987). However, EPS due to the effects of the drugs near term or during delivery have occasionally been reported in neonates. An exception is prochlorperazine, which is used most often as an anti-emetic, and which has apparently been shown to be teratogenic when the foetus is exposed between the sixth and tenth week of gestation (Loudon, 1987).

Antipsychotics are known to be present in breast milk in amounts (when the mother is on the usual therapeutic doses) that are probably too small to be harmful. During lactation, drowsiness in the infant has been reported when chlorpromazine has been taken by the nursing mother, and lethargy and EPS may occur if high doses of antipsychotics are used. They should therefore be avoided unless absolutely necessary.

Concomitant anticholinergic drugs may present more of a problem than antipsychotics. Infants are sensitive to anticholinergic agents, and typical anticholinergic effects such as dry mouth, retention of urine and constipation may occur if the mother is taking such drugs.

The recommendations in the *British National Formulary* are that antipsychotics be avoided and used only if potential benefit outweighs the risk. Chlorpromazine, sulpiride, clozapine and the new second-generation drugs are specifically listed. For further information see Chapter 16 and Worsley (2000).

Antipsychotics in the presence of physical illness

The main problems of treating physically ill patients with schizophrenia arise as a result of possible drug interactions (see above and Chapter 16).

Heart disease

In the presence of heart disease, a reduction in antipsychotic dose is prudent and usually possible. The phenothiazines and pimozide carry the highest risk of cardiotoxicity (see above) and should be avoided in preference to a butyrophenone or a drug with minimal antimuscarinic effects, such as olanzapine or amisulpride.

Liver disease

With liver disease, similar considerations apply. If phenothiazine-induced hepatotoxicity is suspected, then a challenge with a small, single test dose of a drug from a different chemical group should be followed by liver function tests after a few days. If no increase in levels of liver enzymes occurs, then gradual dose increases can be given, but regular liver function tests should continue. Isolated elevations of hepatic enzymes are not uncommon with both first- and second-generation anti-psychotics. Clinical hepatitis is much rarer but has been reported with sulpiride and clozapine. Depot drugs should be avoided, both because of their persistence and because compromised metabolism in the presence of continued release could lead to the accumulation of dangerous plasma levels.

Diabetes

This is not an uncommon problem, both because of the high prevalence of diabetes in schizophrenia and because of drug-induced effects. There is increasing evidence that glucose tolerance leading to frank diabetes mellitus can be a drug-induced effect of the second-generation anti-psychotics, particularly clozapine and olanzapine (see 'Adverse effects', above). If the cause is idiopathic or the offending drug cannot be changed (e.g. clozapine), symptomatic treatment with dietary intervention, oral hypoglycaemics or, occasionally, insulin will be required. The main points are to be aware of the possible diagnosis and that elixirs contain surprisingly large amounts of carbohydrate, which can destabilise diabetic control.

Epilepsy

If epilepsy develops, there is a risk of increasing the incidence of seizures. However, if there is adequate anticonvulsant 'cover', it is good clinical practice to give an adequate dose of an antipsychotic to control the psychotic symptoms. This is dealt with more fully in Chapter 10.

Breast cancer

There is a theoretical risk of increasing the risk of breast cancer because of the hyperprolactinaemia caused by these drugs, but no association has been found in epidemiological studies. If, however, breast cancer develops in a patient who has schizophrenia, it would be wise to avoid sulpiride, to use minimum doses of another antipsychotic and to monitor prolactin levels.

Alternatives to antipsychotics

When a patient develops an allergic or idiosyncratic reaction to an antipsychotic drug, it is usually possible to change to another anti-psychotic from a different chemical group. Nevertheless, if the NMS develops, all antipsychotics should be avoided, at least until the fever and rigidity have abated. If the patient continues to be psychotically disturbed, the safest first-line treatment should be a benzodiazepine, along the lines discussed above. Other alternatives are lithium, carbamazepine and ECT. Nevertheless, while the first two of these are useful adjuncts to antipsychotics, there is little evidence for their antipsychotic efficacy when used alone (Johnstone et al, 1988). ECT, however, can be a life-saving treatment in such situations (see Chapter 8).

Acknowledgements

JLW's studies are supported by the Stanley Medical Research Institute, the Higher Education Authority, a Galen Fellowship from the Irish Brain Research Foundation and the Royal College of Surgeons in Ireland.

DJK is indebted to Ms Julie Boucher and Mrs Maureen Henderson for typing and collating the manuscript.

References

Abi-Dargham, A., Rodenhiser, J., Printz, D., *et al* (2000) Increased baseline occupancy of D$_2$ receptors by dopamine in schizophrenia. *Proceedings of the National Academy of Sciences*, **97**, 8104–8109.

Adams, C., Duggans, L., Wahlbeck, K., *et al* (1998) The Cochrane Schizophrenia Group. *Schizophrenia Research*, **33**, 185–186.

Adamson, L., Curry, S. H., Bridges, P. K., *et al* (1973) Fluphenazine decanoate trial in chronic in-patient schizophrenics failing to absorb oral chlorpromazine. *Diseases of the Nervous System*, **34**, 181–191.

Adler, L. A., Angrist, B., Reiter, S., *et al* (1989) Neuroleptic-induced akathisia: a review. *Psychopharmacology*, **97**, 1–11.

Agelink, M. W., Majewski, T., Wurthmann, C., *et al* (2001) Effects of newer atypical antipsychotics on autonomic neurocardiac function: a comparison between amisulpride, olanzapine, sertindole, and clozapine. *Journal of Clinical Psychopharmacology*, **21**, 8–13.

Allison, D. B., Fontaine, K. R., Heo, M., *et al* (1999) The distribution of body mass index among individuals with and without schizophrenia. *Journal of Clinical Psychiatry*, **60**, 215–220.

Amidsen, A. (1964) Drug-produced obesity: experiences with chlorpromazine, perphenazine and clopenthixol. *Danish Medical Bulletin*, **11**, 182–189.

Arnt, J. & Skarsfeldt, D. (1998) Do novel antipsychotics have similar pharmacological characteristics? A review of the evidence. *Neuropsychopharmacology*, **18**, 63–101.

Arranz, M. J., Munro, J., Birkett, J., *et al* (2000) Pharmacogenetic prediction of clozapine response. *Lancet*, **355**, 1615–1616.

Ashby, C. R. & Wang, R. Y. (1996) Pharmacological actions of the atypical antipsychotic drug clozapine: a review. *Synapse*, **24**, 349–394.

Baastrup, P. C., Hollnagel, P., Sørensen, R., *et al* (1976) Adverse reactions in treatment with lithium carbonate and haloperidol. *Journal of the American Medical Association*, **236**, 2645–2646.

Balant-Gorgia, A. E. & Balant, L. (1987) Antipsychotic drugs. Clinical pharmacokinetics of potential candidates for plasma concentration monitoring. *Clinical Pharmacokinetics*, **13**, 65–90.

Baldessarini, R. J., Cohen, B. M. & Teicher, M. H. (1988) Significance of neuroleptic dose and plasma level in the pharmacological treatment of psychoses. *Archives of General Psychiatry*, **45**, 79–91.

Ban, T. A. & Lehmann, H. E. (1965) Skin pigmentation, a rare side effect of chlorpromazine. *Canadian Psychiatric Association Journal*, **10**, 112–124.

Ban, T. A., Guy, W. & Wilson, W. H. (1985) Neuroleptic-induced skin pigmentation in chronic hospitalized schizophrenic patients. *Canadian Journal of Psychiatry*, **30**, 406–408.

Barnas, C., Tauscher, J., Kufferle, B., *et al* (1997) [123]I IBZM SPECT imaging of dopamine-2 receptors in psychotic patients treated with zotepine. *European Neuropsychopharmacology*, **7** (suppl. 2), S215.

Barnes, T. R. E. (1987) The present status of tardive dyskinesia and akathisia in the treatment of schizophrenia. *Psychiatric Developments*, **4**, 301–319.

Barnes, T. R. E. (1990) Comment on the WHO Consensus Statement. Prophylactic use of anticholinergics in patients on long-term neuroleptic treatment. *British Journal of Psychiatry*, **156**, 413–414.

Barnes, T. R. E. & McPhillips, M. A. (1999) Critical analysis and comparison of the side-effect and safety profiles of the new antipsychotics. *British Journal of Psychiatry*, **174** (suppl. 38), 34–43.

Bench, C. J., Lammertsma, A. A., Grasby, P. M., *et al.* (1996) The time course of binding to striatal dopamine D2 receptors by the neuroleptic ziprasidone (CP-88,059-01) determined by positron emission tomography. *Psychopharmacology*, **124**, 141–147.

Bernard, C. (1865) *Introduction à la Médecine Expérimentale*. (English translation by H. C. Green, 1957, *An Introduction to the Study of Experimental Medicine*. New York: Dover Publications.)

Bick, P. A. & Hannah, A. L. (1986) Intramuscular lorazepam to restrain violent patients, *Lancet*, *i*, 206.

Bigliani, V., Mulligan, R. S., Acton, P. D., *et al* (1999) In vivo occupancy of striatal and temporal cortical D_2/D_3 dopamine receptors by typical antipsychotic drugs. *British Journal of Psychiatry*, **175**, 231–238.

Bigliani, V., Mulligan, R. S., Acton, P. D., *et al* (2000) Striatal and temporal cortical D_2/D_3 receptor occupancy by olanzapine and sertindole in vivo: a [^{123}I] epidepride single photon emission tomography (SPECT) study. *Psychopharmacology*, **150**, 132–140.

Bjørndal, N., Bjerre, M., Gerlach, J., *et al* (1980) High dosage haloperidol therapy in chronic schizophrenic patients: a double-blind study of clinical response, side effects, serum haloperidol, and serum prolactin. *Psychopharmacology*, **67**, 17–23.

Blake, T.-J., Tillery, C. E. & Reynolds, G. P. (1998) Antipsychotic drug affinities at alpha$_2$-adrenoceptor subtypes in post-mortem human brain. *Journal of Psychopharmacology*, **12**, 151–154.

Bodkin, J. A. (1990) Emerging uses for high potency benzodiazepines in psychotic disorders. *Journal of Clinical Psychiatry*, **51** (suppl.), 41–46.

Browne, F. W. A., Cooper, S. J., Wilson, R., *et al* (1988) Serum haloperidol levels and clinical response in chronic, treatment-resistant schizophrenic patients. *Journal of Psychopharmacology*, **2**, 94–103.

Buckley, N. & McManus, P. (1998). Fatal toxicity of drugs used in the treatment of psychotic illnesses. *British Journal of Psychiatry*, **172**, 461–464.

Bymaster, F. P., Calligaro, D. O., Falcone, J. F., *et al* (1996) Radioreceptor binding profile of the atypical antipsychotic olanzapine. *Neuropsychopharmacology*, **14**, 87–96.

Carlsson, A. & Lindqvist, M. (1963) Effect of chlorpromazine or haloperidol on formation of 3-methoxytyramine and normetanephrine in mouse brain. *Acta Pharmacologica et Toxicologica*, **20**, 140–144.

Carpenter, W. T., Conley, R. & Kirkpatrick, B. (2000) On schizophrenia and new generation drugs. *Neuropsychopharmacology*, **22**, 660–661.

Cassens, G., Inglis, A. K., Appelbaum, P. S., *et al* (1990) Neuroleptics: effects on neuropsychological function in chronic schizophrenic patients. *Schizophrenia Bulletin*, **16**, 477–499.

Clifford, J. J. & Waddington, J. L. (2000) Topographically based search for an 'ethogram' among a series of novel D_4 dopamine receptor agonists and antagonists. *Neuropsychopharmacology*, **22**, 538–544.

Clozapine Study Group (1993) The safety and efficacy of clozapine in severe treatment-resistant schizophrenic patients in the UK. *British Journal of Psychiatry*, **163**, 150–154.

Cohen, H., Loewenthal, U., Matar, M., *et al* (2001) Association of autonomic dysfunction and clozapine. Heart rate variability and risk for sudden death in patients with schizophrenia on long-term psychotropic medication. *British Journal of Psychiatry*, **179**, 167–171.

Committee on Safety of Medicines (1990) Cardiotoxic effects of pimozide. *Current Problems*, **29**, 1–2.

Coppens, H. J., Slooff, C. J., Paans, A. M. J., *et al* (1991) High central D_2-dopamine receptor occupancy as assessed with positron emission tomography in medicated but therapy-resistant schizophrenic patients. *Biological Psychiatry*, **29**, 629–634.

Coukell, A. J., Spencer, C. M. & Benfield, P. (1996) Amisulpride: a review of its pharmacodynamic and pharmacokinetic properties and therapeutic efficacy in the management of schizophrenia. *CNS Drugs*, **6**, 237–256.

Crane, G. E. (1973) Persistent dyskinesia. *British Journal of Psychiatry*, **122**, 395–405.

Crow, T. J., MacMillan, J. F., Johnson, A. L., *et al* (1986) The Northwick Park study of first episodes of schizophrenia. II. A randomised controlled trial of prophylactic neuroleptic treatment. *British Journal of Psychiatry*, **148**, 120–127.

Cunningham Owens, D. G. (1999) *A Guide to the Extrapyramidal Side-effects of Antipsychotic Drugs*. Cambridge: Cambridge University Press.

Cunningham Owens, D. G., Johnstone, E. C. & Frith, C. D. (1982) Spontaneous involuntary disorders of movement: their prevalence, severity, and distribution in chronic schizophrenics with and without treatment with neuroleptics. *Archives of General Psychiatry*, **39**, 452–461.

Daniel, D. G., Wozniak, P., Mack, R. J., *et al* (1998) Long-term efficacy and safety comparison of sertindole and haloperidol in the treatment of schizophrenia. *Psychopharmacology Bulletin*, **34**, 61–69.

Davis, R. & Markham A. (1997) Ziprasidone. *CNS Drugs*, **8**, 153–159.

Deakin, J. F. W. (2000) Glutamate, GABA and cortical circuitry in schizophrenia. In *The Psychopharmacology of Schizophrenia* (eds M. A. Reveley & J. F. W. Deakin), pp. 56–70. London: Arnold.

De Beaurepaire, R., Labelle, A., Naber, D., *et al* (1995) An open trial of the D_1 antagonist SCH 39166 in six cases of acute psychotic states. *Psychopharmacology*, **121**, 323–327.

De Haan, L., Lavalaye, J., Linszen, D., *et al* (2000) Subjective experience and striatal dopamine D_2 receptor occupancy in patients with schizophrenia stabilized by olanzapine or risperidone. *American Journal of Psychiatry*, **157**, 1019–1020.

Den Boer, J. A., van Megen, H. J. G. M., Fleischhacker, W. W., *et al* (1995) Differential effects of the D1–DA receptor antagonist SCH 39166 on positive and negative symptoms of schizophrenia. *Psychopharmacology*, **121**, 317–322.

Depoortere, R., Perrault, G. & Sanger, D. J. (1997) Potentiation of prepulse inhibition of the startle reflex in rats: pharmacological evaluation of the procedure as a model for detecting antipsychotic activity. *Psychopharmacology*, **132**, 366–374.

Dickey, W. (1991) The neuroleptic malignant syndrome. *Progress in Neurobiology*, **36**, 425–436.

Dillner, L. (1993) Inquiry says depot injections can kill. *BMJ*, **307**, 641.

Drake, R. E. & Ehrlich, H. (1985) Suicide attempts associated with akathisia. *American Journal of Psychiatry*, **142**, 499–501.

Dunn, C. J. & Fitton, A. (1996) Sertindole. *CNS Drugs*, **5**, 224–230.

Dursun, S. M., McIntosh, D. & Milliken, H. (1999) Clozapine plus lamotrigine in treatment resistant schizophrenia. *Archives of General Psychiatry*, **56**, 950.

Edwards, J. G. (1986) The untoward effects of antipsychotic drugs: pathogenesis and management. In *The Psychopharmacology and Treatment of Schizophrenia* (British Association for Psychopharmacology Monograph) (eds P. B. Bradley & S. R. Hirsh), pp. 403–441. Oxford: Oxford University Press.

Ehmann, T. S., Delva, J. J. & Beninger, R. J. (1987) Flupenthixol in chronic schizophrenic inpatients: a controlled comparison with haloperidol. *Journal of Clinical Psychopharmacology*, **3**, 173–175.

Ekbom, K. A. (1945) Restless legs. *Acta Psychiatrica Scandinavica*, **158** (suppl. 1), 1–123.

Ellenbroek, B. A. & Cools, A. R. (2000) Animal models for the negative symptoms of schizophrenia. *Behavioural Pharmacology*, **11**, 223–233.

Farde, L., Nordstrom, A. L., Wiesel, F. A., *et al* (1992) Positron emission tomographic analysis of central D_1 and D_2 dopamine receptor occupancy in patients treated with classical neuroleptics and clozapine. *Archives of General Psychiatry*, **49**, 538–544.

Farde, L., Suhara, T., Nyberg, S., *et al* (1997) A PET-study of [^{11}C]FLB 457 binding to extrastriatal D_2-dopamine receptors in healthy subjects and antipsychotic drug-treated patients. *Psychopharmacology*, **133**, 396–404.

Fischman, A. J., Bonab, A. A., Babich, J. W., *et al* (1996) Positron emission tomographic analysis of central 5-hydroxytryptamine$_2$ receptor occupancy in healthy volunteers treated with the novel antipsychotic agent, ziprasidone. *Journal of Pharmacology and Experimental Therapeutics*, **279**, 939–947.

Fitzgerald, P. B., Kapur, S., Remington, G., *et al* (2000) Predicting haloperidol occupancy of central dopamine D_2 receptors from plasma levels. *Psychopharmacology*, **149**, 1–5.

Flaherty, J. A. & Lahmeyer, H. W. (1978) Laryngeal–pharyngeal dystonia as a possible cause of asphyxia with haloperidol treatment. *American Journal of Psychiatry*, **135**, 1414–1415.

Frangou, S. & Byrne, P. (2000) How to manage the first episode of schizophrenia. *BMJ*, **321**, 522–523.

Frangou, S. & Murray, R. M. (2000) Pharmacological treatment strategies. In *Schizophrenia* (2nd edn) (eds S. Frangou & R. Murray), pp. 49–59. London: Martin Dunitz.

Fulton, B. & Goa, K. L. (1997) Olanzapine: a review of its pharmacological properties and therapeutic efficacy in the management of schizophrenia and related psychoses. *Drugs*, **53**, 281–298.

Gazi, L., Bobirnac, I., Danzeisen, M., *et al* (1999) Receptor density as a factor governing the efficacy of the dopamine D_4 receptor ligands, L-745,870 and U-101958 at human recombinant $D_{4.4}$ receptors expressed in CHO cells. *British Journal of Pharmacology*, **128**, 613–620.

Geddes, J., Freemantle, N., Harrison, P., *et al* (2000) Atypical antipsychotics in the treatment of schizophrenia: systematic overview and meta-regression analysis. *BMJ*, **321**, 1371–1376.

Gefvert, O., Bergstrom, M., Langstrom, B., *et al* (1998) Time course of central nervous dopamine-D_2 and 5-HT_2 receptor blockade and plasma drug concentrations after discontinuation of quetiapine (Seroquel®) in patients with schizophrenia. *Psychopharmacology* **135**, 119–126.

Green, M. F. (1996) What are the functional consequences of neurocognitive deficits in schizophrenia? *American Journal of Psychiatry*, **153**, 321–330.

Gunasekara, N. S. & Spencer, C. M. (1998) Quetiapine: a review of its use in schizophrenia. *CNS Drugs*, **9**, 325–340.

Hägg, S., Spigset, O. & Söderström, T. G. (2000) Association of venous thromboembolism and clozapine. *Lancet*, **355**, 1155–1156.

Heaton, R. K. & Crowley, T. J. (1981) Effects of psychiatric disorders and their somatic treatments on neuropsychological test results. In *Handbook of Clinical Neuropsychology* (eds S. B. Fliskov & T. J.Boll), pp. 481–525. New York: Wiley.

Heinz, A., Knable, M. B., Coppola, R., *et al* (1998) Psychomotor slowing, negative symptoms and dopamine receptor availability – an IBZM SPECT study in neuroleptic-treated and drug-free schizophrenic patients. *Schizophrenia Research*, **31**, 19–26.

Hertel, P., Fagerquist, M. V. & Svensson, T. H. (1999) Enhanced cortical dopamine output and antipsychotic-like effects of raclopride by α_2 adrenoceptor blockade. *Science*, **286**, 105–107.

Higgins, G. A. (1998) From rodents to recovery: development of animal models of schizophrenia. *CNS Drugs*, **9**, 59–68.

Hirsch, S. R. & Barnes, T. R. E. (1994) Clinical use of high-dose neuroleptics. *British Journal of Psychiatry*, **164**, 94–96.

Hirsch, S. R., Gaind, R., Rohde, P. D., *et al* (1973) Outpatient maintenance of chronic schizophrenic patients with long-acting fluphenazine: a double-blind placebo trial. *BMJ*, *i*, 633–637.

Hollister, L. E. & Kim, D. Y. (1982) Intensive treatment with haloperidol of treatment-resistant chronic schizophrenic patients. *American Journal of Psychiatry*, **139**, 1466–1468.

Hrib, N. J. (2000) The dopamine D_4 receptor: a controversial therapeutic target. *Drugs of the Future*, **25**, 587–611.

Ipsen, M., Zhang, Y., Dragsted, J., *et al* (1997) The antipsychotic drug sertindole is a specific inhibitor of alpha$_{1A}$-adrenoceptors in rat mesenteric small arteries. *European Journal of Pharmacology*, **336**, 29–35.

Johnson, D. A. W. (1978) Prevalence and treatment of drug-induced extrapyramidal symptoms. *British Journal of Psychiatry*, **132**, 27–30.

Johnson, D. A. W., Pasterski, G., Ludlow, J. M., *et al* (1983) The discontinuance of maintenance neuroleptic therapy in chronic schizophrenic patients: drug and social consequences. *Acta Psychiatrica Scandinavica*, **67**, 339–352.

Johnstone, E. C., Crow, T. J., Frith, C. D., *et al* (1978) Mechanism of the antipsychotic effect in the treatment of acute schizophrenia. *Lancet*, *i*, 848–851.

Johnstone, E. C., Frith, C. D., Crow, T. J., *et al* (1988) The Northwick Park 'Functional' Psychosis Study: diagnosis and treatment response. *Lancet*, *ii*, 119–125.

Jolley, A. G., Hirsch, S. R., Morrison, E., *et al* (1990) Trial of brief intermittent neuroleptic prophylaxis for selected schizophrenic outpatients: clinical and social outcome at two years. *BMJ*, **301**, 837–842.

Kane, J. M. (1999) Pharmacologic treatment of schizophrenia. *Biological Psychiatry*, **46**, 1396–1408.

Kane, J. M. & Lieberman, J. A. (1992) *Adverse Effects of Psychotropic Drugs*. New York: Guilford.

Kane, J. M. & Smith, J. M. (1982) Tardive dyskinesia. Prevalence and risk factors, 1959–1979. *Archives of General Psychiatry*, **39**, 473–481.

Kane, J. M., Honigfeld, G., Singer, J., *et al* (1988) Clozapine for the treatment-resistant schizophrenic. A double-blind comparison with chlorpromazine. *Archives of General Psychiatry*, **45**, 789–796.

Kang, J., Wang, L., Cai, F., *et al* (2000) High affinity blockade of the HERG cardiac K$^+$ channel by the neuroleptic pimozide. *European Journal of Pharmacology*, **392**, 137–140.

Kapur, S. & Remington, G. (1996) Serotonin–dopamine interaction and its relevance to schizophrenia. *American Journal of Psychiatry*, **153**, 466–476.

Kapur, S., Zipursky, R. B. & Remington, G. (1999) Clinical and theoretical implications of 5-HT$_2$ and D$_2$ receptor occupancy of clozapine, risperidone, and olanzapine in schizophrenia. *American Journal of Psychiatry*, **156**, 286–293.

Kapur, S., Zipursky, Jones, C., *et al* (2000*a*) Relationship between dopamine D$_2$ occupancy, clinical response, and side effects: a double-blind PET study of first-episode schizophrenia. *American Journal of Psychiatry*, **157**, 514–520.

Kapur, S., Zipursky, Jones, C., *et al* (2000*b*) A positron emission tomography study of quetiapine in schizophrenia. *Archives of General Psychiatry*, **57**, 553–559.

Karle, J., Clemmesen, L., Hansen, L., *et al* (1995) NNC 01-0687, a selective dopamine D1 receptor antagonist, in the treatment of schizophrenia. *Psychopharmacology*, **121**, 328–329.

Karlsson, P., Smith, L., Farde, L., *et al* (1995) Lack of apparent antipsychotic effect of the D$_1$-dopamine receptor antagonist SCH 39166 in acutely ill schizophrenic patients. *Psychopharmacology*, **121**, 309–316.

Kasper, S., Tauscher, J., Kufferle, B., *et al* (1998) Sertindole and dopamine D$_2$ receptor occupancy in comparison to risperidone, clozapine and haloperidol – a ^{123}I-IBZM SPECT study. *Psychopharmacology*, **136**, 367–373.

Kasper, S., Hale, A., Azorin, J. M., *et al* (1999) Benefit–risk evaluation of olanzapine, risperidone and sertindole in the treatment of schizophrenia. *European Archives of Psychiatry and Clinical Neuroscience*, **249** (suppl. 2), II12–II14.

Kebabian, J. W. & Calne, D. B. (1979) Multiple receptors for dopamine. *Nature*, **277**, 93–96.

Keefe, R. S. E., Silva, S. G., Perkins, D. O., *et al* (1999) The effects of atypical antipsychotic drugs on neurocognitive impairment in schizophrenia: a review and meta-analysis. *Schizophrenia Bulletin*, **25**, 201–222.

Kellam, A. M. P. (1987) The neuroleptic malignant syndrome, so-called: a survey of the world literature. *British Journal of Psychiatry*, **150**, 752–759.

Kemp, R., Hayward, P., Applewhaite, G., *et al* (1996) Compliance therapy in psychotic patients: randomised controlled trial. *BMJ*, **312**, 345–349.

Ketai, R., Matthews, J. & Mozdzen, J. J. (1979) Sudden death in a patient taking haloperidol. *American Journal of Psychiatry*, **136**, 112–113.

Kilian, J. G., Kerr, K., Lawrence, C., *et al* (1999) Myocarditis and cardiomyopathy associated with clozapine. *Lancet*, **354**, 1841–1845.

King, D. J. (1990) The effect of the neuroleptics on cognitive and psychomotor function. *British Journal of Psychiatry*, **157**, 799–811.

King, D. J. (1998) Atypical antipsychotics and the negative symptoms of schizophrenia. *Advances in Psychiatric Treatment*, **4**, 53–61.

King, D. J. & Green, J. F. (1996) Medication and cognitive functioning in schizophrenia. In *Schizophrenia: A Neuropsychological Perspective* (eds C. Pantelis, H. E. Nelson & T. R. E. Barnes), pp. 419–445. Chichester: Wiley.

King, D. J. & Mills, P. J. (1993) Clozapine: the Holywell experience with the first 24 patients. *Irish Journal of Psychological Medicine*, **10**, 30–34.

King, D. J., Blomqvist, M., Cooper, S. J., *et al* (1992) A placebo controlled trial of remoxipride in the prevention of relapse in chronic schizophrenia. *Psychopharmacology*, **107**, 175–179.

Kinon, B. J. & Lieberman, J. A. (1996) Mechanisms of action of atypical antipsychotic drugs: a critical analysis. *Psychopharmacology*, **124**, 2–34.

Kitayama, H., Kiuchi, K., Nejima, J., *et al* (1999) Long-term treatment with antipsychotic drugs in conventional doses prolonged QTc dispersion, but did not increase ventricular tachyarrhythmias in patients with schizophrenia in the absence of cardiac disease. *European Journal of Clinical Pharmacology*, **55**, 259–262.

Klawans, H. L., Goetz, C. & Perlik, S. (1980) Tardive dyskinesia: review and update. *American Journal of Psychiatry*, **137**, 900–908.

Knable, M. B., Heinz, A., Raedler, T., *et al* (1997) Extrapyramidal side effects with risperidone and haloperidol at comparable D_2 receptor occupancy levels. *Psychiatry Research: Neuroimaging*, **75**, 91–101.

Kornhuber, J., Schultz, A., Wiltfang, J., *et al* (1999) Persistence of haloperidol in human brain tissue. *American Journal of Psychiatry*, **156**, 885–890.

Kramer, M. S., Last, B., Getson, A., *et al* (1997) The effects of a selective D_4 dopamine receptor antagonist (L-745,870) in acutely psychotic inpatients with schizophrenia. *Archives of General Psychiatry*, **54**, 567–572.

Kuenstler, U., Juhnhold, U., Knapp, W. H., *et al* (1999) Positive correlation between reduction of handwriting area and D_2 dopamine receptor occupancy during treatment with neuroleptic drugs. *Psychiatry Research: Neuroimaging*, **90**, 31–39.

Kufferle, B., Tauscher, J., Asenbaum, S., *et al* (1997) IBZM SPECT imaging of striatal dopamine-2 receptors in psychotic patients treated with the novel antipsychotic substance quetiapine in comparison to clozapine and haloperidol. *Psychopharmacology*, **133**, 323–328.

Laruelle, M. & Abi-Dargham, A. (1999) Dopamine as the wind of the psychotic fire: new evidence from brain imaging studies. *Journal of Psychopharmacology*, **13**, 358–371.

Lawrie, S. M. (1999) Schizophrenia. In *Clinical Evidence. Issue 2* (ed. F. Godlee), pp. 385–395. London: BMJ Publishing Group.

Leff, J. P. & Wing, J. K. (1971) Trial of maintenance therapy in schizophrenia. *BMJ*, iii, 559–604.

Lehmann, H. E. & Hanrahan, G. E. (1954) Chlorpromazine. New inhibiting agent for psychomotor excitement and manic states. *Archives of Neurology and Psychiatry*, **71**, 227–237.

Lerner, Y., Lwow, E., Levitin, A., *et al* (1979) Acute high-dose parenteral haloperidol treatment of psychosis. *American Journal of Psychiatry*, **136**, 1061–1064.

Leucht, S., Pitschel-Walz, G., Abraham, D., *et al* (1999) Efficacy and extrapyramidal side-effects of the new antipsychotics olanzapine, quetiapine, risperidone and sertindole compared to conventional antipsychotics and placebo. A meta-analysis of randomized controlled trials. *Schizophrenia Research*, **35**, 51–68.

Levant, B. (1997) The D_3 dopamine receptor: neurobiology and potential clinical relevance. *Pharmacology Reviews*, **49**, 231–252.

Levenson, J. L. (1985) Neuroleptic malignant syndrome. *American Journal of Psychiatry*, **142**, 1137–1145.

Leysen, J. E. (2000) Receptor profile of antipsychotics. In *Atypical Antipsychotics* (eds B. A. Ellenbroek & A. R. Cools), pp. 57–81. Basel: Birkhauser.

Lidow, M. S., Williams, G. V. & Goldman-Rakic, P. S. (1998) The cerebral cortex: a case for a common site of action of antipsychotics. *Trends in Pharmacological Sciences*, **19**, 136–140.

Lidsky, T. I. (1995) Reevaluation of the mesolimbic hypothesis of antipsychotic drug action. *Schizophrenia Bulletin*, **21**, 67–74.

Lipska, B. K. & Weinberger, D. R. (2000) To model a psychiatric disorder in animals: schizophrenia as a reality test. *Neuropsychopharmacology*, **23**, 223–239.

Litman, R. E., Su, T. P., Potter, W. Z., *et al* (1996) Idazoxan and response to typical neuroleptics in treatment-resistant schizophrenia. Comparison with the atypical neuroleptic, clozapine. *British Journal of Psychiatry*, **168**, 571–579.

Loebel, A. D., Lieberman, J. A., Alvir, J. M. J., *et al* (1992) Duration of psychosis and outcome in first-episode schizophrenia. *American Journal of Psychiatry*, **149**, 1183–1188.

Loo, H., Poirier-Littre, M.-F., Theron, M., *et al* (1997) Amisulpride versus placebo in the medium-term treatment of the negative symptoms of schizophrenia. *British Journal of Psychiatry*, **170**, 18–22.

Loudon, J. B. (1987) Prescribing in pregnancy: psychotropic drugs. *BMJ*, **294**, 167–169.

Marsden, C. D. & Jenner, P. (1980) The pathophysiology of extrapyramidal side-effects of neuroleptic drugs. *Psychological Medicine*, **10**, 55–72.

Martinot, J. L., Pailliere-Martinot, M. L., Poirier, M. F., *et al* (1996) *In vivo* characteristics of dopamine D_2 receptor occupancy by amisulpride in schizophrenia. *Psychopharmacology*, **124**, 154–158.

Matsumoto, R. R. & Pouw, B. (2000) Correlation between neuroleptic binding to σ_1 and σ_2 receptors and acute dystonic reactions. *European Journal of Pharmacology* **401**, 155–160.

Maudsley Hospital (1999) *Maudsley Prescribing Guidelines* (5th edn) (eds D. Taylor, D. McConnell, H. McConnell, *et al*), pp. 21–37. London: Martin Dunitz.

May, P. R. A. & van Putten, T. (1978) Plasma levels of chlorpromazine in schizophrenia. A critical review of the literature. *Archives of General Psychiatry*, **35**, 1081–1087.

May, P. R. A., Tuma, A. H., Yale, C., *et al* (1976) Schizophrenia – a follow-up study of results of treatment. II. Hospital stay over two to five years. *Archives of General Psychiatry*, **33**, 481–486.

McCreadie, R. G. (2000) Recent advances in the drug treatment of schizophrenia. *Primary Care Psychiatry*, **6**, 9–14.

McEvoy, J. P., Hogarty, G. E. & Steingard, S. (1991) Optimal dose of neuroleptic in acute schizophrenia: a controlled study of the neuroleptic threshold and higher haloperidol dose. *Archives of General Psychiatry*, **48**, 739–745.

McGlashan, T. H. & Johannessen, J. O. (1966) Early detection and intervention with schizophrenia: rationale. *Schizophrenia Bulletin*, **22**, 201–222.

McGorry, P. D., Edwards, J., Mihalopoulos, C., *et al* (1996) EPPIC: an evolving system of early detection and optimal management. *Schizophrenia Bulletin*, **22**, 305–326.

McGrath, J. & Emmerson, W. B. (1999) Treatment of schizophrenia. *BMJ*, **319**, 1045–1048.

Meagher, D., Quinn, J., Murphy, P., *et al* (2001) Relationship of the factor structure of psychopathology in schizophrenia to the timing of initial intervention with antipsychotics. *Schizophrenia Research*, **50**, 95–103.

Medalia, A., Gold, J. & Merriam, A. (1988) The effect of neuroleptics on neuropsychological test results of schizophrenics. *Archives of Clinical Neuropsychology*, **3**, 249–271.

Mehtonen, O. P., Aranko, K., Mälkonen, L., *et al* (1991) A study of sudden death associated with the use of antipsychotic or antidepressant drugs. *Acta Psychiatrica Scandinavica*, **84**, 58–64.

Meisenzahl, E. M., Dresel, S., Frodl, T., *et al* (2000) D$_2$ receptor occupancy under recommended and high doses of olanzapine: an iodine-123-iodobenzamide SPECT study. *Journal of Psychopharmacology*, **14**, 364–370.

Meltzer, H. Y. (1992) Some personal recommendations about using clozaril. *Clozaril Newsletter*, no. 4, 1–3.

Meltzer, H. Y. (1999) The role of serotonin in antipsychotic drug action. *Neuropsychopharmacology*, **21**, 106S–115S.

Meltzer, H. Y. & McGurk, S. (1999) The effect of clozapine, risperidone and olanzapine in cognitive function in schizophrenia. *Schizophrenia Bulletin*, **25**, 233–256.

Meltzer, H. Y., Matsubara, S. & Lee, J-C. (1989) Classification of typical and atypical antipsychotic drugs on the basis of dopamine D-1, D-2 and serotonin2 pKi values. *Journal of Pharmacology and Experimental Therapeutics*, **251**, 238–246.

Millan, M. J., Dekeyne, A., Rivet, J-M., *et al* (2000) S33084, a novel, potent, selective, and competitive antagonist at dopamine D3-receptors: II. Functional and behavioural profile compared with GR218,231 and L741,626. *Journal of Pharmacology and Experimental Therapeutics*, **293**, 1063–1073.

Mir, S. & Taylor, D. (2001) Atypical antipsychotics and hyperglycaemia. *International Clinical Psychopharmacology*, **16**, 63–74.

Missale, C., Nash, S. R., Robinson, S. W., *et al* (1998) Dopamine receptors: from structure to function. *Physiological Review*, **78**, 189–225.

Modestin, J., Krapf, R. & Boker, W. (1981) A fatality during haloperidol treatment: mechanisms of sudden death. *American Journal of Psychiatry*, **138**, 1616–1617.

Mortimer, A. M. (1997) Cognitive function in schizophrenia – do neuroleptics make a difference? *Pharmacology, Biochemistry and Behavior*, **56**, 789–795.

Murdoch, P. S. & Williamson, J. (1982) A danger in making the diagnosis of Parkinson's disease. *Lancet*, *i*, 1212–1213.

National Institute of Mental Health (1964) Phenothiazine treatment in acute schizophrenia. *Archives of General Psychiatry*, **10**, 246–261.

National Institute for Clinical Excellence (2002) Guidance on the use of newer (atypical) antipsychotic drugs for the treatment of schizophrenia. *Technology Appraisal Guidance*, no. 43 (June).

Needham, P. L., Atkinson, J., Skill, M. J., *et al* (1996) Zotepine: preclinical tests predict antipsychotic efficacy and an atypical profile. *Psychopharmacology Bulletin*, **32**, 123–128.

Nemeroff, C. B., DeVane, C. L. & Pollock, B. G. (1996) Newer antidepressants and the cytochrome P450 system. *American Journal of Psychiatry*, **153**, 311–320.

Newman-Tancredi, A., Chaput, C., Verriele, L., *et al* (1996) Clozapine is a partial agonist at cloned, human serotonin 5-HT$_{1A}$ receptors. *Neuropharmacology*, **35**, 119–121.

Niznik, H. B., Sugamori, K. S., Clifford, J. J., *et al* (2002) D$_1$-like dopamine receptors: molecular biology and pharmacology. In *Handbook of Experimental Pharmacology: Dopamine in the CNS* (ed. G. Di Chiara), pp. 121–158. Heidelberg: Springer.

Nordstrom, A. L. & Farde, L. (1998) Plasma prolactin and central D$_2$ receptor occupancy in antipsychotic drug treated patients. *Journal of Clinical Psychopharmacology*, **18**, 305–310.

Nordstrom, A. L., Farde, L., Nyberg, S., *et al* (1995) D_1, D_2, and 5-HT_2 receptor occupancy in relation to clozapine serum concentration: a PET study of schizophrenic patients. *American Journal of Psychiatry*, **152**, 1444–1449.

Nordstrom, A. L., Nyberg, S., Olsson, H., *et al* (1998) Positron emission tomography finding of a high striatal D_2 receptor occupancy in olanzapine-treated patients. *Archives of General Psychiatry*, **55**, 283–284.

Nyberg, S., Farde, L. & Halldin, C. (1997) Delayed normalization of central D_2 dopamine receptor availability after discontinuation of haloperidol decanoate. *Archives of General Psychiatry*, **54**, 953–958.

Nyberg, S., Dencker, S. J., Malm, U., *et al* (1998) D_2- and 5-HT_2 receptor occupancy in high-dose neuroleptic-treated patients. *International Journal of Neuropsychopharmacology*, **1**, 95–101.

Nyberg, S., Eriksson, B., Oxenstierna, G., *et al* (1999) Suggested minimal effective dose of risperidone based on PET-measured D_2 and $5HT_{2A}$ receptor occupancy in schizophrenic patients. *American Journal of Psychiatry*, **156**, 869–875.

Pearlman, C. A. (1986) Neuroleptic malignant syndrome: a review of the literature. *Journal of Clinical Psychopharmacology*, **6**, 257–273.

Perrault, G. H., Depoortere, R., Morel, E., *et al* (1997) Psychopharmacological profile of amisulpride: an antipsychotic drug with presynaptic D_2/D_3 dopamine receptor antagonist activity and limbic selectivity. *Journal of Pharmacology and Experimental Therapeutics*, **280**, 73–82.

Pezawas, L., Quiner, S., Moertl, D., *et al* (2000) Efficacy, cardiac safety and tolerability of sertindole: a drug surveillance study. *International Clinical Psychopharmacology*, **15**, 207–214.

Pickar, D., Su, T.-P., Weinberger, D. R., *et al* (1996) Individual variation in D_2 dopamine receptor occupancy in clozapine-treated patients. *American Journal of Psychiatry*, **153**, 1571–1578.

Pilowsky, L. S., Ring, H., Shine, P. J., *et al* (1992) Rapid tranquillisation. A survey of emergency prescribing in a general psychiatric hospital. *British Journal of Psychiatry*, **160**, 831–835.

Pilowsky, L. S., Mulligan, R. S., Acton, P. D., *et al* (1997a) Limbic selectivity of clozapine. *Lancet*, **350**, 490–491.

Pilowsky, L. S., O'Connell, P., Davies, N., *et al* (1997b) In vivo effects on striatal dopamine D_2 receptor binding by the novel atypical antipsychotic drug sertindole – a ^{123}I IBZM single photon emission tomography (SPET) study. *Psychopharmacology*, **130**, 152–158.

Poyurovsky, M. & Weizman, A. (2001) Serotonin-based pharmacotherapy for acute neuroleptic-induced akathisia: a new approach to an old problem. *British Journal of Psychiatry*, **179**, 4–8.

Prakash, A. & Lamb, H. M. (1998) Zotepine: a review of its pharmacodynamic and pharmacokinetic properties and therapeutic efficacy in the management of schizophrenia. *CNS Drugs*, **9**, 153–175.

Prinssen, E. P. M., Kleven, M. S. & Koek, W. (1999) Interactions between neuroleptics and 5-HT_{1A} ligands in preclinical behavioral models for antipsychotic and extrapyramidal effects. *Psychopharmacology*, **144**, 20–29.

Quitkin, F., Rifkin, A. & Klein, D. F. (1975) Very high dose v. standard dosage fluphenazine in schizophrenia. A double-blind study of nonchronic treatment-refractory patients. *Archives of General Psychiatry*, **32**, 1276–1281.

Raedler, T. J., Knable, M. B., Lafargue, T., *et al* (1999) In vivo determination of striatal dopamine D_2 receptor occupancy in patients treated with olanzapine. *Psychiatry Research: Neuroimaging*, **90**, 81–90.

Raedler, T. J., Knable, M. B., Jones, D. W., *et al* (2000) In vivo olanzapine occupancy of muscarinic acetylcholine receptors in patients with schizophrenia. *Neuropsychopharmacology*, **23**, 56–68.

376

Rampe, D., Murawsky, M. K., Grau, J., *et al* (1998) The antipsychotic agent sertindole is a high affinity antagonist of the human cardiac potassium channel HERG. *Journal of Pharmacology and Experimental Therapeutics*, **286**, 788–793.

Reilly, J. G., Ayis, S. A., Ferrier, I. N., *et al* (2000) QTc-interval abnormalities and psychotropic drug therapy in psychiatric patients. *Lancet*, **355**, 1048–1052.

Remington, G. & Kapur, S. (2000) Atypical antipsychotics: are some more atypical than others? *Psychopharmacology*, **148**, 3–15.

Reynolds, G. P., Cowey, L., Rossor, M. N., *et al* (1982) Thioridazine is not specific for limbic dopamine receptors. *Lancet*, **ii**, 499–500.

Reynolds, G. P., Zhang, Z-J. & Zhang, X-B. (2002) Association of antipsychotic drug-induced weight gain with a 5-HT$_{2C}$ receptor gene polymorphism. *Lancet*, **359**, 2086–2087.

Richelson, E. & Nelson, A. (1984) Antagonism by neuroleptics of neurotransmitter receptors of normal human brain *in vitro*. *European Journal of Pharmacology*, **103**, 197–204.

Rifkin, A., Quitkin, F., Carrillo, C., *et al* (1971) Very high dosage fluphenazine for nonchronic treatment-refactory patients. *Archives of General Psychiatry*, **25**, 398–403.

Rifkin, A., Doddi, S., Karajgi, B., *et al* (1991) Dosage of haloperidol for schizophrenia. *Archives of General Psychiatry*, **48**, 166–170.

Rollema, H., Lu, Y., Schmidt, A. W., *et al* (1997) Clozapine increases dopamine release in prefrontal cortex by 5-HT$_{1A}$ receptor activation. *European Journal of Pharmacology*, **338**, R3–R5.

Rosenheck, R., Dunn, L., Peszke, M., *et al* (1999) Impact of clozapine on negative symptoms and on the deficit syndrome in refractory schizophrenia. *American Journal of Psychiatry*, **156**, 88–93.

Royal College of Psychiatrists (1997) *The Association Between Antipsychotic Drugs and Sudden Death* (Council Report CR57). London: Royal College of Psychiatrists.

Sams-Dodd, F. (1999) Phencyclidine in the social interaction test: an animal model of schizophrenia with face and predictive validity. *Reviews in the Neurosciences*, **10**, 59–90.

Sanchez, C., Arnt, J., Dragsted, N., *et al* (1991) Neurochemical and in vivo pharmacological profile of sertindole, a limbic-selective neuroleptic compound. *Drug Development Research*, **22**, 239–250.

Schlegel, S., Schlosser, R., Hiemke, C., *et al* (1996) Prolactin plasma levels and D$_2$-dopamine receptor occupancy measured with IBZM-SPECT. *Psychopharmacology*, **124**, 285–287.

Schoemaker, H., Claustre, Y., Fage, D., *et al* (1997) Neurochemical characteristics of amisulpride, an atypical dopamine D$_2$/D$_3$ receptor antagonist with both presynaptic and limbic selectivity. *Journal of Pharmacology and Experimental Therapeutics*, **280**, 83–97.

Schotte, A., Janssen, P. F., Gommeren, W., *et al* (1996) Risperidone compared with new and reference antipsychotic drugs: in vitro and in vivo receptor binding. *Psychopharmacology*, **124**, 57–73.

Seeman, P. (1980) Brain dopamine receptors. *Pharmacological Reviews*, **32**, 229–313.

Seeman, P. (1992) Dopamine receptor sequences: therapeutic levels of neuroleptics occupy D$_2$ receptors, clozapine occupies D$_4$. *Neuropsychopharmacology*, **7**, 261–284.

Seeman, P. & Tallerico, T. (1998) Antipsychotic drugs which elicit little or no Parkinsonism bind more loosely than dopamine to brain D$_2$ receptors, yet occupy high levels of these receptors. *Molecular Psychiatry*, **3**, 123–134.

Seeman, P. & Tallerico, T. (1999) Rapid release of antipsychotic drugs from dopamine D$_2$ receptors: an explanation for low receptor occupancy and early clinical relapse upon withdrawal of clozapine or quetiapine. *American Journal of Psychiatry*, **156**, 876–884.

Seeman, P. & Ulpian, C. (1983) Neuroleptics have identical potencies in human brain limbic and putamen regions. *European Journal of Pharmacology*, **94**, 145–148.

Seeman, P., Corbett, R. & Van Tol, H. H. M. (1997) Atypical neuroleptics have low affinity for dopamine D_2 receptors or are selective for D_4 receptors. *Neuropsychopharmacology*, **16**, 93–110.

Sekine, Y., Rikihisa, T., Ogata, H., *et al* (1999) Correlations between in vitro affinity of antipsychotics to various central neurotransmitter receptors and clinical incidence of their adverse drug reactions. *European Journal of Clinical Pharmacology*, **55**, 583–587.

Shalev, A., Hermesh, H. & Munitz, H. (1989) Mortality from neuroleptic malignant syndrome. *Journal of Clinical Psychiatry*, **50**, 18–25.

Sharma, T. (1999) Cognitive effects of conventional and atypical antipsychotics in schizophrenia. *British Journal of Psychiatry*, **174** (suppl. 38), 44–51.

Silke, B., Campbell, C. & King, D. J. (2002) The potential cardiotoxicity of antipsychotic drugs as assessed by heart rate variability. *Journal of Psychopharmacology*, **16**, 355–360.

Simpson, G. M., Josiassen, R. C., Stanilla, J. K., *et al* (1999) Double-blind study of clozapine dose response in chronic schizophrenia. *American Journal of Psychiatry*, **156**, 1744–1750.

Sokoloff, P., Martres, M.-P., Giros, B., *et al* (1992) The third dopamine receptor (D_3) as a novel target for antipsychotics. *Biochemical Pharmacology*, **43**, 659–666.

Sprouse, J. S., Reynolds, L. S., Braselton, J. P., *et al* (1999) Comparison of the novel antipsychotic ziprasidone with clozapine and olanzapine: inhibition of dorsal raphe cell firing and the role of 5-HT_{1A} receptor activation. *Neuropsychopharmacology*, **21**, 622–631.

Sugamori, K. S., Hamadanizadeh, S. A., Scheideler, M. A., *et al* (1998) Functional differentiation of multiple dopamine D_1-like receptors by NNC 01-0012. *Journal of Neurochemistry*, **71**, 1685–1693.

Swerdlow, N. R., Varty, G. B. & Geyer, M. A. (1998) Discrepant findings of clozapine effects on prepulse inhibition of startle: is it the route or the rat? *Neuropsychopharmacology*, **18**, 50–56.

Tarazi, F. I. & Baldessarini, R. J. (1999) Dopamine D_4 receptors: significance for molecular psychiatry at the millennium. *Molecular Psychiatry*, **4**, 529–538.

Tauscher, J., Kufferle, B., Asenbaum, S., *et al* (1999) In vivo ^{123}I IBZM SPECT imaging of striatal dopamine-2 receptor occupancy in schizophrenic patients treated with olanzapine in comparison to clozapine and haloperidol. *Psychopharmacology*, **141**, 175–181.

Taylor, D. (2000) Low dose typical antipsychotics – a brief evaluation. *Psychiatric Bulletin*, **24**, 465–468.

Thompson, C. (1994) The use of high-dose antipsychotic medication. *British Journal of Psychiatry*, **164**, 448–458.

Thompson, T. R., Lal, S., Yassa, R., *et al* (1988) Resolution of chlorpromazine-induced pigmentation with haloperidol substitution. *Acta Psychiatrica Scandinavica*, **78**, 763–765.

Travis, M. J., Busatto, G. F., Pilowsky, L. S., *et al* (1997) Serotonin: 5-HT_{2A} receptor occupancy *in vivo* and response to the new antipsychotics olanzapine and sertindole. *British Journal of Psychiatry*, **171**, 290–291.

Travis, M. J., Busatto, G. F., Pilowsky, L. S., *et al* (1998) 5-HT_{2A} receptor blockade in patients with schizophrenia treated with risperidone or clozapine. A SPET study using the novel 5-HT_{2A} ligand ^{123}I-5-I-R-91150. *British Journal of Psychiatry*, **173**, 236–241.

Trichard, C., Paillere-Martinot, M. L., Attar-Levy, D., *et al* (1998) Binding of antipsychotic drugs to cortical 5-HT_{2A} receptors: a PET study of chlorpromazine, clozapine, and amisulpride in schizophrenic patients. *American Journal of Psychiatry*, **155**, 505–508.

Truffinet, P., Tamminga, C. A., Fabre, L. F., *et al* (1999) Placebo-controlled study of the D_4/5-HT_{2A} antagonist fananserin in the treatment of schizophrenia. *American Journal of Psychiatry*, **156**, 419–425.

van Putten, T., Marder, S. R. & Mintz, J. (1990) A controlled dose comparison of haloperidol in newly admitted schizophrenic patients. *Archives of General Psychiatry*, **47**, 754–758.

Van Tol, H. H. M., Bunzow, J. R., Guan, H.-C., *et al* (1991) Cloning of the gene for a human dopamine D$_4$ receptor with high affinity for the antipsychotic clozapine. *Nature*, **350**, 610–614.

Volavka, J., Cooper, T., Czobor, P., *et al* (1992) Haloperidol blood levels and clinical effects. *Archives of General Psychiatry*, **49**, 354–361.

Waddington, J. L. (1987) Tardive dyskinesia in schizophrenia and other disorders: associations with ageing, cognitive dysfunction and structural brain pathology in relation to neuroleptic exposure. *Human Psychopharmacology*, **2**, 11–22.

Waddington, J. L. (1992) Mechanisms of neuroleptic-induced extrapyramidal side effects. In *Adverse Effects of Psychotropic Drugs* (eds J. M. Kane & J. A. Lieberman), pp. 246–265. New York: Guilford Press.

Waddington, J. L. (1993) Pre- and postsynaptic D-1 to D-5 dopamine receptor mechanisms in relation to antipsychotic activity. In *Antipsychotic Drugs and Their Side Effects* (ed. T. R. E. Barnes), pp. 65–85. London: Academic Press.

Waddington, J. L. & Casey, D. E. (2000) Comparative pharmacology of classical and novel (second-generation) antipsychotics. In *Schizophrenia and Mood Disorders: The New Drug Therapies in Clinical Practice* (eds P. F. Buckley & J. L. Waddington), pp. 3–13. Oxford: Butterworth Heinemann.

Waddington, J. L. & Morgan, M. M. (2001) Pathobiology of schizophrenia: implications for clinical management and treatment. In *Comprehensive Care of Schizophrenia: A Handbook of Clinical Management and Treatment* (eds R. M. Murray & J. A. Lieberman), pp. 27–35. London: Martin Dunitz.

Waddington, J. L. & O'Callaghan, E. (1997) What makes an antipsychotic 'atypical'? *CNS Drugs*, **7**, 341–346.

Waddington, J. L. & Youssef, H. A. (1986) Late onset involuntary movements in chronic schizophrenia: relationship of 'tardive' dyskinesia to intellectual impairment and negative symptoms. *British Journal of Psychiatry*, **149**, 616–620.

Waddington, J. L., Daly, S. A., McCauley, P. G., *et al* (1994) Levels of functional interaction between 'D-1-like' and 'D-2-like' dopamine receptor systems. In *Dopamine Receptors* (ed. H. B. Niznik), pp. 511–537. New York: Marcel Dekker.

Waddington, J. L., Scully, P. J. & O'Callaghan, E. (1997) The new antipsychotics, and their potential for early intervention in schizophrenia. *Schizophrenia Research*, **28**, 207–222.

Waddington, J. L., Deveney, A. M., Clifford, J. J., *et al* (1998) D$_1$-like dopamine receptors: regulation of psychomotor behavior, D$_1$-like: D$_2$-like interactions and effects of D$_{1A}$ targeted gene deletion. In *Dopamine Receptor Subtypes* (eds P. Jenner & R. Demirdamar), pp. 45–63. Amsterdam: IOS Press.

Waddington, J. L., Kapur, S. & Remington, G. (2003) The neuroscience and clinical psychopharmacology of first- and second-generation antipsychotic drugs in schizophrenia. In *Schizophrenia* (2nd edn) (eds S. R. Hirsch & D. R. Weinberger), pp. 421–441. Blackwell: Oxford.

Wadenberg, M. L. (1996) Serotonergic mechanisms in neuroleptic-induced catalepsy in the rat. *Neuroscience and Biobehavioral Reviews*, **20**, 325–339.

Wahlbeck, K., Cheine, M., Essali, A., *et al* (1999) Evidence of clozapine's effectiveness in schizophrenia: a systematic review and meta-analysis of randomized trials. *American Journal of Psychiatry*, **156**, 990–999.

Warner, J. P., Barnes, T. R. E. & Henry, J. A. (1996) Electrocardiographic changes in patients receiving neuroleptic medication. *Acta Psychiatrica Scandinavica*, **93**, 311–313.

Wolkin, A., Barouche, F., Wolf, A. P., *et al* (1989) Dopamine blockade and clinical response: evidence for two biological subgroups of schizophrenia. *American Journal of Psychiatry*, **146**, 905–908.

Worsley, A. J. (2000) Psychiatric disorders. In *Therapeutics in Pregnancy and Lactation* (eds A. Lee, S. Inch & D. Finnegan), pp. 101–116. Oxford: Radcliffe Medical Press.

Wykes, T., Sturt, E. & Katz, R. (1990) The prediction of rehabilitative success after three years. The use of social, symptom and cognitive variables. *British Journal of Psychiatry*, **157**, 865–870.

Young, C. D., Meltzer, H. Y. & Deutch, A. Y. (1998) Effects of desmethylclozapine on fos protein expression in the forebrain: in vivo biological activity of the clozapine metabolite. *Neuropsychopharmacology*, **19**, 99–103.

Youngren, K. D., Inglis, F. M., Pivirotto, P. J., *et al* (1999) Clozapine preferentially increases dopamine release in the Rhesus monkey prefrontal cortex compared with the caudate nucleus. *Neuropsychopharmacology*, **20**, 403–412.

Zarifian, E., Scatton, B., Bianchetti, G., *et al* (1982) High doses of haloperidol in schizophrenia. A clinical, biochemical, and pharmacokinetic study. *Archives of General Psychiatry*, **39**, 212–215.

Zimbroff, D. L., Ane, J. M., Tamminga, C. A., *et al* (1997) Controlled, dose–response study of sertindole and haloperidol in the treatment of schizophrenia. *American Journal of Psychiatry*, **154**, 782–791.

Zornberg, G. L. & Jick, H. (2000) Antipsychotic drug use and risk of first-time idiopathic venous thromboembolism: a case-control study. *Lancet*, **356**, 1219–1223.

Further reading

Barnes, T. R. E. & McPhillips, M. A. (1999) Critical analysis and comparison of the side-effect and safety profiles of the new antipsychotics. *British Journal of Psychiatry*, **174** (suppl. 38), 34–43.

Buckley, P. F. & Waddington, J. L. (eds) (2000) *Schizophrenia and Mood Disorders: The New Drug Therapies in Clinical Practice*. Oxford: Butterworth Heinemann.

Cunningham Owens, D. G. (1999) *A Guide to the Extrapyramidal Side-effects of Antipsychotic Drugs*. Cambridge: Cambridge University Press.

Kupfer, D. J. & Sartorius, N. (eds) (2002) The usefulness and use of second-generation antipsychotic medications. *Current Opinion in Psychiatry*, **15** (suppl. 1), S1–S51.

Leonard, B. E. (1997) *Fundamentals of Psychopharmacology* (2nd edn). Chichester: Wiley.

Miyamoto, S., Duncan, G. E., Goff, D. C., *et al* (2002) Therapeutics of schizophrenia. In *Neuropsychopharmacology: The Fifth Generation of Progress* (eds K. L. Davis, D. Charney, J. T. Coyle, *et al*), pp. 775–807. Philadelphia: Lippincott, Williams & Wilkins.

Reveley, M. A. & Deakin, J. F. W. (2000) *The Psychopharmacology of Schizophrenia*. London: Arnold.

CHAPTER 10

Anti-epileptic drugs

Robert J. McClelland and James I. Morrow

The nature and causes of epilepsy

Definitions

The Commission on Epidemiology and Prognosis of the International League Against Epilepsy (1993) defined epilepsy as a condition characterised by recurrent, that is two or more, epileptic seizures unprovoked by any immediately identifiable cause. An epileptic seizure is an intermittent, stereotyped disturbance of behaviour, emotion, motor function or sensation that is presumed to result from an abnormal and excessive discharge of cortical neurons. Epilepsy is a clinical manifestation of diverse underlying conditions, a final common pathway, at the basis of which there are recurrent, paroxysmal, disorderly discharges of cerebral neurons.

Pathophysiology

Several discrete abnormalities in nerve cell physiology are now believed to underlie the epileptic process. The relative contribution of each of these mechanisms varies between the different kinds of epilepsy. This is of relevance to the modes of action of the different anticonvulsant drugs. In the epilepsies that begin focally, small recurring depolarisations in the 'epileptic' neuron, termed paroxysmal depolarisation shifts (PDS), are a characteristic feature of the neuron between seizure episodes (Matsumoto & Ajmone-Marsan, 1964). The development of seizures depends on an impairment in the balance between excitation and inhibition, reflecting net balances in Na^+, Ca^{2+}, K^+ and Cl^- ion currents. Fundamental to epileptogenesis is an imbalance in favour of excitation

---

The authors pay tribute to George Fenton, the original author of this chapter, who died in 2001. George was an international expert on the psychiatric aspects of epilepsy, whose obvious academic abilities were always tempered by his unique human touch.

in a given neural population. This may be the result of specific disease processes, such as gliosis, or as part of a genetically expressed imbalance.

During the seizure itself, prolonged membrane depolarisations occur. The PDS appear to be triggered by burster cells. While such cells normally occur among cortical neurons, it has been shown that a small down-regulation of K^+ currents may turn ordinary cells into burster cells. These cells in turn recruit other cells into inter-ictal discharge, particularly if excitatory coupling is increased (Connors & Gutnick, 1984). Positive feedback loops are probably involved in seizure development (Jones & Lambert, 1990).

The epileptigenic process can spread to recruit large populations of normal nerve cells, and even the whole cortex of both cerebral hemispheres. When the discharging area is extensive, a clinical seizure occurs. The clinical phenomena of the fit reflect the function of the area of brain affected, through excitation or inhibition of the populations of neurons involved.

In primary generalised non-convulsive seizures (e.g. absence seizures) the fundamental abnormality appears to be depolarising after potentials in nerve cells (Coulter *et al*, 1989). Different strands of evidence point to either a cortical origin or thalamic origin in different forms of primary generalised epilepsy. Again, an imbalance of excitation over inhibition occurs (Gloor, 1988). This in turn increases the sensitivity of cortical neurons, with lateral synchronisation of cortical columns leading to the generation of generalised seizures with the characteristic spike-wave discharge observed in the electroencephalogram (EEG). The predominant expression of primary generalised epilepsy in childhood is consistent with the evidence of relatively late maturation of inhibitory systems within the central nervous system (CNS) (Luhmann & Prince, 1991).

Seizure termination

During seizures, several mechanisms are initiated which ultimately lead to a termination of seizures. These include acidification of the extracellular fluid, activation of the Na^+ pump and the release of adenosine triphosphate (ATP) and related substances. All of these activate K^+ conductances, which restores the balance of repolarisation and depolarisation.

Classification of seizures

The present internationally agreed classification of seizures categorises seizures as either partial (focal or localisation-related) or generalised (Commission on Classification and Terminology of the International League Against Epilepsy, 1981). Generalised seizures involve large areas of the brain, usually bilateral in their initial manifestations, which include impairment of consciousness, absence seizures, in which there is only impairment of consciousness, and generalised tonic/clonic seizures.

Partial seizures arise from specific locations within the cerebral cortex and are further subclassified according to whether consciousness is retained (simple partial seizure) or impaired (complex partial seizure) or spreads to involve the entire cortex, causing a generalised seizure (when it is termed a secondary generalised seizure). When the abnormal neuronal discharge remains confined to a specific cortical area, it may elicit a conscious sensation or motor phenomena, which may be described by the patient as a warning or aura. Such phenomena are manifestations of a simple partial seizure, which may lead to either a complex partial seizure or secondary generalisation, or both.

Classification of epilepsies

The Commission on Classification and Terminology of the International League Against Epilepsy (1989) defined an epileptic syndrome as follows:

'an epileptic disorder characterised by a cluster of cells customarily occurring together; these include such items as type of seizure, aetiology, anatomy, precipitating factors, age of onset, severity, chronicity, diurnal and circadian cycling and sometimes prognosis.'

In spite of this all-embracing attempt at categorisation, two main divisions continue to be widely used: first, whether the associated seizures are generalised from onset or partial in type; second, whether the epilepsy has a known aetiology (symptomatic), is idiopathic (no evidence of structural pathology) or is of unknown cause (Box 10.1). Within general adult psychiatry late-onset epileptic seizures are predominantly partial in type and symptomatic in origin.

The fundamental basis for this categorisation is the differentiation between partial and generalised seizures. Given that both may ultimately be manifest as a generalised seizure, the separation is crucially based on the early seizure manifestation or the EEG. Approximately 40% of adults presenting with partial epilepsy of late onset have an underlying cerebral tumour (Sander *et al*, 1990) and cerebrovascular disease is estimated to account for 50% of those developing epilepsy after the age of 50 (Shorvon *et al*, 1994).

Epidemiology, natural history, aetiology

Incidence rates for epilepsy in various studies range between 20 and 50 per 100 000 per year, with a lifetime cumulative incidence of around 3% (Hauser & Kurland, 1975; Shorvon, 1990). Point prevalence rates in the

---

Box 10.1 Summary of the international classification of epilepsies and epileptic syndromes

1   Localisation-related (focal, local, partial) epilepsies and syndromes
1.1   Idiopathic
        Benign childhood epilepsy with centrotemporal spikes
        Childhood epilepsy with occipital paroxysms
        Primary reading epilepsy
1.2   Symptomatic
1.2.1   Epilepsy characterised by simple partial seizures
1.2.2   Characterised by complex partial seizures
1.2.3   Characterised by secondarily generalised seizures
1.3   Unknown as to whether the syndrome is idiopathic or symptomatic

2   Generalised epilepsies and syndromes
2.1   Idiopathic
2.2   Cryptogenic or symptomatic
2.3   Symptomatic
2.3.1   Non-specific aetiology:
        Early myoclonic encephalopathy
2.3.2   Specific syndromes: epileptic seizures may complicate many disease
        states.
        Under this heading are included those diseases in which seizures are a
        presenting or predominant feature.

3   Epilepsies and syndromes undermined, whether focal or generalised
3.1   With both generalised and focal seizures: neonatal seizures

4   Special syndromes
4.1   Situation-related seizures
        Febrile convulsions
        Isolated seizures or isolated status epilepticus
        Seizures occurring only when there is an acute metabolic or toxic event,
        due to, for example, alcohol, drugs, eclampsia, non-ketotic hyper-
        glycaemia, uraemia, etc.

Source: Commission on Classification and Terminology of the International League Against Epilepsy (1989).

---

general population are much higher (4–10 per 1000 for active epilepsy), with a lifetime prevalence (a measure of the number of people in a population who have ever had epilepsy) of between 2% and 5%. The difference between prevalence and incidence reflects the temporary nature of the condition in many people.

Incidence and prevalence vary with age, being highest in early childhood, falling dramatically in early adult life, and rising again among those over 50 years of age. As many as 1 in 20 people in the general population will have had an epileptic seizure at some time in their life, and 1 in 200 will have recurring seizures (epilepsy). Epilepsy is slightly more common in males and in the lower socio-economic groups.

The standardised mortality rate is high. In about 25% of people who have ever had epilepsy, death may be related to a seizure (status epilepticus), accidental injury or sudden unexplained death. Suicide and cerebral tumours are also over-represented as causes of death.

Genetic factors are predominant in the primary generalised epilepsies, for which an autosomal dominant inheritance with age-specific penetrance is proposed, although a polygenic inheritance is also possible. Epilepsy is an important feature of more than 140 single-gene disorders, mostly autosomal recessive in character, and for two-thirds of these mental retardation, with or without epilepsy, is also characteristic. Nonspecific genetic factors also increase the susceptibility to symptomatic epilepsy in patients with acquired cerebral lesions.

Chronic lesions, both diffuse and focal, of the cerebral cortex have a much higher probability of causing (acquired) epilepsy than do subcortical lesions. The precise area in which the cortical lesion occurs determines its degree of epileptogenicity. The frontal and occipital polar regions are areas of low epileptic propensity, while the central area, near the Rolandic fissure, the medial hemispheric regions, and the temporal lobe, appear to be particularly epileptogenic, regardless of the underlying pathology.

Virtually any cerebral pathology can cause epilepsy, including heredofamilial diseases (e.g. tuberose sclerosis, the leucodystrophies, the lipodoses, Lafora's disease and phenylketonuria), metabolic brain disease, perinatal brain damage, anoxic brain damage due to severe infantile convulsions, intracranial infections (abscess, encephalitis and meningitis), head injury, cerebrovascular disorders, cerebral tumours and degenerative diseases of the brain.

Around three-quarters of people with epilepsy have no evidence of an underlying structural lesion of the CNS. The most complete data available are the thorough studies in Rochester, Minnesota, from 1935 to 1967 (Hauser & Kurland, 1975). Of this sample of 516 patients, only 23% had epilepsy of known cause: 2% birth injury, 4% congenital abnormalities, 4% postnatal head injuries, 3% infections, 5% vascular lesions, 4% cerebral tumours and 0.6% degenerative lesions.

The neuropathology of specimens taken from patients undergoing anterior temporal lobectomy for intractable temporal lobe epilepsy is of special interest to psychiatrists. About 50% show mesial temporal sclerosis, with loss of nerve cells in the amygdala and hippocampal areas accompanied by fibrosis, gliosis and atrophy, possibly due to hypoxia caused by severe infantile convulsions. Another 20% have small, circumscribed foci of abnormal (alien) tissue (hamartomas), probably of congenital or developmental origin. The presence of the latter was thought to be associated with schizophrenia-like psychoses

(Falconer, 1973). Recent work suggests that this relationship relates specifically to a subset of such alien-tissue lesions. These are ganglio-gliomas (clumps of abnormal glia and neurons resembling ganglion cells and showing abnormal shape, orientation or processes), which differ from the other alien-tissue lesions in having a mesial medial temporal lobe location, an early age at first fit, and a strong association with the development of a schizophrenia-like psychosis (Roberts *et al*, 1990).

A number of factors may precipitate a fit in susceptible people or may exacerabate established epilepsy, for example sleep deprivation, hyper-ventilation, hypoglycaemia, antidepressant and neuroleptic drugs, alcohol and drug withdrawal, high fever, anoxia, and the stimuli of reflex epilepsy. Reflex epilepsy – fits occurring as a direct reflex response to a specific stimulus – is experienced by 1–6% of people with epilepsy. The most common stimulus modality is the visual one, although every sensory system has been incriminated. Various types of mental and motor activity may also trigger fits.

Complex partial and secondarily generalised seizures account for about 60% of active cases of epilepsy, primary generalised seizures about 30% and generalised absence (petit mal) and myoclonus less than 5% (Hauser & Kurland, 1975; Juul-Jensen & Foldsprang, 1983). In the UK National General Practice Study of Epilepsy (Sander *et al*, 1990) – a prospective cohort population study – a secondarily generalised seizure was the first fit in 36%, a primary generalised tonic/clonic seizure in 33%, a simple partial seizure in 4%, an absence seizure in 1% and myoclonus in 1%. About a third of active cases have less than one seizure a year, a third 1–12 seizures a year, a third more than one seizure a month.

Earlier, hospital-based data suggested a poor prognosis, with two-thirds of patients with epilepsy having a chronic course. However, more recent, community-based studies indicate that the earlier findings were biased by an excess of refractory cases referred for tertiary hospital treatment (Rodin, 1968). One large general-practice study has shown that in 65% of people with epilepsy, the seizure disorder lasted for less than 5 years followed by long-term remission; a further 13% remitted and then relapsed; only 22% had chronic unremitting epilepsy (Goodridge & Shorvon, 1983*a,b*). Hence, people developing epilepsy for the first time can be subdivided into two distinct groups:

(1) almost 80% who have a mild seizure disorder of limited duration
(2) just over 20% who develop a chronic, potentially disabling intractable epilepsy and a formidable array of possible epilepsy-related and psychosocial handicaps that may impair psychosocial adjustment (Table 10.1).

Table 10.1 Consequences of epilepsy

Possible feature of epilepsy	Consequence
Occurrence of seizures	
Frequent fits	Trauma to body and brain
	Restriction of activities
	Anxiety and loss of internal locus of control, and 'learned helplessness'
	Discrimination/stigma by peers and general public
Cerebral dysfunction	
Diffuse brain damage	Low IQ
	Impaired impulse control
Focal temporal lobe damage	More severe epilepsy
	Specific learning deficits
	Reduced impulse control
	Possibly enhanced sensory–limbic connections with altered interpretation of environmental stimuli
Frequent epileptic discharges:	
clinical	Restricted social, educational and work opportunities
subclinical	Impaired information processing
Medication	Cognition impaired
	Dysphoria
	Reduced impulse control
	Low levels of folate, calcium and sex hormones
Family attitudes	
Parental over-protectiveness	Undue dependence on family
	Reduced peer group interaction
	Limited development of social skills
	Problems on becoming independent as a teenager
	Lifelong passive dependent attitudes
Perceptions of person's potential too low or too high	Problems at school and at work
Discrimination	
On the part of peers, teachers, employers, general public	Problems finding friends and appropriate educational, leisure and work opportunities, low self-esteem, depression/self-pity, paranoid attitudes, stigma
Self-perception	Low self-esteem, learned helplessness, external locus of control, dependent attitudes, limited social skills, limited social orbit, depression/pessimism, paranoid attitudes

Psychiatric disorders of epilepsy

The handicaps associated with epilepsy have been summarised in Table 10.1. The psychiatric disorders can be divided into the following three main groups, according to whether or not a direct link can be established between clinical seizures and mental state or behaviour (Fenton, 1981):

(1) disorders due to the brain disease causing the fits
(2) disorders temporally related to seizures
(3) inter-ictal disorders not temporally related to seizures.

Disorders due to the brain disease causing the fits

Here, the seizures and the neuropsychiatric or developmental disorder are both a reflection of underlying cerebral pathology, such as that underlying mental handicap, the specific epileptic syndromes (West's syndrome, etc.), focal brain disease and the dementias.

Disorders temporally related to seizures

Pre-ictal

Prodromal irritability and dysphoria in the hours or days preceding fits are not accompanied by clouding of consciousness. They resolve after the seizure. Little is known about their prevalence and pathogenesis.

Ictal

Ictal disorders comprise paroxysmal disturbances of higher cerebral function during clinical seizures, that is, partial seizures with psychic manifestations including automatisms, absence (petit mal) and complex partial status epilepticus.

Post-ictal

These disorders immediately follow the termination of the clinical seizure and often merge imperceptibly with its resolution. The predominant feature is clouding of consciousness due to post-seizure depression of cortical function following one or more generalised convulsions. The EEG is usually dominated by diffuse slow frequencies in the theta and delta range. If the disorder is brief (minutes only), automatic behaviour is manifest. When prolonged for hours or days, the clinical picture is that of an acute confusional state. Paranoid and other psychotic phenomena may occur (ictal-related psychosis). Complete recovery is the rule.

Inter-ictal disorders not temporally related to seizures

Here it is assumed that the epilepsy or the cerebral epileptogenic lesion has played a role in the genesis of the psychiatric disorder. Although the illness is unrelated in time to the seizure, the onset, intensity and course may be influenced by fit frequency. There is commonly an exacerbation of fits, less often and more controversially a reduction in fit frequency, so that there is an inverse relation between fits and mental state (Flor-Henry, 1976; Wolf, 1991).

The inter-ictal disorders invariably occur in clear consciousness. The range and type of mental state phenomena and behaviour disturbance do not differ significantly from those found in psychiatric patients without epilepsy.

The clinical features the patient develops are strongly influenced by age. Children and adolescents present with behaviour difficulties. Adults tend to develop mild affective symptoms. Personality disorder, unless a direct result of a focal brain lesion, is usually a reflection of lifelong disturbance, featuring early onset of fits, brain damage and a history of maladjustment, with behaviour and neurotic problems in childhood. The aetiology of all non-psychotic inter-ictal disorders in both children and adults with epilepsy is multi-factorial. The mental state and behavioural disturbances in any one individual are the final manifestation of an interaction between a range of epilepsy-related and psychosocial factors.

The link between temporal lobe dysfunction and psychopathology has been established in children, but is not beyond challenge in adults. Factors strongly related to well-being are the patients' perception of themselves and of their epilepsy, time since diagnosis, a diagnosis of 'absence' seizures, and being employed full time (Collings, 1990). Psychosocial predictors of psychopathology in adults with epilepsy are increased perceived stigma, more stressful life events, poor adjustment to epilepsy, financial stress, vocational problems, external locus of control and earlier onset of epilepsy (Hermann *et al*, 1990).

The characteristic 'epileptic personality traits' (e.g. slowness in speech and thought, circumstantial speech, religiosity, unstable mood, irritability and impulsivity) are rare (occuring in about 4% of people with epilepsy). They result from multiple acquired handicaps, both biological and psychosocial, and are not specific to epilepsy.

A specific temporal lobe behavioural syndrome has been hypothesised (Gerschwind, 1979). Its characteristics are an excessive tendency to adhere to each thought, feeling or action (viscosity), irritability and deepened emotionality (hyperemotionality), and decreased sexual interest and arousal (hyposexuality). The hypothesis is that the chronic activation of limbic structures due to repeated and intermittent epileptic discharges has had a kindling effect, with increased limbic reactivity leading to enhanced affective labelling of previously neutral stimuli, events or concepts due to the induction of new synaptic connections between the primary sensory cortex and mesial limbic structures. However, the evidence for the specificity of this syndrome is weak, and attempts to identify it among patients with temporal lobe epilepsy have not been consistently successful (Hermann & Whitman, 1984).

Complaints of reduced libido and impotence are common in male patients with intractable epilepsy. The causes are complex. In many cases poor sexual skills are a reflection of poor social skills in immature, dependent persons, who have led sheltered and restricted lives, with little opportunity to relate to the opposite sex because of frequent fits, parental overprotection and too much medication. Another factor is anticonvulsant induction of liver enzymes, with consequent rapid metabolism of testosterone and low free testosterone serum levels. The latter correlate with ratings of low sex drive in epilepsy (Toone, 1986).

Although the prevalence of epilepsy among imprisoned male offenders has been shown to be three times higher than in the general population (Gunn & Fenton, 1969), violent offences are no more common among epileptic prisoners than in other prisoners; nor is there any direct association between violence and temporal lobe epilepsy. Most reports relating temporal lobe epilepsy to a propensity for violent behaviour have been biased by the selection of patients with intractable epilepsy complicated by an early onset of fits, organic brain disease, low IQ, and personality and behaviour disorder. Serious violence during an epileptic automatism is also rare, since the concomitant clouding of consciousness means that well structured, goal-directed behaviour is difficult to initiate and maintain (Fenton, 1993).

In contrast to the ictal-related psychoses, the inter-ictal psychoses occur in a setting of clear consciousness. The symptoms resemble those of affective, schizoaffective or schizophrenia-like psychoses, and are thought to have a special relationship with temporal lobe dysfunction (Flor-Henry, 1976). Such psychoses may be either short lived or chronic.

Short-lived psychotic episodes

These include:

(1) very transient schizophrenia-like psychoses preceded by an exacerbation of fits, lasting only a few days, with rapid remission (these are presumably due to brief, subclinical limbic dysfunction)

(2) affective or schizoaffective states lasting weeks or months and running a course similar to unipolar affective disorder; mania can occur but is rare, and occasionally paranoid symptoms are predominant (Betts, 1981; Palha, 1985).

In contrast to the states of clouded consciousness, the onset of these short-lived affective/schizoaffective psychoses is rarely heralded by fits, but is occasionally terminated by a generalised convulsion (Dongier, 1959). Indeed, there may be a reduction of seizure frequency immediately before the onset of the psychosis (Betts, 1981). The earlier reports of an association with non-dominant temporal lobe epileptogenic lesions have not been confirmed (Toone, 1991). Their frequency among patients admitted for epilepsy to mental hospitals is around 20% (Betts, 1981).

It should also be noted that one side-effect of the anticonvulsant drugs vigabatrin and topiramate is psychosis. If a patient recently prescribed either of these drugs develops psychotic or paranoid symptoms, then drug-induced side-effects should be considered and the medication withdrawn.

Chronic schizophrenia-like psychoses

Slater *et al* (1963) published the first detailed study of the schizophrenia-like psychoses of epilepsy. They provided some epidemiological evidence that the occurrence of the two conditions was not coincidental. Two-thirds of those with the condition had temporal lobe dysfunction, and the psychosis developed on average 14 years after the onset of the epilepsy.

The predominant clinical picture is of a paranoid schizophrenia-like state, with delusions of reference and persecution and visual hallucinations being more common than in 'non-epileptic' schizophrenia. Catatonic symptoms are less frequent. Affect tends to be well preserved and the progress of the disorder benign, with little social deterioration. Further contrasts with non-epileptic schizophrenia are the relative lack of schizoid premorbid personality traits and of a family history of schizophrenia.

There appears to be an excess of females and of sinistrality in the schizophrenia-like psychosis of epilepsy. There is an association with temporal lobe hamartomatous lesions, especially gangliomas located in the mesial temporal structures. Slater and his colleagues regarded this disorder as symptomatic schizophrenia due to the temporal lobe dysfunction, a view generally accepted since.

There is a relation to dominant temporal lobe epileptogenic involvement, although this is by no means invariable and may be restricted to those with nuclear schizophrenia (Trimble, 1991). Toone (1991) provides a brief but informative review of this complex subject.

Assessment of the relationship between epilepsy and psychiatric disorder

A conventional psychiatric diagnostic formulation should first be carried out. This will include diagnosis of the presenting psychiatric syndrome and an evaluation of the relative importance of genetic, organic, environmental and personality factors, and current situational problems in the genesis of the illness. Then the following sequence of questions concerning the interaction between the fits and mental state must be considered.

(1) If there is a direct temporal relationship, then the mental state changes are a direct reflection of the cortical and subcortical dysfunction caused by the epileptogenic discharges –
   (a) pre-ictal – usually dysphoric symptoms
   (b) ictal – complex partial seizures, absence, or complex partial status
   (c) post-ictal – automatisms or confusional states.

(2) If there is no direct relationship in time to the fits, the phenomenology of the consequent inter-ictal disorder is likely to resemble that of a functional psychiatric illness and the causation will be multifactorial. The respective roles of the following factors must be considered –
   (a) the influence of the underlying epileptogenic lesion on the person's cognitive function, behaviour and emotional state, because of its extent (diffuse) or location (temporal lobe) or because of the frequency of subclinical seizure discharges
   (b) the relation between seizure type and frequency and the mental state disturbance
   (c) the effects of the anticonvulsant medication on the person's behaviour, mental processes, and neurological, metabolic and haematological status
   (d) the effects of having fits and being labelled epileptic on the person's emotional development and acquisition of social, academic and vocational skills.

The impact of all these personal and social factors on the development of the person's social competence and capacity to cope with current life events should be evaluated. The person's style of reacting to the problems of living with a chronic handicap should also be noted, for example the use of the sick role, aggressive acting out behaviour, and the ego defence mechanisms of denial, projection and reaction formation.

Of course, all the factors that influence the development of the inter-ictal disorders may also play a role in determining the psychological adjustment of the person who presents with a mental disturbance directly related to seizure occurrence.

Principles of drug treatment of epilepsy

The use of a single anti-epileptic drug (monotherapy) is to be preferred in all cases, since drug interactions are common with polytherapy (combined therapy with two or more drugs). Polytherapy can also lead to unpredictable side-effects. In new cases, monotherapy will produce an immediate remission of seizures in up to 50% of patients and around 80% will have entered remission within 4 years of starting treatment.

The chosen first-line drug (see below) should be introduced at low dosage; this dosage may then be gradually increased in order to reduce the risk of immediate side-effects, such as undue sedation. The drug needs to be continued for a trial period long enough to assess its efficacy. A rough rule is to continue with it for long enough to cover the time scale of occurrence of three to five seizures or a cluster of seizures, or for at least 2 months, whichever is the longer (Shorvon, 1990). The trial period should be with the drug at full dosage. Serum concentrations may be useful with some drugs as a rough guide to dosage schedules, but in many cases dosage may be simply gauged on clinical grounds with respect to the continuation or absence of seizures and the presence or absence of side-effects.

If seizure control remains a problem at the end of the trial period or there are unacceptable side-effects, the first drug may be gradually replaced by another first-line agent, which again should be tried for an adequate trial period. The process can be repeated using other drugs as necessary. Table 10.2 shows adult dosage guidelines for the most commonly used agents.

Selecting the first-line drug

The choice of first-line drug depends, in part, on the type of seizure. This may be ascertained from the clinical features and the EEG findings. The drug must be matched to the individual patient in terms of potential adverse effects and ease of use (Feely, 1999).

For tonic/clonic seizures of a primary generalised or secondary generalised nature, sodium valproate, carbamazepine or lamotrigine would be considered first-line agents, as they would for partial seizures with or without secondary generalisation. For absence seizures (which are generally found in children), sodium valproate, lamotrigine or ethosuximide would be considered first-line agents. For myoclonic epilepsies, the commonest of which is juvenile myoclonic epilepsy, sodium valproate and lamotrigine would be regarded as the drugs of first choice.

Phenytoin, because it is available for parenteral administration, is generally considered the first-line drug for patients with status epilepticus. Otherwise, because of its adverse effects, its role as a first-line agent in the longer-term treatment of epilepsy has come under scrutiny and most would now regard it as a second-line agent.

Selecting a second-line drug

Phenytoin is most useful for patients with partial epilepsy with or without secondary generalisation. Its major role continues to be in the treatment of status epilepticus.

Table 10.2 Adult dosage guidelines for the most commonly used agents

Drug	Indications	Starting dose (mg)	Commonest daily dose (mg)	Standard maintenance dose (mg)	Doses per day
Carbamazepine	Partial and generalised tonic/clonic seizures	200	600	600–1600	1–4
Clobazam	Partial and generalised seizures	10	20	10–40	1–4
Clonazepam	Myoclonic and generalised tonic/clonic seizures	0.5	4	2–8	1–4
Ethosuximide	Absence seizures	500	1000	500–2000	1–4
Gabapentin	Add-on therapy for partial and generalised tonic/clonic seizures	300	1600	900–3600	3
Lamotrigine	All generalised seizures/partial seizures	25[a]	200	100–600	1 or 2[a]
Levetiracetam	Add-on therapy for partial and generalised tonic/clonic seizures	1000	1000	1000–3000	2
Oxcarbazepine	Partial and generalised tonic/clonic seizures	600	600	600–2400	2–4
Phenobarbitone	Partial and generalised tonic/clonic, myoclonic, clonic and tonic seizures, and status epilepticus	60	120	60–240	1 or 2
Phenytoin	Partial and generalised tonic/clonic seizures	200	300	100–500	1 or 2
Sodium valproate	All generalised seizures and partial seizures	500	1000	500–3000	1 or 2
Tiagabine	Add-on therapy for partial and generalised tonic/clonic seizures	10	30	30–45	3
Topiramate	Add-on therapy for partial and generalised tonic/clonic seizures	25	200	100–600	2
Vigabatrin	Add-on therapy for partial and generalised tonic/clonic seizures	500	2000	1000–4000	2

[a]On alternative days if added to sodium valproate.

Gabapentin is a more recently introduced agent licensed for the add-on therapy of partial epilepsies with or without secondary generalisation. It is often required in high dosages (up to and sometimes exceeding 3.6 g per day). Its mode of action is not wholly understood.

Topiramate has a number of modes of action. It is a useful add-on treatment for the refractory epilepsies and appears to have a broad spectrum of action.

Tiagabine is a gamma-aminobutyric acid (GABA) reuptake inhibitor and is licensed for the add-on treatment of partial epilepsies with or without secondary generalisation.

The most recently introduced agent is levetiracetam. This drug is licensed for the add-on treatment in patients with refractory epilepsy and appears to have a broad spectrum of action.

The benzodiazepines clonazepam and clobazam are occasionally used for the treatment of epilepsy; however, because of tolerance, these drugs are rarely of value in the long term. Clobazam in particular has a place for the intermittent treatment of seizures in patients who have clusters of attacks or catamenia epilepsy.

Primidone and phenobarbitone are now considered third-line agents because of their high levels of sedation.

Vigabatrin, a relatively recently introduced agent which acts on GABA-transaminase and therefore increases GABA levels, is licensed as an add-on treatment for patients with refractory seizures with or without secondary generalisation. It has proved a very effective agent for some patients. However, recent concern over visual field constriction has very much limited the use of this drug and patients receiving vigabatrin are recommended to have visual field testing every six months.

What to do if seizures are resistant to monotherapy

If the patient's seizures prove resistant to monotherapy with one of the first-line drugs, possible reasons for the failure should be sought before the therapy is changed. Poor compliance is not uncommon, and can be ascertained by estimation of serum concentrations.

Failure to respond to adequate anti-epileptic drug therapy in spite of optimal serum levels is a reason for reviewing the diagnosis. Recent research has revealed that as many as 20% of patients referred to special epilepsy clinics and receiving anti-epileptic drug therapy do not have epilepsy. Common misdiagnoses are syncope, cardiac arrhythmias and non-epileptic seizures/pseudo-seizures. Non-epileptic seizures/pseudo-seizures are psychologically or behaviourally mediated attacks, which may superficially resemble epileptic seizures and which may be very difficult to differentiate from true epileptic attacks. Video EEG monitoring has facilitated diagnosis in this regard.

When considering diagnosis, the seizure type also needs to be addressed, as lack of response to treatment may be due to a failure to recognise certain seizure types and therefore prescription of the wrong anti-epileptic drug therapy. Absence seizures and myoclonic seizures will not respond to treatment with carbamazepine, for example. Another reason for failure to respond may be that there is an underlying structural cause for the epilepsy and one may consider a computerised tomography (CT) scan or magnetic resonance imaging (MRI) scan to exclude such an aetiology. MRI scans in particular are felt to have a higher diagnostic yield than CT, although MRI is less widely available than CT.

Polypharmacy

More than 25% of people with epilepsy appear to remain refractory to therapy with a single anti-epileptic drug. Many of these patients have partial seizures and many will have an underlying anatomical abnormality. Current evidence suggests that the addition of a second drug is successful in only around 10% of such patients (Schmidt & Gram, 1995). However, it is likely that the combination of drugs with similar or overlapping modes of action may be responsible for this poor outcome. The advent of some of the newer anti-epileptic agents with defined modes of action suggests that rational polytherapy – the employment of agents with differing modes of action – may prove beneficial (Dichter & Brodie, 1996). Combining multiple drugs, however, increases the likelihood of drug interactions and consequent adverse effects.

Dosage schedules and pharmacokinetics

Table 10.2 outlines the dosage schedules. Phenytoin may generally be given once daily. Sodium valproate, carbamazepine, lamotrigine, topiramate, levetiracetam, phenobarbitone, primidone (not shown) and clonazepam are generally given twice daily. Gabapentin and tiagabine are recommended to be given three times per day.

For details of the clinical pharmacology of the established drugs, the reader is referred to Brodie & Dichter (1997). The pharmacokinetic properties of the commonly used anti-epileptic drugs are summarised in Table 10.3.

When are plasma concentrations useful?

With the exception of phenytoin, it is generally not important for the clinician to determine the plasma concentrations of anticonvulsants: levels above the limit are not necessarily associated with toxicity and many patients are well controlled despite concentrations below the

Table 10.3 Pharmacokinetic properties of the commonly used anti-epileptic drugs

Drug	Absorption (bioavailability)	Protein binding (% bound)	Elimination half-life (hours)	Route of elimination	Comments
Carbamzepine	Slow (75–85%)	70–78	8–24	Hepatic metabolism: CNZ 10,11 epoxide active metabolite	Enzyme inducer; auto-induction of metabolism
Clobazam	Rapid (90–100%)	87–90	10–30	Hepatic metabolism; N-desmethylclobazam active metabolite	Tolerance possible; exacerbation on withdrawal
Clonazepam	Rapid (80–90%)	80–90	30–40	Hepatic metabolism	Sedative; tolerance; withdrawal exacerbations
Ethosuximide	Rapid (90–95%)	0	20–60	Hepatic metabolism – 25% excreted unchanged	More rapid clearance in children
Gabapentin	Rapid (50–60%)	0	5–7	Largely excreted unchanged	Similar absorption with high dosage
Lamotrigine	Rapid (95–100%)	55	22–36	Hepatic metabolism to glucuronide conjugate	Metabolism induced or inhibited by other anti-convulsant drugs
Phenobarbitone	Slow (95–100%)	48–54	72–144	Hepatic metabolism – 25% excreted unchanged	Enzyme inducer; sedative
Phenytoin	Slow (85–95%)	90–93	9–40	Saturable hepatic metabolism	Enzyme inducer; elimination half-life concentration dependent
Sodium valproate	Rapid (100%)	88–92	7–17	Hepatic metabolism, active metabolites	Enzyme inhibitor; concentration dependent protein binding
Vigabatrin	Rapid (60–80%)	0	5–7	Largely excreted unchanged	Long acting due to irreversible binding to GABA aminotransferase

lower limit of the range. Drug levels are primarily indicated as a measure of compliance. Estimations of the plasma level of the anti-convulsant may be indicated in the following situations:

(1) to monitor phenytoin therapy because of its zero-order kinetics
(2) when there is a high probability of drug interactions due to polytherapy or the concomitant prescription of another type of drug known to interfere with the anti-epileptic drug's metabolism (in which case, however, free levels may be useful, as there may be a displacement of drug from plasma protein binding)
(3) for patients such as those with severe learning disability, in whom communication problems make the clinical detection of toxicity difficult
(4) for patients with a renal/hepatic disease.

First-line anticonvulsants

Carbamazepine

The first clinical studies of carbamazepine in epilepsy were not carried out until 1963. Over the years it has become one of the most widely used treatments for partial and tonic/clonic seizures. Carbamazepine, however, is not effective in the treatment of absence of myoclonic seizures.

The drug acts by preventing repetitive firing of sodium-dependent action potentials in depolarised neurons. Carbamazepine should be introduced at a low dosage, 100–200 mg daily, and increased slowly, in increments of 100–200 mg, every 2 weeks, to a maintenance dose of 600–1600 mg daily. A slow incremental increase in dosage allows tolerance to develop to the CNS side-effects of this drug.

Carbamazepine can cause a range of idiosyncratic reactions, the most common of which is rash. This may occur in around 10% of patients (*Lancet*, 1999). More severe skin eruptions, including the Stevens–Johnston syndrome, have also been reported. A reversible leucopenia is not uncommon with carbamazepine therapy, but it does not usually require discontinuation of therapy unless it is accompanied by evidence of infection or a falling white cell count.

Idiosyncratic reactions to carbamazepine include hyponatraemia (as a result of an antidiuretic hormone-like action of the drug), which may result in an increase in seizure frequency.

Dose-related side-effects are also common with carbamazepine. These include diplopia, dizziness, nausea, vomiting and sedation. These effects may be intermittent if high peak plasma concentrations occur. The use of the retard (i.e. slow-release) version may reduce some of these peak effects. As carbamazepine induces hepatic enzymes, interaction with commonly used drugs such as warfarin and the oral contraceptive pill may occur.

Sodium valproate

Sodium valporate has a broad spectrum of action and is considered a first-line drug for myoclonic and absence seizures as well as tonic/clonic seizures and partial seizures. It is available in both parenteral and oral forms. The starting dose for adults and adolescents is 400 mg daily in divided doses, which is then increased every 1–2 weeks to, for most adults, 1000–2000 mg daily. The drug's mode of action is uncertain. It has been shown to enhance GABA function but it also inhibits excitatory transmitters and reduces the threshold for calcium and potassium conductance.

Sodium valporate does not exhibit a clear-cut concentration–efficacy or concentration–toxicity relationship, and the daily variations in concentration at a given dose are wide. Routine blood monitoring is therefore not generally helpful, except as a measure of compliance.

The most common side-effects of sodium valporate are dose related and include tremor, weight gain and thinning or loss of hair (usually temporary). There is some recent evidence to suggest that there may be a link with the development of polycystic ovaries (Isojarvi et al, 1993).

Idiosyncratic reactions such as hepatic toxicity affects fewer than 1 in 20 000 treated individuals. It is more common in children under the age of 3 years receiving anti-epileptic polypharmacy, some of whom may have a coexisting metabolic defect. Hyperammonaemia without hepatic damage can be demonstrated in approximately 20% of all patients receiving valproic acid (Patsalos et al, 1993). It is usually transient but can occasionally present as confusion, nausea, vomiting and clouding of consciousness. Other sporadic problems include thrombocytopenia and pancreatitis.

Sodium valproate does not interfere with the contraceptive pill, but it has been associated with an increased risk of teratogenicity: cases of spina bifida are said to occur in 1–2% of the offspring of mothers exposed to sodium valproate during pregnancy.

Lamotrigine

Lamotrigine is a relatively recently introduced anti-epileptic agent which is now in increasing in use as a first-line agent. It has a spectrum of action similar to that of sodium valproate and is effective against myoclonic and absence seizures as well as tonic/clonic seizures and partial seizures.

Its mode of action is thought to be through the stabilisation of neuronal membranes by its blocking voltage-dependent sodium channel conductance.

Lamotrigine is generally well tolerated and may produce less sedation than some of the older agents. Rash is a common idiosyncratic reaction (approximately 5% of patients) and is particularly common in patients pre-treated with sodium valproate. Slow introduction of lamotrigine may reduce this risk. In monotherapy lamotrigine is usually started at 25 mg once daily and increased at fortnightly intervals by 25 mg, until a maintenance dose is reached of 100–600 mg per day. For patients already receiving sodium valproate, introduction of 25 mg on alternate days for the first 2 weeks is generally recommended.

Some patients experience insomnia with lamotrigine and so if the dose is given once daily it is generally recommended that it is taken in the morning. Other side-effects are generally mild; these include diplopia, headache, ataxia, dizziness, nervousness and nausea.

Concomitant anti-epileptic drugs may alter the metabolism of lamotrigine; hepatic-inducing agents may reduce the half-life and higher doses may therefore be required. Sodium valproate appears to inhibit its metabolism and therefore slower introduction and lower final doses should be employed. Lamotrigine does not interfere with the oral contraceptive pill. Animal studies suggest less risk of teratogenicity with lamotrigine than with some of the conventional agents; human data are lacking.

Ethosuximide

Ethosuximide retains a limited place as a first-line anti-epileptic drug. It is useful principally against absence seizures but may have some effect against myoclonic seizures. It is not effective against partial seizures or tonic/clonic seizures. Its use is therefore confined largely to children. The drug is thought to act by inhibiting low-threshold calcium currents in the thalamus. In children over 6 years of age, 500 mg per day is a reasonable starting dose, with increments added as necessary to a maximum of 2 g daily.

The side-effects of ethosuximide are generally dose related and usually involve the gastrointestinal tract (nausea, vomiting, abdominal pain) or the CNS (lethargy, dizziness and ataxia). Routine drug monitoring is not necessary.

Second-line anticonvulsants

Phenytoin

Phenytoin is a useful drug against partial seizures and tonic/clonic seizures, whether primary or secondary generalised. It exerts its influence mainly through the blocking of sodium channels. Phenytoin has zero-order kinetics at therapeutic dosage, that is, as the concentration rises, the capacity of the hepatic enzyme system to metabolise the drug becomes saturated. When this occurs, small increments in dosage can result in large rises in serum levels. In addition, phenytoin is commonly involved in drug interactions, as it is a potent hepatic enzyme inducer.

Phenytoin can produce a range of dose-related and idiosyncratic adverse effects. Of the latter, cosmetic changes (e.g. gum hyperplasia, acne, hirsutism, facial coarsening), although often mild, can be troublesome. Symptoms of neurotoxicity (drowsiness, dysarthria, tremor, ataxia and cognitive difficulties) become increasingly likely as the concentration of the drug rises. Permanent cerebellar damage (Botez *et al*, 1998) may be a consequence of chronic toxicity. Phenytoin is available in a parenteral form and is a particularly useful agent in the treatment of status epilepticus when given by slow intravenous injection (with electrocardiographic monitoring) at a dose of 15 mg/kg at a rate of not more than 50 mg per minute (in adults). Intramuscular use of phenytoin is not recommended. Fos-phenytoin, which is a recently introduced pro-drug of phenytoin, can be given more rapidly and is said to cause fewer reactions at the injection site when given intravenously; it can also be given by intramuscular injection, although absorption from this site is considered too slow for the treatment of status epilepticus.

Vigabatrin

Vigabatrin was licensed in the UK in 1989 for the 'add on' treatment of refractory partial epilepsies. It is not thought to be effective against primary generalised seizures. Vigabatrin is a GABA transaminase inhibitor and has been shown to raise the levels of the inhibitory neurotransmitter GABA in both brain and cerebrospinal fluid. Preliminary studies of this drug suggested that approximately half the patients exposed to it would experience a 50% or greater reduction in seizure frequency. After it obtained its licence and was more widely used, it became clear that the drug was associated with the development of psychosis in a proportion of patients (Sander *et al*, 1991). Subsequently its use has become limited by its association with visual field constriction (Committee on Safety of Medicines & Medicines Control Agency, 1998). Typically vigabatrin results in a loss to a nasal visual field. This may occur in up to 30% of patients exposed to vigabatrin, although many remain asymptomatic. It is therefore recommended that patients taking vigabatrin therapy have regular visual field examination.

Gabapentin

The structure of gabapentin is similar to that of GABA. It freely crosses the blood–brain barrier, although it does not appear to attach to GABA receptor sites and its exact mode of action is essentially unknown. It has been shown in clinical trials, however, to be a useful adjunctive treatment in partial seizures. It has not been shown to be effective in seizures of a generalised type. Initial trials (UK Gabapentin Study Group, 1990) suggested a dosage in the order of 900–1600 mg; however, subsequent and more widespread use of the drug suggested that higher doses (up to 3600 mg, or even higher) may be required to achieve a therapeutic result.

The drug is excreted largely unchanged in the urine and has the advantage of interacting with very few drugs. Initial studies suggested that it is also well tolerated and has few adverse effects. However, with the increasing realisation that higher doses are required, adverse effects may be encountered more frequently than was initially suggested. Drowsiness and cognitive effects are the most frequently reported.

Topiramate

Topiramate has recently been licensed in the UK for use as add-on treatment for refractory epilepsy. It does not as yet have a monotherapy licence. It is effective against both partial seizures and primary generalised seizures. Clinical studies have suggested that topiramate appears to be a highly effective drug against refractory partial seizures (Faught et al, 1996).

Topiramate has a number of mechanisms of action: it inhibits sodium conductance, enhances GABA activity and inhibits glutamate receptors. It is a mild hepatic enzyme inducer and therefore there is the potential for drug interactions, particularly with the oral contraceptive pill.

Common adverse effects include drowsiness, effects on cognition and weight loss. An association with renal stones has been found in clinical trials. However, topiramate has been associated with the development of psychosis in a number of patients with epilepsy. The occurrence of adverse effects may be reduced by a slow and cautious introduction of the drug, starting at a dose of 25 mg daily and increasing by 25 mg per week or fortnight until the therapeutic range of 100–600 mg daily is reached.

Tiagabine

Tiabagine is a GABA reuptake inhibitor. It has been shown to be effective as add-on therapy against partial seizures in particular. It does not cause hepatic enzyme induction, and therefore is less liable for interaction with other drugs, including the oral contraceptive pill. Visual field constriction found with vigabatrin has not been demonstrated with tiagabine.

Oxcarbazepine

Oxcarbazepine is a drug that is structurally related to carbamazepine. Not all patients who are allergic to carbamazepine will prove to be allergic to oxcarbazepine. Oxcarbazepine is thought to have a number of advantages over carbamazepine, which include less sedation. However, it is a hepatic enzyme inducer (although weaker than carbamazepine) and therefore may still interact with other drugs, including the oral contraceptive pill (Shorvon, 2000).

Levetiracetam

Levetiracetam is the most recently introduced drug for add-on treatment in refractory epilepsy. It seems to have a broad spectrum of action. Trials have shown that 41% of patients on 3000 mg per day have achieved a 50% or greater seizure reduction. The therapeutic dose range is 1000–3000 mg per day. The drug is excreted through the kidney and caution is advised in patients with renal impairment. It is generally held to be well tolerated; the most commonly encountered side-effects are drowsiness and dizziness.

Clobazam

The benzodiazepine clobazam is occasionally used alone but is more commonly used as add-on treatment in refractory epilepsies. In common with the other benzodiazepines, clobazam works at the benzodiazepine binding site of the GABA receptor complex, and therefore enhances the inhibitory neurotransmitter effects of GABA. The problem as with all benzodiazepines is the development of tolerance. Benzodiazepines also tend to be the most sedative anti-epileptic agents.

The widest use of benzodiazepines, including clobazam, is for catamenial epilepsy, where seizures can be predicted in relation to menstruation, and in patients who have clusters of attacks. In both cases seizures may be avoided or aborted by the intermittent use of clobazam (Feely & Gibson, 1984).

Drug interactions

This topic is discussed in detail by Richens & Robinson (1992).

Enzyme induction

Liver enzyme induction can increase the rate of metabolism of many drugs and so reduce their plasma levels and hence efficacy. Phenytoin, phenobarbitone, primidone and carbamazepine are potent enzyme inducers. The newer agents, topiramate and oxcarbazepine, are also recognised to be hepatic enzyme inducers. These drugs may lower the plasma levels of each other as well of other drugs, such as sodium valproate and lamotrigine. Other commonly used drugs that may be affected are oral anticoagulants and the contraceptive pill. With regard to the latter, for women taking hepatic enzyme-inducing agents it is generally recommended that the dose of oestrogen in the pill is increased to 50 μg; however, even then, contraception cannot be guaranteed and other methods should be advised.

Enzyme inhibition

Enzyme inhibition can decrease the rate of metabolism and raise plasma levels of the relevant drug. Inhibition of metabolism of carbamazepine with consequent toxicity has been reported with cimetidine, danazole, dextropropoxyphane (in Co-Proxamol), diltiazem, erythromycin, verapamil and viloxazine. Sodium valproate may inhibit the metabolism of carbamazepine and its active epoxide metabolite. It may also inhibit the metabolism of phenytoin, phenobarbitone and ethosuximide, increasing their plasma concentrations. However, in recent years the most significant interaction is between sodium valproate and lamotrigine. The introduction of lamotrigine should be much slower in patients being treated with sodium valproate and the final dose lower. If sodium valproate is subsequently withdrawn, the dose of lamotrigine may need to be increased.

Saturable enzyme inhibitors such as allopurinol, choramphenicol, cimetidine, imipramine, metronidazole and sulfonamides can increase plasma phenytoin levels and precipitate toxicity.

Displacement from plasma protein binding sites

The most important example of displacement from binding sites resulting in an increase in free drug is that of phenytoin by sodium valproate. This can result in toxicity, and, if not recognised, chronic toxicity from phenytoin can cause permanent cerebellar damage.

Adverse effects of anti-epileptic drug treatment

The principal adverse effects of the first-line agents are summarised in Table 10.4. They are also described in detail by Chadwick (1991).

Acute dose-related adverse effects

Any of the anti-epileptic drugs may be associated with decreased concentration, sedation, fatigue, drowsiness and dizziness. These effects are less likely with sodium valproate and perhaps lamotrigine than with many of the other drugs and can be limited by a slow introduction of the offending drug.

Table 10.4 Side-effects of first-line anticonvulsants

Carbamazepine	Sodium valproate	Lamotrigine	Ethosuximide
Predictable			
Diplopia*	Tremor*	Dizziness*	Nausea*
Dizziness*	Weight gain*	Nausea*	Anorexia
Nausea*	Hair loss*	Insomnia*	Vomiting
Drowsiness	Anorexia	Agitation	Drowsiness
Headache	Dyspepsia	Irritability	Headache
Hyponatraemia	Nausea		Lethargy
Hypocalcaemia	Vomiting		
Orafacial	Rash		
dyskinesia	Peripheral oedema		
Cardiac	Drowsiness		
arrhythmia			
Idiosyncratic			
Morbiliform rash*	Acute pancreatitis	Rash*	Rash
Agranulocytosis	Hepatotoxicity	Stevens–Johnson	Erythema
Aplastic anaemia	Thrombocytopenia	syndrome	multiforme
Hepatotoxicity	Hyperammonaemia	Disseminated intra-	Stevens–Johnson
Photosensitivity	Stupor	vascular coagulation	syndrome
Lupus-like	Encephalopathy		Lupus-like
syndrome			syndrome
Thrombocytopenia			Agranulocytosis
Pseudolymphoma			Aplastic anaemia

*Most common side-effects.

Acute idiosyncratic adverse effects

The most common acute idiosyncratic side-effect is a maculopapular skin eruption, which usually occurs within the first 4 weeks of the start of treatment. There is some evidence to suggest that the incidence of rash may be reduced by slower introduction of the drug. Skin reactions are most common with carbamazepine, lamotrigine and phenytoin. The onset of a rash will require withdrawal of the drug. Occasionally an exfoliative dermatitis or the Stevens–Johnson syndrome may occur. Aplastic anaemia is a rare complication of most anti-epileptic drugs. An acute hepatitis with pyrexia, lymphadenopathy and skin eruption may occur with phenytoin. Usually changes will reverse on withdrawal of the drug, but fatal cases have been reported.

A more serious hazard is acute liver failure in children – more often those taking polytherapy regimens that include sodium valproate. It tends to occur after 3–6 months of treatment. The incidence is highest in patients with Lennox–Gastaut syndrome or other epileptic syndromes involving brain damage and learning disability. In some cases a metabolic abnormality may be responsible.

Longer-term adverse effects

Neuropsychological effects

A pseudo-dementia with declining cognitive function and increasing frequency and severity of seizures may be seen in younger people with learning disability and epilepsy treated with phenytoin. It is usually associated with toxic serum concentrations of the drug. Chronic confusional states may also be associated with sodium valproate toxicity.

Cerebellar atrophy with loss of Purkinge cells has been seen in patients with chronic epilepsy and has been linked to the long-term use of phenytoin in high doses. Motor sensory neuropathy has also been linked with chronic usage of some of the anti-epileptic agents, including phenytoin.

Changes in mood and irritability have been linked with most of the anti-epileptic agents. Some more serious psychiatric reactions, including psychoses, have been linked with the newer agents, in particular vigabatrin and topiramate. A recent review of the neuropsychological effects of the various drugs may be found in Kwan & Brodie (2001).

Skin disorders

Acne and hirsuitism can be troublesome side-effects of phenytoin and carbamazepine. Hair loss may occur with sodium valproate.

Haematological disorders

The mean red cell volume tends to rise following phenytoin therapy; there is also an association with low serum folate levels, sometimes leading to a macrocytic anaemia. The cause remains uncertain. Thrombocytopenia may occur with sodium valproate therapy. An asymptomatic low white cell count is commonly found in patients taking carbamazepine.

Endocrine effects

Hepatic enzyme induction by anti-epileptic drugs may increase the metabolism of steroids, including the contraceptive pill, and thereby give higher risks of breakthrough bleeding and contraceptive failure. A similar effect on vitamin D metabolism may be responsible for osteo-malacia. Patients with epilepsy are recognised as being at increased risk of osteoporosis and this risk may be higher in patients taking hepatic enzyme-inducing agents. Plasma thyroxine levels may be lowered by the hepatic enzyme induction of anti-epileptic agents.

Effects on connective tissues

Gum hyperplasia occurs in up to 50% of patients treated with phenytoin and is exacerbated by poor dental hygiene. Coarsening of the facial features (e.g. thickening of the lips, widening of the nose) and thickening of the subcutaneous tissues have also been reported in patients with severe epilepsy. These changes may be drug related.

Effects on the reproductive system

Patients with epilepsy are recognised to be less fertile than the general population. The causes of this are largely psychosocial. However, there have been reports of a link with anti-epileptic drug therapy and the polycystic ovary syndrome. This problem has been primarily linked to sodium valproate therapy (Isojarvi *et al*, 1993) and may lead to increased rates of infertility.

It is recognised that patients with epilepsy have a two to three times increased risk of foetal malformation. Spina bifida has been associated with sodium valproate at a rate of 1–2% and with carbamazepine at a rate of 0.5–1%. Cleft lip, cardiac abnormalities and genito-urinary abnormalities are also relatively frequently reported. The relative rates of teratogenetic effects between the drugs is essentially unknown, although all have been associated with increased risk. Animal studies have suggested that the newer agents (lamotrigine and gabapentin) may be safer than the older agents, although human data are as yet lacking and a number of prospective registries have been established to monitor pregnancy outcomes. Polytherapy, however, carries a higher risk than monotherapy. Folic acid (5 mg) has been recommended pre-conceptually in order to minimise the risk of spina bifida.

It is important in the management of women with epilepsy to offer pre-conceptual counselling, at which time the diagnosis may be reviewed, and the need for drug therapy re-evaluated and withdrawn if possible. Drug withdrawal (see below), however, has to be tempered with the risk of seizures recurring during pregnancy. There is some anecdotal evidence to suggest that seizures, at least in the latter parts of pregnancy, may result in foetal distress. There is always the risk of trauma to the women involved but the increased risk of teratogenic effects due to seizures is essentially unknown.

Stopping anti-epileptic medication

After a minimum period of 2 years of freedom from seizures, drug withdrawal may be considered. However, in every case the advantages of drug withdrawal must be balanced against the risks, particularly risks of seizure recurrence, which will have consequences for vehicle driving and may prejudice employment as well as threaten self-esteem (Chadwick, 1991). The relapse rate is high, around 20% in children and 40% in adults. It has been shown that most seizures will occur either during the withdrawal phase or within 6–12 months of complete cessation.

Good prognostic factors are considered to be a single seizure type, especially primary generalised seizures (excluding myoclonic seizures), the absence of a neuropsychiatric deficit or underlying brain pathology, a relatively short duration of seizures and a mild seizure disorder in terms of number and frequency of seizures before remission. Conversely, adverse factors are considered to be a variety of different seizures, the presence of myoclonic seizures or partial seizures without secondary generalisation, the presence of cerebral pathology or any psychiatric disorder, a long duration of epilepsy and frequent seizures before remission. The predictive value of an EEG remains controversial. It has been thought to be useful in childhood epilepsy but less so in adults.

If drugs are to be withdrawn, one drug should be withdrawn at a time and a 3-month dose-reduction phase leading to withdrawal should be considered a *minimum* for each drug.

Driving and epilepsy

It has been estimated that the rate of road traffic accidents is increased 1.3–2-fold in patients with epilepsy. The UK legislation regarding epilepsy at present states that patients are to be considered ineligible to drive until they demonstrate a 12-month period of freedom from epileptic seizures. If, however, patients continue to experience seizures but have an established pattern of nocturnal seizures (i.e. while sleeping) over a 3-year period, they may also be considered eligible to drive.

If drugs are to be withdrawn, it is recommended that patients cease driving during the time of withdrawal and for 6 months afterwards, because of the risk of seizure recurrence.

Licences for heavy-goods vehicles or public-service vehicles are issued only if patients can demonstrate 10 years' freedom from seizures and have been off all anti-epileptic medication for a similar period.

The surgical treatment of epilepsy

A number of surgical treatments have been gaining in popularity over the past two decades. These include:

(1) the removal of an epileptogenic focus (most commonly, temporal lobectomy)
(2) corpus callosotomy
(3) vagus nerve stimulation.

Removal of an epileptogenic focus

The removal of an epileptogenic focus may be considered if:

(1) the patient is seriously handicapped by frequent seizures
(2) the epilepsy has proved refractory to drug treatment

(3)   there is clinical, radiological and EEG evidence that the seizures arise consistently from a defined area of the cortex that can be excised without causing the patient disability.

The most commonly performed operation is temporal lobectomy. A good summary of indications for this form of treatment may be found in the guidelines for the management of adults with poorly controlled epilepsy issued by the Royal College of Physicians *et al* (1997). Patients must be carefully assessed before surgery. They must have been given an adequate period of time on medical treatment and have proved to be refractory to it. A single focus should be suggested by the clinical description of the seizures and from EEG localisation. This will usually require prolonged EEG recordings, with perhaps the use of foramen ovale or depth electrodes.

In recent years the use of MRI scanning has proved invaluable in locating areas of abnormality and in particular the presence of hippocampal sclerosis. The presence of hippocampal sclerosis with a concordant history and EEG findings are generally good prognostic indicators of a favourable outcome.

Full neuropsychological assessment should take place pre-operatively and this should include WADA testing, the injection of amylobarbitol into the carotid artery on the affected side to determine localisation of speech and language and to test memory function on the affected side.

Temporal lobectomy is associated with low mortality and morbidity rates and has been proven to be successful in abolishing seizures in approximately 70% of patients.

Corpus callosotomy

Corpus callosotomy may restrict the spread of seizure activity from a partial onset, thus reducing the number of generalised tonic/clonic seizures, although patients may continue to have minor seizures. It is a less satisfactory operation than temporal lobectomy and rarely will result in freedom from seizures. Nevertheless, it may prove useful in patients with multiple epileptogenic foci.

Vagus nerve stimulation

Stimulation of the vagus nerve has been shown to reduce seizure frequency (Benmenachen *et al*, 1994). The device is surgically implanted in the chest wall and an electrode is attached to the left vagus nerve. This device intermittently stimulates afferent fibres which, through neuronal or chemical connections, appear to reduce the propensity to seizures. The device is programmed to fire intermittently, usually for 30 seconds every 5 minutes, although these parameters may be altered, as may the strength of the stimulus.

The use of the device has been reported in a number of trials worldwide and it has been shown to produce an overall reduction in seizure frequency of approximately 30%. The device is generally well tolerated and side-effects are generally mild – usually consisting of transient coughing or hoarseness when the device fires (Ramsay *et al*, 1994). Its use is reserved at present for patients with drug-refractory epilepsy who are not considered candidates for more definitive surgical treatment.

References

Benmenachen, E., Manon-Espaillat, R., Ristanovic, R., *et al* (1994) Vagus nerve stimulation for the treatment of partial seizures. A controlled study of effect on seizures. *Epilepsia*, **35**, 616–626.

Betts, T. A. (1981) Epilepsy and the mental hospital. In *Epilepsy and Psychiatry* (eds E. H. Reynolds & M. R. Trimble), pp. 175–184. Edinburgh: Churchill Livingstone.

Botez, M. I., Ezzedine, A. & Vezina, J. L. (1998) Cerebellar atrophy in epileptic patients. *Canadian Journal of Neurological Science*, **15**, 299–303.

Brodie, M. J. & Dichter, M. A. (1997) Established anti-epileptic drugs. *Seizure*, **6**, 159–174.

Chadwick, D. (1991) The medical treatment of epilepsy. In *Clinical Neurology* (eds M. Swash & J. Oxbury), pp. 276–297. Edinburgh: Churchill Livingstone.

Collings, J. A. (1990) Psychosocial wellbeing and epilepsy: an empirical study. *Epilepsia*, **31**, 418–426.

Commission on Classification and Terminology of the International League Against Epilepsy (1981) Proposal for revised clinical electroencephalographic classification of epileptic seizures. *Epilepsia*, **22**, 489–501.

Commission on Classification and Terminology of the International League Against Epilepsy (1989) Proposal for revised classification of epilepsies and epileptic seizures. *Epilepsia*, **30**, 389–399.

Commission on Epidemiology and Prognosis of the International League Against Epilepsy (1993) Guidelines for epidemiological studies on epilepsy. *Epilepsia*, **34**, 592–586.

Committee on Safety of Medicines & Medicines Control Agency (1998) Vigabatrin (Sabril) and visual field defects. *Current Problems in Pharmacovigilance*, **24**, 1.

Connors, B. W. & Gutnick, M. J. (1984) Cellular mechanisms of neocortical epilepto-genesis in an acute experimental model. In *Electrophysiology of Epilepsy* (eds P. A. Schwartzkroin & H. V. Wheal), pp. 79–105. New York: Academic Press.

Coulter, D. A., Huguenard, J. R. & Prince, D. A. (1989) Specific petit mal anti-convulsants reduce calcium currents in thalamic neurons. *Neuroscience Letters*, **98**, 74–78.

Dichter, M. A. & Brodie, M. J. (1996) New anti-epileptic drugs. *New England Journal of Medicine*, **336**, 1583–1590.

Dongier, S. (1959) Statistical study of clinical and electroencephalographic manifest-ations of 536 psychotic episodes in 516 epileptics between clinical seizures. *Epilepsia*, **1**, 117–142.

Falconer, M. A. (1973) Reversability by temporal lobe resection of the behavioural abnormalities of temporal lobe epilepsy. *New England Journal of Medicine*, **289**, 450–455.

Faught, E., Wilder, B. J., Ramsay, R. A., *et al* (1996) Topiramate placebo controlled dose-ranging trial in refractory partial epilepsy using 200, 400, and 600 mg daily dosages. *Neurology*, **46**, 1684–1690.

Feely, M. (1999) Drug treatment of epilepsy. *BMJ*, **318**, 106–109.

Feely, M. & Gibson, J. (1984) Intermittent clobazam for catamenial epilepsy: tolerance avoided. *Journal of Neurology, Neurosurgery and Psychiatry*, **27**, 1279–1282.

Fenton, G. W. (1981) Psychiatric disorders of epilepsy: classification and phenomenology. In *Epilepsy and Psychiatry* (eds E. H. Reynolds & M. R. Trimble), pp. 12–26. Edinburgh: Churchill Livingstone.

Fenton, G. W. (1993) Epilepsy and psychiatric disorder. In *Companion to Psychiatric Studies* (eds R. E. Kendell & A. K. Zeally), pp. 343–357. Edinburgh: Churchill Livingstone.

Flor-Henry, P. (1976) Epilepsy and psychopathology. In *Recent Advances in Clinical Psychiatry* (ed. K. Granville-Grossman), pp. 262–295. Edinburgh: Churchill Livingstone.

Gerschwind, N. (1979) Behavioural changes in temporal lobe epilepsy. *Psychological Medicine*, **9**, 217–219.

Gloor, P. (1988) Neurophysiological mechanism of generalised spike and wave discharge and its implications for understanding absence seizures. In *Elements of Petit Mal Epilepsy* (eds M. S. Myslobodsky & A. F. Mirsky), pp. 159–210. New York: Peter Lang.

Goodridge, D. M. G. & Shorvon, S. D. (1983a) Epileptic seizures in a population of 6000. 1: Demography, diagnosis and classification. *BMJ*, **287**, 641–644.

Goodridge, D. M. G. & Shorvon, S. D. (1983b) Epileptic seizures in a population of 6000. 2: Treatment and prognosis. *BMJ*, **287**, 645–647.

Gunn, J. & Fenton, G. (1969) Epilepsy in prisons: a diagnostic survey. *BMJ*, *iv*, 325–328.

Hauser, W. A. & Kurland, L. C. (1975) The epidemiology of epilepsy in Rochester, Minnesota, 1935 through 1967. *Epilepsia*, **16**, 1–66.

Hermann, B. P. & Whitman, S. (1984) Behavioural and personality correlates of epilepsy: a review, methodological critique and conceptual model. *Psychological Bulletin*, **95**, 451–497.

Hermann, B. P. & Whitman, S., Wyler, A. R., *et al* (1990) Psychosocial predictors of psychopathology in epilepsy. *British Journal of Psychiatry*, **156**, 98–105.

Isojarvi, J. L., Laatikainen, T. J., Pakarinen, A. J., *et al* (1993) Polycystic ovaries and hyperandrogenism in women taking valproate for epilepsy. *New England Journal of Medicine*, **329**, 1383–1388.

Jones, R. S. G. & Lambert, J. D. C. (1990) Synchronous discharges in the rat entorhinal cortex in vitro: site of initiation and the role of excitatory amino and receptors. *Neuroscience*, **34**, 657–670.

Juul-Jensen, P. & Foldsprang, A. (1983) Natural history of epileptic seizures. *Epilepsia*, **24**, 297–310.

Kwan, P. & Brodie, M. J. (2001) Neuropsychological effects of epilepsy and anti-epileptic drugs. *Lancet*, **357**, 216–222.

Lancet (1999) Editorial. Carbamazepine update. *Lancet*, *ii*, 595–597.

Luhmann, H. J. & Prince, D. A. (1991) Postnatal maturation of the GABAergic system in rat neocortex. *Journal of Neurophysiology*, **65**, 247–263.

Matsumoto, H. & Ajmone-Marsan, C. (1964) Cortical cellular phenomena in experimental epilepsy: interictal manifestations. *Experimental Neurology*, **9**, 286–304.

Palha, A. J. P. (1985) *A Epilepsia Em Psiquiatria*. Doctoral dissertation, Faculty of Medicine, University of Oporto.

Patsalos, P. N., Wilson, S. J., Popovik, M., *et al* (1993) The prevalence of valproic acid associated hyperammonaemia in patients with intractable epilepsy resident in the Chalfont Centre for Epilepsy. *Journal of Epilepsy*, **6**, 228–232.

Ramsay, R. E., Uthman, B. M., Augustinsson, L. E., *et al* (1994) Vagus nerve stimulation for treatment of partial seizures. Safety, side effects and tolerability. *Epilepsia*, **35**, 627–636.

Richens, A. & Robinson, M. K. (1992) Anticonvulsant pharmacokinetics. In *Diseases of the Nervous System. Clinical Neurobiology* (eds A. K. Ashbury, G. M. McKhann & W. I. Macdonald), pp. 1000–1007. Philadelphia: W. B. Saunders.

411

Roberts, G. W., Done, D. J., Bruton, C., *et al* (1990) A 'mock-up' of schizophrenia temporal lobe epilepsy and schizophrenia-like psychoses. *Biological Psychiatry*, **28**, 127–143.

Rodin, E. A. (1968) *The Prognosis of Patients with Epilepsy.* Springfield: Thomas.

Royal College of Physicians, Institute of Neurology & National Society for Epilepsy (1997) *Adults with Poorly Controlled Epilepsy. Clinical Guidelines for Treatment.* London: Royal College of Physicians.

Sander, J. W. A. S., Hart, Y. M., Johnson, A. L., *et al* (1990) National General Practice Study of Epilepsy: newly diagnosed epileptic seizures in a general population. *Lancet*, **336**, 1267–1271.

Sander, J. W. A. S., Hart, Y. M., Trimble, M. R., *et al* (1991) Vigabatrin and psychosis. *Journal of Neurology, Neurosurgery and Psychiatry*, **54**, 435–439.

Schmidt, D. & Gram, L. (1995) Monotherapy versus polytherapy in epilepsy. A reappraisal. *CNS Drugs*, **3**, 194–208.

Shorvon, S. D. (1990) Epidemiology, classification, natural history and genetics of epilepsy. *Lancet*, **336**, 93–96.

Shorvon, S. D. (2000) Oxcarbazepine: a review. *Seizure*, **9**, 75–79.

Shorvon, S. D., Fish, D. R., Bydder, G., *et al* (eds) (1994) *Magnetic Resonance Scanning and Epilepsy.* New York: Plenum Press.

Slater, E., Beard, A. W. & Glitheroe, E. (1963) The schizophrenia-like psychoses of epilepsy. *British Journal of Psychiatry*, **109**, 95–150.

Toone, B. K. (1986) Hyposexuality among male epileptic patients: clinical and hormonal correlates. In *Aspects of Epilepsy and Psychiatry* (eds M. R. Trimble & T. G. Bolwig), pp. 61–74. Chichester: Wiley.

Toone, B. K. (1991) The psychoses of epilepsy. *Journal of the Royal Society of Medicine*, **84**, 457–459.

Trimble, M. R. (1991) *The Psychoses of Epilepsy.* New York: Raven Press.

UK Gabapentin Study Group (1990) Gabapentin in partial epilepsy. *Lancet*, **335**, 114–117

Wolf, P. (1991) Acute behavioral symptomatology at disappearance of epileptiform EEG abnormality. Paradoxical or 'forced' normalisation. *Advances in Neurology*, **55**, 127–142.

Part III
Special therapeutic areas

CHAPTER 11

The psychopharmacology of childhood and adolescence

Peter Hill and Nicolette Adrian

General principles

The use of medication in child and adolescent psychiatry is less prevalent than in adult psychiatry and most cases of psychiatric disorder in the young will not require it. Much psychiatric pathology in young people is effectively the result of distorted psychological development or a reaction to adverse circumstances within the child's family or school. It follows that psychological interventions to promote development or healthier adaptation, and social measures to reduce adverse circumstances or relationships, are the commonest form of treatment. Medication is nearly always deployed alongside psychosocial interventions and integrated into a total treatment package; it is exceptional for it to be the only form of intervention.

Most of the conditions for which medication is useful affect older children and adolescents (see Table 11.1), and it is unusual to prescribe for pre-school children. The reaction of very young children to psychotropic medication is often unpredictable. Furthermore, some drugs (e.g. fluoxetine) can, in animal studies, result in enduring physical change to the immature brain and the implications of this are unclear. Caution is advisable.

As an extension of this, it is necessary to be clear for whose benefit medication is being prescribed. In the disruptive behaviour disorders of childhood, there may be requests from parents and teachers to use medication to make the child easier to manage. If this results in improved family relationships or greater academic achievement, then it would be justified, but enabling an easier life for adult caregivers is insufficient reason to prescribe.

There is a common misunderstanding about drugs that are not 'licensed' for children, this term being used in pharmaceutical company literature, data sheets and formularies. A licence is a marketing authorisation granted by a national standards body (the Medicines and Healthcare Products Regulatory Agency (MHRA) in the UK; the Food

Table 11.1 Summary of drug use in child and adolescent psychiatry

Category	Drugs	Indications
Stimulants	Methylphenidate Dexamfetamine Pemoline	ADHD, head injury, narcolepsy
Serotonin reuptake inhibitors Selective	Citalopram Escitalopram Fluoxetine Fluvoxamine Paroxetine Sertraline	Anxiety, OCD, depression, self-injury, bulimic symptoms
Less selective	Clomipramine	
Other antidepressants	Imipramine Nortriptyline Desipramine Clomipramine Trazodone Bupropion Venlafaxine	Mainly in ADHD
Lithium and mood stabilisers	Carbamazepine Valproate Lamotrigine Gabapentin Topiramate	Juvenile bipolar disorder or other unstable mood underlying aggression
Antipsychotics	Typicals Atypicals (especially risperidone) and clozapine	Schizophrenia, rage outbursts and Tourette's
Adrenergic blockers	Clonidine	Tourette's, ADHD, PTSD, sleep disorders, self-injury
Hypnotics	Diphenhydramine Promethazine Trimeprazine Melatonin Chloral derivatives	Insomnia
Miscellaneous	Propanolol Desmopressin Laxatives Diazepam Atomoxetine	Rage Enuresis Faecal soiling Parasomnias ADHD

ADHD, attention-deficit hyperactivity disorder; OCD, obsessive–compulsive disorder; PTSD, post-traumatic stress disorder.

and Drugs Administration in the USA) to a company entitling it to promote the drug for a specified indication. This will be granted only if there is enough information about safety. Most companies do not test new drugs on children and in the UK there is no requirement for them to do so, although recent developments in the USA will mean new drugs there will have to be tested on people of all ages. Obtaining a marketing authorisation is expensive and commercial interests mean that the cost needs to be set against the likely profits from widening the indications or age range for the product. The low rate of use of drugs for children's psychiatric disorders means that the market for psychoactive medicines for children is only occasionally large enough to be commercially viable and it is thus unusual for marketing authorisation to be sought. In other words, few psychiatric drugs will be licensed for children.

This is not a situation unique to psychiatry. Various studies have demonstrated that nearly half the children in neonatal and paediatric general wards will are prescribed unlicensed ('off-label') medications.

A pharmaceutical company cannot promote a drug for which no marketing authorisation has been granted. This means that it will have to write 'not recommended for children' in the informative literature or advertising. Matters in the UK became confused some years ago when some National Health Service (NHS) trusts, alarmed about possible litigation, issued policies that forbade the use of 'unlicensed' medication, and there are signs that some of the new primary care trusts are taking the same line. Some doctors have a mistaken impression that they are simply not allowed to prescribe unlicensed medication. General guidance from the Department of Health in England and Wales has, however, been that a consultant may initiate off-label prescription and reasonably expect a general practitioner to issue maintenance prescriptions so long as the child is under the care of the consultant. However, the prescribing doctor is the one who carries responsibility and some general practitioners are wary of prescribing unlicensed medication. To ensure that guidelines for responsible practice exist in this area, the Royal College of Paediatrics and Child Health (2003) has issued a formulary (*Medicines for Children*), which contains a detailed section on psychiatric drugs. The construction of this manual involved very extensive peer-group consultation as well as expert advice and can confidently be referred to as accepted guidance on good prescribing for children.

Children (here taken to include school-age adolescents) often need lower doses of medication than adults do, but a common error is to reduce the dose too much. In general paediatrics, doses are commonly calculated according to body weight or surface area. In a pre-pubertal child this is a useful contribution to estimating a starting dose, but it is usual in psychopharmacological practice subsequently to titrate the dose against symptoms or functioning and dose-related adverse effects so that an optimal dose is arrived at. By their early teens, young people usually need adult doses. Although not yet fully grown, their livers are healthy and fit, so that much of an orally administered drug will be broken down by first-pass metabolism before it reaches the brain. The frequency of dosing may need to be greater than that for adults.

The practice of titrating dose, and sometimes frequency of administration, requires the goals of treatment to be clarified in advance. It also leads to the extensive use of rating scales to be completed by the child, parents or teachers, in order to obtain some reliable information about therapeutic response and sometimes adverse effects. The scores or other results on such rating scales can be obtained remotely by telephone, post or e-mail. This should not wholly substitute for personal review, however, or else opportunities to detect adverse effects or responses not included in scales are lost, as is the opportunity to promote adherence.

As a general rule, children do not relish the task of taking regular medication. To many adolescents it is an unwelcome imposition. This is particularly true if a decision about prescribing is made simply on the basis of a discussion with parents. Adherence can be promoted by an individual discussion with the individual child patient about why the medication is needed and what adverse effects can be expected. This is particularly important when there is likely to be little subjective symptom improvement, as would be the case, for instance, after the first dose of an antidepressant, or with a prophylactic medication, such as lithium. Child patients should be involved in the decisions about optimal dosing and their view sought as to progress. These discussions form the necessary basis for informed consent and are good practice in any case, even with children too young to be fully competent to grant or withhold consent. They can be supplemented by handouts describing the drug in question, which can be more positive and informative than the data sheets supplied by the manufacturers. If these are tailored separately for children, teenagers, parents and teachers their value is even greater.

Not all children find swallowing tablets and capsules easy, and liquid preparations of medicines are often not available. It may be necessary to teach a child how to swallow a tablet using a graded series of small cake decorations and sweets, ensuring that swallowing a solid item is always followed by a drink; tablets retained in the oesophagus are all too common a cause of a failed dose. Parents need to keep medications safe and secure and should supervise the taking of them. This is particularly important with controlled drugs such as the stimulants. Schools and particularly the school doctor should be informed (provided that parents agree) if a child is taking psychiatric medication and staff must be actively involved in the storage and administration of medication to be taken during the day. This is not easy and many adolescents resent having to turn up for a midday dose to be given. Sometimes negotiation with the school to facilitate this in the least embarrassing way is necessary.

Knowing when to stop medication is not always easy. Treatment success commonly involves a suppression of signs or symptoms, and discontinuing medication too early will result in relapse. It is, of course, for such reasons that medication is normally prescribed (as 'water wings') alongside psychological measures, which might, for instance, promote coping skills (as in learning to swim). For many indications, especially attention-deficit hyperactivity disorder (ADHD), obsessive–compulsive disorder (OCD), affective disorders and psychosis, medication will need to be taken for months or years, possibly into adulthood. In very general terms it is wise to consider discontinuing medication every 12 months or so, and to test whether it is still needed.

Paediatric variations in pharmacokinetics

Generally, drug response varies with age, weight, sex, disease state, absorption, distribution, metabolism and excretion: thus developmental factors that influence these things are important to consider. The process of development is not linear across systems and children are not, pharmacologically, scaled-down adults. For ethical reasons to do with consent, however, most pharmacokinetic and pharmacodynamic studies are done with adults.

The extent and rate of absorption of a drug after its oral administration is determined by gastrointestinal factors, which resemble the adult profile after the first year of life. The rate of absorption may be slightly faster in children and peak levels reached earlier. This is less of a concern for drugs that have long absorption times. Some paediatric medicines are administered as liquids, which are more quickly absorbed than pills.

Distribution is influenced by the size of the body water and fat compartments and the binding capacity of plasma and tissue proteins. Fat distribution varies across childhood, rising during the first year, falling towards puberty and increasing thereafter to adulthood. Large fat stores slow the elimination of fat-soluble drugs (e.g. fluoxetine) from the body.

Hepatic metabolism gradually develops in the first year, is highest in early childhood and is twice that of adults in middle childhood (6–12 years). It plateaus to adult values in the early teens. A transient decrease in metabolism has been reported for some medications in the few months before puberty, possibly due to the competition with sex hormones for hepatic enzymes. Thus, for hepatically metabolised drugs (e.g. most antidepressants), children may require higher doses per kilogram of body weight than adults. Renal function also develops at different rates but resembles that of adults by the first year.

Of the Caucasian population, 5–10% show slow hepatic metabolism of a number of drugs as a normal variant. This too is a consideration in children.

The clinical response to and side-effect profile of a drug can be altered by developmental immaturity. Children may display a different drug receptor sensitivity to adults. Animal studies suggest that the noradrenergic system does not develop fully until early adulthood, so serotonergic drugs may be more effective in this age group. Effective plasma ranges in children may be different to those in adults; for example, children require a slightly lower range for chlorpromazine, haloperidol and phenytoin. Such differences may be due to decreased protein binding and increased free fraction of drug rather than increased receptor sensitivity.

Therapeutic drug monitoring is the measurement of drug levels in body fluids (predominantly blood) and the use of these levels to adjust dose. In child and adolescent psychopharmacology, therapeutic ranges have been suggested for lithium, imipramine and nortriptyline and the anticonvulsants used for mood stabilisation, such as valproate and carbamazepine. It is hardly ever used for other medications.

Stimulants

A key area in which psychopharmacology of the young differs from adult practice is stimulant medication in the treatment of ADHD or hyper-kinetic disorder. The stimulants include methylphenidate (Equasym, Ritalin), dexamfetamine (Dexedrine) and pemoline, although the last is available only on a named-patient basis and not generally available in the NHS because of concerns about liver damage. Methylphenidate is the most widely used and the most thoroughly researched, so that much of what is written here applies to it specifically. Conversely, pemoline is not considered in detail. Both methylphenidate and dexamfetamine are controlled drugs in all countries of the world because of fears of misuse and in the UK are 'Schedule 2' controlled drugs. They have been extensively reviewed (see e.g. Wilens & Biederman, 1992; Greenhill et al, 1999; Santosh & Taylor, 2000) and much of what is said here, when unreferenced, is based on evidence cited in such reviews.

Methylphenidate is a piperidine derivative, not an amphetamine (as is often casually asserted). For practical purposes, only its d-isomer is clinically effective. Like dexamfetamine, it acts to increase the amount of noradrenaline and dopamine at synaptic clefts, particularly in the orbitofrontal cortex and the striatum. These are areas of reduced metabolic activity in children with ADHD. The positive effects of stimulant medication are not confined to sufferers from ADHD and can be seen in normal children (Rapoport *et al*, 1978). The end result is to increase the level of activation of the central nervous system (CNS) in those areas. It is currently thought that its most important action is to promote dopaminergic activity, via the release of dopamine from axon terminals and the inhibition of the dopamine transporter (DAT) which takes dopamine from the extracellular synaptic space back into intracellular stores. The level of synaptic dopamine is thus increased (Volkov *et al*, 1998).

Overall, this enhances alertness, focused concentration, and persistence of voluntary activity and self-control. These effects can be conceptualised as inhibiting impulsiveness and promoting cognitive executive function: the capacity to select, activate, monitor, regulate and adjust voluntary activity according to anticipated goals. Promoting orbitofrontal activity enables children to envisage the probable rewards or beneficial outcomes and evaluate their own activities to achieve these. In addition, methylphenidate can be shown to enhance working (short-term) memory.

Stimulants are given orally and are absorbed promptly. They show little plasma protein binding, cross the blood–brain barrier readily and are eliminated from the body by widespread tissue metabolism to ritalinic acid (methylphenidate) or benzoic acid (dexamfetamine), and subsequently by urinary excretion. Dexamfetamine itself can be excreted directly into the urine, and if this is acidified, the majority of the drug can be lost in this way. There is very little, if any, induction of liver enzymes and neither sensitisation nor tolerance over months or years has been demonstrated. When medication seems less effective than before in a particular patient, adherence is likely to be imperfect. There may be some tachyphylaxis (increasing tolerance to sequential doses) during the day (several doses are required – see below), but this disappears overnight, before the first dose of the next day.

Methylphenidate reaches maximal plasma level in about 2 hours, about 30 minutes ahead of dexamfetamine. Its half-life is about 3 hours, approximately 1 hour less than that of dexamfetamine. The desired behavioural effects can be seen in 30–60 minutes with both drugs, peak at 1–3 hours and last about 3.5 hours for methylphenidate, a little longer for dexamfetamine. An adverse effect on sleep onset can be seen for about 5 hours. The drugs are almost completely eliminated from the body within 24 hours. There is substantial variation between individuals as far as these figures are concerned. The rate of uptake seems more significant than absolute plasma levels and there is no point in estimating these.

For practical purposes, a clinical effect can be seen very promptly but the duration of effect is brief, so that several doses a day are required. By tradition, dexamfetamine provides 'smoother' control of inattention or hyperactivity, lessening the 'roller coaster' effect of methylphenidate (swinging from restrained behaviour to excitability as each dose is absorbed and deactivated). Recently formulated sustained-release preparations of methylphenidate use waxed beads of methylphenidate (Equasym XL) or a sophisticated osmotic release (OROS) technology (Concerta XL); both preparations provide 8–12 hours of cover from a single morning dose. At the time of writing no sustained-release preparations of dexamfetamine were ordinarily available in the UK.

There are important inter-individual differences between children in their response to stimulant medication. These do not seem to stem from any particular factor and probably represent a combination of elements: context, desired effect, maturity and comorbid conditions.

Psychological effects

Stimulants promote stimulus discrimination, concentration, cognitive focus and persistence of effort. At the same time they reduce distractibility, irrelevant motor activity, noisiness, excitability and impulsive behaviour (risky actions initiated suddenly and without consideration of adverse consequences) (Rapoport *et al*, 1980). Effectively, they promote central regulation of the allocation of mental effort. Many children report subjective calmness after taking a stimulant, although a few complain of non-vertiginous 'dizziness' or 'feeling strange'. A few, probably mainly those with lower intelligence or autistic spectrum disorders, become obviously tearful and miserable, particularly on higher doses. This may be reflected by misleading gains on rating scales for hyperactivity because the child is quiet and withdrawn.

The positive effects of stimulants are most noticeable in structured, cognitively demanding settings, notably the classroom. This means that information obtained directly from school is crucial in monitoring treatment. Theoretically, stimulants should enhance academic learning. Evidence for this is not very strong outside the laboratory, although such effects can often be demonstrated for an individual child if appropriate baseline measures are taken. Although there have been concerns that learning during stimulant administration may be state dependent, so that the results of learning are manifest only under the same conditions as when it was first acquired, the evidence that this occurs is not convincing.

Children treated with stimulants become more likely to comply with instructions given by parents and teachers, possibly because they are more likely to envisage eventual reward, as a result of enhanced orbitofrontal cerebral activity. They are also more likely to succeed, since they are less distractible and more focused and persistent, as well as being less excitable. This also seems to improve their ability to cooperate with peers. The ultimate effect of these changes is secondarily to change the behaviour of teachers, peers and parents, so that they become less censorious and hostile, and to lower their expressed emotion. This has a beneficial effect on the likelihood of future compliance and self-esteem and probably reduces the rate of antisocial behaviour.

Since the beneficial effects of stimulants can be seen in normal children (Rapoport *et al*, 1978, 1980), improvement on medication does not provide confirmation of, for instance, the diagnoses of hyperkinetic disorder or ADHD.

At higher doses, children tend to become 'over-focused' and perseverative. They sit quietly and initiate little activity. They may perform the same action repeatedly, even to the extent of a motor stereotypy, and the term 'zombified' is applied informally by parents and teachers. This state of mind is transient and dose related. More persistent is the occasional occurrence of auditory hallucinations in clear consciousness, which can be seen at therapeutic dose ranges. Although many books refer to psychosis as an occasional toxic effect, something that obviously occurs with high doses used in illicit self-administration, we have never seen a full-blown psychotic disorder in clinical practice result from prescribed stimulant medication.

Two concerns about unwanted psychological effects arise frequently in clinical work. One is the risk of dependency, particularly because substance misuse is common in association with ADHD, independently of treatment. In that the beneficial effects of stimulants are transient for each dose, clearly there is a need to continue taking medication to produce an effect, yet there is no tendency for the dose to escalate with time (Safer & Allen, 1989). Nor do children and young teenagers experience much, if anything, in the way of euphoria with methylphenidate, although the picture with dexamfetamine is less clear. Recreational use of methylphenidate is virtually unknown in young people with ADHD; indeed, the usual problem is getting them to take their tablets. There have been a very few reports of misuse by 'snorting' crushed tablets, yet in our experience teenagers who have tried this are unwilling to try it again. Nor does stimulant medication seem to increase the likelihood of cocaine misuse later on in life; indeed, it seems to reduce it (Biederman *et al*, 1999). Healthy teenagers will sometimes procure stimulants in order to stay awake all night, but this does not seem to be an issue with patients. One issue to consider, however, is the possibility that stimulants may be misused by other family members, especially to lose weight.

A more subtle yet unfounded concern is that the practice of taking stimulant medication will lead children to attribute their improvement to the drug and minimising the contribution of their own efforts, so that self-esteem is impaired. In practice the reverse seems to be true and one of the effects of medication seems to be an enhancement of self-esteem.

Physical effects

These are usually experienced as unwanted effects and all apply only during the few hours following each dose. At therapeutic doses, mild stimulation of heart rate (about 10 beats per minute) and an increase in both systolic and diastolic blood pressure (about 5 mmHg) are usual. Diminished appetite can lead to a reduction in weight gain with growth or, rarely, to weight loss. It is unusual for height to be affected (Kramer *et al*, 2000), and if it is there is a rebound in growth on discontinuation of treatment. In longer-term studies of children prescribed stimulants, findings are contradictory as to whether adult height is affected. If it is, it is only by 1–2 cm.

Stimulants, by their nature, will cause insomnia and, for each dose, this effect lasts longer than the promotional effect on cognitive executive function. In the same vein, some increase in neurophysiological activity and reactivity can be seen on routine EEG and evoked potentials, although whether this results in a lowering of the threshold for seizures is disputed. Well-controlled epilepsy is not destabilised by therapeutic doses (Feldman *et al*, 1989) but status epilepticus can be precipitated when seizures are poorly controlled. In spite of clinical anecdote that dexamfetamine is less ictogenic, it is not clear that there is any difference between methylphenidate and dexamfetamine in this respect.

It is commonly reported that stimulants worsen or precipitate tics. Often it is difficult to disentangle spontaneously occurring tics, which are common in childhood, particularly in boys, from medication-related tics. This is particularly true of Tourette's syndrome, in which hyperactivity may precede the development of tics by several months or years. Although Tourette's syndrome is frequently cited as a contraindication, only a minority of ticqueurs experience their tics worsening while they are on methylphenidate (Tourette's Syndrome Study Group, 2002). Tics need not be a contraindication for stimulant prescription, provided that there is close surveillance (Castellanos, 1999).

A minority of children, perhaps about a quarter, will experience headaches or epigastric pain through an unknown mechanism. Occasionally one sees a child whose pre-existing headaches are alleviated by methylphenidate.

A desirable physical effect, observed anecdotally, is the ability of stimulants to improve motor planning and coordination of complex fine-motor skills. Handwriting in particular often improves.

Adverse physical effects that are idiosyncratic include skin rashes and a lowering of white cell count, theoretically a harbinger of agranulocytosis. Both reverse on discontinuation. Whether the latter risk should lead to routine blood counts is arguable. General experience is that the leucopenia is mild and does not appear to impair immunity, so that the major centres for the treatment of ADHD in the UK do not carry out routine counts, since these have an adverse effect on acceptance of treatment. It may be more satisfactory practice to have a low threshold for suspecting agranulocytosis and ask parents to report severe sore throats, and to carry out a white cell count if one occurs.

Clinical practice

The main indication for stimulant medication is inattentive, impulsive restlessness, as in ADHD or hyperkinetic disorder (here taken as synonymous), in childhood or school-age teenagers. There is no doubt that stimulants have a powerful effect on the key features of ADHD, with an effect size of between 0.8 and 1.2, depending upon which variable is considered (see Joughin & Zwi, 1999). The effect is temporary, lasting 3–4 hours after each dose. With this in mind, it is not surprising that long-term benefit has not been established. Most clinicians see stimulant medication as providing a 'window of opportunity' for the child, a near-normal period during which there can be better social interactions and improved learning, and it is these that may have beneficial long-term consequences.

For such reasons it has become the orthodoxy to combine psychological and educational provisions with medication in the treatment of ADHD (*Drugs and Therapeutics Bulletin*, 2001; Scottish Intercollegiate Guidelines Network, 2001), although the report by the National Institute for Clinical Excellence, while in line with such practice, equivocates somewhat on this issue (National Institute for Clinical Excellence, 2000). Specifically, it recommends that methylphenidate should be used as part of a comprehensive treatment programme, which 'could but does not need to include specific psychological treatment'. This reflects the fact that it has been hard to demonstrate that medication enhances the effect of psychosocial interventions, and the large MTA study did not show this (MTA Co-operative Group, 1999a,b), although parallel psychosocial interventions allowed lower doses of stimulants to be used in the group that had both sorts of treatment applied. It also follows that treatment should be prolonged, yet there are no controlled studies of stimulant medication that extend beyond 18 months.

It is thought unwise for non-experts in the field to use stimulant medication with children under 6 years of age. The validity of the ADHD diagnosis is poor in pre-school children, which probably explains why, although effectiveness has been demonstrated in 4- to 5-year-olds, their response to stimulant medication is rather more erratic (Firestone *et al*, 1988). Correspondingly, relatively little is known about the optimal treatment of ADHD in adults, even though methylphenidate is effective. In both instances, if medication is thought necessary, a specialist centre should be contacted.

Given the considerable differences between children, it is now accepted that titration rather than a fixed (mg/kg) dose is appropriate. Details of this approach are given in various protocols (Pliszka *et al*, 2000; Hill & Taylor, 2001). Although there is no marked difference in effectiveness when methylphenidate and dexamfetamine are compared, methylphenidate is preferred as the initial agent because more is known about it and because of the impression that it presents fewer adverse effects in routine clinical practice. A dose of 5 mg two or three times a day is a starting point. The spacing of such doses is at approximately 3.5-hour intervals, with the last dose not usually after 4.00 p.m., because of the usual unwanted effect of onset insomnia. A common regimen is doses at 7.30–8.00 a.m., 11.00 a.m.–12.00 midday and 3.00–4.00 p.m., with the administrative arrangements at school being the key variable. Children should not be allowed to keep their own tablets because of the drug's controlled status and the risk that the pills may be forcibly taken from them by other children. Some practitioners prefer to start with 5 mg in the morning only and then contrast behaviour in mornings and afternoons to test for an effect.

A positive response can be expected in most children with un-complicated ADHD and will be greater in those whose parents provide both structure and encouragement, in children with the more severe degrees of inattentiveness and hyperactivity.

Doses can then be increased, in accordance with the child's results on rating scales completed by both parents and teachers, such as the Conners Rating Scale (Revised), SNAP–IV, DuPaul or Brown – see Hill & Cameron (1999) for sources. Baseline records of academic achievement are used to assess academic progress. Titration is against behavioural improvement, academic gains and adverse effects. An eventual maximum dose is likely to be less than 60 mg/day in three or four divided doses or as a sustained-release preparation given once daily in the morning. Higher doses are sometimes required but should be implemented only in consultation with a tertiary-care expert service.

If the child does not respond to methylphenidate, the diagnosis should be reviewed and adherence to the prescribed regimen questioned. True non-responders with non-comorbid, mainstream ADHD are very unusual in our experience. A few children whose ADHD does not respond to methylphenidate will respond to dexamfetamine (used in doses half that of methylphenidate, i.e. 2.5–30 mg daily in divided doses). There is no reason to combine stimulants in the treatment of an individual.

Once an optimal dose has been established, rating scale monitoring should be carried out every 6 months. Medication should be discontinued from time to time, certainly after the first year, to test whether it is still required. In practice, many children drop out after a few years, but for those who do not it is usually possible to discontinue medication in the mid-teens. Some will need treatment into adult life, but what proportion and for how long are scientifically undetermined.

Conditions comorbid with ADHD may complicate matters, and this is well discussed by Pliszka *et al* (2000). The ADHD pattern of difficulties associated with autistic spectrum (pervasive developmental) disorders responds less predictably to stimulants, as is the case when it is associated with general learning disability (severe mental retardation). When it is associated with Tourette's syndrome it responds well but sometimes at the expense of a temporary worsening of tics. These are interventions best implemented in specialist centres.

Anxiety is often worsened by stimulants, so that their use becomes counterproductive. Substance misuse would ordinarily be a contraindication unless the prescriber is very experienced and there is good supervision of the patient. Well-controlled epilepsy and simple tics are no longer thought to be contraindications, although a measure of caution is required. The same is true for short stature. Fortunately, ADHD and eating disorders rarely coincide, as it would be risky to provide a patient who has an eating disorder with a pill that reduces appetite. The inattentiveness associated with schizophrenia should not be treated with stimulants, as these are likely to worsen hallucinations. Aggressive behaviour coexistent with ADHD often seems to respond to the co-prescription of clonidine or risperidone alongside a stimulant.

Other uses of stimulants are less well established scientifically – generally having been tested only in small or open trials. Pathological inattentiveness not associated with hyperactive, impulsive behaviour (ADHD, predominantly inattentive type, for which there is no specific ICD–10 equivalent) will usually improve with stimulants. Narcolepsy will usually respond (although Kleine–Levin syndrome will not). Conduct disorder with aggressive behaviour will sometimes respond, especially if there is explosive rage (Taylor *et al*, 1987; Klein *et al*, 1997). Abulia or overactive, disinhibited behaviour following closed head injury may respond favourably, although not predictably.

Atomoxetine, a noradrenaline transporter inhibitor, has recently been granted a licence in the USA for the treatment of ADHD and at the time of writing a licence was being sought in the UK. It has not been classed as a stimulant and is not a controlled drug in the USA. It can be given once daily. These appear to be practical advantages but precisely what its role will be in the treatment of ADHD has yet to be determined.

It appears only slightly less powerful than methylphenidate, does not cause insomnia yet does cause nausea in a few and can impair weight gain at least in the first year of administration.

Selective serotonin reuptake inhibitors (SSRIs)

The SSRIs are being increasingly considered as first-line medications for several conditions in child and adolescent psychiatry, as a result of their relatively good tolerability and safety. For these reasons, this group is a better alternative to tricyclics that have serotonergic activity such as clomipramine. However, as in most child psychiatric disorders, there are few published controlled trials to provide clinical guidelines, and so many protocols are derived from experience with adults. While case reports and open trials have demonstrated the efficacy of the SSRIs, the results from placebo-controlled trials generally suggest that effect size may be rather smaller than has been otherwise reported. Clinical evidence suggests that, generally speaking, no particular SSRI is superior in efficacy to any other (although substituting another if the first does not work is sometimes effective) and initial choice is largely based on side-effect profile and pharmacokinetic parameters. For instance, the long half-life of fluoxetine may be advantageous in terms of compliance but less favourable if side-effects are likely to be problematic.

Having made the general point about choice between SSRIs being limited by sparse efficacy data (mainly from open-label trials) in childhood and adolescence, there are a few pointers from published randomised controlled trials (RCTs). Fluoxetine has been shown to be effective in depression (Emslie *et al*, 1997), OCD (Geller *et al*, 2001; Riddle *et al*, 1992) and selective mutism (Black & Uhde, 1994). Sertraline is effective in OCD (March *et al*, 1998) and anxiety disorders (Rynn *et al*, 2001). Fluvoxamine is also effective in anxiety disorders (Vitiello, 2000; Isaacs, 2001; Riddle *et al*, 2001). Paroxetine is superior to placebo in OCD (Geller *et al*, 2002) but its effect on depression is less clear – data from unpublished RCTs sponsored by the manufacturer fail to support its effectiveness in child and adolescent depression (although the quality of the trials that failed to show an effect is marginal), leading to a caution against its use for this indication in the UK (e.g. MHRA, 2003*a*).

Side-effects of SSRIs

The frequency of reported side-effects with SSRIs in clinical trials with children and adolescents varies widely. The most commonly reported have been insomnia, gastrointestinal effects and headache.

Fluoxetine is the SSRI used in most clinical trials and case reports. Reports indicate that it can precipitate hypomania in some children and adolescents. Clinical experience and some single case reports indicate that the same holds true for the other SSRIs, but few data are available on relative frequency and SSRIs are overall less likely to precipitate mania than are other antidepressants. More common, however, appears to be a milder, less impairing behavioural activation syndrome of social disinhibition and fatuousness, accompanied by apparent motor excitement, which reverses on dose reduction or cessation of medication. Children also seem to be more sensitive to sedative effects.

There have also been occasional reports of bleeding tendencies, galactorrhoea and hyperprolactinaemia in children. The MHRA's caution about SSRIs in depression (e.g. MHRA, 2003a,b) hinges on a significantly higher rate of reported ideas of self-harm. Yet in the studies perused by that body the rate of such ideation was below the rates reported in the general population (which is odd) and there was no increase in actual self-harm in the active treatment groups.

The best tolerance of unwanted effects has been reported in trials that kept initial doses low and built up dose slowly. This strategy may be particularly useful in younger children, anxious children and those who may be at particular risk of hypomania or behavioural activation – that is, those with ADHD with emotional instability, major depression with psychotic features or a family history of bipolar disorder.

Co-administration with foods and medications, particularly over-the-counter antihistamines that are metabolised through the cyto-chrome P450 system (see Chapter 16), may alter the side-effect profile of SSRIs because of competition for the pathway. For instance, SSRIs given alongside St John's wort, a herbal remedy for depression, may result in a serotonin toxicity syndrome.

As with adults, SSRIs seem relatively safe in overdose at up to over 40 times the average dose, although toxic thresholds have not yet been defined.

SSRIs in depression

The first goal in treatment of depression in children is the safe and prompt resolution of the current episode and the second is to prevent recurrence. Pharmacological treatments are used in conjunction with interventions designed to improve interpersonal, social and academic functioning (see Park & Goodyer, 2000). By and large, SSRIs are the most widely used first-line medication in the treatment of depression in children and adolescents, although evidence from the most tightly controlled trials suggests that medication may not be completely effective in this age group. As is often found, controlled studies yield smaller effect sizes than open trials – see Riddle *et al* (2001) for an overview.

SSRIs in OCD

About 1% of the child and adolescent population have OCD. Children and adolescents tend to report similar symptoms to adults and their disorder may persist into adulthood.

The efficacy of fluoxetine, sertraline and paroxetine has been demonstrated in placebo-controlled trials.

Symptom reduction may begin only after 6 weeks of pharmacotherapy. As in adults, the majority of patients relapse after stopping medication and the addition of cognitive–behavioural therapy may be effective in prolonging remissions.

SSRIs in anxiety disorders

The hard evidence base is limited to RCTs with fluvoxamine, sertraline, paroxetine and (if selective mutism is construed as an anxiety disorder) fluoxetine. A common assertion is that SSRIs should be used as part of a multi-modal approach to treat a variety of anxiety disorders in children, including generalised anxiety disorder, panic disorder, social phobia, school refusal and elective mutism. Significant improvement is seen by about 10 weeks. In anxious patients treatment should be started in low doses and built up, to avoid confusion between panic symptoms and side-effects. Effective doses may be higher than those used to treat depression.

SSRIs in eating disorders

There is some evidence that SSRIs can be effective in the treatment of bulimia nervosa in adults. However, response to pharmacological treatment is only partially effective and cognitive–behavioural therapy (with or without SSRIs) is superior to medication alone.

The mechanism of action may be different in bulimia nervosa and depression, as the average dose of fluoxetine used to treat bulimia is higher than that used for depression. The presence of depressive symptoms does not predict the response of bulimia to antidepressant medication.

The SSRIs should be avoided when there is concomitant substance misuse (including of diet pills), poor physiological status, non-compliance or purging, which will adversely affect compliance and absorption.

In general, pharmacotherapy is not of proven benefit as a direct treatment of anorexia nervosa, although SSRIs can be effective to treat a comorbid depressive illness or to target bulimic symptoms.

SSRIs and neurodevelopmental disorders

There is a lack of data from RCTs. Although SSRIs are ineffective in treating the core phenomena of the pervasive developmental disorders, it is believed on the basis of open trials that they might be helpful in improving the global clinical picture in children with autism who have prominent obsessive–compulsive symptoms, anxiety or ritualistic ('obsessional') behaviour. Adolescents with Asperger syndrome and other non-autistic pervasive developmental disorders are prone to depression and an SSRI can be an effective treatment where environmental or circumstantial triggers cannot be identified and ameliorated.

The SSRIs can treat the obsessive–compulsive symptoms commonly associated with Tourette's syndrome, although their effect on tics is usually marginal and probably secondary to decreased arousal following resolution of the obsessions.

The SSRIs are of no demonstrated benefit in the treatment of ADHD in childhood, although some adult sufferers claim relief from unstable and rapidly fluctuating mood. Anecdotal evidence suggests they may be usefully combined with stimulants in the treatment of a minority of affected children who have comorbid anxiety.

SSRIs and other disorders

Case reports suggest that fluoxetine (20–80 mg) may sometimes be beneficial in the treatment of obsessive eating associated with Prader–Willi syndrome, and self-injurious behaviours seen in Lesch–Nyhan syndrome or associated with severe learning difficulties. Perhaps as an extension of this, other mildly self-injurious behaviours such as trichotillomania (compulsive hair pulling), are also responsive, probably through anxiolytic or anti-obsessive actions.

There is no convincing evidence for the treatment of chronic fatigue syndrome with an SSRI unless there is a comorbid depressive disorder.

Tricyclic/heterocyclic antidepressants

Following a meta-analysis by Hazell et al (1995) which failed to demonstrate effectiveness of tricyclic antidepressants in child or adolescent depression, the use of non-SSRI antidepressants for depression has fallen, although they continue to find favour for a number of other clinical indications.

In general, the properties of heterocyclic antidepressants are the same as in adults, and the adverse effects and the differences between various drugs show the same pattern. Amitriptyline, trimipramine and trazodone are the most sedative; amitriptyline, clomipramine and imipramine the most anticholinergic and so forth. Half-lives are a little shorter in children but have not usually been determined with sufficient accuracy for clinical use. Because children metabolise drugs more rapidly, doses (mg/kg) are higher than in adults. Plasma levels do not show a definite relationship to therapeutic potency, but there is a trend in several studies for responders to have higher levels. There is tremendous variation between individuals in what plasma level results from a particular dose, so that mg/kg dosing is unreliable and it is better to titrate, starting with a low dose, such as the equivalent of 25 mg of imipramine.

A concern about adverse cardiac effects limits their use. Cardio-vascular effects are mainly:

(1) delayed repolarisation of the myocardium, with slowing of intra-cardiac conduction, prolongation of PR and QT intervals and an increase in QRS duration
(2) elevation of blood pressure, both systolic and diastolic
(3) tachycardia.

In virtually all children prescribed therapeutic doses of heterocyclic antidepressants, the increases still result in electrocardiogram (ECG) variables being within normal limits. The risk is that in children with a familial predisposition to long QT intervals, heterocyclic antidepressants can precipitate a particular form of ventricular tachycardia (*torsade de pointes*). This is more likely when the P450 cytochrome system is competed for by other medication, such as non-sedating antihistamines, macrolide antibiotics or imidazole antifungal agents, thus raising blood levels. With this in mind, before prescribing a heterocyclic antidepressant it is wise to ask about a family history of sudden death, whether other medication is being taken and whether there have been palpitations and syncope. The American Heart Association (Gutgesell *et al*, 1999) states that it is 'prudent' to record a preliminary ECG (to detect familial long QT syndrome) and to repeat this when steady state is reached. This seems a little alarmist, given the extensive past prescription of imipramine for enuresis without apparent mortality at low doses. Our personal preference is for initial and follow-up ECGs to be undertaken when the equivalent dose of imipramine exceeds 75 mg/day. Thresholds for concern are:

(1) heart rate > 130 bpm
(2) PR > 200 ms
(3) QRS > 120 ms
(4) QTc > 450 ms

Imipramine is demonstrably effective in the treatment of ADHD and is generally regarded as a second-line treatment – for when stimulants have been unsuccessful or cannot be prescribed. In similar vein, nortriptyline has also been shown to be effective. In all cases there is a general impression that hyperactivity responds rather better than inattentiveness. In comparison with the other non-SSRI antidepressants, imipramine appears to be relatively safe, as it has been used for years in the past for the symptomatic treatment of enuresis with little known risk to patients (although their siblings have been known to drink its liquid formulation by mistake and have thus fallen victim to accidental poisoning). The dose for imipramine is generally 50–75 mg/day, but a few authorities think that higher doses (up to 200 mg/day) are more beneficial.

Imipramine is no longer considered a first-line treatment for enuresis. It is effective in symptom suppression but relapse occurs on discontinuation. It is less effective than an enuresis alarm and as a symptomatic treatment desmopressin is generally preferred, since it is safer.

In the treatment of anxiety, indifferent results and failure to replicate findings have led to heterocyclic antidepressants being abandoned in favour of SSRIs in particular.

Imipramine and trimipramine are occasionally used in the treatment of sleep disorders. Imipramine can suppress rapid-eye-movement (REM) sleep and thus reduce recurrent nightmares arising out of horrific experiences. It can also suppress night-terrors, although diazepam is more widely used for this purpose. Indeed, imipramine may produce unsettled sleep in pre-school children. Trimipramine is sometimes used to treat onset insomnia in adolescents. These uses are based on open trials or clinical recommendation.

Clomipramine

The potential of clomipramine, a tertiary-amine tricyclic antidepressant, to potentiate serotonin as well as block acetylcholine and noradrenaline led to its use in OCD. Controlled assessment has demonstrated an effect in children and adolescents with OCD. The high level of anticholinergic and sedative side-effects with the doses usually required (up to 250 mg/day) means that SSRIs are usually preferred, although clomipramine can be useful in some children who do not respond to these.

Trichotillomania will also often respond to clomipramine, but yet again SSRIs and behavioural intervention are generally preferred as an initial intervention.

Bupropion

The atypical (propiophenone) antidepressant bupropion is an effective antidepressant in adults but has not been evaluated in child or adolescent depression. It is, however, of demonstrable benefit in ADHD, according to two RCTs in children and one open trial in adults. In one of these trials (Barrickman *et al*, 1995) it was no less powerful than methylphenidate. It promotes dopamine neurotransmission more than the other antidepressants. Like the stimulants, it tends to reduce appetite and can cause onset insomnia. It is not a controlled drug, does not produce euphoria and can be given in a slow-release form, so that a single dose provides all-day cover. This means that patients do not have to remember to turn up to collect their medication during the school day (something they find difficult) and there is no risk of misuse by teenagers.

For years it was not available in the UK (in spite of being made by a UK company), but it has now been released as Zyban, with a marketing authorisation for smoking cessation. This, together with the statement that it is 'not recommended' (by the manufacturer) for children, and adverse publicity following two deaths in young adults (one from status epilepticus in a patient with undisclosed epilepsy, one from an intentional overdose) has led general practitioners to be wary of its use. At a specialist level, however, it seems to be of particular value for the reasons cited in the paragraph above. The fatalities among those (adults) using the drug seem to have been mainly in older people who were heavy smokers, but in one case a young adult woman died who had failed to inform the prescribing doctor that she had frequent seizures. Bupropion is ictogenic and should not be prescribed to people with epilepsy. There have been no deaths in children or adolescents. Families should be advised not to be distracted by the literature about smoking cessation that comes with the packaging in the UK.

Other antidepressants

Trazodone is sometimes prescribed to help children taking stimulants settle at night, as it has a sedative effect. There is no formal scientific test of this practice. It has also been claimed that it augments haloperidol in the treatment of Tourette's syndrome. The rare possibility of priapism should indicate caution in its prescription for boys.

Several small open trials have shown a beneficial effect for venlafaxine in adult ADHD and there has thus been occasional prescription of it for adolescents with ADHD. In line with its original development as an antidepressant, it is used in resistant adolescent depression, although the manufacturers and the MHRA cautions against its use in this age group.

Antipsychotics

Antipsychotics are dealt with in Chapter 9 and only issues relevant to children and adolescents are addressed here. There are no antipsychotics that cannot be used in childhood and none is confined to child and adolescent psychiatry.

Most recent interest has been in the so-called atypical antipsychotics ('atypicals'). The main reason for this is that children with chronic conditions requiring maintenance medication will be taking medication for longer than an adult. The fact that atypicals have a lower rate of extrapyramidal side-effects than classical antipsychotics has led to a view that they should be the antipsychotic medication of first choice in the young, even though there is no evidence that they are more efficacious (with the exception of clozapine). Recent concern about the impact of weight gain, hyperglycaemia and hyperlipidaemia associated with many atypicals indicates that this view cannot go absolutely unchallenged.

Adolescents are often treated with one of the atypicals – olanzapine, risperidone, amisulpride, quetiapine, sertindole or zotepine – when they suffer a first episode of schizophrenia. There is, however, a striking paucity of studies of antipsychotics in childhood and adolescents and such practice derives predominantly from studies in adults. There are a few open-label studies; otherwise, studies have been confined to classical antipsychotics (haloperidol, thiothixene, thioridazine) and clozapine, which generally demonstrate effectiveness, although rather less so than in adults.

The status of clozapine is comparable to that in adult practice. It is effective in childhood and adolescence but is usually reserved for those patients who have failed to respond to other antipsychotics. It has been pointed out, though, that 'there are theoretical arguments for its use first-line in young patients' (Santosh & Heyman, 2002).

Classical antipsychotics will retain a role when rapid tranquillisation is required (mania and confusional states), when they are often used in combination with a benzodiazepine, or when a depot preparation is needed. Nevertheless, mania in adolescence can be treated successfully with olanzapine or risperidone.

Psychosis is the clearest indication for antipsychotic treatment in the young, but antipsychotics have also been used widely in Tourette's syndrome, particularly haloperidol, pimozide, sulpiride and risperidone. Similar concerns about the risk of extrapyramidal side-effects emerging with long-term use has led to an interest in the role of atypicals to control both tics and rage.

The third major area of application of antipsychotics is in the management of hyperarousal and aggression in children who have pervasive developmental disorders or general learning disability. Haloperidol is often chosen and there is some evidence to support its role.

In recent years there has been enthusiasm for the use of risperidone and sometimes olanzapine as a treatment for impulsive, aggressive behaviour, particularly when associated with ADHD. Formal study of this has been confined to a few open-label trials and anecdotal papers. Our experience in a tertiary-care centre has been favourable, but whether it is actually superior to the older practice of thioridazine used in a similar way remains to be established. There does not seem to be any indication that antipsychotics alone are useful in treating core ADHD symptoms.

Risperidone has also attracted interest by virtue of single-case or small-scale studies in anorexia nervosa and Prader–Willi syndrome, and may have a role in potentiating SSRIs in resistant OCD.

The choice of atypical antipsychotics is on the basis of relative frequency of side-effects. Risperidone and olanzapine are frequently selected but there are grounds for thinking that amisulpride would be a logical choice if it is, as asserted, less prone to produce weight gain. It does, however, raise prolactin levels.

Clonidine

The action of clonidine is complex. It is a noradrenergic agonist at α_2 receptors, which are found in the locus coeruleus and the cerebral cortex. In the neurons of the locus coeruleus, the main noradrenergic complex in the brain-stem, the α_2 receptors are presynaptic and form part of a feedback loop, so that stimulation of them inhibits noradrenaline release at the synapse downstream from them. Where α_2 receptors are postsynaptic, as in the frontal cortex, the action is to promote noradrenergic activity. As a rough rule of thumb, low doses of clonidine stimulate presynaptic receptors and diminish noradrenergic activity, while higher doses stimulate postsynaptic receptors and promote noradrenergic activity. Yet higher doses also stimulate a different subtype of α_2 receptors in the thalamus and cause drowsiness. Not surprisingly, this means that the ultimate clinical action of clonidine in an individual can be hard to predict, so that the usual approach is to titrate slowly from a low starting dose.

The unwanted effects are predominantly drowsiness (which tends to wear off after about 10 days), a mild bradycardia and a slight lowering of blood pressure. Sudden discontinuation carries a theoretical risk of rebound hypertension, but we have never seen this ourselves. Nevertheless, parents should be warned not suddenly to stop giving the child the tablets. Children taking the drug occasionally develop cold extremities or disturbed sleep.

For several years the combination of clonidine and a stimulant was thought to be dangerous, since they have opposing effects on the heart. Early reports of deaths were subsequently seen as alarmist. The combination is now widely used. It is good practice to obtain a baseline ECG if this combination is to be used, although this is probably not necessary if clonidine alone is to be used in a child with a clinically normal cardiovascular system. It would be wise not to use clonidine in an individual with known cardiovascular problems or a strong family history suggestive of cardiac arrythmias.

Clonidine's widest use is in the treatment of ADHD. It has a demonstrable though less powerful and less predictable effect than the stimulants in reducing hyperactivity but is rather less effective in promoting concentration. A meta-analysis (Connor et al, 1999) suggests an effect size of 0.6 in treating ADHD symptoms, which is less than the effect sizes obtained for stimulants (0.8–1.2). Importantly, it will also reduce aggressive impulsive behaviour and, unlike the stimulants, does not cause anorexia or onset insomnia. It is not a controlled drug.

It may be used as an alternative to stimulants or given alongside a stimulant to enhance control without too much in the way of stimulant side-effects. It can be given in divided doses during the day (usual total daily dose 3–5 μg/kg or about 75–150 μg a day) or as a single dose of about 50–75 μg in the late afternoon to improve symptom control during a period when it is often impossible to give a dose of stimulants (because they can cause insomnia). The sedative effect often seen with single doses over 100 μg at night can be used to promote sleep.

It is the commonest drug worldwide for the treatment of severe tic disorders, particularly Tourette's syndrome, although evidence for its effectiveness comes principally from one RCT. There have been negative trials which were probably underpowered since only just over half of children will respond, and even in these effects are considerably greater on motor rather than vocal tics. In children and adolescents it is given as 50 μg two or three times a day, titrating upwards until control or unremitting drowsiness supervenes. This tends to be above 5 μg/kg daily.

Other indications for clonidine, which rest on open trials or case reports, include self-injurious behaviour in a setting of pervasive developmental disorders, post-traumatic stress disorder and various forms of sleep disturbance. Guanfacine, which is generally similar but with less sedative action, is not yet routinely available in the UK.

Desmopressin acetate

Desmopressin acetate is an antidiuretic hormone analogue. The drug decreases urinary flow rate by increasing renal absorption of water without affecting sodium, potassium or creatinine concentrations.

It is administered as a nasal spray or tablets at a starting dose of 20 μg per day, given half an hour before bedtime. Side-effects are rare. Increased blood pressure has been reported with doses over 40 μg/day, which are not recommended. Dose-related effects on plasma factor VIII and plasma aggregation have also been reported and it can cause electrolyte chaos in children with cystic fibrosis.

Laxatives

Although not technically a psychopharmacological intervention, the pharmacological management of faecal retention and constipation is a common reason for child and adolescent psychiatrists to prescribe for children. The initial management of faecal soiling associated with faecal retention is to remove accumulated faeces in the rectum by diet: increasing fluid and fibre intake by advising more fruit, cereals and vegetables. If this fails, then soft or firm faeces can be shifted by an osmotic laxative such as lactulose (10–15 ml twice daily for children over 5 years) more effectively than by senna. Should lactulose prove insufficient, then a stimulant laxative such as senna (Senokot 5 ml each morning) or bisacodyl (Dulcolax 5–10 mg orally at night) can be added. Hard faeces, particularly if rectal distension is marked, need docusate (5–10 ml three times daily), which is a stool-softening agent as well as a stimulant laxative. Bowel evacuation with powerful stimulant laxatives such as picosulphate or magnesium citrate sachets taken orally, or sodium citrate micro-enemas, will be required only if the above fails. Treatment also involves advice and often a behavioural incentive programme. In secondary care, several months of treatment is usually required before the rectum returns to normal functioning.

Melatonin

Melatonin, a serotonin derivative produced in the pineal gland, is associated with the regulation of circadian rhythm. As it is an endogenous substance, it is not licensed for use as a medicine in the UK but can be prescribed on a named-patient basis or other special arrangement.

Reports have centred on its use to attempt to alleviate jet lag in adults (unsuccessful in controlled trial) and the treatment of chronic sleep disturbance in children and adolescents with multiple neurological disability, with and without visual disturbance. It may be useful for children who cannot interpret the cues for synchronising the sleep–wake cycle: trials in children have shown it to be effective in this regard and to have minimal side-effects. Despite reports of a mild anticonvulsant effect in animal studies and in humans, there has been a report of increased seizure activity in four of six children, which paralleled melatonin administration. It should therefore be used with caution in children with poorly controlled epilepsy.

After other causes of sleep disturbance have been excluded, melatonin may be given as a single night-time dose of 3–6 mg (or a maximum of 9 mg) half an hour before bedtime on an empty stomach. The half-life is between 4 and 8 hours, and it is hepatically metabolised. It should be used for a 2- to 3-month period in conjunction with a sleep hygiene programme.

Drugs that may be indicated for various conditions or symptoms: a rational approach to their use

This section is by no means a complete guide to the treatment of child and adolescent psychiatric disorder. Rather, it is an attempt to suggest what medication may be selected and in what order. As far as possible it is based on evidence, but, with the exception of ADHD, trials of medication have not been of sufficient number or quality to allow more than an indication as to what seems sensible to us.

ADHD or hyperkinetic disorder

Not all children with ADHD need medication, but most with hyperkinetic disorder (equivalent to severe ADHD, combined type) do. Medication should not be introduced until parental and school handling have been optimised and should not ordinarily be used for pre-school children. In other words, certain conditions should be met (Hill & Taylor, 2001). Management involves more than medication (Taylor *et al*, 1998).

The first choice of medication is ordinarily methylphenidate, titrated against effect and tolerance, using information obtained from both home and school. A starting dose of 5 mg in the morning and at midday can be increased progressively to 20 mg three times daily, the third dose normally in mid-afternoon. Because the duration of effect of each dose is short, it is sometimes helpful to prescribe a morning dose only in order to observe any contrast between mornings and afternoons. Failure to obtain satisfactory benefit from methylphenidate leads to reappraisal of the diagnosis and, if confirmed, a trial of dexamfetamine (doses of which are half those of methylphenidate, i.e. starting at 2.5 mg and increasing to 30 mg daily in divided doses). If neither stimulant can be tolerated or fails to achieve the desired effect, then imipramine (50–75 mg daily) or bupropion (150 mg of slow-release preparation daily) can be considered as alternatives. It may be that atomoxetine will, when released, become the preferred alternative to stimulants.

Associated aggressive behaviour may not respond to the above, in which case clonidine can be added in divided doses starting at 25 µg two or three times a day and titrating upwards until enduring drowsiness supervenes (usually above 200 µg a day).

Particularly with higher doses of stimulants, difficulty settling to sleep becomes an issue for the child, so that a problem emerges regarding how to balance a need to control ADHD symptoms in the evening with wakefulness at bedtime. Clonidine (25–75 µg, as a single dose) can be given on return from school to mitigate ADHD symptoms in the evening. If the problem is confined to difficulty getting off to sleep, and if simple sleep hygiene measures (specified bedtime, settled, quiet routine, warm milky drink, etc.) fail, a higher single dose (50–150 µg) can be given in the late evening to facilitate settling. Alternatively, a straightforward sedative antihistamine (diphenhydramine, promethazine) may be useful. Some authorities use trazodone for the same effect, although there is a risk of priapism in boys. It is best to avoid using tricyclic antidepressants (trimipramine, amitriptyline, imipramine) for the same purpose, as they will increase the blood levels of stimulants, sometimes unpredictably.

At the time of writing, the status of long-acting stimulant medication in the UK is changing, as new preparations of methylphenidate are becoming available in the next year or so. Concerta XL has already been widely prescribed.

Depression

The pharmacological treatment of depression in late childhood or adolescence takes its place as a component of overall treatment (see e.g. Park & Goodyer, 2000). Although the effectivness of SSRIs as antidepressants is disputed (Riddle, 2001; Jureidini et al, 2004), an SSRI should be selected, probably fluoxetine (e.g. MHRA, 2003b), in the first place. Alternatively, a useful algorithm is provided by Hughes et al (1999). Dosing should ordinarily start at half the adult dose, but, at least in teenagers, should subsequently be increased to adult dose levels (e.g. 20–40 mg a day for fluoxetine). Social disinhibition or hypomanic symptoms may be dose responsive and subside if the dose is reduced, but sometimes the medication has to be discontinued. In our experience it is sometimes the case that a similar reaction does not recur if another SSRI is substituted.

Failure to respond to one SSRI is probably an indication to try another, even though evidence for efficacy is sparse and needs to be contrasted with a possibly higher rate of adverse effects than placebo. Although this may seem to have no basis in logic, clinical experience indicates that it is worthwhile. Should this prove ineffective, the subsequent choice is open and there is little hard evidence from studies on children and adolescents to provide guidance.

Obsessive–compulsive disorder

The SSRIs have replaced clomipramine as the pharmacological treatment of first choice. There is probably nothing to choose between the SSRIs in terms of effectiveness and once again the choice is made on the grounds of personal preference. If one SSRI fails to provide sufficient benefit, another can be substituted. If this is insufficient, clomipramine may produce improvement, doses starting at 25 mg daily and increasing on a weekly basis until relief is obtained or side-effects prove intolerable. In childhood, sedation, feelings of hotness, dry mouth, tremor and constipation are most frequently encountered.

Because relapse on discontinuation is common, it is usually considered good practice to combine cognitive–behavioural treatment with medication.

Bipolar disorder

Lithium is the standby for prophylaxis and the treatment of acute mania. Thereafter little hard evidence is available to guide choice. Carbamazepine and valproate are known to be effective and are used quite widely in prophylaxis but whether they are superior to vigabatrin or gabapentin in the young is not known. Topiramate is rarely used because of a belief that it may cause depression and weight loss.

Aggression and rage

Both are common in a childhood population, so much so that it would be remarkable to consider medication as a first move; hardly ever would rage in a pre-school child be treated pharmacologically. Aggressive behaviour, when premeditated, is unlikely to respond to medication, but when part of an angry, impulsive outburst (especially if characterised as episodic dyscontrol) may be ameliorated. Particularly if such outbursts accompany ADHD, stimulant medication prescribed for the main condition may be effective. Thereafter, no priority can easily be established for which agents to select.

Clonidine (50 to about 300 μg a day in divided doses) is sometimes useful, although not predictably so. Risperidone (0.5–3 mg daily), on anecdotal evidence (including our own experience), can be dramatically effective but at the expense of weight gain and largely unknown long-term effects if taken for any length of time.

A few children with episodic rage will be calmed but not sedated by a beta-blocker, of which propanolol is the commonest to be employed. The dose is titrated against both effect and the possibility of a lowering of blood pressure and is likely to be between 100 and 200 mg daily.

Even in children who present no evidence of a seizure disorder, anticonvulsants are quite often recommended for a reduction of aggressive or angry outbursts. There is evidence that valproate is sometimes effective, but at least one controlled study has failed to show that carbamazepine is useful.

Although lithium can be shown to be effective in children with explosive, aggressive rages, the need for blood level monitoring rather subtracts from its general usefulness.

Schizophrenia

Current thinking is that an atypical antipsychotic should be the first agent to be tried because of the smaller risk of extrapyramidal side-effects in both the short and long term. There is no evidence that one is superior to another, with the exception of clozapine. It is thought by some that the balance of adverse effects favours amisulpride. If the first antipsychotic fails or is not tolerated, another should be substituted. If this does not work sufficiently well, it should be discontinued in favour of clozapine.

Pervasive developmental (autistic spectrum) disorders

There is no direct treatment for these conditions. Initial hopes that secretin would prove effective have been dashed. Stereotypies associated with autism may be helped by haloperidol, clomipramine or risperidone, and aggressive outbursts that do not respond to behaviour therapy may be eased by one of the agents mentioned above.

Self-injurious behaviour associated with general learning disability

A host of agents have been employed for this challenging set of behaviours. On the basis of small studies, clonidine, SSRIs and antipsychotics are worth trying, but behavioural treatments need to be considered as well, especially because of the possibility of detecting remediable environmental triggers.

Anxiety disorders

The range of conditions and situations in which disproportionate anxiety occurs is heterogeneous. In general, removing stressors and promoting coping through cognitive–behavioural measures are indicated.

If medication is indicated, SSRIs are now regarded as the first choice. There is little evidence that any one is superior to the others, although paroxetine, sertraline, fluvoxamine and fluoxetine have some RCT evidence in their favour. Rather higher doses are needed than are generally employed for antidepressant treatment. Clonazepam has been enjoying something of a vogue recently as a short-term measure, either alone or in conjunction with an SSRI, although the data to support this are rather thin.

Enuresis

The primary treatments for enuresis are behavioural. Medication plays a small part by providing temporary suppression of urinary incontinence. Natural remission of the problem may take place while this is effected but more usually there is relapse on discontinuation. Desmopressin is the treatment of choice, except in the setting of cystic fibrosis. Imipramine or viloxazine are alternatives, but are generally considered to be less safe.

Faecal soiling

A sequence of laxatives was outlined earlier in the chapter. Lactulose will usually prove effective, with senna added if required. If this is insufficient, picosulphate can be substituted and micro-enemas deployed only if this fails.

Sleep problems and disorders

Difficulties settling a small child to sleep are best dealt with behaviourally, but occasionally a sedative antihistamine is used to provide respite for exhausted parents. Promethazine or diphenhydramine are available over the counter. Trimeprazine is more powerful but may very occasionally cause respiratory arrest, so that close observation of a trial dose is wise. Melatonin is increasingly popular with neurologically impaired children of school age or those on stimulant treatment, although empirical evidence is sparse.

Parasomnias may respond to a week's worth of anticipatory waking 15 minutes before their occurrence if their time can be predicted. This is not always possible and a benzodiazepine will reduce stage IV sleep and make their occurrence much less likely. It can often be discontinued without relapse after several weeks.

Tourette's syndrome

Helping a child adapt to having a chronic, fluctuating disorder is more important than suppressing tics. When symptoms are of especial concern, many children and their families find that rage attacks and accompanying symptoms of hyperactivity and inattention are more significant problems than tics.

In the Tourette's clinic at Great Ormond Street Hospital for Children we use clonidine as a first-line pharmacological treatment, starting usually at 50 µg twice daily and titrating upwards until enduring drowsiness supervenes, usually at 200–300 µg daily. A little more than half of all children will respond satisfactorily to this.

Failure to provide sufficient benefit leads us to try either sulpiride or risperidone. The latter seems particularly useful in rage control. Our third line is haloperidol, retained until last because of the relatively high risk of extrapyramidal side-effects and the fact that a number of children voice their dislike of feeling tranquillised. Although it is effective, we do not often use pimozide, because of the risks of extrapyramidal side-effects and cardiac complications.

In those children with associated ADHD symptoms, some will improve with clonidine. If not, cautious use of methylphenidate seems helpful. In those children whose tics worsen on this, supportive encouragement to continue for two whole months often results in the exacerbation subsiding. A few find that methylphenidate ameliorates their tics.

Associated obsessive–compulsive symptoms usually respond to an SSRI (and/or cognitive–behavioural therapy).

References

Barrickman, L., Perry, P. & Allen A. (1995) Bupropion versus methylphenidate in the treatment of attention-deficit hyperactivity disorder. *Journal of the American Academy of Child and Adolescent Psychiatry*, **34**, 649–657.

Biederman, J., Wilens, T., Mick, E., *et al* (1999) Pharmacotherapy of attention-deficit hyperactivity disorder reduces risk for substance use disorder. *Pediatrics*, **104**, e20.

Black, B. & Uhde, T. W. (1994) Treatment of elective mutism with fluoxetine: a double-blind, placebo-controlled study. *Journal of the American Academy of Child and Adolescent Psychiatry*, **33**, 1000–1006.

Castellanos, F. X. (1999) Stimulants and tic disorders: from dogma to data. *Archives of General Psychiatry*, **56**, 337–338.

Connor, D. F., Fletcher, K. E. & Swanson, J. M. (1999) A meta-analysis of clonidine for symptoms of attention deficit hyperactivity disorder. *Journal of the American Academy of Child and Adolescent Psychiatry*, **38**, 1551–1559.

Drugs and Therapeutics Bulletin (2001) Stimulant drugs for severe hyperactivity in childhood. *Drugs and Therapeutics Bulletin*, **39**, 52–54.

Emslie, G. J., Rush, A. J., Weinberg, W. A., *et al* (1997) A double-blind, randomized, placebo-controlled trial of fluoxetine in children and adolescents with depression. *Archives of General Psychiatry*, **54**, 1031–1037.

Feldman, H., Crumrine, P., Handen, B. L., *et al* (1989) Methylphenidate in children with seizures and attention-deficit disorder. *American Journal of Disabilities of Children*, **143**, 1081–1086.

Firestone, P., Musten, L. M., Pisterman, S., *et al* (1988) Short-term side effects of stimulant medication are increased in preschool children with attention-deficit/hyperactivity disorder: a double-blind placebo-controlled study. *Journal of Child and Adolescent Psychopharmacology*, **8**, 13–25.

Geller, D. A., Hoog, S. L. & Heiligenstein, J. H. (2001) Fluoxetine treatment for obsessive–compulsive disorder in children and adolescents: a placebo-controlled clinical trial. *Journal of the American Academy of Child and Adolescent Psychiatry*, **40**, 773–779.

Geller, D. A., Wagner, K. D., Emslie, G. J., *et al* (2002) Efficacy of paroxetine in pediatric OCD: results of a multicenter study (Abstract). *New Research Abstracts, Annual Meeting of the American Psychiatric Association 2002*. Washington, DC: APA. http://www.psych.org/edu/other_res/lib_archives/archives/meetings/2002nra.htm.

Greenhill, L., Halperin, J. M. & Abikoff, H. (1999) Stimulant medications. *Journal of the American Academy of Child and Adolescent Psychiatry*, **38**, 503–512.

Gutgesell, H., Atkins, D., Barst, R., *et al* (1999) AHA scientific statement: cardiovascular monitoring of children and adolescents receiving psychotropic drugs. *Journal of the American Academy of Child and Adolescent Psychiatry*, **38**, 1047–1050.

Hazell, P., Heathcote, D., Robertson, J., *et al* (1995) Efficacy of tricyclic drugs in treating child and adolescent depression: a meta-analysis. *BMJ*, **310**, 897–901.

Hill, P. & Cameron, M. (1999) Recognising hyperactivity: a guide for the cautious clinician. *Child Psychology and Psychiatry Review*, **4**, 50–60.

Hill, P. & Taylor, E. (2001) An auditable protocol for treating attention deficit/hyperactivity disorder. *Archives of Disease in Childhood*, **84**, 404–409.

Hughes, C. W., Emslie, G. J., Crismon, M. L., *et al* (1999) The Texas children's medication algorithm project: report of the Texas consensus panel on medication treatment of childhood major depressive disorder. *Journal of the American Academy of Child and Adolescent Psychiatry*, **38**, 1442–1454.

Isaacs, E. (2001) Fluvoxamine for the treatment of anxiety disorders in children and adolescents. *New England Journal of Medicine*, **344**, 1279–1285.

Joughin, C. & Zwi, M. (eds) (1999) *Focus on the Use of Stimulants in Children with ADHD: Primary Evidence-Based Briefing.* London: Royal College of Psychiatrists' Research Unit.

Jureidini, J. J., Doecke, C. J., Mansfield, P. R., *et al* (2004) Efficacy and safety of antidepressants for children and adolescents. *BMJ*, **328**, 879–883.

Klein, R. G., Abikoff, H., Klass, E., *et al* (1997) Clinical efficacy of methylphenidate in conduct disorder with and without attention deficit hyperactivity disorder. *Archives of General Psychiatry*, **54**, 1073–1080.

Kramer, J. R., Loney, J., Ponto, L. B., *et al* (2000) Predictors of adult height and weight in boys treated with methylphenidate for childhood behavior problems. *Journal of the American Academy of Child and Adolescent Psychiatry*, **39**, 517–524.

March, J. S., Biederman, J., Wolkow, R., *et al* (1998) Sertraline in children and adolescents with obsessive–compulsive disorder: a multicenter randomized controlled trial. *Journal of the American Medical Association*, **280**, 1752–1756.

MHRA (2003*a*) *10 June 2003. Message from Professor G. Duff, Chairman of Committee on Safety of Medicines. Safety of Seroxat (paroxetine) in Children and Adolescents under 18 Years – Contraindication in the Treatment of Depressive Illness.* http://medicines.mhra. gov.uk (accessed from Committee on Safety of Medicines' homepage, Messages to health professionals, Important safety messages issued in 2003).

MHRA (2003*b*) *10 December 2003. Selective Serotonin Reuptake Inhibitors (SSRIs) – Use in Children and Adolescents with Major Depressive Disorder.* http://medicines.mhra.gov.uk (accessed from Committee on Safety of Medicines' homepage, Messages to health professionals, Important safety messages issued in 2003).

MTA Co-operative Group (1999*a*) A 14-month randomized clinical trial of treatment strategies for attention-deficit/hyperactivity disorder. *Archives of General Psychiatry*, **56**, 1073–1086.

MTA Co-operative Group (1999*b*) Moderators and mediators of treatment response for children with attention-deficit/hyperactivity disorder: the multi-modal treatment study of children with attention-deficit/hyperactivity disorder. *Archives of General Psychiatry*, **56**, 1088–1096.

National Institute for Clinical Excellence (2000). *Guidance on the Use of Methylphenidate (Ritalin, Equasym) for Attention Deficit/Hyperactivity Disorder (ADHD) in Childhood.* Technology Appraisal Guidance No. 13. London: NICE (available at www.nice.org.uk).

Park, R. & Goodyer, I. (2000) Clinical guidelines for depressive disorders in childhood and adolescence. *European Journal of Child and Adolescent Psychiatry*, **9**, 147–161.

Pliszka, S., Greenhill, L., Crismon, M. L., *et al* (2000) The Texas children's medication algorithm project: report of the Texas consensus conference panel on medication treatment of childhood attention-deficit/hyperactivity disorder. *Journal of the American Academy of Child and Adolescent Psychiatry*, **39**, 908–919.

Rapoport, J. L., Buchsbaum, M. S., Zahn, T. P., *et al* (1978) Dextroamphetamine. Cognitive and behavioral effects in normal prepubertal boys. *Science*, **199**, 560–563.

Rapoport, J. L., Buchsbaum, M. S., Weingartner, H., *et al* (1980) Dextroamphetamine. Its cognitive and behavioral effects in normal and hyperactive boys and normal men. *Archives of General Psychiatry*, **37**, 933–943.

Riddle, M. A. (2001) Pediatric psychopharmacology. *Journal of Child Psychology and Psychiatry*, **42**, 73–90.

Riddle, M. A., Scahill, L., King, R., *et al* (1992) Double-blind cross-over trial of fluoxetine and placebo in children and adolescents with obsessive–compulsive disorder. *Journal of the American Academy of Child and Adolescent Psychiatry*, **31**, 1062–1069.

Riddle, M. A., Reeve, E. A., Yaryura-Tobias, J. A., et al (2001) Fluvoxanine for children and adolescents with obsessive–compulsive disorder: a randomized, controlled, multicenter trial. *Journal of the American Academy of Child and Adolescent Psychiatry*, **40**, 222–229.

Royal College of Paediatrics and Child Health (2003) *Medicines for Children* (2nd edn). London: Royal College of Paediatrics and Child Health.

Rynn, M. A., Siqueland, L. & Rickels, K. (2001) Placebo-controlled trial of sertraline in the treatment of children with generalized anxiety disorder. *American Journal of Psychiatry*, **158**, 2008–2014.

Safer, D. & Allen, R. P. (1989) Absence of tolerance to the behavioral effects of methylphenidate in hyperactive and inattentive children. *Journal of Pediatrics*, **115**, 1003–1008.

Santosh, P. & Heyman, I. (2002) Pharmacological and other physical treatments. In *Child and Adolescent Psychiatry* (4th edn) (eds M. Rutter & E. Taylor), pp. 998–1018. Oxford: Blackwell Scientific.

Santosh, P. & Taylor, E. (2000) Stimulant drugs. *European Journal of Child and Adolescent Psychiatry*, **9**, 27–43.

Scottish Intercollegiate Guidelines Network (SIGN) (2001) *Attention Deficit and Hyperkinetic Disorders in Children and Young People*. SIGN publication no. 52. Available at http://www.sign.ac.uk.

Taylor, E., Schachar, R., Thorley, G., et al (1987) Which boys respond to stimulant medication? A controlled trial of methylphenidate in boys with disruptive behaviour. *Psychological Medicine*, **17**, 121–143.

Taylor, E., Sergeant, J., Doepfner, M., et al (1998) Guidelines for treatment of hyperkinetic disorders. *European Journal of Child and Adolescent Psychiatry*, **7**, 184–200.

Tourette's Syndrome Study Group (2002) Treatment of ADHD in children with tics. *Neurology*, **58**, 527–536.

Vitiello, B. (2000) A multi-site double-blind placebo-controlled trial of fluvoxamine for children and adolescents with anxiety disorders. *Journal of Child and Adolescent Psychopharmacology*, **10**, 257–258.

Volkov, N. D., Wang, G. J., Fowler, J. S., et al (1998) Dopamine transporter occupancies in the human brain induced by therapeutic doses of oral methylphenidate. *American Journal of Psychiatry*, **155**, 1325–1331.

Wilens, T. & Biederman, J. (1992) The stimulants. *Psychiatric Clinics of North America*, **15**, 191–222.

CHAPTER 12

Psychopharmacology in the elderly

Stephen Curran and John P. Wattis

The proportion of people aged 65 years or more in the UK population is gradually rising and is currently estimated to be 15%. This is expected to continue to rise and by 2025 the number aged 85 years or more is set to increase by at least 50% (Braithwaite, 1998). Life expectancy is increasing and it is now common to talk about 'young old' and 'old old' (Wheatley & Smith, 1998). The National Service Framework for Older People (Department of Health, 2001) distinguishes three groups:

(1)   entering old age – this is a socially constructed definition that embraces those aged 50 and upwards who have completed their careers and reached 'retirement age'
(2)   transitional phase – those in transition between a healthy, active life and frailty
(3)   frail older people – these people are vulnerable because of health problems or social care needs.

As people become older they have an increased prevalence of a range of physical illnesses and so often take numerous medications, which increases the scope for adverse side-effects and drug interactions. Psychiatric disorders are also common in old age. The prevalence of dementia increases from approximately 0.7% in those aged 60–64 years, doubling every 5 years to reach nearly 40% of those aged 90–95 years (Demirovic, 1998). Depression is also common. In community samples the prevalence of mild depression is around 11% (Alexopoulous, 1992), but this rises to approximately 45% in samples of hospitalised elderly patients with physical illness (Koenig *et al*, 1988). Paranoid disorders are also very common in older people. It has been estimated that approximately 10% of all psychiatric first admissions of people over the age of 60 years are for late-onset paranoid disorders (Naguib & Levy, 1995). Other notable disorders in older people include acute confusional states, neurotic disorders and personality disorders (Wattis & Curran, 2001).

The treatment of older people with mental illness invariably needs an integrated approach, with pharmacological, social and psychological approaches working together. However, this chapter focuses on the pharmacological approaches. In general, the pharmacological evidence base is much better for younger patients. In particular, many clinical trials exclude older people and this means it becomes necessary to extrapolate the findings to older people, which can be problematic. Older people may be excluded because it is harder to control for confounding variables such as concurrent diseases and the medications needed to treat them. This must always be borne in mind when interpreting data from studies in younger people for use in older people. There is a need for more research on the use of psychotropic drugs in this vulnerable group.

Age-related brain changes

A wide range of changes occur in the central nervous system with increasing age. Overall brain weight and volume decrease and there is widening of both sulci and ventricles. There is also dendritic loss as well as increasing numbers of senile plaques and tangles. A wide variety of substances are deposited, including lipofuscin, aluminium, copper and iron. The brain weight decreases by 10% in old age and about 100 000 neurons are lost per day. During the first 50 years grey matter is lost at a greater rate than white, whereas in the second 50 years the loss of white matter is greater (Esiri & Morris, 1997). These observations have important implications, since these changes are also seen in early Alzheimer's disease and in the early stages it may be difficult to distinguish between them. However, not all parts of the brain age at the same rate (Esiri & Morris, 1997): some regions (e.g. the hippocampus, locus coeruleus and substantia nigra) have a high neuronal loss, whereas other areas (e.g. the nucleus basalis, deep cerebellar nuclei and area 17 in the occipital cortex) are not associated with significant cell loss with increasing age.

There are also reductions in synaptic transmission with increasing age, although methodological factors confuse interpretation. Variations in laboratory methods, problems in applying animal models to humans and artefacts introduced after death, such as degeneration, all complicate interpretation. For these reasons few studies have conclusively demonstrated changes in neurotransmitter systems with increasing age and no consistent pattern has emerged. However, with increasing age, reductions in acetylcholine, dopamine, noradrenaline and serotonin (and other neurotransmitters) are thought to occur (Whitehouse, 1994) and these are often further reduced when pathology is present (e.g. acetylcholine in Alzheimer's disease) (Esiri & McShane, 1997).

Pharmacokinetic effects of psychotropic drugs in older people

Older people are more sensitive to the side-effects of drugs and experience adverse events more frequently than younger patients. Pharmacodynamic and pharmacokinetic changes with increasing age both play a part in explaining increased drug sensitivity (Lader, 1994). Pharmacodynamic changes include increased receptor sensitivity and a reduction in total receptor numbers with increasing age. Changes in drug distribution, metabolism and excretion are the main pharmacokinetic factors involved. A shift in body composition, with a relative reduction in total body water compared with fat, alters the distribution of lipid-soluble drugs in particular. As a result, the half-life of many lipid-soluble psychotropic drugs is prolonged. Hepatic metabolism of psychotropic drugs is reduced because of decreased hepatic blood flow and slowed enzyme metabolism. Glomerular filtration rate declines by 50% between young adulthood and the age of 70 (Lader, 1994), which is of particular importance in explaining the increased risk of lithium toxicity in older patients.

The general clinical impression that older people are more sensitive to adverse effects and experience more of these compared with younger people has been supported by a number of studies. Hurwitz (1969) reported a higher level of drug interactions in in-patients and studies of out-patients have reported similar findings (Learoyd, 1972). There have also been reports of increased side-effects associated with benzodiazepines and tricyclic antidepressants (TCAs) in older compared with younger people (Ray et al, 1992).

In relation to absorption there is reduced gastric acid production, gastric emptying, gastrointestinal motility and absorptive gut surface area. These changes may reduce the rate of absorption of some drugs.

Issues regarding distribution are also important. There is a reduced total body mass and this has the effect of increasing the dose per unit body weight. There is also a reduction in the lean body mass, an increase in the proportion of fat and overall reduced body water. This results in increased blood levels for water-soluble drugs and a reduction in blood levels for lipid-soluble drugs. There is also a reduction in plasma albumin and therefore reduced plasma binding and an increase in the free fraction.

There are also important hepatic and renal changes. In particular there are reductions in renal blood flow, glomerular filtration rate and tubular secretion. These changes have the effect of reducing the excretion of polar and water-soluble molecules. There are also reductions in liver mass and altered enzyme activity, with the result that there is reduced hepatic clearance and increased first-pass bioavailability for some drugs (Braithwaite, 1998).

Table 12.1 Age-related changes in pharmacokinetics

Drug group	Comments
Benzodiazepines	With diazepam there is increased plasma half-life. Triazolam causes significantly greater impairment of psychomotor performance in older people. Very little research has been done on other benzodiazepines. Significantly smaller (50%) doses are often needed.
Non-benzodiazepine anxiolytics	Buspirone is a relatively new non-benzodiazepine anxiolytic. No differences have been identified between younger and older patients.
Non-benzodiazepine hypnotics	Zopiclone is a relatively new non-benzodiazepine hypnotic. Preliminary studies have shown that older patients have much higher total plasma concentrations of zopiclone.
Antidepressants Tricyclics	Most research has focused on amitriptyline, nortriptyline, imipramine and desipramine. Large variations in plasma drug concentrations have been observed for similar doses and this variation is greater in older people. Reduced clearance and increased half-lives are also observed.
Trazodone	Clearance is reduced in older people and its half-life is increased.
Selective serotonin reuptake inhibitors	Age-related increases in plasma concentrations have been reported for citalopram, paroxetine, fluoxetine and sertraline. They all inhibit hepatic microsomal cytochrome enzymes. Citalopram and sertraline weakly inhibit CYP 2D6, whereas fluoxetine, fluvoxamine and paroxetine are potent inhibitors of CYP 2D6. There is therefore a strong potential for drug interactions.
Lithium	Lithium is associated with a high incidence of side-effects in older people. Lithium clearance is reduced. Smaller doses are needed to achieve the same therapeutic benefit.
Antipsychotics	There is very little information available on the changes in pharmacokinetics with increasing age. This is partly because these drugs (particularly classical antipsychotics, such as chlorpromazine and haloperidol) are associated with significant side-effects in older people. Studies examining the use of antipsychotics tend to exclude older people.

Based on Braithwaite (1998).

In summary, the important pharmacokinetic and pharmacodynamic changes with increasing age include:

(1) increased risk of side-effects and drug interactions
(2) increased receptor sensitivity
(3) decreased receptor numbers
(4) the half-life of lipid-soluble drugs is prolonged

(5)   increased blood levels of water-soluble drugs
(6)   decreased plasma albumin
(7)   decreased gastric acid production and emptying
(8)   reduced hepatic metabolism
(9)   decreased glomerular filtration rate.

The effects of these changes with increasing age on some of the commonly prescribed drugs are summarised in Table 12.1.

Side-effects of psychotropic drugs in older people

Mental illness is common in older people, especially the very old, and psychotropic drugs are commonly prescribed. Older people are more likely to have a range of physical illnesses and psychotropic drugs may exacerbate these. These conditions may be cardiovascular (e.g. arrhythmias and hypertension), endocrine (e.g. diabetes), gastrointestinal (e.g. constipation, malnutrition), urological (e.g. prostatic hypertrophy), neurological (e.g. dementia, seizure disorders) or ophthalmic (e.g. glaucoma) (Smith, 1998). These disorders can cause particular risks for older patients treated with psychotropic drugs but an awareness of them can lead to more focused prescribing.

The side-effects of psychotropic drugs can be categorised according to their effects on neurotransmitter systems. They may be anticholinergic (e.g. reduced salivation, sweating and gastric acid, increased intra-ocular pressure, blurred vision, urinary retention, tachycardia, impotence and delirium), antidopaminergic (extrapyramidal side-effects, galactorrhoea, gynaecomastia and pigmentation), antihistaminic (sedation, hypotension and weight gain) and anti-α_1 adrenergic (tachycardia, arrhythmia, angina, insomnia and tremor) (Smith, 1998). Knowledge of the mechanism of action of particular psychotropic drugs will enable the prescriber to predict likely side-effects in older people with specific physical illnesses and thus avoid them. In addition, knowledge of drug interactions should reduce side-effects through more focused prescribing. Some of the more important side-effects and drug interactions are summarised in Table 12.2.

Assessment of and information for older people prescribed psychotropic drugs

Older people should be thoroughly assessed before they are prescribed psychotropic drugs. The main reasons for this include:

(1)   the greater incidence of physical illnesses
(2)   their greater sensitivity to side-effects
(3)   the increased likelihood of drug interactions.

Table 12.2 Common adverse drug reactions and interactions[1]

Drug	Comments
Benzodiazepines	Increased drowsiness with sedative drugs (e.g. alcohol, antihistamines, tricyclic antidepressants, phenothiazines) Reduced absorption when co-administered with antacids and anticholinergic drugs Cimetidine inhibits the metabolism of long-acting benzodiazepines Increased clearance by smoking (nicotine) Potentiation of phenytoin by diazepam and chlordiazepoxide Antagonism of L-dopa by diazepam, nitrazepam and chlordiazepoxide
Diazepam	Clearance reduced by propranolol; levels increased by fluoxetine; diazepam increases zotepine levels by approximately 10%
Antidepressants	
Tricyclic antidepressants	Increased drowsiness with sedative drugs; enhanced anticholinergic effects with anticholinergic drugs; increased levels with haloperidol; reduced levels with high-fibre diet; reduced metabolism with cimetidine; increased metabolism of imipramine, doxepin and amitriptyline by carbamazepine; raised phenytoin levels with imipramine
Citalopram	Increased risk of hyponatraemia and serotonin syndrome with buspirone
Fluoxetine	Carbamazepine levels increased; cardiac arrhythmias with cisapride; increased risk of serotonin syndrome with lithium; phenytoin levels increased; increased risk of cardiotoxicity with terfenadine
Paroxetine	Reduced bioavailability with cimetidine and phenytoin
Sertraline	Possible cardiac arrhythmias with cisapride; raised phenytoin levels
Mirtazepine	Increased sedation with benzodiazepines
Moclobemide	Increased half-life with cimetidine
Reboxetine	Increased risk of hypokalaemia with diuretics; avoid with erythromycin and flecainide
Venlafaxine	Increased diazepam clearance; reduced clearance with cimetidine; serious adverse reaction with selegiline
Antipsychotics	Increased drowsiness with sedative drugs; enhanced anticholinergic effects with anticholinergic drugs
Chlorpromazine	Enhanced effect of hypotensives; reduced absorption with antacids; reduced levels with cimetidine; reduced metabolism of sodium valproate
Haloperidol	Reduced absorption by antacids; levels decreased by rifampicin
Risperidone	Clearance increased by carbamazepine
Olanzapine	Clearance increased by carbamazepine
Quetiapine	Levels reduced by carbamazepine; levels increased with erythromycin; slightly raised lithium levels; levels reduced by phenytoin
Antidementia drugs	Antagonism of anticholinergic medication; exacerbation of succinylcholine-type muscle relaxation during anaesthesia
Donepezil	Increased risk of developing ulcers with non-steroidal anti-inflammatory drugs
Rivastigmine	None reported
Galantamine	Plasma levels increased by paroxetine; clearance reduced by paroxetine and fluoxetine

1. This list is not exhaustive and prescribers should seek up-to-date information from drug data sheets when in doubt.

Based on Carvajal & Arias (2000), Cowen (2000) and Jefferson (2000).

The patient's physical health and current medications (including over-the-counter drugs) will need to be reviewed. For specific treatments an accurate diagnosis is essential. In the case of the antidementia drugs in the UK (see below) the guidelines produced by National Institute for Clinical Excellence (2001) specify a severity range as well as a diagnosis.

The assessment is also an important opportunity to develop a trusting relationship, and to improve understanding of and compliance with treatment. The assessor will also need to consider whether the patient is able safely to take medication or whether special arrangements are needed.

Patients should be given adequate information about the drugs they are taking. The following points should be covered (*Drug and Therapeutics Bulletin*, 1981):

(1)   the name of the medicine
(2)   the aim of the treatment (relief of symptoms, cure, prevention of relapse or prophylaxis)
(3)   how the patient will know whether the drug is working or not
(4)   when and how to take it
(5)   what to do if a dose is missed
(6)   how long to take it
(7)   the possible side-effects
(8)   any likely effects on performance (e.g. driving ability)
(9)   any interactions with other drugs.

Some patients, especially those with dementia or communication difficulties, may not be able to give real consent. The doctor's ethical obligation is to act in the patient's best interest. This principle is particularly important when the patient's ability to exercise autonomy is diminished. Where appropriate, recourse may be made to the mental health legislation. However, in England and Wales patients with dementia who lack capacity can be treated or admitted to hospital without the need to use mental health legislation, provided that the health care professionals involved and the patient's family agree that this is the most appropriate course of action and that the patient is not actively refusing medication or trying to leave hospital.

Use of antipsychotics in older people

Clinical use and efficacy

Classical antipsychotics have had a profound impact on the treatment of schizophrenia and related disorders. There is good evidence for their clinical effectiveness. Thornley *et al* (1997), in a review of 144 studies, found that chlorpromazine significantly reduced the relapse rate in schizophrenia, and improved positive symptoms and functioning. However, it was associated with significant side-effects, including sedation, acute movement disorders, parkinsonism, weight gain and seizures. Prescribing practices have altered over time and low doses (with fewer side-effects) are now considered as effective as high doses (see Chapter 9).

More recently a heterogeneous group of drugs has been introduced and designated 'atypical'. Atypical antipsychotics are at least as effective as classical antipsychotics but are associated with significantly fewer side-effects (Brown et al, 1999; Fleischhacker, 1999; Hawkins et al, 1999). Although atypical antipsychotics in general have fewer side-effects, particularly extrapyramidal side-effects (EPS), they may be associated with a number of important side-effects, such as neutropenia and gastrointestinal obstruction with clozapine (Committee on Safety of Medicines, 1999). There is also a growing body of evidence that atypical antipsychotics may be cost-effective (Almond & O'Donnell, 2000).

The classical antipsychotics are particularly associated with EPS. Age and length of treatment may be risk factors for some EPS, including tardive dyskinesia. Compared with atypical antipsychotics, they may be particularly dangerous in high doses (Tyson et al, 1999). Side-effects are usually dose related and can easily be detected with careful monitoring (Chaplin et al, 1999). However, classical antipsychotics have an important role to play in a number of clinical situations, for example with patients who require intramuscular medication (Schultz & McGorry, 2000).

Although many randomised controlled trials have examined the efficacy of antipsychotic medication in younger patients with schizophrenia and related disorders, there is a relative paucity of studies in patients with late-onset schizophrenia. However, there have been numerous case reports and open studies (Tram et al, 1994). Although data are limited, several studies have supported the use of atypical antipsychotics in older people with schizophrenia, including clozapine, risperidone, olanzapine, quetiapine and ziprasidone (Sajatovic et al, 2000).

Risperidone is effective and well tolerated in older people with psychotic symptoms (Czobor et al, 1995; Davidson et al, 2000) and it is also effective for the management of aggression in patients with dementia. However, there has been concern expressed about a possible increased risk of stroke in older patients taking risperidone (Frenchman & Prince, 1997; De Deyn et al, 1999; De Deyn & Katz, 2000).

Olanzapine is well tolerated in older people and there is some evidence that it is effective in the management of behavioural disturbance in patients with Alzheimer's disease (Street et al, 2000a,b) and schizophrenia (Taylor et al, 1996; Jones & Tollefson, 1998). A rapid-action intramuscular preparation has been developed and preliminary findings have shown it to be safe and well tolerated, and to have significant clinical benefit in the management of agitated patients with dementia (Jones *et al*, 2000).

Recent guidance published by the Committee on Safety of Medicines recommends that risperidone and olanzapine should not be used for the treatment of behavioural symptoms of dementia. In addition, the use of risperidone for the management of acute psychotic conditions in elderly patients who also have dementia should be limited to short term and should be under specialist advice. Further information can be found on the Medicines and Healthcare Products Regulatory Agency's website (http://medicines.mhra.gov.uk).

Quetiapine is also effective and well tolerated in older people with psychotic disorders, including schizophrenia and related disorders, affective disorders and dementia (McManus *et al*, 1999). In a review by Stark (2000: pp. 4–12), quetiapine-treated patients were more likely to continue with treatment, and they had a lower incidence of movement disorders compared with patients receiving classical antipsychotics.

Zotepine is licensed for use in the elderly. The starting dose should be 25 mg twice daily and titration should be gradual. Most clinical trials carried out with zotepine have included patients up to 65 years of age. Shahpesandy *et al* (2000) reported a study that compared the efficacy and tolerability of zotepine with those of risperidone in the treatment of psychotic disorders in older people. Fourteen patients received risperidone (1 mg/day) and 10 received zotepine (average 60 mg/day) over 42 days. There was no difference between the effect of zotepine and risperidone on scores on the Positive and Negative Symptom Scale but 37.5% of patients on risperidone experienced EPS, compared with 20% of those taking zotepine.

Dementia

A comprehensive review of the use of antipsychotic agents in patients with dementia has been published by Defilippi & Crismon (2000).

The management of psychotic symptoms in patients with Lewy-body dementia can be difficult because of the increased risk of EPS. The atypicals are preferred but should be prescribed cautiously, usually starting with a low dose. There is also limited evidence that olanzapine is effective and safe in reducing psychotic symptoms in patients with Lewy-body dementia (Clark *et al*, 2000). In addition, in a recent double-blind, randomised, placebo-controlled study involving 29 patients with Lewy-body dementia, olanzapine (5 and 10 mg) significantly reduced psychotic symptoms without worsening parkinsonism (Cummings *et al*, 2002). There is also limited evidence of benefit and safety for clozapine (Geroldi *et al*, 1997) and risperidone (Tarsy *et al*, 2002), but considerably more research is needed. However, antipsychotic drugs should generally be avoided in these patients. If they are used, the newer drugs are preferable, and patients should be started on a small dose, increased cautiously (at intervals of no greater than once daily initially). Some have advocated cholinesterase inhibitors instead and rivastigmine was well tolerated in one study (McKeith *et al*, 2000).

Delirium

Delirium is a complex neuropsychiatric syndrome with an acute onset and fluctuating course with generalised cognitive impairment, disturbed sleep–wake cycle and disturbed activity levels and perception. It occurs in approximately 15–20% of all patients admitted to general hospital and is particularly common in older patients but is frequently not diagnosed (Conn & Lieff, 2001). Physical illness, drugs (including benzodiazepines and anticholinergics) and environmental factors can all contribute to the development of delirium and management must redress all the various contributory factors. However, in older people infections account for 43% of cases of delirium and cerebrovascular disease accounts for another 25% (Rahkonen *et al*, 2000). In addition, it is important to diagnose and treat delirium because it has a high mortality (Rahkonen *et al*, 2000).

Drugs with anticholinergic side-effects are a recognised cause of delirium and should be avoided (Han *et al*, 2001). Most published research has found significant benefit for haloperidol (an intramuscular dose of 0.5–10 mg) for severe disturbance. Old age psychiatrists would generally be reluctant to use single intramuscular doses of more than 2.5 mg and total daily doses of more than 5 mg. Although there is good evidence for the use of haloperidol in the management of delirium, the very high doses (100 mg delivered intravenously every 24 hours) recommended by Meagher (2001) are potentially very dangerous and should be avoided in older people. It is surprising that the same authors recommend droperidol, considering that it is cardiotoxic and that it has been withdrawn. There have also been a small number of case reports of benefit with oral olanzapine (5–10 mg) and risperidone (1.5–4 mg), but these are usually unsuitable for the severely disturbed patient. Lorazepam (up to 2 mg intramuscularly in 24 hours) can also be given if EPS are anticipated or occur. Since antipsychotics can cause severe reactions in patients with Lewy-body dementia (see above) they should generally be avoided for delirium in these patients.

Choosing an antipsychotic

The choice of antipsychotic in older people should be individualised and should take account of the patient's physical health and concomitant medications, as well as the drug's likely side-effects. Most of the currently available antipsychotics are empirically equivalent in terms of their clinical efficacy, but they vary greatly in terms of their side-effects, some of which are particularly troublesome in older people.

The daily dose should be slowly titrated upwards until a therapeutic effect is observed or intolerance to side-effects occurs. After a desired response is achieved, one should gradually reduce the dose to maintain the elderly patient on the minimum effective dose. Although guidelines on the use of antipsychotics in older people do not exist, the following general principles of prescribing antipsychotics would be appropriate:

(1)   use one antipsychotic drug
(2)   adjust the dose according to the individual patient's response
(3)   use anticholinergics with great care
(4)   use for the minimum period
(5)   discontinue gradually
(6)   ensure there is appropriate follow-up of patients after they stop taking the drug (Taylor et al, 1999).

The American Psychiatric Association (1997) has published detailed guidelines for the use of antipsychotics in patients with schizophrenia. For patients with acute schizophrenia, first-line treatment with either a classical or atypical antipsychotic is recommended (not clozapine). If there are 'intolerable' side-effects, it is recommended that an atypical antipsychotic should be used. If there is no response, it is recommended that an antipsychotic from a different group be used. The guidelines note that the choice of antipsychotic is frequently guided by the patient's tolerance to side-effects. Clozapine should be reserved for treatment-resistant cases of schizophrenia. No specific guidance is available for the use of antipsychotics in older people.

Adverse drug reactions

Some of the commoner side-effects involve anticholinergic effects (e.g. dry mouth, urinary retention, exacerbation of glaucoma, cardiotoxicity), EPS, α-adrenergic blockade (e.g. orthostatic hypotension), antihistamine effects (e.g. sedation) and effects on the central nervous system (CNS) (e.g. sedation, impaired psychomotor function and reduced convulsion threshold). These can all cause significant problems in older people, among whom side-effects with chlorpromazine and haloperidol are more common than with atypical antipsychotics (Carvajal & Arias, 1999).

Concern has often been expressed about the effect of antipsychotic drugs on cardiac function and Reilly et al (2000) examined the effect of a range of antipsychotic drugs on abnormalities of the QT interval. The two drugs with significant associations with QT lengthening were droperidol and thioridazine, and this was particularly true among elderly patients. Droperidol has been withdrawn and the use of thioridazine has been severely restricted in the UK.

Atypical antipsychotic drugs have an overall improved side-effect profile compared with classical antipsychotics, but they are by no means devoid of side-effects. Individual drugs should be prescribed in the light of the patient's general medical heath and use of other drugs, to minimise side-effects and avoid potentially serious drug interactions.

For a detailed discussion of antipsychotics and the treatment of schizophrenia see Chapter 9.

Antidepressants

Most drug trials that have compared the efficacy of antidepressants have excluded patients over the age of 65 and those with significant physical illness. This has resulted in a relative lack of evidence on which to base decisions when treating patients over the age of 65.

When prescribing an antidepressant to an older patient, the maxim 'start low and go slow' is good advice (Baldwin & Burns, 1998). A small starting dose and a gradual increase in dose are necessary if troublesome side-effects are to be avoided. Although the elderly as a group are more sensitive to medication, there is wide inter-subject variation in drug metabolism, with up to a tenfold variation in plasma levels between patients given the same dose of antidepressant (Bertilsson & Dahl, 1996). For this reason some older patients can tolerate a dose of antidepressant equivalent to that used in younger patients, provided increases in dose are carried out gradually.

Clinical efficacy

The selective serotonin reuptake inhibitors (SSRIs) are now commonly prescribed for older people. Between 1993 and 1997 in Ontario, the proportion of older people being treated with antidepressants increased, and during the same period the proportion being prescribed an SSRI increased from 9.6% to 45.1%. There was a significant reduction in the prescribing of TCAs (Mamdani et al, 2000). Livingston & Livingston (1999) reviewed five double-blind randomised controlled trials that compared TCAs with newer antidepressants (SSRIs and venlafaxine) in patients over the age of 65. All five trials found that TCAs and the newer antidepressants were equally effective. However, none of the trials included enough subjects to detect small differences in efficacy and patients with significant physical illness were excluded. In a more recent double-blind, randomised study involving 210 elderly patients with depression treated for 12 weeks with sertraline (50–150 mg/day) or nortriptyline (25–100 mg/day), no significant differences were found between the two drugs (Bondareff et al, 2000). Karlsson et al (2000) examined citalopram (20–40 mg/day) and mianserin (30–60 mg/day) in a 12-week double-blind randomised study that involved 336 elderly depressed patients with or without dementia. The two treatments were equally effective and well tolerated, although fatigue was more frequent with mianserin. However, there is evidence that TCAs are more effective than SSRIs in treating patients with severe melancholic-type depression characterised by anhedonia, diurnal mood variation, early-morning wakening and psychomotor retardation or agitation (Roose et al, 1994).

There is also good evidence that other drugs are effective in older people with depression. In an 8-week double-blind randomised trial that involved 347 elderly patients, reboxetine (4–6 mg/day) was found to be as effective as imipramine (50–100 mg/day) but with significantly less hypotension and fewer serious adverse events (Katona et al, 1999). In a more recent open-label study that involved 160 older people with depressive disorder or dysthymia, 104 patients completed a 52-week treatment period of reboxetine. After 2 weeks 15.1% reported feeling 'much' or 'very much' improved. This increased to 88.7% by week 6 and 95.2% by week 52, and the treatment was well tolerated (Aguglia, 2000).

Two studies have examined the use of mirtazapine in older people. Halikas (1995) compared mirtazapine (maximum 35 mg/day) and trazodone (maximum 280 mg/day) in a 6-week, randomised, double-blind, placebo-controlled study that involved 150 patients with depression aged 55 years or older. Both drugs significantly improved depression scores compared with placebo by week 2. In addition, both drugs were associated with a significantly higher frequency of dry mouth compared with placebo, but patients treated with trazodone also experienced a significantly higher frequency of dizziness and blurred vision. A further double-blind, randomised, multi-centre study compared mirtazapine (maximum 45 mg/day) with amitriptyline (30–90 mg/day) in 115 patients aged 60 years or more with depression. The depression scores and frequency of adverse events were not significantly different in the two groups (Hoyberg et al, 1996).

In younger patients, the monoamine oxidase inhibitors (MAOIs) have traditionally been recommended for depression with associated anxiety. Unfortunately, the traditional MAOIs can cause marked postural hypotension and should be used with great caution in older people. However, moclobemide, a reversible inhibitor of monoamine oxidase (RIMA), requires little or no dietary restrictions. It is well tolerated in the elderly and may be a useful alternative for depressed patients with prominent anxiety and an absence of melancholic features (Tourigny-Rivard, 1997).

Patients suffering from severe depression associated with mood-congruent delusions require a different treatment from the outset. In this group of patients, antidepressants used alone are less likely to be effective and a combination of antidepressant with an antipsychotic is usually necessary (Spiker et al, 1985). Delusional depression in the elderly seems to be more resistant to pharmacotherapy than in younger patients and electroconvulsive therapy (ECT) may be the treatment of choice in this group of patients (Flint & Rifat, 1998).

Depression is also common in early Alzheimer's disease. In a 12-week, double-blind, placebo-controlled study of 22 patients with depression and Alzheimer's disease treated with sertraline (in normal therapeutic doses), depression significantly improved, particularly during the third week (Lyketsos *et al*, 2000).

Treatment duration

The elderly are at high risk of recurrence following a depressive episode – it may be as high as 70% within 2 years of remission (Flint, 1992). Continuation treatment for 6 months after full remission is now standard practice in patients under 65 years of age. Flint (1992) cites evidence to support using continuation treatment beyond 6 months in the elderly. First, naturalistic studies of untreated depression in the elderly suggest a duration of 12–48 months. Second, the risk of recurrence after a single depressive episode in the elderly is high and about the same as that for younger patients with a history of recurrent depression. Last, with further episodes there is a tendency to shorter periods of remission, longer duration of episodes and increasing treatment resistance.

One of the few placebo-controlled trials of maintenance anti-depressants for patients over the age of 65 showed that, compared with placebo, those treated with dothiepin (75 mg daily) were 2.5 times less likely to have a recurrence of their depressive illness (Old Age Depression Interest Group, 1993). More recently Flint & Rifat (2000) found that 70% of patients with unipolar depression who were maintained on an antidepressant at full dose remained well at 4 years.

Adverse effects

Meta-analyses of the drop-out rates from trials comparing anti-depressants suggest that SSRIs are better tolerated than the older TCAs, as 10% fewer patients taking the former are withdrawn from trials (Anderson & Tomenson, 1995). However, this does not seem to be the case for trials in which SSRIs were compared with newer TCAs or heterocyclic antidepressants (e.g. trazodone), where there was no difference in the rates of patient withdrawal (Song *et al*, 1993). These findings have been confirmed in a more recent meta-analysis of patients withdrawn from trials (Hoptopf *et al*, 1997). The importance of this analysis is that Hoptopf *et al* examined 11 trials that included elderly patients and found that drop-out rates did not differ significantly from those of younger patients. One of the difficulties in interpreting the clinical significance of drop-out rates from randomised controlled trials of antidepressants is that they give no indication of the *seriousness* of the events that led to antidepressants being withdrawn.

Table 12.3 Common and important side-effects of tricyclic antidepressants and selective serotonin reuptake inhibitors

Tricyclic antidepressants	Selective serotonin reuptake inhibitors
α₁-adrenergic receptor blockade	*5-HT₃ receptor stimulation*
Postural hypotension	Nausea
Dizziness	Headache
	Gastrointestinal upset
Muscarinic receptor blockade	*5-HT₂ receptor stimulation*
Constipation	Agitation
Blurred vision	Akathisia
Dry mouth	Insomnia
Urinary retention	Sexual dysfunction
Delirium	
Tachycardia	
Heart block	
Histamine receptor blockade	
Weight gain	
Drowsiness	

Hyponatraemia is a side-effect of both drugs; it is more common in the elderly. Presents with vague symptoms which may be attributed to depression, e.g. lassitude and headaches.

Given equal efficacy, the choice of first-line antidepressants in the elderly is strongly influenced in favour of those antidepressants least likely to cause troublesome side-effects. SSRIs are not without potentially hazardous side-effects in the elderly, such as hyponatraemia. However, one reason for favouring SSRIs as first-line antidepressants over the older TCAs for the elderly is the latter's toxicity in overdose (either deliberate or accidental). The risk results from the propensity of the older TCAs to cause cardiac arrhythmias or seizures at toxic levels (Edwards, 1995). Dothiepin seems to be particularly risky in overdose (Buckley *et al*, 1994).

Nortriptyline is well tolerated in elderly patients and those with cardiovascular disease (Roose *et al*, 1994). In addition, lofepramine is a useful alternative TCA. It is well tolerated and free of cardiotoxicity and it remains a popular antidepressant for the treatment of depression in older people.

A summary of some of the side-effects of TCAs and SSRIs is summarised in Table 12.3.

Treatment resistance

In about one-third of patients there will be an inadequate response to the first antidepressant used (Flint, 1995). In younger patients a 4-

461

week trial of antidepressant is generally considered adequate; thereafter, if there is no response, a change to a different class of antidepressant is advised (Spigset & Martensson, 1999). Quitkin *et al* (1984) have shown that improvement can be delayed for 4–6 weeks, and a trial of 8 weeks may be necessary for a response to occur in the elderly (Georgetas & McCue, 1989). The likelihood of obtaining a response by extending the use of an antidepressant beyond 4 weeks has to be weighed against the distress and risks of persistent depression for each patient. It may be necessary to give ECT if the response to antidepressants is delayed or slow and there is concern about suicide risk.

If there has been no or only partial response to two antidepressants from different classes, augmentation should be considered. A number of augmentation strategies have been advocated, including use of lithium, tri-iodothyronine, anti-epileptic drugs and antidepressant combinations. Evidence for the efficacy of augmentation mainly comes from studies in younger patients.

The few studies that have included elderly patients have used lithium augmentation (Flint, 1995). In a survey of patients over 65 years of age who were prescribed lithium, Head & Dening (1998) found that 38% had the prescription for a depressive illness. Prospective controlled trials of lithium use for elderly patients with depression have reported response rates of about 20% (Flint & Rifat, 1994), which is less than the response rate in younger patients (about 35%).

Elderly patients are sensitive to the side-effects of lithium and are at greater risk of neurotoxicity. The elderly may experience lithium toxicity when plasma levels are within the therapeutic range. In addition, up to 50% of elderly patients will experience side-effects with lithium (Flint & Rifat, 1994), including polydipsia, polyuria, tremor, dry mouth and nausea. The elderly may respond to lower plasma concentrations of lithium than younger patients, although Flint (1995) suggests that levels of greater than 0.5 mmol/l are necessary. In a review of lithium use in elderly people, Foster (1992) suggested an ideal range of 0.4–0.7 mmol/l. Once-daily dosing minimises side-effects.

Initial reports of lithium augmentation suggested that a response occurs within a few days, but 3–4 weeks is considered a minimum trial. It is important to monitor elderly patients on lithium and to measure lithium levels every 3 months if dose and physical health are stable (Jefferson, 2000). Four to seven days after a patient starts on lithium or after any change in dose, plasma concentrations should be checked, and then checked weekly until they are stable. Closer monitoring may be warranted for some elderly patients, particularly those with a history of heart disease or renal impairment. To reduce the risk of toxicity it is important to give patients and carers clear and preferably written information about lithium to ensure that this information is understood.

Toxicity can occur if the risks of drug–lithium interactions are not fully recognised. Lithium levels will need to be checked. Commonly prescribed drugs in the elderly that may lead to an increase in lithium concentration are angiotensin-converting enzyme (ACE) inhibitors, thiazide diuretics (as they cause a 25% reduction in lithium excretion) and non-steroidal anti-inflammatory drugs (NSAIDs) (Bazire, 2000). Patients should be warned not to buy ibuprofen over the counter without discussing this with their general practitioner.

There is little evidence to guide clinicians on how long lithium augmentation should be continued once a response has been achieved. Risks of long-term lithium maintenance have to be weighed against the risks of recurrence of a mood disorder for each patient. Maintenance treatment with lithium is associated with hypothyroidism, so regular monitoring of thyroid function is necessary. In one survey, 25% of patients on maintenance lithium were also taking thyroxine (Head & Dening, 1998). Urea and electrolytes with serum creatinine should also be monitored. Therapeutic levels of lithium are thought not to lead to renal impairment, but episodes of toxicity may cause renal damage. Renal impairment due to other causes significantly increases the risk of toxicity.

The addition of tri-iodothyronine (T3) to antidepressant medication at doses of 25–50 µg/day is a strategy that has been used in younger patients with treatment-resistant depression. A meta-analysis of eight controlled studies that mainly involved younger patients showed that T3 augmentation produced twice as many responses as were found in the control group (Aronson et al, 1996). There have been no controlled studies of T3 augmentation in elderly patients (Flint, 1995) and so routine use in the elderly cannot be justified, although it may be of benefit in individual cases. T3 augmentation should be used with caution in the elderly, especially those with cardiovascular disease. If this strategy is adopted, small doses of T3 should be used and thyroid function regularly monitored.

Open studies and case series have reported responses in elderly patients to augmentation with carbamazepine and sodium valproate in treatment-resistant depression (Flint, 1995). The use of carbamazepine and sodium valproate as mood stabilisers in bipolar affective disorder is well established, but as yet there is no evidence of their efficacy from randomised controlled studies of treatment-resistant depression in the elderly. They should therefore be used with caution. Carbamazepine has limiting side-effects in the elderly, including drowsiness, nausea and ataxia; regular blood tests are necessary, as there is a risk of blood dyscrasias. Sodium valproate seems to be better tolerated in the elderly (Flint, 1995). There is clearly a need for more detailed research in this area.

For a detailed discussion of antidepressants and lithium see Chapters 6 and 7, respectively.

Bipolar affective disorder

Most patients with mania in late life have 'converted' to bipolarity after many years of repeated episodes of depression, or have developed mania secondary to an underlying brain disease (e.g. cerebrovascular disease). The prognosis of mania is generally worse than that of depression and patients experience a higher prevalence of cognitive dysfunction, more persistent symptoms and greater mortality (Shulman & Herrmann, 1999). Management of older patients with bipolar disease is usually with mood stabilisers such as lithium and valproate, with appropriate monitoring; valproate is better-tolerated (Shulman & Herrmann, 1999). The use of antipsychotics is frequently unavoidable during the initial stabilisation phase but evidence for the efficacy of individual anti-psychotics in older patients is notably absent. The atypical antipsychotics are preferred by some clinicians because they have fewer anticholinergic effects and EPS but their clinical efficacy has not been properly established. As yet, there has been very little pharmacological research that has focused specifically on older people and guidelines for the treatment of older people with mania need to be clearer and evidence based (Snowdon, 2000).

Hypnotics and sedatives

Hypnotics and anxiolytics are commonly prescribed for older people. The 'ideal' hypnotic would be one that rapidly induces sleep, keeps the patient asleep without disrupting sleep architecture, has no side-effects, produces no following-morning sedation, does not cause dependence or rebound insomnia and is safe in patients with medical conditions and in overdose. Although the 'newer' drugs such as zolpidem, zopiclone and zaleplon satisfy many of these criteria to varying degrees, it is unlikely that we shall ever have the 'perfect' hypnotic.

Insomnia is a common disorder and assessment should include a detailed history, a physical examination and appropriate investigations to determine the cause before a hypnotic drug is prescribed. Psychiatric disorders are often causes of insomnia. Other causes include physical illness (particularly painful conditions), jet lag and related phenomena, and poor conditions for promoting sleep. A large number of drugs, non-prescribed as well as prescribed, can also cause insomnia: the former include decongestants, caffeine, nicotine and alcohol, and the latter β-agonists, aminophylline, beta-blockers, corticosteroids, calcium-channel blockers and diuretics. Thus, underlying physical and psychological conditions, poor sleep hygiene and drug use should be reviewed before a hypnotic drug is prescribed (Curran, 1996).

Barbiturates

These are now rarely prescribed but may occasionally be taken by older people who have done so for many years. They are rapidly absorbed and quickly enter the CNS. For phenobarbitone, the half-life is 30–90 hours. Barbiturates produce a general depression of CNS activity and enhance the activity of gamma-aminobutyric acid (GABA) at its receptor. They are very toxic, especially in older people, and side-effects include impaired psychomotor function, impaired cognition, vertigo, nausea, vomiting, diarrhoea, tolerance, cross-tolerance and physical dependence. They are now obsolete as anxiolytics and hypnotics, and have largely been superseded by other drugs for these indications and in the management of epilepsy.

Benzodiazepines

These were first identified in 1957. Chlordiazepoxide became available in 1960 and diazepam in 1962. They are less potent than barbiturates. Initially, physical dependence was not thought to be a problem but in the early 1970s reports began to appear of a withdrawal syndrome.

These drugs are the most commonly prescribed psychotropic drugs in the elderly. In one survey, 17.3% of elderly patients in primary care were taking a benzodiazepine and half these patients were taking long-acting ones; there were twice as many women as men taking these drugs (Kirby *et al*, 1999). Drugs with a long half-life are associated with significant next-day sedation and psychomotor impairment.

Diazepam is commonly prescribed and is typical of the long-acting benzodiazepines used in older people. It has a high bioavailability. It reaches peak concentrations in 30–90 minutes and has a half-life of 30–100 hours in the elderly. However, the benzodiazepines have a wide range of half-lives (Table 12.4).

Table 12.4 Half-lives of some common benzodiazepines

Drug	$t_{1/2}$ (hours)*
Diazepam	20–100
Chlordiazepoxide	5–30
Alprazolam	5–15
Oxazepam	5–15
Lorazepam	7–35
Nitrazepam	20–50
Temazepam	4–20
Triazolam	2–5

*Half-lives tend to be in the upper end of the range for older people.
Adapted from Racagni *et al* (1997).

The benzodiazepines have a number of side-effects. These can be classified as *common* (sedation, dizziness, psychomotor impairment), *occasional* (dry mouth, blurred vision, gastrointestinal upset, ataxia, headache, hypotension) and *rare* (amnesia, restlessness, skin rash). The increased prevalence of these in older people has been reported by a number of authors. One study retrospectively examined adverse reactions to hypnotics over a 3-year period in a 1000-bed US teaching hospital (Mendelson *et al*, 1996). Confusion and hypotension were reported as the most common side-effects. Overall, the rate of side-effects was very low (0.05%), which confirms that these drugs are safe when used appropriately. However, although the overall number of adverse reactions was low, the vast majority of these were reported in patients over the age of 55 years.

A further retrospective study (Mendelson, 1996) in the US examined the relationship between falls in hospital and hypnotic medication among older people. Patients who had fallen were compared with a control group matched for age, gender, medical specialty and period of admission. Patients who fell were four times more likely to have received benzodiazepines. This is important, since falls induced by benzo-diazepines have important medical, social and financial implications. There has also been a recent report of an increased risk of road traffic accidents in older people taking benzodiazepines (Barbone *et al*, 1998). In addition, in a Swedish study of 548 suicides in older people between 1992 and 1996, a benzodiazepine was the sole agent in 72% of cases, and 90% of these were either flunitrazepam or nitrazepam (Carlsten *et al*, 2003). Benzodiazepines are common in drug-poisoning suicides by elderly people and should be prescribed with caution for this age group.

Tolerance to and dependence on benzodiazepines are important issues with older people, as they are often very reluctant to stop their medication, but long-term use should be avoided. This area has been poorly studied but once older people have become dependent on benzodiazepines it can be very difficult to discontinue these drugs. The mechanism includes a combination of pharmacokinetic (induction of metabolism) and pharmacodynamic effects (reduction in the number of benzodiazepine receptor sites/sensitivity and uncoupling of the func-tional link between the benzodiazepine and $GABA_A$ receptors). Physical (physiological) dependence is usually secondary to the development of tolerance. Benzodiazepine withdrawal symptoms include tremor, muscle pains, sleep disturbance, headache, nausea, sweating, perceptual disturbances, psychotic reactions and seizures. Older people can be particularly sensitive to withdrawal symptoms, especially if they have been taking drugs for many years. The general principles of management are the same as for younger patients, with the exception that a longer time is usually needed to get the patient off the drug. Occasionally withdrawal is not possible if the patient has been on it for many years.

Buspirone

Buspirone is an azaspirodecanedione that has no affinity for the benzodiazepine receptor complex. It is devoid of anticonvulsant, muscle-relaxant or sedative effects, is an agonist at 5-HT_{1A} receptors and is mainly used as an anxiolytic. It has a slow mode of onset and may take 2–3 weeks to reduce anxiety levels sufficiently for this to be clinically observed. It is generally well tolerated and has a low propensity for tolerance and dependence but it is not widely used with the elderly (Curran & Musa, 2000).

Zopiclone, zolpidem and zaleplon

Zopiclone and zolpidem are relatively new hypnotic drugs and are widely used in older people (Racagni *et al*, 1997); zaleplon has become available more recently. Benzodiazepines act non-selectively at two central receptor sites, namely Ω_1 and Ω_2 receptors. The sedative action of benzodiazepines involves the Ω_1 receptors, whereas Ω_2 receptors are responsible for their effects on memory and cognitive functioning. Zolpidem, zopiclone and zaleplon are selective compounds that interact preferentially with Ω_1 receptors (Terzano *et al*, 2003).

Zopiclone (a cyclopyrrolone) is well tolerated and has few side-effects (although there have been a few reports of memory disturbance with higher doses, but considerably less than with benzodiazepines). For these reasons it is commonly prescribed for elderly patients.

In one recent double-blind, randomised, four-way, cross-over study the effects of zolpidem (5 mg), zopiclone (3.75 mg), lormetazepam (1 mg) and placebo on memory were evaluated in 48 healthy elderly volunteers. The medication was administered at night and effects were assessed the following morning (9 hours later). The ability to recall five digits was not impaired in any of the treatments groups, but for six or more digits significant impairments were observed in the lormetazepam and zopiclone groups (Allain *et al*, 2003).

Following a single oral dose the peak plasma concentration is reached within 0.5–1.5 hours and more than 93% is absorbed. The half-life is approximately 3–6 hours, but this increases to 8 hours in the elderly (Racagni *et al*, 1997). There has also been a report of a 72-year-old woman with cancer who died after ingesting approximately 200–350 mg of zopiclone (Bromness *et al*, 2001).

Zolpidem (an imidazopyridine) is a chemically novel non-benzodiazepine hypnotic agent. It interacts with the benzodiazepine Ω_1 receptor, especially in the cortex, cerebellum, substantia nigra and pallidum. It is devoid of muscle-relaxant properties. It is readily absorbed, has a bioavailability of approximately 70%, and reaches peak plasma concentrations in approximately 2 hours. The elimination half-life is

1.4–2.5 hours in young healthy volunteers, but this increases in older people (Racagni *et al*, 1997).

In one study the hypnotic effects of zolpidem (10 mg), temazepam (15 mg) and placebo were compared in healthy adults (including older people) in a multi-centre study. Medications were administered 15 minutes before lights out, which was followed by polysomnographic monitoring for 7.5 hours. Subjective questionnaires and performance tests, including the digit symbol substitution test and symbol copying test, were administered at study entry and after waking. Six hundred and thirty subjects completed the study. Neither active agent significantly reduced objective sleep latency relative to placebo but zolpidem reduced awakenings compared with temazepam. Both agents improved sleep efficiency and most subjective sleep measures relative to placebo, with zolpidem superior on five of six subjective outcome measures compared with temazepam. Results on the symbol copying test, morning sleepiness and morning concentration were not altered by any treatment. Zolpidem provided greater subjective hypnotic efficacy than temazepam in this model of transient insomnia, and reduced the number of polysomnographically recorded awakenings (Erman *et al*, 2001).

However, there has been a recent report of zolpidem dependence in a 67-year-old Caucasian woman. The insomnia had been managed with zolpidem, 10 mg at bedtime, but she had increased her dose to 100 mg daily for 18 months. She experienced severe generalised tremor, psychomotor agitation, facial flushing and anxiety. These symptoms persistent despite treatment with benzodiazepines; a tapering dose of zolpidem was initiated and after taking 15 mg of zolpidem her symptoms completely subsided within 30 minutes (Madrak & Rosenberg, 2001).

There has also been a recent case of delirium in an 86-year-old woman admitted to hospital with headaches and diplopia. On day 3, the patient received 5 mg zolpidem and, approximately 2 hours later, became restless, disorientated and physically agitated. The zolpidem was stopped, she was treated with haloperidol and needed restraining for her own safety. The patient's symptoms resolved by day 5 and she had no recollection of the incident. However, no challenge was attempted (Brodeur & Stirling, 2001).

Zaleplon (a pyrazolopyrimidine) is a relatively new short-acting, non-benzodiazepine hypnotic with a half-life of approximately 1 hour. In older people it significantly reduces sleep latency and improves the subjective quality of sleep. It also appears to be well tolerated, but Hedner *et al* (2000) found mild rebound insomnia after 2 weeks of a 10 mg dose. However, in a review, Israel & Kramer (2002) reported that zaleplon has a rapid onset of action and elimination and is well tolerated in both young and older patients.

For a detailed discussion of anxiolytics, sedatives and hypnotics see Chapter 5.

Antidementia drugs

Drugs affecting the cholinergic system

Since the 1970s, deficits in the cholinergic system have been reported in patients with Alzheimer's disease and most of the research treatment strategies have focused on this neurotransmitter system. Acetyl co-enzyme A and choline are used to synthesise acetylcholine (ACh) by choline acetyl transferase (CAT), concentrations of which are reduced in Alzheimer's disease. ACh is eventually metabolised by acetyl-cholinesterase. ACh activity can therefore be increased by a number of different methods, including increasing the availability of precursor, inhibiting the breakdown of ACh by acetylcholinesterase and by direct and indirect agonists.

Precursor loading

This involves 'loading' with the components used to synthesise ACh, namely acetyl co-enzyme A and choline. Loading with choline has been tried but there is little evidence that it is efficacious in humans when used alone. There have also been attempts to increase levels of acetyl co-enzyme A using L-acetylcarnitine. Pettegrew *et al* (1995) examined L-acetylcarnitine in a double-blind placebo-controlled study in seven patients and five controls with Alzheimer's disease, over 12 months. Patients treated with L-acetylcarnitine showed significantly less deterioration in their scores on the Mini-Mental State Examination (MMSE). There is thus some evidence that precursor loading with L-acetylcarnitine may benefit patients with Alzheimer's disease, but data are very limited.

Direct agonists

Acetylcholine acts on both muscarinic and nicotinic brain receptors. Continuous intravenous infusion of arecoline (a muscarinic and nicotinic agonist) produced significant improvements over 2 weeks in five out of nine patients with Alzheimer's disease, but the drug's use in humans has been limited by the need for parenteral administration. Xanomeline (an M_1 receptor agonist and analogue of arecoline) also produced significant improvements on a number of measures, including cognitive function and behavioural disturbance, in a double-blind placebo-controlled study of 300 patients with Alzheimer's disease, over 6 months (De Deyn *et al*, 1991). However, further clinical data are needed.

Patients with Alzheimer's disease have large reductions in nicotinic cholinergic receptors in both the neocortex and hippocampus. In addition, nicotine is also neuroprotective for both cholinergic and dopaminergic receptors (James & Nordberg, 1995). People who smoke may therefore have a reduced risk of developing Alzheimer's disease (van Duijn & Hofman, 1991), although the risk of multi-infarct dementia is increased. A few studies have suggested there is clinical benefit from the subcutaneous administration of nicotine in patients with Alzheimer's disease. There have also been some encouraging results with the transdermal administration of nicotine. In one recent study, Wilson *et al* (1995) examined the use of nicotine and placebo patches in patients with moderate Alzheimer's disease. Patients treated with nicotine displayed significant reductions in learning errors, which remained low during the 1 week wash-out period. Although these results are preliminary, they are encouraging and nicotine may prove to be an important treatment in the future. However, a more recent double-blind placebo-controlled study of nicotine patches in 18 patients with Alzheimer's disease found no significant benefit on memory function (Snaedal *et al*, 1996).

Indirect agonists

This group of drugs has not produced any promising results. These drugs enhance the release of ACh. In animal models, 4-aminopyridine has been shown to protect against impaired learning due to aluminium toxicity (Yokel *et al*, 1994), but further preclinical and clinical work is needed with these compounds.

Cholinesterase inhibitors

These drugs are effective for the management of cognitive deficits in patients with Alzheimer's disease and a common feature of these drugs is inhibition of acetylcholinesterase.

Acetylcholinesterase is a 76 kD protein that metabolises ACh by hydrolysing it to choline and acetate. It is found in cholinergic synapses in the periphery and CNS. This enzyme has a number of asymmetric forms, which have a variable number of catalytic subunits; for example, the G1 and G4 forms have respectively one and four catalytic subunits. In patients with Alzheimer's disease there is a selective reduction in the G4 form, which is associated with the presynaptic region, but the G1 form (associated with postsynaptic regions) remains unchanged (Weinstock, 1999). In addition, rivastigmine is more selective (4–5 times more so) for the G1 molecular form than for the G4 form, while donepezil appears to have a similar effect on both forms (Barner & Gray, 1998). These different forms have some practical significance because G4 is the main form found in the presynaptic membrane at the neuro-muscular junction and inhibition at this site leads to muscle cramps. Because rivastigmine is more selective for the G1 form muscle cramps are reported less frequently with rivastigmine (Weinstock, 1999).

Butyrylcholinesterase has a similar structure to acetylcholinesterase. It is synthesised by the liver and secreted into the plasma. It is also found in the gastrointestinal tract and comprises 1–10% of the total amount of cholinesterase in the CNS, where it is present in glial cells. The precise role of butyrylcholinesterase is unclear, but it is thought to be involved in the deactivation of a number of chemicals, including ACh.

Some cholinesterase inhibitors, such as physostigmine, tacrine (tetrahydroaminoacridine, THA) and rivastigmine, inhibit both acetylcholinesterase and butyrylcholinesterase, whereas others are selective inhibitors of the former. For example donepezil is 30 times and galantamine six times more selective in inhibiting acetylcholinesterase than butyrylcholinesterase (Fulton & Benfield, 1996; Doody, 1999).

Physostigmine was one of the first drugs in this group to be investigated. When given intravenously, it appears to improve memory consistently (Davis & Mohs, 1982), but when given orally its effect is brief and irregular. Burns *et al* (1995) reported significant improvements in eight out of ten studies. However, physostigmine has a short half-life, a narrow therapeutic index and poor oral absorption, which make it unsuitable for routine clinical use. More recently, extended-release physostigmine was evaluated in a multi-centre, double-blind study that lasted 12 weeks and involved 850 patients with mild to moderate Alzheimer's disease. Physostigmine significantly improved a global clinical rating and cognitive function compared with placebo but nausea and vomiting were experienced in nearly half the patients (van Dyck *et al*, 2000).

Tacrine was first developed approximately 50 years ago during research on antiseptics. The first report of its clinical effectiveness in Alzheimer's disease was by Summers *et al* (1986). They investigated THA in 17 patients with moderate to severe Alzheimer's disease. The study involved three phases: an initial open phase on medication, a second phase that was a double-blind, placebo-controlled, cross-over design and a third phase, a follow-up on medication for approximately 12 months. Patients taking THA significantly improved compared with baseline and the placebo group. In addition, no serious side-effects were reported. However, this study has since been extensively criticised. In a review of ten studies, Burns *et al* (1995) found significant clinical benefit in nine, but the high prevalence of hepatic side-effects has significantly reduced the clinical usefulness of this drug.

More recently three cholinesterase inhibitors, donepezil, rivastigmine and galantamine, have become available. A number of studies have demonstrated clinical benefit in patients with mild to moderate Alzheimer's disease.

Donepezil is a reversible non-competitive piperidine-type cholinesterase inhibitor. It is selective for acetylcholinesterase rather than butyrylcholinesterase. It is well absorbed after oral administration and this is not affected by food. The maximum plasma concentration is achieved after 3 hours, steady state after 14–22 days and the plasma half-life is 70 hours. It is largely metabolised by P450 isoenzymes, especially 3A4 and 2D6 (Dooley & Lamb, 2000). A number of studies have shown that it gives significant improvements in cognition over 3 months (Rogers *et al*, 1998*a*; Evans *et al*, 2000) and 6 months (Rogers *et al*, 1998*b*; Burns *et al*, 1999). Other studies have shown that significant benefit is still present after 98 weeks and that clinical progression of the disease is slowed down (Rogers & Friedhoff, 1998). Several studies have found clinical benefit in routine clinical practice (Cameron *et al*, 2000; Matthews *et al*, 2000) and a number of review articles have been published (Weinstock, 1999; Dooley & Lamb, 2000).

Rivastigmine is a long-acting, reversible and non-competitive carbamate acetylcholinesterase inhibitor. It is rapidly absorbed, although its absorption is slowed by food. At least 95% of an oral dose is absorbed but because of a high first-pass metabolism the bioavailability is only about 35%. It has a half-life of about 1–1½ hours (Polinski, 1998), although inhibition of acetylcholinesterase lasts for up to 11–12 hours. Recent research suggests that rivastigmine has a low propensity to interact with a wide range of drugs used in older people (Grossberg *et al*, 2000). A number of short-term randomised studies have demonstrated significant clinical benefits, particularly on cognitive function (e.g. Rosler *et al*, 1999). A number of good reviews report the pharmaco-kinetic properties and data from volunteer studies (Polinski, 1998; Birks *et al*, 2000).

Galantamine is a competitive reversible inhibitor of ACh. It also acts as an allosteric modulator of nicotinic receptors in the brain. It is rapidly absorbed; peak plasma concentrations are attained approximately 1 hour after oral administration. The rate of absorption is reduced by food. The bioavailability is approximately 90% and steady-state plasma concentrations are achieved within 3 days. Galantamine is mainly eliminated by cytochrome 450 isoenzymes (mainly 2D6 and 3A4) in the liver and the half-life is approximately 11 hours (Scott & Goa, 2000). Several short-term randomised studies have demonstrated its clinical efficacy in patients with mild to moderate Alzheimer's disease (Raskind *et al*, 2000; Tariot *et al*, 2000; Wilcock *et al*, 2000) and some useful reviews report its pharmacokinetic and pharmacodynamic properties (Blesa, 2000; Maelicke, 2000; Scott & Goa, 2000).

These three drugs are well tolerated but some of the more commonly observed side-effects are summarised in Table 12.5 (Weinstock, 1999).

Drugs affecting the NMDA system

There is increasing evidence that cortical dementia results in part from excitotoxicity caused by sustained elevations of glutamate or increased sensitivity to glutamate, which lead to neuronal degeneration

Table 12.5 Comparison of side-effects of cholinesterase inhibitors

Side-effects	Rivastigmine	Donepezil	Galantamine
Nausea	+++	+++	++
Vomiting	++	++	++
Diarrhoea	++	++	+
Dizziness	++	+	+
Headache	+	−	−
Abdominal pain	+	−	−
Anorexia	+	+	−
Fatigue	+	+	+
Muscle cramps	−	+	−
Agitation	−	−	+

+++, common; ++, occasional; +, rare; −, none reported.

(Cacabelos *et al*, 1999). Glutamate is the principal excitatory amino acid neurotransmitter in cortical and hippocampal neurons (Danysz *et al*, 2000).

One of the major excitatory amino acid receptors activated by glutamate is the N-methyl-D-aspartate (NMDA) receptor (Danysz *et al*, 2000) and this is thought to be one of the central mechanisms responsible for learning and memory (Malenka & Nicoll, 1999). However, excessive stimulation of NMDA receptors by glutamate may lead to functional disturbance of the signalling pathways and neuronal damage (Cacabelos *et al*, 1999). Agents such as memantine block pathological but not physiological stimulation of NMDA receptors.

Within the therapeutic range, memantine is fairly selective for NMDA receptors in the brain and has no significant affinity for most other CNS receptors, including other glutamate receptors – α-amino-3-hydroxy-5-methyl-4-isoxazoleproprionate (AMPA) and kainite (KA) (Danysz *et al*, 1997). The NMDA-sensitive glutamate receptors are ion channels formed as tetrameric complexes activated by glutamate and glycine. The channel is permeable to calcium, sodium and potassium ions and it is blocked by magnesium. The NMDA receptor is composed of four subunits. There are different types of subunit and these are currently classified as GLU_{N1}, GLU_{N2A}, GLU_{N2B}, GLU_{N2C}, GLU_{N2D}, GLU_{N3A} and GLU_{N3B}. GLU_{N1} and GLU_{N2} constitute the two major subunit families. Functional NMDA receptors in the adult mammalian CNS are formed by a combination of GLU_{N1} and GLU_{N2} subunits. GLU_{N3} subunits are mainly seen in the developing CNS. The GLU_{N1} form has eight variants (Zukin & Bennett, 1995) and the GLU_{N2} subfamily consists of four individual subunits. The different NMDA receptors are produced by varying combinations of GLU_{N1} and GLU_{N2} subunits and these differ in their magnesium sensitivity and pharmacological profiles (Sucher *et al*, 1996).

Table 12.6 Incidence (%) of side-effects with memantine, compared with placebo

Adverse event	Memantine (*n* = 299)	Placebo (*n* = 288)
Agitation	9.0	17.4
Diarrhoea	5.4	4.9
Insomnia	5.4	4.9
Dizziness	5.0	2.8
Headache	5.0	3.1
Hallucinations	5.0	2.1
Falls	4.7	4.9
Constipation	4.0	4.5

Memantine's mechanism of NMDA receptor block is uncompetitive because the binding site is accessible only if the receptor is activated. The memantine binding site is located within the ion channel and overlaps with the binding sites for other uncompetitive inhibitors, such as Mg^{2+} (Parsons *et al*, 1993). In contrast, high-affinity uncompetitive NMDA inhibitors include phencyclidine (PCP). Removal of memantine from the channel is slower than for Mg^{2+} but substantially faster than for PCP.

A recent randomised, double-blind, placebo-controlled study that involved 252 patients with moderate to severe Alzheimer's disease demonstrated significant benefit for patients treated with memantine (20 mg daily) for 28 weeks, in terms of global change, activities of daily living and severity of impairment (Reisberg *et al*, 2003). There have been a number of smaller studies and benefit has also been found in patients with vascular dementia. A detailed review of the clinical data has been published (Jarvis & Figgitt, 2003). In clinical trials, the overall incidence rate of side-effects did not differ from placebo treatment (Jarvis & Figgitt, 2003) (Table 12.6).

Other mechanisms

Attempts to modify other neurotransmitter systems, including the noradrenaline, serotonin and dopamine systems, have been tried, with variable benefit. Other strategies that have been tried with limited success include excitatory amino acids (e.g. D-cycloserine, a glutamate agonist), cerebroactive compounds (e.g. piracetam, which increases the availability of adenosine triphosphate), nerve growth factor and ACE inhibitors. There have been slightly more promising results with anti-inflammatory drugs (Gasiorowski *et al*, 1995) and hormone replacement therapy (Henderson *et al*, 1996), but, in summary, only the cholinesterase inhibitors have been clinically successful. A helpful critical review of treatment strategies for the management of patients with Alzheimer's disease has been published by Hopker (1999).

NICE guidelines

The National Institute for Clinical Excellence (NICE) (2001) has published guidance on the use of antidementia drugs. Broadly speaking, treatment should meet the following criteria:

(1) Patients should have mild to moderate Alzheimer's disease (they should score between 12 and 26 on the MMSE test of cognition).

(2) Assessment should take place in a specialist clinic before the drug is prescribed and include tests of cognition, global and behavioural function, and activities of daily living.

(3) Only specialists (old age psychiatrists, neurologists and physicians specialising in care of the elderly) should initiate treatment.

(4) A carer or care worker who is in contact with the patient should ensure adequate compliance.

(5) A further assessment should be made, usually 2–4 months after the maintenance dose of the drug is reached. Following this assessment the drug should be continued only if there has been improvement or no deterioration in MMSE score, together with evidence of global improvement on the behavioural or functional assessment.

(6) Patients who continue on the drug should be reviewed (cognition, global functioning and behavioural assessment) every 6 months.

These guidelines, however, make a number of assumptions. Patients must have a diagnosis of mild to moderate Alzheimer's disease before treatment can be commenced. However, in the early stages of the disease, diagnosis can be very difficult because of the overlap with normal ageing. In addition, there is no currently available diagnostic test and although neuroimaging techniques have shown some promising results, these are of little practical value when one considers the large number of community-based patients who have not been diagnosed with Alzheimer's disease. Genetic tests may be helpful in the future to assist with diagnosis, but these give no indication about when a person is about to develop the condition. The concept of preclinical treatment is of theoretical interest, but there are clear ethical and financial concerns about treating patients at this stage, as it could be many years before the condition is expressed.

It is not clear from the NICE guidelines how clinical 'benefit' should be determined. This is reasonably clear if there is evidence of improvement compared with baseline. Benefit might also be present if there has been no change or if the decline has been less than would have been predicted. The last point in particular can be very difficult to determine with accuracy in individual patients. The guidelines recommend that cognition, behaviour, global functioning and activities of daily living should all be assessed but they do not specify which of the many available instruments should be used. In fact, there is no national or international agreement about which instruments should be used to evaluate antidementia drugs and what level of change must be present for 'benefit' to be shown. The available data on antidementia drugs are very encouraging. However, there needs to be agreement about which measures of efficacy should be used in clinical practice and 'benefit' needs to be clearly defined.

Prospects for antidementia treatments

More work is needed to identify subgroups of patients who may benefit from treatment, especially those with severe dementia with psychotic symptoms and behavioural disturbance. For example, patients with Lewy-body dementia appear to have a much better response to anti-dementia drugs than those with Alzheimer's disease (Samuel et al, 2000). In the future, cholinesterase inhibitors will probably be used in a variety of other clinical situations. There is increasing evidence for their use in the management of psychotic and Parkinsonian symptoms in dementia and especially in patients with Lewy-body dementia (McKeith et al, 2000). There has also been some limited evidence for benefit with donepezil in Lewy-body dementia (Lanctot & Herrmann, 2000), but the total number of patients treated remains small.

Pharmacogenetics is a rapidly developing field and the use of genetics in the future to help predict which patients are most likely to benefit from treatment will become increasingly important.

Antidementia drugs are increasingly being used and the issue of their cost-effectiveness has inevitably been raised. Statistical analysis reveals that between three and seven patients need to be treated with them in order for one of them to experience an amelioration of clinical symptoms or postponement of deterioration (Livingston & Katona, 2000). None the less, the general consensus (including NICE, 2001) is that when patients are carefully selected and monitored these are cost-effective drugs.

In Alzheimer's disease there are multiple neurotransmitter deficits and it is surprising that there has not been more research into combination therapies. This would need careful evaluation, in part because it is contrary to the general view that we should be avoiding polypharmacy in older people.

Conclusions

Psychotropic drugs are commonly prescribed for older people. They should be used with great caution in older people because of their increased susceptibility to side-effects and drug interactions, but sub-therapeutic doses should be avoided. Although pharmacological considerations are important, developing a good relationship with older people and adopting a multi-professional approach to treatment are vital if patients are to make genuine therapeutic progress. Patients will need a careful assessment before they start treatment, and the pharmaco-kinetic and pharmacodynamic changes associated with increasing age will need to be taken into consideration when psychotropic drugs are prescribed for older people.

References

Aguglia, E. (2000) Reboxetine in the maintenance therapy of depressive disorder in the elderly: a long-term open study. *International Journal of Geriatric Psychiatry*, **15**, 784–793.

Alexopoulous, G. S. (1992) Geriatric depression reaches maturity. *International Journal of Geriatric Psychiatry*, **7**, 305–306.

Allain, H., Bentue-Ferrer, D., Tarral, A., *et al* (2003) Effects on postural oscillation and memory function of a single dose of zolpidem 5 mg, zopiclone 3.75 mg and lormetazepam 1 mg in elderly healthy subjects. A randomised, cross-over, double-blind study versus placebo. *European Journal of Clinical Pharmacology*, **59**, 179–188.

Almond, S. & O'Donnell, O. (2000) Cost analysis of the treatment of schizophrenia in the UK. A simulation model comparing olanzapine, risperidone and haloperidol. *Pharmacoeconomics*, **17**, 383–389.

American Psychiatric Association (1997) *Practice Guidelines for the Treatment of Patients with Schizophrenia* (1st edn). Washington, DC: APA.

Anderson, I. M. & Tomenson, B. M. (1995) Treatment discontinuation with selective serotonin reuptake inhibitors compared with tricyclic antidepressants: a meta-analysis. *BMJ*, **310**, 1433–1438.

Aronson, R., Offman, H. J., Joffe, R. T., *et al* (1996) Triiodothyronine augmentation in the treatment of refractory depression: a meta-analysis. *Archives of General Psychiatry*, **53**, 842–848.

Baldwin, R. & Burns, A. (1998) Pharmacological treatments. In *Seminars in Old Age Psychiatry* (eds R. Butler & B. Pitt), pp. 247–264. London: Gaskell.

Barbone, F., McMahon, A. D. & Davey, P. G. (1998) Use of benzodiazepines increased road traffic accidents whereas use of tricyclic antidepressants and SSRIs did not. *Lancet*, **352**, 1331–1336.

Barner, E. L. & Gray, S. L. (1998) Donepezil use in Alzheimer's disease. *Annals of Pharmacotherapy*, **32**, 70–77.

Bazire, S. (2000) *Psychotropic Drug Directory*. Exeter: Quay Books.

Bertilsson, L. & Dahl, M. L. (1996) Polymorphic drug oxidation: relevance to treatment of psychiatric disorders. *CNS Drugs*, **3**, 200–223.

Birks, J., Iakovidou, V. & Tsolaki, M. (2000) Review: rivastigmine may improve cognitive outcomes in Alzheimer's disease. *Evidence-Based Mental Health*, **3**, 10.

Blesa, R. (2000) Galantamine: therapeutic effects beyond cognition. *Dementia and Geriatric Cognitive Disorders*, **11** (suppl. 1), 28–34.

Bondareff, W., Alpert, M., Friedhoff, A. J., *et al* (2000) Comparison of sertraline and nortriptyline in the treatment of major depressive disorder in late life. *American Journal of Psychiatry*, **157**, 729–736.

Braithwaite, R. A. (1998) Pharmacokinetics of psychotropic drugs in the elderly. In *Psychopharmacology of Cognitive and Psychiatric Disorders in the Elderly* (eds D. Wheatley & D. Smith), pp. 22–35. London: Chapman and Hall Medical.

Brodeur, M. R. & Stirling, A. L. (2001) Delirium associated with zolpidem. *Annals of Pharmacotherapy*, **35**, 1562–1564.

Bromness, J. G., Arnestad, M., Karinen, R., *et al* (2001) Fatal overdose of zopiclone in an elderly woman with bronchogenic carcinoma. *Journal of Forensic Sciences*, **46**, 1247–1249.

Brown, C. S., Markowitz, J. S., Moore, T. R., *et al* (1999) Atypical antipsychotics. Part II – adverse effects, drug interactions and costs. *Annals of Pharmacotherapy*, **33**, 210–217.

Buckley, N. A., Dawson, A. H., Whyte, I. M., *et al* (1994) Greater toxicity in overdose of dothiepin than other tricyclic antidepressants. *Lancet*, **343**, 159–162.

Burns, A., Howard, R. & Pettit, W. (1995) *Alzheimer's Disease: A Medical Companion*, pp. 85–103. Oxford: Blackwell Science.

Burns, A., Rossor, M., Hecker, J., *et al* (1999) The effects of donepezil in Alzheimer's disease – results from a multinational trial. *Dementia*, **10**, 237–244.

Cacabelos, R., Takeda, M. & Winblad, B. (1999) The glutamatergic system and neurodegeneration in dementia: preventive strategies in Alzheimer's disease. *International Journal of Geriatric Psychiatry*, **14**, 3–47.

Cameron, I., Curran, S., Newton, P., *et al* (2000) Use of donepezil in routine clinical practice. *International Journal of Geriatric Psychiatry*, **15**, 887–891.

Carlsten, A., Waern, M., Holmgren, P., *et al* (2003) The role of benzodiazepines in elderly suicides. *Scandinavian Journal of Public Health*, **31**, 224–228.

Carvajal, A. & Arias, L. H. M. (1999) Antipsychotic drugs. In *Side-effects of Drugs*, Vol. 22 (ed. J. K. Aronson), pp. 45–80. Oxford: Elsevier.

Carvajal, A. & Arias, L. H. M. (2000) Antipsychotic drugs. In *Side-effects of Drugs, Vol. 23* (ed. J. K. Aronson), pp. 48–82. Oxford: Elsevier.

Chaplin, R., Gordon, J. & Burns, T. (1999) Early detection of antipsychotic side-effects. *Psychiatric Bulletin*, **23**, 657–660.

Clark, W. S., Street, J. S., Sanger, T. M., *et al* (2000) *Reduction of Psychotic Symptoms in Patients with Lewy Body-Like Symptoms Treated with Olanzapine*. London: British Gerontological Society.

Committee on Safety of Medicines (1999) Clozapine and gastrointestinal obstruction. *Current Problems in Pharmacovigilance*, **25**, 5–6.

Conn, D. K. & Lieff, S. (2001) Diagnosing and managing delirium in the elderly. *Canadian Family Physician*, **47**, 101–108.

Cowen, P. J. (2000) Antidepressant drugs. In *Side-effects of Drugs, Vol. 23* (ed. J. K. Aronson), pp. 15–22. Oxford: Elsevier.

Cummings, J. L., Street, J., Masterman, D., *et al* (2002) Efficacy of olanzapine in the treatment of psychosis in dementia with Lewy bodies. *Dementia and Geriatric Cognitive Disorders*, **13**, 67–73.

Curran, S. (1996) Hypnotics and sedatives. In *Side-effects of Drugs, Vol. 19* (ed. J. K. Aronson & C. J. van Boxtel), pp. 33–39. Amsterdam: Elsevier.

Curran, S. & Musa, S. (2000) Hypnotics and sedatives. In *Side-effects of Drugs, Vol. 23* (ed. J. K. Aronson), pp. 44–47. Oxford: Elsevier.

Czobor, P., Volavka, J. & Meibach, R. C. (1995) Effect of risperidone on hostility in schizophrenia. *Journal of Clinical Psychopharmacology*, **15**, 243–249.

Danysz, W., Parsons, C. G., Kornhuber, J., *et al* (1997) Aminoadamantanes as NMDA receptor antagonists and antiparkinsonian agents – preclinical studies. *Neuroscience Behaviour Reviews*, **21**, 455–468.

Danysz, W., Parsons, C. G., Mobius, H. J., *et al* (2000) Neuroprotective and symptomatological action of memantine relevant for Alzheimer's disease – a unified hypothesis on the mechanism of action. *Neurotoxicity Research*, **2**, 85–97.

Davidson, M., Harvey, P. D., Vervarcke, J., *et al* (2000) A long-term, multicentre, open-label study of risperidone in elderly patients with psychosis. *International Journal of Geriatric Psychiatry*, **15**, 506–514.

Davis, K. & Mohs, R. (1982) Enhancement of memory processes in Alzheimer's disease with multiple-dose intravenous physostigmine. *American Journal of Psychiatry*, **139**, 1421–1424.

De Deyn, P. P. & Katz, I. R. (2000) Control of aggression and agitation in patients with dementia: efficacy and safety of risperidone. *International Journal of Geriatric Psychiatry*, **15**, S14–S22.

De Deyn, Verslegers, W., Saerens, J., *et al* (1991) Treatment strategies in Alzheimer's disease. In *Diagnostic and Therapeutic Assessments in Alzheimer's Disease* (eds C. G. Gottfries, R. Levy, G. Clincke, *et al*), pp. 177–194. Petersfield: Wrighton Biomedical Publishing.

De Deyn, Rabheru, K., Rasmussen, A., *et al* (1999) A randomised trial of risperidone, placebo and haloperidol for behavioural symptoms of dementia. *Neurology*, **53**, 946–955.

Defilippi, J. L. & Crismon, L. (2000) Antipsychotic agents in patients with dementia. *Pharmacotherapy*, **20**, 23–33.

Demirovic, J. (1998) Epidemiology of Alzheimer's disease. In *Advances in the Diagnosis and Treatment of Alzheimer's Disease* (eds V. Kumar & C. Eisdorfer), pp. 3–30. New York: Springer.

Department of Health (2001) *National Service Framework for Older People*. London: DoH.

Doody, R. S. (1999) Clinical profile of donepezil in the treatment of Alzheimer's disease. *Gerontology*, **45**, 23–32.

Dooley, M. & Lamb, H. M. (2000) Donepezil: a review of its use in Alzheimer's disease. *Drugs and Aging*, **16**, 199–226.

Drug and Therapeutics Bulletin (1981) What should we tell patients about their medicines? *Drug and Therapeutics Bulletin*, **19**, 73–74.

Edwards, J. G. (1995) Editorial. Suicide and antidepressants. *BMJ*, **310**, 205–206.

Erman, M. K., Erwin, C. W., Gengo, F. M., *et al* (2001) Comparative efficacy of zolpidem and temazepam in transient insomnia. *Human Psychopharmacology*, **16**, 169–176.

Esiri, M. M. & McShane, R. H. (1997) Parkinson's disease and dementia. In *The Neuropathology of Dementia* (eds M. M. Esiri & J. H. Morris), pp. 174–193. Cambridge: Cambridge University Press.

Esiri, M. M. & Morris, J. H. (1997) Practical approach to pathological diagnosis. In *The Neuropathology of Dementia* (eds M. M. Esiri & J. H. Morris), pp. 36–69. Cambridge: Cambridge University Press.

Evans, M., Ellis, A., Watson, D., *et al* (2000) Sustained cognitive improvement following treatment of Alzheimer's disease with donepezil. *International Journal of Geriatric Psychiatry*, **15**, 50–53.

Fleischhacker, W. W. (1999) The psychopharmacology of schizophrenia. *Current Opinion in Psychiatry*, **12**, 53–59.

Flint, A. J. (1992) The optimum duration of antidepressant treatment in the elderly. *International Journal of Geriatric Psychiatry*, **7**, 617–619.

Flint, A. J. (1995) Augmentation strategies in geriatric depression. *International Journal of Geriatric Psychiatry*, **10**, 137–146.

Flint, A. J. & Rifat, S. L. (1994) A prospective study of lithium augmentation in antidepressant-resistant geriatric depression. *Journal of Clinical Psychopharmacology*, **14**, 353–356.

Flint, A. J. & Rifat, S. L. (1998) The treatment of psychotic depression in later life: a comparison of pharmacotherapy and ECT. *International Journal of Geriatric Psychiatry*, **13**, 23–28.

Flint, A. J. & Rifat, S. L. (2000) Maintenance treatment for recurrent depression in late life. *American Journal of Geriatric Psychiatry*, **8**, 112–116.

Foster, J. R. (1992) Use of lithium in elderly psychiatric patients: a review of the literature. *Lithium*, **3**, 77–93.

Frenchman, I. B. & Prince, T. (1997) Clinical experience with risperidone, haloperidol and thioridazine for dementia-associated behavioural disturbances. *International Psychogeriatrics*, **9**, 431–435.

Fulton, B. & Benfield, P. (1996) Galantamine. *Drugs and Aging*, **9**, 60–65.

Gasiorowski, K., Leszek, J. & Kiejna, A. (1995) Anti-inflammatory therapy of Alzheimer's disease: current concepts. *International Psychogeriatrics. Proceedings of the 7th International Psychogeriatric Association Congress, Sydney*, p. 94. New York: Springer.

Georgetas, A. & McCue, R. (1989) The additional benefit of extending an anti-depressant trial past seven weeks in the depressed elderly. *International Journal of Geriatric Psychiatry*, **4**, 191–195.

Geroldi, C., Frisoni, G. B., Bianchetti, A., *et al* (1997) Drug treatment in Lewy body dementia. *Dementia and Geriatric Cognitive Disorders*, **8**, 188–197.

Grossberg, G. T., Stahelin, H. B., Messina, J. C., *et al* (2000) Lack of adverse pharmacodynamic drug interactions with rivastigmine and twenty-two classes of medication. *International Journal of Geriatric Psychiatry*, **15**, 242–247.

Halikas, J. A. (1995) Org 3770 (mirtazapine) versus trazodone: a placebo controlled trial in depressed elderly patients. *Human Psychopharmacology*, **10**, S125–S133.

Han, L., McCusker, J., Cole, M., *et al* (2001) Use of medications with anticholinergic effect predicts clinical severity of delirium symptoms in older medical inpatients. *Archives of Internal Medicine*, **161**, 1099–1105.

Hawkins, K. A., Mohamed, S. & Woods, S. W. (1999) Will the novel antipsychotics significantly ameliorate neuropsychological deficits and improve adaptive functioning in schizophrenia? *Psychological Medicine*, **29**, 1–8.

Head, L. & Dening, T. (1998) Lithium in the over-65's: who is taking it and who is monitoring it? *International Journal of Geriatric Psychiatry*, **13**, 164–171.

Hedner, J., Yaeche, R., Emilien, G., *et al* (2000) Zaleplon shortens subjective sleep latency and improves subjective sleep quality in elderly patients with insomnia. *International Journal of Geriatric Psychiatry*, **15**, 704–712.

Henderson, V. W., Watt, L. & Buckwalter, J. G. (1996) Cognitive skills associated with oestrogen replacement in women with Alzheimer's disease. *Psychoneuroendocrinology*, **21**, 421–430.

Hopker, S. (1999) *Drug Treatments and Dementia*. London: Jessica Kingsley.

Hotopf, M., Hardy, R. & Lewis, G. (1997) Discontinuation rates of SSRIs and tricyclic antidepressants: a meta-analysis and investigation of heterogeneity. *British Journal of Psychiatry*, **170**, 120–127.

Hoyberg, O. J., Maragakis, B., Mullin, J., *et al* (1996) A double-blind multicentre comparison of mirtazapine and amitriptyline in elderly depressed patients. *Acta Psychiatrica Scandinavica*, **93**, 184–190.

Hurwitz, N. (1969) Predisposing factors in adverse reactions to drugs. *BMJ*, *i*, 536–540.

Israel, A. G. & Kramer, J. A. (2002) Safety of zaleplon in the treatment of insomnia. *Annals of Pharmacotherapy*, **36**, 852–859.

James, J. R. & Nordberg, A. (1995) Genetic and environmental aspects of the role of nicotinic receptors in neurodegenerative disorders: emphasis on Alzheimer's disease and Parkinson's disease. *Behaviour Genetics*, **25**, 149–159.

Jarvis, B. & Figgitt, D. P. (2003) Memantine. *Drugs and Aging*, **20**, 465–476.

Jefferson, J. W. (2000) Lithium. In *Side-effects of Drugs, Vol. 23* (ed. J. K. Aronson), pp. 23–3. Oxford: Elsevier.

Jones, B. & Tollefson, G. (1998) Olanzapine versus risperidone and haloperidol in the treatment of schizophrenia. *Schizophrenia Research*, **29**, 1–2.

Jones, B., Wang, H., David, S. R., *et al* (2000) A double-blind, placebo-controlled study of short-acting intramuscular olanzapine and lorazepam in acutely agitated patients with dementia. *Proceedings of the 39th Annual Meeting of the American College of Neuropsychopharmacology (ACNP)*, p. 190. San Juan, Puerto Rico: ACNP.

Karlsson, I., Godderis, J., De Mendonca Lima, C. A., *et al* (2000) A randomised, double-blind comparison of the efficacy and safety of citalopram compared to mianserin in elderly, depressed patients with or without mild to moderate dementia. *International Journal of Geriatric Psychiatry*, **15**, 295–305.

Katona, C., Bercoff, E., Chiu, E., *et al* (1999) Reboxetine versus imipramine in the treatment of elderly patients with depressive disorders: a double-blind randomised trial. *Journal of Affective Disorders*, **55**, 203–213.

Kirby, M., Denihan, A., Bruce, I., *et al* (1999) Benzodiazepine use among the elderly in the community. *International Journal of Geriatric Psychiatry*, **14**, 280–284.

Koenig, H. G., Meador, K. G., Cohen, H. J., *et al* (1988) Depression in elderly hospitalised patients with medical illness. *Archives of Internal Medicine*, **148**, 1929–1936.

Lader, M. (1994) Neuropharmacology and pharmacokinetics of psychotropic drugs in old age. In *Principles and Practice of Geriatric Psychiatry* (eds J. Copeland, M. Abou-Saleh & D. Blazer), pp. 79–82. Chichester: John Wiley.

Lanctot, K. L. & Herrmann, N. (2000) Donepezil for behavioural disorders associated with Lewy bodies: a case series. *International Journal of Geriatric Psychiatry*, **15**, 338–345.

Learoyd, B. M. (1972) Psychotropic drugs and the elderly patient. *Medical Journal of Australia*, *i*, 1131–1133.

Livingston, G. & Katona, C. (2000) How useful are cholinesterase inhibitors in the treatment of Alzheimer's disease? A number to treat analysis. *International Journal of Geriatric Psychiatry*, **15**, 203–207.

Livingston, M. G. & Livingston, H. M. (1999) Editorial. New antidepressants for old people? *BMJ*, **318**, 1640–1641.

Lyketsos, C. G., Sheppard, J. M. E., Steele, C. D., *et al* (2000) Randomised, placebo-controlled, double-blind clinical trail of sertraline in the treatment of depression complicating Alzheimer's disease: initial results from the depression in Alzheimer's disease study. *American Journal of Psychiatry*, **157**, 1686–1689.

Madrak, L. N. & Rosenberg, M. (2001) Zolpidem abuse. *American Journal of Psychiatry*, **158**, 1330–1331.

Maelicke, A. (2000) Allosteric modulation of nicotinic receptors as a treatment strategy for Alzheimer's disease. *Dementia and Geriatric Cognitive Disorders*, **11** (suppl. 1), 11–18.

Malenka, R. C. & Nicoll, R. A. (1999) Long-term potentiation – a decade of progress? *Science*, **285**, 1870–1874.

Mamdani, M. M., Parikh, S. V., Austin, P. C., *et al* (2000) Use of antidepressants among elderly subjects: trends and contributing factors. *American Journal of Psychiatry*, **157**, 360–367.

Matthews, H. P., Korbey, J., Wilkinson, D. G., *et al* (2000) Donepezil in Alzheimer's disease: eighteen month results from Southampton Memory Clinic. *International Journal of Geriatric Psychiatry*, **15**, 713–720.

McKeith, I. G., Grace, J. B., Walker, Z., *et al* (2000) Rivastigmine in the treatment of dementia with Lewy bodies: preliminary findings from an open trial. *International Journal of Geriatric Psychiatry*, **15**, 387–392.

McManus, D. Q., Arvanitis, L. A. & Kowalcyk, B. B. (1999) Quetiapine, a novel antipsychotic: experience in elderly patients with psychotic disorders. *Journal of Clinical Psychiatry*, **60**, 292–298.

Meagher, D. J. (2001) Delirium: optimising management. *BMJ*, **322**, 144–149.

Mendelson, W. B. (1996) The use of sedative/hypnotic medication and its correlation with falling down in hospital. *Sleep*, **19**, 698–701.

Mendelson, W. B., Thompson, C. & Franko, T. (1996) Adverse reactions to sedative/hypnotics: three years' experience. *Sleep*, **19**, 702–706.

Naguib, M. & Levy, R. (1995) Paranoid states in the elderly and late paraphrenia. In *Psychiatry in the Elderly* (eds R. Jacoby & C. Oppenheimer), pp. 758–778. Oxford: Oxford University Press.

National Institute for Clinical Excellence (2001) *Guidance on the Use of Donepezil, Rivastigmine and Galantamine for the Treatment of Alzheimer's Disease*. Technology Appraisal Guidance Number 19. London: NICE. Available at www.nice.org.uk.

Old Age Depression Interest Group (OADIG) (1993) How long should the elderly take antidepressants? A double-blind placebo-controlled study of continuation/prophylaxis therapy with dothiepin. *British Journal of Psychiatry*, **162**, 175–182.

Parsons, C. G., Gruner, R., Rozental, J., *et al* (1993) Patch clamp studies on the kinetics and selectivity of N-methyl-D-aspartate receptor antagonism by memantine. *Neuropharmacology*, **32**, 1337–1350.

Pettegrew, J. W., Klunk, W. E., Panchalingam, K., *et al* (1995) Clinical and neurochemical effects of acetyl-L-carnitine in Alzheimer's disease. *Neurobiology of Aging*, **16**, 1–4.

Polinski, R. J. (1998) Clinical pharmacology of rivastigmine: a new-generation acetylcholinesterase inhibitor for the treatment of Alzheimer's disease. *Clinical Therapeutics*, **20**, 634–647.

Quitkin, F. M., Robkin, J. G., Ross, D., *et al* (1984) Duration of antidepressant drug treatment. *Archives of General Psychiatry*, **41**, 238–245.

Racagni, G., Masotto, C. & Steardo, L. (1997) *Pharmacology of Anxiolytic Drugs*. Seattle, WA: Hogrefe and Huber.

Rahkonen, T., Makela, H., Paanila, S., *et al* (2000) Delirium in elderly people without severe predisposing disorders: aetiology and one-year prognosis after discharge. *International Psychogeriatrics*, **12**, 437–481.

Raskind, M. A., Peskind, E. R., Wessel, T., *et al* (2000) Galantamine in Alzheimer's disease. A 6-month randomised, placebo-controlled trail with a 6-month extension. *Neurology*, **54**, 2261–2268.

Ray, W. A., Fought, R. L. & Decker, M. D. (1992) Psychoactive drugs and risk of injurious motor vehicle crashes in elderly drivers. *American Journal of Epidemiology*, **136**, 873–883.

Reilly, J. G., Ayis, S. A., Ferrier, I. N., *et al* (2000) QTc-interval abnormalities and psychotropic drug therapy in psychiatric patients. *Lancet*, **355**, 1048–1052.

Reisberg, B., Doody, R., Stoffler, A., *et al* (2003) Memantine in moderate-to-severe Alzheimer's disease. *New England Journal of Medicine*, **348**, 1333–1341.

Rogers, S. L. & Friedhoff, L. T. (1998) Long-term efficacy and safety of donepezil in the treatment of Alzheimer's disease: an interim analysis of the results of a US multicentre open label extension study. *European Neuropsychopharmacology*, **8**, 67–75.

Rogers, S. L., Doody, R. S., Mohs, R. C., *et al* (1998a) Donepezil improves cognition and global function in Alzheimer's disease. *Archives of Internal Medicine*, **158**, 1021–1031.

Rogers, S. L., Farlow, M. R., Doody, R. S., *et al* (1998b) A 24-week, double-blind, placebo-controlled trial of donepezil in patients with Alzheimer's disease. *Neurology*, **50**, 136–145.

Roose, S. P., Glassman, A. H., Attia, E., *et al* (1994) Comparative efficacy of selective serotonin reuptake inhibitors and tricyclics in the treatment of melancholia. *American Journal of Psychiatry*, **151**, 1735–1739.

Rosler, M., Anand, R., Cicin-Sain, A., *et al* (1999) Efficacy and safety of rivastigmine in patients with Alzheimer's disease: international randomised controlled trial. *BMJ*, **318**, 633–638.

Sajatovic, M., Madhusoodanan, S. & Buckley, P. (2000) Schizophrenia in the elderly: guidelines for management. *CNS Drugs*, **13**, 103–115.

Samuel, W., Caligiuri, M., Galasko, D., *et al* (2000) Better cognitive and psychopathologic response to donepezil in patients prospectively diagnosed as dementia with Lewy bodies: a preliminary study. *International Journal of Geriatric Psychiatry*, **15**, 794–802.

Schultz, C. & McGorry, P. (2000) Traditional antipsychotic medications: contemporary clinical use. In *Schizophrenia and Mood Disorders* (eds P. F. Buckley & J. L. Waddington), pp. 14–20. Oxford: Butterworth Heinemann.

Scott, L. J. & Goa, K. L. (2000) Galantamine: a review of its use in Alzheimer's disease. *Drugs*, **60**, 1095–1122.

Shahpesandy, H. M., Medvecky, M., Doci, I., *et al* (2000) Zotepine versus risperidone in the treatment of psychotic disorders in the elderly. *Homeostasis*, **40**, 243–244.

Shulman, K. I. & Herrmann, N. (1999) The nature and management of mania in old age. *Psychiatric Clinics of North America*, **22**, 649–665.

Smith, D. (1998) Side-effects of psychotropic drugs. In *Psychopharmacology of Cognitive and Psychiatric Disorders in the Elderly* (eds D. Wheatley & D. Smith), pp. 36–54. London: Chapman and Hall Medical.

Snaedal, J., Johannesson, T., Jonsson, J. E., *et al* (1996) The effects of nicotine in dermal plaster on cognitive functions in patients with Alzheimer's disease. *Dementia*, **7**, 47–52.

Snowdon, J. (2000) The relevance of guidelines for treatment mania in old age. *International Journal of Geriatric Psychiatry*, **15**, 779–783.

Song, F., Freemantle, N., Sheldon, T. A., *et al* (1993) Selective serotonin reuptake inhibitors: meta-analysis of efficacy and acceptability. *BMJ*, **306**, 683–687.

Spigset, O. & Martensson, B. (1999) Drug treatment of depression. *BMJ*, **318**, 1188–1191.

Spiker, D. G., Weiss, J. C., Dealy, R. S., *et al* (1985) The pharmacological treatment of delusional depression. *American Journal of Psychiatry*, **142**, 430–436.

Stark, C. (2000) *Schizophrenia: Public Health Aspects*. Guildford: A&M Publishing.

Street, J. S., Clark, W. S., Gannon, K. S., *et al* (2000a) Olanzapine treatment of psychotic and behavioural symptoms in patients with Alzheimer's disease in nursing care facilities. *Archives of General Psychiatry*, **57**, 968–976.

Street, J. S., Clark, W. S., Kadman, D. L., *et al* (2000b) *Long-Term Efficacy of Olanzapine in the Control of Psychotic and Behavioural Symptoms in Nursing Home Patients with Alzheimer's Disease*. London: British Gerontological Society.

Sucher, N. J., Awobuluyi, M., Choi, Y. B., *et al* (1996) NMDA receptors: from genes to channels. *Trends in Pharmacological Science*, **17**, 348–355.

Summers, W., Haovskil, M. & Marsh, G. (1986) Oral THA in the long term treatment of senile dementia, Alzheimer type. *New England Journal of Medicine*, **315**, 1241–1245.

Tariot, P. N., Solomon, P. R., Morris, J. C., *et al* (2000) A 5-month, randomised, placebo-controlled trial of galantamine in AD. *Neurology*, **54**, 2269–2276.

Tarsy, D., Baldessarini, R. J. & Tarazi, F. I. (2002) Effects of newer antipsychotics on extrapyramidal function. *CNS Drugs*, **16**, 23–45.

Taylor, D., McConnell, D., McConnell, H., *et al* (1999) *The Bethlem and Maudsley NHS Trust Prescribing Guidelines*. London: Martin Dunitz.

Taylor, N., Beuzen, J. N., Wesnes, K., *et al* (1996) The effect of olanzapine on cognition and psychomotor function in healthy elderly volunteers. *Schizophrenia Research*, **18**, 131.

Terzano, M. G., Rossi, M., Palomba, V., *et al* (2003) New drugs for insomnia: comparative tolerability of zopiclone, zolpidem and zaleplon. *Drug Safety*, **26**, 261–282.

Thornley, B., Adams, C. E. & Awad, G. (1997) Chlorpromazine versus placebo for those with schizophrenia. Cochrane review. *Cochrane Library*, issue 3.

Tourigny-Rivard, M. F. (1997) Pharmacotherapy of affective disorders in old age. *Canadian Journal of Psychiatry*, **42** (suppl. 1), 10–18.

Tram, K., Tran-Johnson, M., Harris, M. J., *et al* (1994) Pharmacological treatment of schizophrenia and delusional disorder of late life. In *Principles and Practice of Geriatric Psychiatry* (eds J. R. M. Copeland, M. T. Abou-Saleh & D. G. Blazer), pp. 685–692. Chichester: John Wiley.

Tyson, P. J., Mortimer, A. M. & Wheeler, J. A. (1999) High-dose antipsychotic treatment in clinical practice. A review audit and survey of consultant psychiatrist opinions. *Psychiatric Bulletin*, **23**, 661–664.

van Duijn, C. M. & Hofman, A. (1991) Relation between nicotine intake and Alzheimer's disease. *BMJ*, **302**, 1491–1494.

van Dyck, C. H., Newhouse, P., Falk, W. E., *et al* (2000) Extended-release physostigmine in Alzheimer's disease: a multi-centre, double-blind, 12-week study with dose enrichment. *Archives of General Psychiatry*, **57**, 157–164.

Wattis, J. P. W. & Curran, S. (2001) *Practical Psychiatry of Old Age* (3rd edn). Oxford: Radcliffe Medical.

Weinstock, M. (1999) Selectivity of cholinesterase inhibition: clinical implications for the treatment of Alzheimer's disease. *CNS Drugs*, **12**, 307–323.

Wheatley, D. & Smith, D. (1998) *Psychopharmacology of Cognitive and Psychiatric Disorders in the Elderly*. London: Chapman and Hall Medical.

Whitehouse, P. J. (1994) Neurochemistry of ageing. In *Principles and Practice of Geriatric Psychiatry* (eds J. R. M. Copeland, M. T. Abou-Saleh & D. G. Blazer), pp. 61–63. Chichester: John Wiley.

Wilcock, G. K., Lilienfeld, S. & Gaens, E. (2000) Efficacy and safety of galantamine in patients with mild to moderate Alzheimer's disease: multicentre randomised controlled trial. *BMJ*, **321**, 1145–1449.

Wilson, A. L., McCarten, J. R., Langley, L. K., *et al* (1995) Transdermal nicotine administration in Alzheimer's disease: effects on cognition, behavior and cardiac function. In *Research Advances in Alzheimer's Disease and Related Disorders* (eds K. Iqbal, J. Mortimer, B. Winblad & H. Wisniewski), pp. 305–314. Chichester: John Wiley.

Yokel, R. A., Allen, D. D. & Meyer, J. J. (1994) Studies of aluminium neurobehavioural toxicity in the intact mammal. *Cellular and Molecular Neurobiology*, **14**, 791–808.

Zukin, R. S. & Bennett, M. V. L. (1995) Alternative spliced isoforms of the NMDAR1 receptor subunits. *Trends in Neuroscience*, **18**, 306–331.

CHAPTER 13

Pharmacological aspects of drugs of misuse

Brian E. Leonard

The human race has always shown a surprising ingenuity for finding drugs that have a pleasurable effect. Alcohol in its various forms is perhaps the oldest drug to be used for its effects on the brain, closely followed by various naturally occurring hallucinogens; for example, fungi have long been known to be an important component of religious ritual in many societies. Other drugs, some of which have had therapeutic uses, include the opioid analgesics such as morphine and codeine, cannabis, cocaine (until recently in a relatively crude form extracted from the leaf of the Andean coca plant) and the milder stimulants, caffeine and nicotine. The use of extracts of opium, coca leaves and khat, a plant growing in some Middle Eastern countries that contains several stimulants, has had social importance in some non-industrialised societies, where such substances are commonly used as social alternatives to alcohol and also have a role in counteracting hunger and fatigue. Most societies in which these drugs are used recognise their potential dangers to health should they be consumed to excess. Thus both the non-medical use of drugs and the related problem of drug misuse have been widely recognised since antiquity. This chapter concentrates on the psychopharmacological properties of drugs of misuse.

Definitions

The term 'drug misuse' refers to the use of any drug in a manner that is at variance with the approved use in that particular culture. Thus the term refers to socially disapproved use and is not descriptive of a particular pattern of misuse. For example, chewing the leaves of *Catha edulis*, or khat (the main active ingredients of which are cathanine and cathadrine), is socially acceptable in the Yemen and other Middle Eastern countries, where there is little evidence that, within the confines of that culture, it is misused or that it causes major health problems. In most European countries, however, its use is illegal (but not in the UK) and it is treated as a criminal offence to be in possession of this substance. Conversely, alcohol is a major health hazard in most industrialised countries, where it is socially accepted, but is banned in many Muslim countries, and there are often dire consequences for those who transgress the ban.

'Non-medical drug use' covers, for example, the occasional use of alcohol and the regular use of the opioid analgesics. This term includes the occasional recreational use of licit and illicit drugs for their pleasurable effects (e.g. the use of amphetamines or cannabis) and outside their approved medical indications.

'Drug dependence' is defined as a syndrome in which someone continues to take the drug because of the reinforcing effect that is derived from it. This behaviour occurs despite the adverse social or medical consequences it may have; the dependent person is motivated to continue taking the drug for his/her continued well-being. Often the dose of the drug must be increased to maintain its desired effect. This leads to a change in the behaviour of the dependent person, which varies from a mild desire to obtain the drug to a craving or compulsion. With some drugs of misuse, for example the opioids, physical and psychological dependence on the drug may occur, so that lifestyle becomes dominated by the need to secure further supplies of the drug.

The term 'addiction' is so non-specific that it should no longer be used. When used, it suggests that the person is severely dependent on a drug of misuse.

Drug dependence and withdrawal

Three factors are generally involved in drug dependence: tolerance, physical dependence, and psychological dependence.

Tolerance

Tolerance means that an increasing amount of the drug must be administered to obtain the required pharmacological effect; tolerance may occur as a result of the drug being more rapidly metabolised, so-called *metabolic tolerance*, or through a drug-induced insensitivity of the receptors or target sites upon which it acts within the brain, termed *tissue tolerance*, Thus tolerance should be considered a general phenomenon that is not restricted to drugs of misuse. For example, tolerance is known to develop to anticholinergic agents.

Regarding drugs of misuse, tissue tolerance commonly occurs to the opioids, alcohol and the sedatives of the benzodiazepine type. Tolerance does not develop to all drugs of misuse, however. Thus the amphetamines maintain their stimulant and euphoriant effects for a prolonged period of administration without any need to increase the dose appreciably.

Psychological tolerance is the term used to describe the reduction in the desired psychological effects of the drug; this may not be paralleled by an increase in the metabolic tolerance.

Physical dependence

This term is used to describe the phenomenon in which abnormal behavioural and autonomic symptoms occur when the drug is abruptly withdrawn or its effects are terminated by the administration of a specific antagonist. Most drugs of misuse produce some physical dependence, although withdrawal symptoms are relatively mild following the abrupt withdrawal of cannabis, the stimulants and cocaine.

The nature of the withdrawal symptoms depends upon the neuro-transmitter systems that are the target of the drug. Thus cocaine and the amphetamines alleviate fatigue, cause anorexia and elevate mood; withdrawal therefore results in feelings of fatigue, hyperphagia and depression. Abrupt withdrawal from the sedatives, such as barbiturates or following high doses of benzodiazepines, can be associated with anxiety, insomnia and spontaneous seizures.

It must be emphasised that the relationship between tolerance, physical dependence and compulsive drug use is complex and depends on both the category of drug and the personality of the misuser. For example, it appears that the majority of patients prescribed benzo-diazepines even for many months experience relatively minor withdrawal symptoms when the drugs are abruptly stopped; others, however, experience severe anxiety states and have extreme difficulty in stopping the drug.

Psychological dependence

Psychological dependence occurs with most drugs of misuse. Such drugs produce an immediate pleasurable effect and, after their continuous administration, the individual experiences dysphoria and intense craving should the drug be abruptly stopped. Many drugs of misuse cause both physical and psychological dependence.

Cross-dependence

Cross-dependence arises when a drug can suppress the symptoms of withdrawal due to another drug. For example, the effects of alcohol withdrawal can be suppressed by the administration of a benzodiazepine. As both drugs affect the gamma-aminobutyric acid (GABA) system – they enhance GABAergic transmission – albeit by different mechanisms, a benzodiazepine can prevent the withdrawal symptoms that arise following the abrupt cessation of alcohol. However, cross-tolerance and cross-dependence can occur only between drugs with a similar mechanism of action at the cellular level. For example, benzodiazepines cannot directly suppress the effects of morphine withdrawal.

Withdrawal syndrome

The occurrence of the withdrawal syndrome after the abrupt termination of administration of the drug is the only objective evidence of physical dependence. The symptoms of withdrawal have at least two origins:

(1) the abrupt removal of the drug of dependence
(2) the hyperarousal of the brain due to readaptation following the absence of the drug.

The pharmacokinetic properties of the drug are of major importance in determining the amplitude and duration of the withdrawal syndrome. The symptoms of drug withdrawal are characteristic for the specific category of the drug and are usually the opposite of those produced when the drug is first administered. For example, an opioid agonist such as morphine produces constricted pupils and bradycardia, but on abrupt withdrawal dilated pupils and tachycardia occur.

Tolerance, physical dependence and withdrawal are natural consequences of the properties of drugs of dependence. They can be produced in experimental animals as readily as they can in humans but the symptoms do not always imply that the individual is dependent on a drug of misuse. For example, a patient with hypertension who is receiving a b-adrenoceptor antagonist such as propranolol will probably exhibit a withdrawal syndrome consisting of a rebound hypertension when the drug is abruptly withdrawn.

Are there some basic neuronal mechanisms that are affected by all drugs of misuse?

Recently, many of the molecular targets for drugs of misuse have been identified and cloned. In addition, it has been possible to integrate this information into a system that extends from the neuron to the behavioural consequences that follow prolonged drug misuse.

Converging evidence suggested that all drugs of misuse affect the dopaminergic system in the brain. It was suggested that although the different classes of drugs of misuse (e.g. stimulants, depressants, hallucinogens, opiates, cannabinoids) influence many different neurotransmitter systems within the brain, all drugs of misuse appear to enhance, directly or indirectly, dopaminergic function in the limbic system. For example, it is known that opiates act as agonists at opioid receptors but that these receptors also increase the activity of the mesolimbic dopaminergic system. This pathway projects to the pre-frontal cortex and also to the striatum. The nucleus accumbens, located near the striatum, is of primary importance in mediating the rewarding effects of stimulants such as cocaine and the amphetamines; this is associated with an increase in the concentration of dopamine in this region of the brain.

The relevance of such changes is suggested by results of studies in which rats self-administer amphetamine to the nucleus accumbens and increase the amount of drug administered when the dopamine receptors are partially blocked by a neuroleptic. Such positive reinforcement is evidence that dopamine is the neurotransmitter involved in the behaviour of reward and this is supported by the observation that lesions of the dopaminergic system completely block the self-admini-stration of amphetamine. Other experimental studies have shown that other types of misused drugs, such as nicotine, the opiates and alcohol, also induce positive behavioural reinforcement by enhancing dopamine release in the mesolimbic pathway, while abrupt withdrawal of such drugs leads to a dramatic reduction in the concentration of dopamine in the nucleus accumbens. Thus it appears that the reinforcing effects of drugs of misuse partly depend on the functioning of the mesolimbic dopaminergic system, which normally mediates the motivational properties of food and sex.

Other aspects of the dopaminergic system have also been implicated in drug dependence. For example, different allelic forms of the D_2 receptor gene have been implicated in predisposing some individuals to drug misuse. In addition, the dopamine transporter is undoubtedly involved in the stimulant action of cocaine and of the amphetamines. The importance of the dopaminergic system is further suggested by studies of 'knock-out' mice which lack the D_2 receptor. These mice show a reduction in the amount of cocaine they self-administer. Interestingly, in brain imaging studies, it has been shown that the subjective responses to cocaine do not correlate with its action on the dopamine transporter. Thus the simplistic view that enhanced meso-limbic dopaminergic function explains all aspects of drug dependence must be treated with caution.

Of the other transmitters believed to be involved in drug misuse, serotonin has achieved some prominence. There is physiological evidence to suggest that serotonergic and dopaminergic systems are mutually inhibitory. Cocaine, like the selective serotonin reuptake inhibitors (SSRIs) (e.g. fluoxetine and citalopram), blocks the serotonin transporter. Again, it seems improbable that the serotonergic system provides the common neurochemical pathway. Thus mice lacking the $5\text{-}HT_{1B}$ receptor self-administer cocaine more readily than do normal mice but paradoxically $5\text{-}HT_{1B}$ receptor agonists have the same effect.

489

The question arises regarding the existence of a final common pathway by which all drugs of misuse produce their pharmacological effects. One possibility is that they all increase the intracellular activity of cAMP-dependent kinase and thereby increases gene transcriptase activity. This kinase enhances the formation of cyclic adenosine monophosphate (cAMP) response element binding protein (CREB), which switches on the early genes *c-fos* and *c-jun*. It is speculated that the vulnerability of an individual to drug misuse may be linked neurodevelopmentally to a genetic predisposition to an enhanced response to the reinforcing properties of these drugs.

Attempts to develop novel drugs to treat dependence usually focus on the reward region of the brain, namely the dopamine-rich median forebrain bundle. However, it is now apparent that, at least in the rat, the reward region functions independently of the area concerned with craving. When rats become dependent on cocaine and are then withdrawn from the drug, they will increase their electrical self-stimulation of the median forebrain bundle to a greater extent than they do when cocaine is administered. By contrast, stimulation of the ventral subiculum, a glutamate-rich region of the hippocampus, has been shown to produce behaviour associated with craving for cocaine. Thus, while it would appear that stimulation of either the median forebrain bundle or ventral subiculum leads to dopamine release, it is only when the stimulus originates in the hippocampus that the stimulus triggers the memory that is integral to craving. It therefore appears that drug dependence entails two separate processes, one that involves neuro-adaptive changes that are a direct result of the drug and another that involves the establishment of memory traces and is located in the hippocampus.

It is well known that, despite the widespread availability of drugs of dependence, particularly alcohol and nicotine, the majority of individuals do not misuse them. The neurophysiological explanation is that inhibitory mechanisms within the brain normally hold potentially maladaptive behaviour in check. Such a mechanism is usually attributed to the neural networks that involve the prefrontal cortex and striatum. In fact, some of the behavioural and cognitive characteristics of drug misuse, such as impulsivity, risk taking and poor decision making, resemble the changes that follow damage to the ventromedial prefrontal cortex. For example, in decision-making tasks, chronic amphetamine misusers perform similarly to patients with damage to the prefrontal cortex. However, opiate misusers show only part of this deficit. These differences appear to be related to the fact that chronically administered amphetamine causes a reduction in the serotonin content of the orbitofrontal cortex; similar changes have been reported to occur in those misusing methylene-dioxymethamphetamine (MDMA, 'ecstasy').

These general comments on the cellular basis of drug misuse and dependence, while emphasising the common features that may be ascribed to all drugs of misuse, also indicate that there are differences that may be of primary importance in predisposing the individual to prolonged drug misuse.

Sedative drugs of misuse

Alcohol, the barbiturates and the benzodiazepines are included in this group, all of which facilitate GABAergic activity.

Alcohol

The use of alcohol (ethanol) prepared from the fermentation of sugars, starches and other carbohydrates dates back to the beginning of recorded history.

Alcohol is the most important drug of dependence in all industrialised countries, and the clinical and social problems that arise from its widespread misuse are legion. In the USA, the total annual economic cost of alcoholism and its related disorders has been estimated to be approximately $80 billion, and this does not take into account the human cost, which is impossible to quantify. It has been calculated that the lifetime prevalence of alcohol misuse and alcohol dependence (alcoholism) in the USA is 5–10% for men and 3–5% for women.

The American Psychiatric Association (1994) defines 'alcohol misuse' as a condition whereby social life is impaired for at least 1 month as a result of alcohol. 'Alcoholism' is defined as the occurrence of tolerance and physical dependence as a result of prolonged alcohol misuse.

It has been calculated that alcoholism now rivals heart disease and cancer as the major health problem in industrialised countries, with 9% of men and 5% of women currently at risk. In lifetime prevalence rates, alcoholism now ranks first of all psychiatric disorders. However, it is not yet possible to identify any biological, psychological, social or cultural variable that is predictive of alcohol misuse or alcoholism.

There is some epidemiological evidence to show that there is a family predisposition to alcoholism. The incidence of the illness is four times greater in the offspring of parents who were alcohol dependent, and the rate among identical twins is greater than among non-identical twins. Many animal studies also show that some inbred strains have an increased sensitivity to the effects of alcohol and have a greater alcohol intake when given a free choice. From the numerous animal and human studies it has been concluded that alcoholism is a polygenic and multifactorial problem in which genetic factors contribute to the risk of developing the illness.

Recent epidemiological evidence shows that very moderate alcohol consumption, amounting to under three units per day for men and two units for women (one unit being equivalent to about 0.25 litres of beer, one glass of wine or spirits), may protect against myocardial infarction. However, regular consumption of alcohol above 21 units per week for men and 14 units for women predisposes to brain, liver, heart and gastrointestinal tract malfunction. Additional health problems arise as a consequence of the multiple drug misuse that many people who are dependent on alcohol exhibit, particularly of tobacco, minor tranquillisers, sedatives and caffeine.

Pharmacokinetics

Alcohol is readily absorbed from an empty gastrointestinal tract; the rate of absorption is impeded by food. It is widely distributed throughout the body according to the water content of the tissue, and easily penetrates both the blood–brain and placental barriers. More than 90% of the drug is oxidised in the liver to carbon dioxide and water by dehydrogenases, while the remainder is excreted unchanged through the lungs, skin and kidneys. The rate of oxidation is dependent on the degree of tolerance of the individual, the non-tolerant person oxidising approximately 10–15 ml of absolute alcohol per hour. The alcohol-metabolising system is thus easily saturated and its elimination is governed by 'zero-order' kinetics (see Chapter 3).

The daily intake of one or two units of alcohol rapidly leads to tissue tolerance, which is not as extensive as that observed after the administration of any of the opiates and is readily lost after a few days of abstinence.

Psychological tolerance to alcohol develops at a faster rate than metabolic tolerance. Thus death from alcohol overdose can occur in a psychologically tolerant person following only a moderate increase in alcohol intake above that normally consumed.

A 'reverse tolerance' has also been described, whereby a person who is alcohol dependent who takes a small quantity of alcohol may become intoxicated, aggressive and antisocial. This occurs in those who have brain or liver damage and therefore show an enhanced sensitivity to the disinhibiting actions of the drug or a decreased metabolism.

Cross-tolerance also readily occurs between alcohol and other central depressants, for example the benzodiazepines and the barbiturates.

Mode of action

Meyer, in 1901, was the first to suggest that alcohol acts like general anaesthetics by dissolving into cell membranes and thereby disrupting the lipid network that comprises the cell wall. It is now known that, at pharmacologically relevant concentrations (in the range 25–100 mmol/l), alcohol increases the fluidity of cell membranes following its acute administration, these changes correlating with the sedative effects of the drug. This suggests that alcohol produces its effects in a relatively non-specific manner, but it is now known that the nerve membrane is structurally and functionally heterogeneous and that specific regions of the membrane are more sensitive to the disordering effects of the drug than other regions. Thus alcohol may affect the calcium flux across the nerve membrane or, by disrupting the phosphatidyl inositol system intracellularly, affect the intraneuronal availability of calcium. This could have a profound effect upon neuro-transmitter release.

While there is little evidence to suggest that alcohol produces its pharmacological effect via a specific 'alcohol receptor', some lipids do show a particular vulnerability to the disorganising effects of the drug. For example, alcohol selectively inhibits monoamine oxidase-B (MAO-B), and not the A form, in human platelets and brain; similarly, it inhibits sodium/potassium-dependent adenosine triphosphatase in the neuronal membrane but not in the glial membrane.

With regard to its effect on neurotransmitter function, alcohol increases adenylate cyclase activity, possibly via the membrane-bound G-protein complex. The effect of alcohol on the second messenger system appears to depend on its location: the noradrenaline-linked cyclase in the cortex seems to be directly affected by the drug, whereas the dopamine-linked enzyme in the basal ganglia appears to be altered by a combination of changes in the membrane fluidity and those in the G-protein–cyclase complex.

As alcohol has pronounced sedative properties, it is not surprising to find that it facilitates central inhibitory transmission. It has been shown that alcohol has a direct effect on a portion of the GABA–benzodiazepine complex that controls the chloride ion channel. In clinical studies (Suzdak et al, 1986) it has been shown that such inhibitory effects may be reversed by some partial inverse benzodiazepine receptor agonists, but their development as therapeutic agents has been discontinued because they do not reverse other detrimental effects of alcohol on brain function.

Alcohol tolerance has been explained in terms of the adaptational changes in lipids in the nerve membranes. Thus acute alcohol admini-stration is associated with enhanced membrane fluidity due to the disordering effects of the drug, whereas after chronic administration the membranes become more rigid owing to an increased replacement of the unsaturated by saturated fatty acids. Nevertheless, it seems unlikely that such changes are due to a single type of lipid and more likely that different populations of lipids within the nerve membrane show adaptational changes at different rates.

Another approach that has been used to elucidate the biochemical mechanisms associated with tolerance in animals has been to use specific neurotoxins to lesion the noradrenergic and serotonergic systems. Thus lesions of the central noradrenergic system block the development of both environmentally dependent and independent tolerance. (Environmentally dependent tolerance describes the situation in which tolerance to alcohol develops more rapidly when the drug is consumed or administered in the same environment.) Lesions of the serotonergic system are associated only with a block of the environmentally dependent tolerance. The results of such studies suggest that tolerance is a phenomenon that can be separated from the development of physical dependence, and may not therefore be a part of a unitary mechanism for all drugs of misuse.

With regard to the neurotransmitter correlates of alcohol withdrawal and dependence, there is evidence of decreased GABA–benzodiazepine receptor function following chronic alcohol administration, which may be causally related to dependence. Changes in the number of cholinergic muscarinic receptors in the cortex and hippocampus have been reported to occur in alcohol-dependent animals, which return to control levels following withdrawal, but the precise significance of this is unknown.

Experimental studies have also suggested that alcohol may reduce N-methyl-D-aspartate (NMDA) receptor function following acute administration, and following withdrawal of alcohol the functioning of these receptors is enhanced.

Drugs that interact with alcohol

Disulfiram (Antabuse) and calcium carbide are sometimes used to facilitate abstinence for people with alcohol problems, after their detoxification. The rationale behind the use of disulfiram is that it inhibits liver aldehyde dehydrogenase. Any alcohol consumed will lead to an elevation in blood acetaldehyde levels and the aversive toxic effects of acetaldehyde will become apparent. These include facial flushing, nausea, vomiting, gastrointestinal distress and potentially hazardous hypotension and tachycardia. It should be noted that drugs that may be given for other medical conditions can also inhibit liver aldehyde dehydrogenase and cause the Antabuse reaction. These include the sulphonylurea antihyperglycaemics metronidazole and furazolidone (both antimicrobial agents). It must also be emphasised that alcohol will potentiate the action of any drug that has a sedative effect.

Activating drugs and the treatment of alcohol dependence

The aversive effects of alcohol withdrawal are associated with decreased mesolimbic dopaminergic activity and increased extracellular glutamate in the nucleus accumbens. The recently introduced anti-craving drug acamprosate has been shown to reduce the enhanced glutamate release that follows abrupt alcohol withdrawal. In addition, the neuronal hyperexcitability that occurs during alcohol withdrawal is accompanied by an increased expression of the immediate–early gene *c-fos* in several regions of the rat brain; acamprosate has been shown to suppress the elevated *c-fos* expression in these structures. Unlike the sedative drugs, such as the benzodiazepines, which by enhancing GABAergic function are cross-tolerant with alcohol, acamprosate has no effect on the GABAergic system but acts primarily by modulating the activity of the glutamatergic system. In neocortical neurons, for example, it has been shown that acamprosate reduces the activation of excitatory glutamatergic synapses and the depolarising responses evoked by the iontophoretic application of glutamate and NMDA, without changing the membrane potential or the input resistance of the cells. In the hippocampus, the NMDA-initiated changes following the block of transmission have been shown to be enhanced by acamprosate. These effects suggest that acamprosate may act postsynaptically to modulate excitatory transmission in both the neocortex and hippocampus. In addition to the specific changes in the glutamatergic–NMDA system, acamprosate interacts with voltage-gated calcium channels and inhibits the up-regulation of calcium channels in alcohol-withdrawn rats.

In a large double-blind, placebo-controlled European study (Sass *et al*, 1996), acamprosate was shown to be effective in the treatment of alcoholism. Thus at the end of a 1-year period of treatment followed by a 1-year period without medication, 39% of the acamprosate-treated group were still abstinent compared with 17% of the placebo-treated group. Its main clinical effect would appear to be due to its anti-craving properties, as it does not interfere with the pharmacokinetics or pharmacodynamics of alcohol. Furthermore, it does not have any reinforcing effects or discriminative stimulus properties of its own. Acamprosate has now been registered for the treatment of alcoholism in most European counties.

Numerous pharmacological and behavioural studies suggest that alcohol interacts with endogenous opioids. Earlier studies had suggested that the main condensation product of alcohol-derived acetaldehyde and dopamine, tetrahydro-isoquinoline, may stimulate opioid receptors, but *in vivo* evidence is lacking. However, experimental studies have shown that transgenic mice lacking beta-endorphin show a reduction in voluntary consumption when compared with wild-type mice, which suggests that a high alcohol intake is associated with an enhancement of endogenous opioid activity. These findings support the hypothesis that drugs that block the opioid receptors will decrease alcohol intake. Numerous experimental and clinical studies have indicated that the opiate antagonist naltrexone reduces alcohol intake and the drug has now been registered in many countries as an adjunct for the treatment of alcoholism. However, there is evidence that its ability to facilitate abstinence when compared with placebo diminishes over time.

The mechanism of action of naltrexone in the reduction of alcohol consumption is complex, but experimental studies show that opiate antagonists have direct effects on alcohol-seeking behaviour. A possible site for this action could be the mesolimbic dopaminergic reward circuit, in which opioid receptors are located. The activity of endogenous opioids in the ventral tegmental area, the site of origin of the A10 mesolimbic dopaminergic neurons, blocks the activity of the GABAergic interneurons that impinge on the A10 neurons, which leads to disinhibition. Thus, an increase in the endogenous opioid system induced by alcohol would indirectly enhance dopamine release in the mesolimbic system and thereby induce the reward-enhancing effects of the drug. Naltrexone and other antagonists have been shown to antagonise these effects. As naltrexone and other antagonists such as naloxone block the opiate receptors and have been shown in both experimental and clinical studies to suppress alcohol-induced reinforcement, it can be assumed that the activation of the endogenous opioid system is crucially involved in the mediation of alcohol reinforcement.

In summary, naltrexone and acamprosate act via different mechanisms. Naltrexone interferes with the positive reinforcement effects of alcohol and attenuates the effects of conditioned stimuli that had been previously paired with the positive reinforcing effects of alcohol. Acamprosate appears to act by reducing neuronal hyperexcitability and probably inhibits reactivity induced by stimuli that are paired with alcohol withdrawal, an action that may explain the anti-craving action of the drug. While both drugs have been shown to prevent relapse after long abstinence periods, there is no evidence that these drugs also reverse the lasting changes in sensitivity to alcohol. Other compounds that act on NMDA receptors, such as the non-competitive antagonist memantine, appear to hold promise for the treatment of alcoholism in the future.

Anxiolytics and sedatives

The pharmacological properties of these drugs are dealt with in Chapter 5, and therefore only their propensity to cause physical and psychological dependence is considered here. Because of their lack of efficacy, and particularly because of their toxicity, barbiturates should never be used now as anxiolytic or sedative drugs. For this reason, emphasis is placed here on the benzodiazepines, which are not only effective but also relatively safe. Nevertheless, problems have arisen regarding their ability to cause dependence, and so this aspect of their pharmacology must be considered (Lader, 1983; Nutt, 1986).

Considering their widespread use, intentional misuse of prescribed benzodiazepines is relatively rare. Normally, following the administration of a benzodiazepine for several weeks, there is little tolerance or difficulty in stopping the drug when the condition no longer warrants its use.

However, following prolonged treatment (several months for example) tolerance often develops and the abrupt cessation of treatment results in withdrawal symptoms. These consist of: anxiety; agitation; increased sensitivity to light and sound; paraesthesias; muscle cramps; myoclonic jerks; sleep disturbance; and dizziness. These effects are usually short lived and the timing of their onset following withdrawal of the benzodiazepine depends on the half-life of the drug. Following the long-term administration of a high dose of a benzodiazepine, however, seizures and delirium can also occur.

It is often difficult to distinguish withdrawal symptoms from the reappearance of the underlying anxiety state for which the benzodiazepine was originally prescribed. Furthermore, some patients may increase the dose of these drugs over time, particularly if they are taking them for the treatment of insomnia, as tolerance often develops to their sedative effects. However, there is little evidence to suggest that tolerance develops as quickly to the anxiolytic effects of the benzodiazepines and most patients continue to take their medication for years without increasing the dose. The American Psychiatric Association (1990) formed a task force that reviewed these issues and published guidelines for the correct medical use of the benzodiazepines. It recommended intermittent use of these drugs when possible, to reduce the occurrence of tolerance and dependence. Patients with a history of alcohol or drug misuse have an increased risk of developing benzodiazepine misuse and therefore their use in such patients should be avoided.

The benzodiazepines are the most widely used drugs for the management of insomnia, anxiety, muscle spasticity and seizures. About 12% of the adult population in the USA have used such drugs on more than one occasion during the past year for the treatment of insomnia, while approximately 2.4% of adults have taken such drugs continuously for 4 months or longer. Figures from European countries vary, some being higher and some lower than those reported in the USA, but in all cases detailed studies of the prescribing of benzodiazepines show that they are being used appropriately in these countries. Nevertheless, despite this, there has been concern over the dependence potential of these drugs following their therapeutic use, and this has led to restrictions on their use and the recognition of the need to limit administration to less than 6 weeks in most cases.

Opioid analgesics as drugs of misuse

The medical use of opium as a pain-relieving drug dates back to the third century. Arab physicians used extracts of the opium poppy to treat diarrhoea and probably introduced it to the Far East. However, because of its erratic absorption from the gastrointestinal tract, its use as an effective analgesic became possible only with the introduction of the hypodermic syringe, invented in the mid-19th century and in mass production by the mid-20th.

Opium is obtained from the dried juice from the seed capsule of the opium poppy, *Papaver somniferum*. The dried juice contains up to 17% morphine and 4% codeine by weight, as well as other, non-addictive alkaloids that lack analgesic activity, such as noscapine, papaverine and thebaine. Papaveretum is a standardised preparation of opium that is 50% morphine.

The term 'opioid' is used to designate a group of drugs that have opium-like or morphine-like properties. The term 'opiate analgesic' is often used as an alternative. The term 'narcotic analgesic' is now obsolete; it was formerly used to describe potent opiate analgesics that had sedative properties.

The opioids produce their pharmacological effects by interacting with a closely related group of peptide receptors. This suggests that endogenous opioid-like polypeptides exist, which presumably have a physiological function.

In recent years there has been a major research effort, so far without success, to produce potent, centrally acting analgesics that do not have the potential for misuse. The discovery of various types of opioid receptor, which may have different effects on central neurotransmitter function, could lead to the development of such a drug. In the meantime, the most widely used opioids – morphine, heroin (diacetylmorphine) and codeine – are therapeutically effective but are liable to be misused and produce dependence. The structure of some of the morphine-like analgesics and their antagonists is shown in Fig. 13.1.

Substitution of an allyl group on the nitrogen atom of morphine produces drugs that act as antagonists, such substances thereby reversing the analgesia, euphoria and respiratory depressant effects of such agonists as morphine and heroin. The structurally related antagonist naltrexone is frequently used as an antagonist of morphine and related opioid agonists. Other structural analogues of morphine, such as nalorphine, act as partial agonists. When nalorphine, for example, is injected into an animal, it will produce analgesia, but will also counteract such an effect of morphine should this pure agonist be given concurrently. All the opioids exert their pharmacological effects by binding to specific receptors located in the brain and on peripheral organs. The seminal studies of Kosterlitz and Hughes in the 1970s (see Hughes *et al*, 1975) clearly demonstrated the relationship between opioid receptor occupancy and the ability of a drug to inhibit electrically stimulated contractions of the guinea pig ileum *in vitro*.

Later studies showed that the opiates have a high affinity for specific binding sites in the brain and gastrointestinal tract; this affinity is both saturable and stereospecific. However, there does not appear to be a direct relationship between the affinity of an agonist for the central opioid receptors and its analgesic potency. This can be partly explained by the relative lack of accessibility of many opiates to the brain, owing to their low lipophilicity, but other factors, such as the differences in their affinity for the various types of opioid receptors, must also be considered. Ligand-binding studies, subcellular fractionation to determine the location of the receptors at the cellular level, and the application of histochemical and immunocytochemical techniques to map the distribution of the receptors in the brain have now enabled a detailed assessment to be made of their distribution, and possible function, in humans and other mammals.

The highest concentration of opioid receptors appears to be in the sensory, limbic and hypothalamic regions of the brain, with particularly high concentrations being found in the amygdala and the peri-aqueductal grey matter. The importance of receptors in these regions was evaluated by applying morphine to these sites using micro-injection. Injection of morphine into the peri-aqueductal grey matter was found to be associated with analgesia, while retrograde amnesia resulted when the drug was applied to the amygdala, and hyperactivity when it was injected into the basal ganglia. The high density of opioid

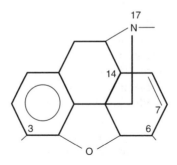

Drug	Chemical groups inserted in positions:		
	3	6	17
Morphine	-OH	-OH	-CH$_3$
Heroin	-OCOCH$_3$	-OCOCH$_3$	-CH$_3$
Levorphanol*	-OH	-H	-CH$_3$
Levallorphan*	-OH	-H	-CH$_2$CH=CH$_2$
Codeine	-OCH$_3$	-OH	-CH$_3$
Hydrocodone**	-OCH$_3$	=O	-CH$_3$
Nalorphine	-OH	-OH	-CHCH=CH$_2$
Naloxone**	-OH	=O	-CHCH=CH$_2$
Naltrexone**	-OH	=O	-CH$_2$-◁
Buprenorphine***	-OH	-OCH$_3$	-CH$_2$-◁
Butorphanol***	-OH	-H	-CH$_2$-◇

* -OH group added to position 14.
** Oxygen bridge missing.
*** Etheno bridge inserted between positions 6 and 14 of rings, plus hydroxy, trimethyl propyl substitution on position 7.

Fig. 13.1   Structure of opiate analgesics and their antagonists (last five listed).

receptors in the spinal cord, particularly the substantia gelatinosa, which is an area that is highly innervated by peripheral type C fibres, accounts for the spinal analgesia that many opiates cause.

Actions of opioids on opioid receptors

The first endogenous ligands for the opioid receptors were isolated by Kosterlitz and Hughes and were found to be the pentapeptides methionine and leucine enkephalin (met- and leu-enkephalin). The structure of these, and related peptides which also act as endogenous ligands for these receptors, are shown in Box 13.1.

Two further families of opioid peptides have since been isolated, namely the endorphins and the dynorphins. Each family of peptides is derived from a distinct precursor polypeptide. These have been identified as:

(1) pro-enkephalin, from which both met- and leu-enkephalin are derived
(2) pro-opiomelanocortin, which gives rise to alpha- and gamma-melanocyte-stimulating hormone (MSH), adrenocorticotrophic hormone (ACTH), beta-lipotropin and met-enkephalin
(3) pro-dynorphin, which produces alpha- and beta-neo-endorphins and leu-enkephalin.

Detailed binding studies in the brain and peripheral tissues have now established that these various opioids interact with different categories of receptors, which have been designated mu, kappa and delta receptors. The synthetic opioid compound N-allylnormetazocine (SKF 10047) has been shown to bind preferentially to another class of receptor, termed the sigma receptor, but it is now recognised that this category of opioid

---

Box 13.1 Structure of some opioid peptides

Leucine enkephalin
Tyr-Gly-Gly-Phe-Leu-OH

Methionine enkephalin
Tyr-Gly-Gly-Phe-Met-OH

Gamma-endorphin
Tyr-Gly-Gly-Phe-Met-Thr-Ser-Glu-Lys-Ser-Gin-Thr-Pro-Leu-Val-Thr-Leu-Phe

Alpha-endorphin
Tyr-Gly-Gly-Phe-Met-Thr-Ser-Glu-Lys-Ser-Gin-Thr-Pro-Leu-Val-Thr

Beta-endorphin
Tyr-Gly-Gly-Phe-Met-Thr-Ser-Glu-Lys-Ser-Gin-Thr-Pro-Leu-Val-Thr-Leu-Phe-Lys-Asn-Ala-Ile-Ile-Lys-Asn-Ala-Tyr-Lys-Lys-Gly-Glu-OH

receptor is not directly associated with the pharmacological activity of the opioid analgesics.

In addition to the opioid peptides that occur in the mammalian brain, it is now evident that morphine, codeine and related benzo-morphans occur naturally, in trace amounts, in the brain, where they exist in a conjugated form, usually bound to brain proteins. The significance of these substances to brain function is unclear.

All opioids produce their effect by activating one or more of the three types of receptors. Thus analgesia involves the activation of the mu receptors that are located mainly at supraspinal sites and kappa receptors in the spinal cord; delta receptors may also be involved but their relative contribution is unclear. Nevertheless, the actions of the opioids on these receptors is complex, as there is evidence that the same substance may act as a full agonist, or as an antagonist at different sites within the brain.

In humans, the changes that result from the activation of different receptors have been inferred from clinical observation and from extrapolation from studies on animals. A summary of the interaction of morphine and a number of synthetic opioids on the three main receptor types is shown in Table 13.1.

To add a further complication to the understanding of ways in which the opioids act, it now appears that the mu receptors may be further subdivided into μ_1 and μ_2 subtypes, the former being high-affinity receptors that mediate supraspinal analgesia, while the latter are of relatively low affinity and are concerned in respiratory depression and in the gastrointestinal effects of the agonists.

Certain benzomorphan analgesics related to pentazocine selectively bind to kappa receptors in the spinal cord, thereby producing analgesia. This analgesia is still present in animals that have been made to tolerate the analgesic effects of morphine, which suggests that there is

Table 13.1 Effects of some opiate agonists and antagonists on opioid receptors in mammalian brain

Opiate agonist or antagonist	Receptor type		
	Mu	Delta	Kappa
Morphine	++	+	+
Butorphanol	−	0	++
Pentazocine	−	0	++
Buprenorphine	+/−	0	−
Naloxone	−	−	−
Nalorphine	−	0	+

Potency of agonist or antagonist shown as + and −, respectively.
0 = inadequate data available; +/− = partial agonist.

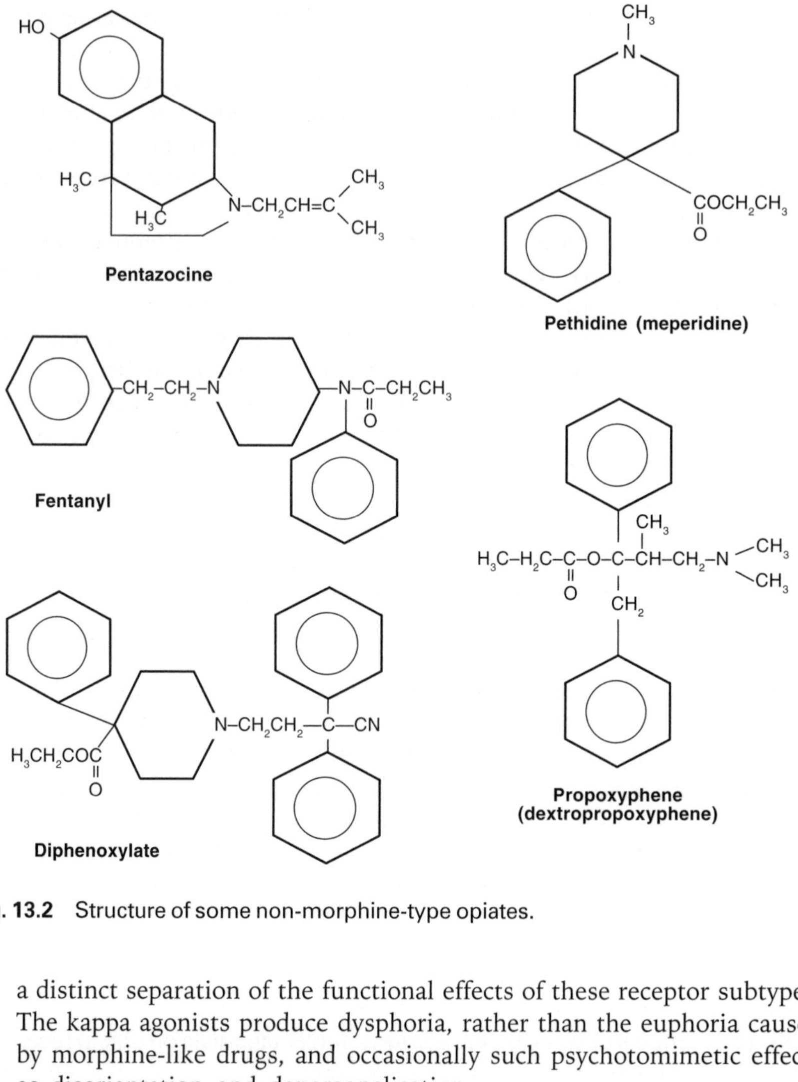

Fig. 13.2 Structure of some non-morphine-type opiates.

a distinct separation of the functional effects of these receptor subtypes. The kappa agonists produce dysphoria, rather than the euphoria caused by morphine-like drugs, and occasionally such psychotomimetic effects as disorientation and depersonalisation.

The precise role of the delta receptors in humans is uncertain, as specific agonists have not yet been developed that cross the blood–brain barrier. The structure of pentazocine and some other opiates is shown in Fig. 13.2.

Mechanism of action

Of all the drugs of misuse, the opiods have had their mechanisms of induced physical dependence most thoroughly studied. There does not appear to be a significant change in the opioid receptor number following chronic drug administration, but there is evidence of a decrease in the functional activity of these receptors, as shown by a decrease in adenylate cyclase activity. This action is mediated by the inhibitory guanine nucleotide binding regulatory protein (Gi). Following abrupt withdrawal of the opioid, the cyclase activity returns to normal. This may be the explanation for the excessive sympathetic activity associated with the abrupt withdrawal of these drugs, particularly as some opiate receptors are located in the locus ceruleus. This relationship between the opioid and adrenergic system in the brain may help to explain why the α_2-adrenoceptor agonist clonidine can attenuate some of the symptoms of opiate withdrawal. Nevertheless, the fact that opiates act on at least two different types of opioid receptors in the brain, the mu and delta receptors, which are widely distributed in the central and peripheral nervous systems, means that the pharmacological effects of these drugs, and the symptoms seen on withdrawal, cannot be entirely ascribed to changes in central noradrenergic transmission.

The mechanism of action of the opioids at their receptor sites is complex and incompletely understood. However, they all share a number of characteristics. Thus they all facilitate inhibitory transmission in the brain and gastrointestinal tract, and appear to be located on presynaptic receptor sites, where they function as heteroreceptors. Furthermore, they all appear to be coupled to guanine nucleotide binding regulatory proteins (G-proteins), and thereby regulate the transmembrane signalling systems. In this way, the opioid receptors can regulate adenylate cyclase, the phosphatidyl inositol system, ion channels, and so on. There is evidence that the mu and delta receptors appear to operate via potassium channels and the adenylate cyclase system, while kappa receptors inhibit voltage-dependent calcium channels.

Pharmacological properties

Drugs in this therapeutic group include morphine, heroine, pethidine, methadone, codeine, dihydrocodeine, dextropropoxyphene, pentazocine, phenazocine, levorphanol and buprenorphine. The principal antagonists in clinical use are naloxone and naltrexone.

All agonists in this therapeutic group decrease the sensation of painful stimuli, which is their main clinical application. They tend to subdue dull, persistent pain rather than sharp pain, but this difference is to some extent dose dependent. The major difference between the non-opioid analgesics such as aspirin and the opiates is that the former reduce the perception of peripherally mediated pain, by reducing the synthesis of local hormones that activate the pain fibres, whereas the latter attenuate the affective reaction to pain without affecting the perception of pain. This clearly suggests that the site of action of the opiate analgesics is in the central nervous system.

503

Euphoria is a common side-effect of most opiates after chronic use, and undoubtedly this effect contributes to their dependence-producing tendency. This may play an important part in modifying the response of the patient to chronic pain. Many opiates also produce sedation, particularly after acute administration.

The opiates reduce anxiety, possibly through their sedative effects, and induce nausea and vomiting. These effects are more marked after acute administration. The emetic effect is due to their stimulant effects on the chemoreceptor trigger zone in the area postrema on the floor of the fourth ventricle, an effect that has been ascribed to an activation of dopamine receptors. The emetic effect is particularly pronounced in the case of the non-analgesic analogue of morphine, apomorphine, which has been used experimentally in the treatment of parkinsonism and to induce emesis following a drug overdose.

The opiates cause constipation by inducing spasm of the stomach and intestines, presumably by the stimulation of opioid receptors in the myenteric plexus and reducing the release of acetylcholine. This property can be used therapeutically for the symptomatic relief of diarrhoea. Biliary colic and severe epigastric pain can occur because of the contraction of the sphincter of Oddi and the resulting increase in pressure in the biliary ducts.

One of the serious complications of the use of the opiate analgesics, even at therapeutic doses, is respiratory depression, an effect that is further complicated by the ability of these drugs to decrease the sensitivity of the respiratory centre to carbon dioxide. The administration of oxygen to a patient whose respiration has been depressed by the opiates is therefore counterproductive and may lead to total respiratory paralysis.

Many opiate analgesics are effective cough suppressants (also called anti-tussives), although only codeine and dihydrocodeine are generally used for this purpose. As there is a dissociation between the anti-tussive and analgesic action of the opiates, dextromethorphan and noscapine are now commonly used as cough suppressants because of their efficacy and lack of dependence-producing properties.

Miosis is a characteristic symptom of opiate administration, and while tolerance develops to many of the pharmacological effects of this class of drug, tolerance to the miotic effects occurs at a much slower rate. Miosis is due to an excitatory action of the autonomic segment of the nucleus of the oculomotor nerve, an effect attributed to the stimulation of the mu receptors. In general, it would appear that the actions of morphine and its analogues on the brain, spinal cord and gastrointestinal tract are due to stimulation of the mu receptors.

Tolerance and dependence

An acute dose of 100–200 mg morphine, or its equivalent, in the non-tolerant adult can lead to respiratory depression, coma and death.

In the tolerant individual, single doses of more than ten times this amount are tolerated and have little visible effect. The development of tolerance to the opiates does not appear to be due to enhanced metabolism (metabolic tolerance) but is probably due to opioid receptor insensitivity (tissue tolerance). A dependent person therefore ultimately requires high doses of the opiate to prevent withdrawal effects.

Cross-tolerance occurs between all opiates that act primarily via the mu receptors. This is the basis of methadone substitution therapy, which is commonly used to withdraw people who are dependent on heroin or morphine; methadone is used because of its relatively long half-life (about 12 hours) and its ease of administration in an oral form. Cross-tolerance does not occur between the opiates and other classes of dependence-producing drugs, such as the barbiturates, alcohol or the amphetamines, that act through different mechanisms.

A sudden reduction in plasma opiate levels, or the administration of an opiate antagonist such as naloxone, leads to withdrawal symptoms. These include restlessness, craving, lacrimation, perspiration, fever, chills, vomiting, joint pain, piloerection and mydriasis. These effects are maximal 2–3 days after the abrupt withdrawal of heroin, morphine or related drugs, but are slower in onset and less severe in the case of drugs like methadone, which have a longer half-life and whose tissue concentration therefore decreases more slowly.

Endogenous opioids and the pain response

It has long been known that stress can elevate the pain threshold. In rodents this may be quantified by measuring the increase in the pain threshold following prolonged unavoidable foot shock. Under conditions of environmental stress, the pain threshold has also been shown to increase in humans. Such effects have been attributed to a rise in opioid peptides in the cerebrospinal fluid (CSF). Conversely, in chronic pain syndromes, the CSF concentration of the endorphins decreases.

Although the physiological basis of acupuncture is incompletely understood, it is now apparent that the endogenous opioid systems are activated by such techniques. Furthermore, when acupuncture is simulated in animals there is a decrease in the pain response to noxious peripheral stimuli, which can be reversed by naloxone.

From such studies, it may be concluded that physical stress leads to an activation of endogenous opioid systems, which raises the pain threshold. The euphoriant effect of physical exercise may also be attributed to the effects of these opioids acting on limbic regions of the brain.

The discovery that the opioid peptides cause analgesia and have anti-tussive and antidiarrhoeal effects led to the widespread search for synthetic peptides that could be administered orally but that would not have the dependence-producing effects of morphine and related drugs. Synthetic peptides modelled on the endogenous opioids have been synthesised that have longer half-lives than the endogenous substance and that are resistant to the enkephalinases, which rapidly degrade the endogenous opioids. Unfortunately, to date, all of the experimental and clinical studies have been disappointing, as it has been found that morphine-dependent animals show cross-tolerance with all such compounds.

The endogenous opioid peptides have a range of affinities for the different types of opioid receptor. Some met-enkephalin derivatives, for example, show affinity for mu and delta receptors, whereas other peptides, derived from pro-enkephalin, show a preference for the delta sites. All peptides from prodynorphin act predominantly on kappa sites, while beta-endorphin behaves like the enkephalins and shows selectivity for the mu and delta sites.

Perhaps it may be possible to use this diversity and selectivity of action to develop new synthetic opiates that will have therapeutic advantages over morphine and its analogues, which, in one form or another, have been used for nearly 2000 years.

Nicotine as a drug of misuse

Nicotine is an alkaloid derived from the leaves of *Nicotiana* species. Tabacco originated in South America, where it has been smoked by the native population for hundreds of years. It was introduced into Western Europe in the 16th century, but shortly after its introduction into Great Britain it was condemned as a habit 'injurious to the lung' by King James I.

Nicotine has both stimulant and depressant actions on the brain. The stimulant and rewarding action is attributed to the action of the drug on the nicotinic cholinergic receptors that indirectly increase the release of dopamine from the nucleus accumbens reward system; an increase in dopamine release has been detected in this brain region following the administration of the drug to rats. This action is a common property of most drugs of misuse and has already been covered in detail at the beginning of this chapter. In addition, nicotine indirectly increases the release of endogenous opioids and glucocorticoids, which adds to the complexity of action of the drug.

Because nicotine provides the reinforcement for the smoking of cigarettes in particular, it is arguably the most influential dependence-producing drug. The dependence, both psychological and to a lesser extent physical, is extremely durable, as is exemplified by the failure rate among smokers who try to stop the habit. For example, it has been calculated that although over 80% of smokers wish to stop the habit, only 35% succeed each year. It has been estimated that dependence can occur in individuals who smoke more than five cigarettes per day; most smokers consume about 20 cigarettes per day.

Nicotine is readily absorbed through the skin, mucous membranes and lungs but smoking is the preferred route because of the rapid absorption of the drug across the mucosa of the lung, which produces an effect on the brain within about 7 seconds. Thus each puff of a cigarette produces a discrete reinforcement and it has been calculated that with an average of 10 puffs per cigarette, 20 cigarettes per day will reinforce the habit 200 times daily. In dependent smokers, there is evidence that the urge to smoke correlates with a low blood nicotine concentration and it has been concluded that those who are dependent smoke not only in order to obtain the reinforcing effect of the drug but also to avoid the symptoms of nicotine withdrawal. These withdrawal symptoms include irritability, impatience, hostility, anxiety, dysphoria, difficulty concentrating, restlessness, bradycardia, increased appetite and weight gain.

Smokers who have been abstinent for several weeks, or those who smoke for the first time, often experience nausea after smoking a cigarette, even at low blood nicotine concentrations. This aversive effect is due to the action of the drug on the chemoreceptor trigger zone, whereby it indirectly activates the release of dopamine. Apomorphine and related dopamine agonists also cause nausea by activating the dopaminergic system in this brain region.

The nicotine withdrawal syndrome can be alleviated by nicotine replacement therapy. Several forms of nicotine replacement products are widely available. These are nicotine gum, transdermally delivered nicotine (nicotine patch) and nasal nicotine spray. Both the nicotine gum and the patch have shown efficacy in increasing short-term abstinence rates, reducing the symptoms of nicotine withdrawal and relieving the craving for cigarettes. Nasal nicotine spray appears to be efficacious in sustaining abstinence from smoking and has the advantage over the other nicotine formulations in that the venous pharmacokinetic profile of nicotine administration closely follows that of smoking a cigarette. Unlike the patch or gum, nicotine spray can cause nasal and throat irritation.

Of the more recently introduced methods for smoking cessation, buproprion (an antidepressant with dopaminomimetic properties) has recently been introduced. Clinical trial data, in which the nicotine patch, buproprion at 300 mg, and a combination of the two drugs were compared with placebo treatment, have shown cessation of smoking rates of 36% for the patch, 49% for buproprion and 58% for the combined treatments after 7 weeks of treatment. The placebo response rate was 23%. All subjects received relapse prevention therapy.

Thus buproprion appears to be a reasonably safe and effective treatment for nicotine dependence. It is, however, contraindicated in those subject to epilepsy. Its main side-effects are dry mouth and insomnia.

The psychostimulants: cocaine and the amphetamines

Cocaine is a major alkaloidal component from the Andean bush *Erythroxylum coca*. Leaves of this plant are chewed by Andean Indians to decrease the feeling of hunger and fatigue; there is little evidence that dependence is caused by this means of administration.

A major health problem arises, however, when cocaine is used in industrialised countries. Thus, in the USA, over 20 million people are estimated to use the drug, by nasal administration ('snorting'), injection of the salts, or smoking the free alkaloid ('crack').

The subjective effects of all the psychostimulants depend on personality, the environment in which it is administered, the dose of the drug and the route of administration. For example, moderate doses of D-amphetamine (10–20 mg) in a normal person will produce euphoria, a sense of increased energy and alertness, anorexia, insomnia and an improvement in the conduct of repetitive tasks. Some people become anxious, irritable and talkative. As the dose of amphetamine is increased, the symptoms become more marked and the influence of the environment less pronounced.

Most psychostimulants produce qualitatively similar effects, and include such drugs as methylamphetamine, phenmetrazine, methyl-phenidate and diethylproprion. The shrub khat, from Yemen and other Middle Eastern countries, contains the stimulant (–)cathinone, which has properties similar to those of the synthetic psychostimulants.

The main difference between cocaine and the amphetamine-like drugs lies in its shorter duration of action, the half-life for cocaine being about 50 minutes, while that of amphetamine is 10 hours.

Because of its widespread misuse, particularly in the USA, detailed studies have recently been undertaken on the pattern of misuse of cocaine. Some 20% of those experimenting with the drug go on to become regular users (i.e. psychologically dependent). Once dependent, the individual may administer the drug as frequently as every 15 minutes for up to 12 hours at a time. The initial positive social effects, such as increased energy and motivation, eventually give rise to the individual becoming asocial and preoccupied with the drug-induced euphoria. Severe psychological and social impairment finally intervenes. The consequence of long-term misuse is unclear, but it does seem that people taking cocaine by the intranasal route may recover without progressing to other forms of drug misuse.

Mechanisms of action

The reinforcing (i.e. dependence-producing) effects of cocaine are thought to result from its ability to inhibit the reuptake of dopamine into the storage vesicles and transporter, and thereby to increase dopaminergic activity, particularly in the ventral tegmental area and the nucleus accumbens, so enhancing the activity of the dopaminergic system in the mesolimbic area (the reward region) of the brain.

By contrast, the stimulant amphetamines, such as D-amphetamine and methylamphetamine, release dopamine from most brain regions. These drugs also inhibit the reuptake of all biogenic amines, but the effects on the noradrenergic and serotonergic systems do not appear to be directly associated with the dependence potential of the drugs.

Fenfluramine is an amphetamine that selectively stimulates the release of serotonin; it lacks dependence and stimulant properties. This drug is used as an anorexiant, a property that it shares with the stimulant amphetamines.

The structure of some of these stimulants is shown in Fig. 13.3.

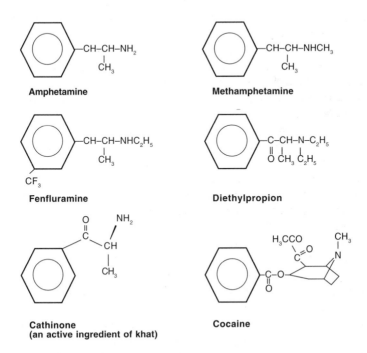

Amphetamine

Methamphetamine

Fenfluramine

Diethylpropion

Cathinone
(an active ingredient of khat)

Cocaine

Fig. 13.3 Chemical structure of some centrally acting stimulants.

Toxicity

Cocaine

The most serious toxic effects of cocaine involve changes in the cardiovascular system. These include cardiac arrhythmias, myocardial ischaemia and infarction, and cerebrovascular spasm, all of which can be largely explained by the facilitation of the action of catecholamines on the cardiovascular system. Another explanation of the cardiotoxicity of cocaine lies in the direct vasconstrictive properties of its major metabolite, norcocaine. It seems likely that the vasconstrictor effects of cocaine are due to a reduction in sodium flux across the cardiac cell wall, as all local anaesthetics block sodium channels but only cocaine causes vasoconstriction. It has been estimated that about 20% of those dying of cocaine overdose show myocarditis at autopsy. Nevertheless, it has also been established that cocaine increases the release of adrenal catecholamines (adrenaline and noradrenaline) and sensitises the cardiac adrenoceptors to their action.

Seizures, possibly due to the local anaesthetic effects of the drug at toxic doses, can occur, particularly in those predisposed to epilepsy. Although such toxic and often fatal effects occur more frequently after intravenous and inhalational administration, nasal administration has also been reported to result in such toxicity, even in young, apparently healthy people.

There is a poor correlation between the euphoriant effects of cocaine and its cardiotoxicity, so that someone who uses the euphoriant effects of the drug to regulate the dose may be unaware of the cardiovascular toxicity. Thus one of the main reasons why the cocaine user may die suddenly is the differential psychological and cardiovascular tolerance. Tolerance develops more rapidly in the brain than the heart, and therefore a slight overdose with the drug can lead to heart failure.

Anxiety and panic attacks may be associated with high doses of cocaine. These effects may be associated with paranoid ideation, visual and tactile hallucinations (called formication) and visual pseudo-hallucinations (seeing snow lights). Ideas of reference, characteristic of stimulant psychosis, also occur.

Similar effects have been reported after misuse of the amphetamines, which, in addition, may be associated with increasing stereotyped behaviour and a full psychotic episode (auditory, visual and tactile hallucinations often unassociated with cardiovascular symptoms) which may be difficult to differentiate from paranoid schizophrenia. This is the basis for using amphetamine as a model for schizophrenia, in both animals and human volunteers. The central effects of high doses of cocaine and the amphetamines may be suppressed by the administration of antipsychotics.

Amphetamines

The toxicity following the administration of high doses of amphetamines arises as a consequence of the release of catecholamines from peripheral and central sympathetic neurons, combined with their reduced metabolism owing to the reduction in their reuptake. The cardiotoxicity is similar to that described for cocaine, in which sympathetic drive to the heart is increased. There is now evidence that high, chronic doses of the amphetamines can cause a degeneration of dopaminergic neurons, possibly because of the formation of an endogenous neurotoxin, 6-hydroxydopamine.

The amphetamines are weak inhibitors of MAO-B, and this may limit the oxidative deamination of 6-hydroxydopamine and thereby lead to its accumulation.

The pronounced anhedonia sometimes seen after chronic amphetamine misuse may be ascribed to a degeneration of dopaminergic neurons in the mesolimbic region of the brain.

Acute intoxication with amphetamine is associated with tremor, confusion, irritability, hallucinations and paranoid behaviour, hypertension, sweating and occasionally cardiac arrhythmias; convulsions and death may occur. The cardiovascular effects of the stimulants may be treated by beta-blockers, or by the combined alpha- and beta-blocker labetalol; calcium-channel antagonists such as nifedipine may correct the arrhythmias, while intravenous diazepam is of value in attenuating seizures.

Tolerance

Tolerance develops to only some of the effects of cocaine, for example the euphoric 'rush' following intravenous administration and some of the cardiovascular effects, but the degree of tolerance is limited. However, most long-term users do require increasing amounts of the drug to produce the same subjective effects to those experienced initially when taking the drug.

Amphetamine users also develop a tolerance to some of the central effects, such as the euphoria and anorexia, which may lead to the escalation of the dose; this may be partly ascribed to enhanced excretion of the drug. Cross-tolerance occurs between the psychostimulants.

Reverse tolerance, or sensitisation, can occur with all the psychostimulants, and may be partly related to enhanced mesolimbic forebrain dopaminergic function. Such increased sensitivity to the effects of these drugs need not depend on the drugs being given daily. The stereotyped behaviour seen in amphetamine misusers may be attributed to the increased activity of the striatal dopaminergic system.

Kindling may account for the lowered seizure threshold following chronic cocaine misuse. This phenomenon has been described elsewhere (e.g. in the use of carbamazepine in the treatment of mania), and occurs when small, subconvulsive doses eventually give rise to spontaneous seizures.

The withdrawal effects that follow the abrupt termination of the administration of psychostimulants comprise depression, anxiety and craving, followed by a general fatigue and disturbed sleep pattern. Hyperphagia and anhedonia are common. In general, the mood returns to normal after several days. There are no grossly observable signs of physical dependence following prolonged psychostimulant misuse. In the USA, desipramine has been found to be beneficial in treating the withdrawal effects from cocaine (so-called 'cocaine crash'). The precise mechanism whereby this tricyclic antidepressant produces such an antagonistic effect is uncertain.

The misuse potential of 'designer' drugs

The term 'designer drug' was first used in the USA to describe a synthetic opioid analogue that was sold to heroin addicts in California in 1980 as a very potent form of heroin (called 'China white', and reputed to be 200 times more potent than morphine). Subsequently the compound was identified as alpha-methyl fentanyl, an analogue of the dissociative analgesic fentanyl. It has been estimated that this compound has caused several hundred deaths through overdose in California alone, the main danger being the narrow margin between the dose producing euphoria and that leading to respiratory depression. People using these fentanyl derivatives show all the features of opiate misuse.

Another synthetic heroin-like compound, sold to heroin-dependent individuals in California in 1982 as 'new heroin', was soon recognised to cause severe Parkinsonian symptoms in young people. Eventually it was discovered that 'new heroin' contained pethidine together with an N-methyl-phenyl-tetrahydropyridine (MPTP) contaminant. It is now established that MPTP is converted to a neurotoxic metabolite, MPP$^+$, by the action of MAO-B in the substantia nigra, where it acts as a neurotoxin and destroys the dopamine cell bodies. MPTP thus acts as a pro-toxin. Its neurotoxicity can be prevented by inhibiting the action of MAO-B by deprenyl, for example, or by the administration of mazindol, which inhibits the dopamine carrier mechanism whereby MPP$^+$ is transported into the dopaminergic neurons. Should MPP$^+$ enter the dopaminergic neurons, irreversible parkinsonism occurs, although it is amenable to treatment with L-dopa. Treatment of rodents and monkeys with MPTP is now used to produce a model of the disease.

The health authorities in many countries are concerned about the widespread use of MDMA ('ecstasy') as a recreational drug. This has reflected the increase in reports in both the medical and popular press of MDMA-related fatalities and severe adverse effects. MDMA is structurally related to methylenedioxyamphetamine (MDA), known among recreational drug users as 'Eve'. Both drugs cause euphoria and are drugs of misuse that are similar to methamphetamine. The acute effects of these drugs in volunteers who have had previous experience of MDMA include symptoms commonly seen after use of stimulants, for example tachycardia, hypertension, dry mouth, mood evaluation and a subjective sense of increased energy. Impaired judgement has also frequently been noticed. Other psychiatric symptoms that have been reported in weekend users of MDMA include a significantly reduced mood during the week following the use of the drug and an impairment of memory, which may reflect the temporary depletion of brain serotonin. Reduced non-rapid-eye-movement sleep and a disturbed sleep pattern have also been described in these users.

In a study of individuals with a history of MDMA misuse, positron emission tomography has shown that there was a decreased global and regional binding of a specific ligand for the serotonin transporter, which suggests that, in humans as in primates and rodents, regular use of MDMA is neurotoxic to serotonergic neurons. The mechanism of this neurotoxicity is unclear but there is experimental evidence to suggest that free radicals, produced by the oxidation of metabolites of MDMA, are implicated. In contrast to these chronic effects of MDMA, the acute effects include both the sympathomimetic effects and those symptoms, such as hyperthermia, hyper-reflexia and myoclonus, which are attributed to the enhanced release of serotonin. Both the acute and chronic effects of MDMA seen in rodents and primates occur at doses commonly taken by recreational drug users (75–150 mg).

The misuse of both MDMA and MDA has been associated with panic disorder, depression and chronic paranoid psychosis. As these conditions may also occur independently of these drugs, it is difficult to prove causality, but it seems reasonable to conclude that some individuals are more vulnerable to such psychiatric disorders, which are exacerbated by these drugs. In addition to the neurological and psychiatric effects that are elicited by these amphetamines, recent evidence suggests that some aspects of cellular immunity are suppressed for several hours after even a single dose of MDMA. At present it is unclear what impact this might have, particularly after regular recreational use, on the resistance of the immune system to infections, but clearly these drugs have effects which far exceed those anticipated from the pharmacology of amphetamine.

In conclusion, recent evidence suggests that MDMA and related compounds do not deserve the widespread belief that they are harmless substances. They present a potentially serious risk of acute toxic reactions that cannot be predicted from the dose taken. The acute

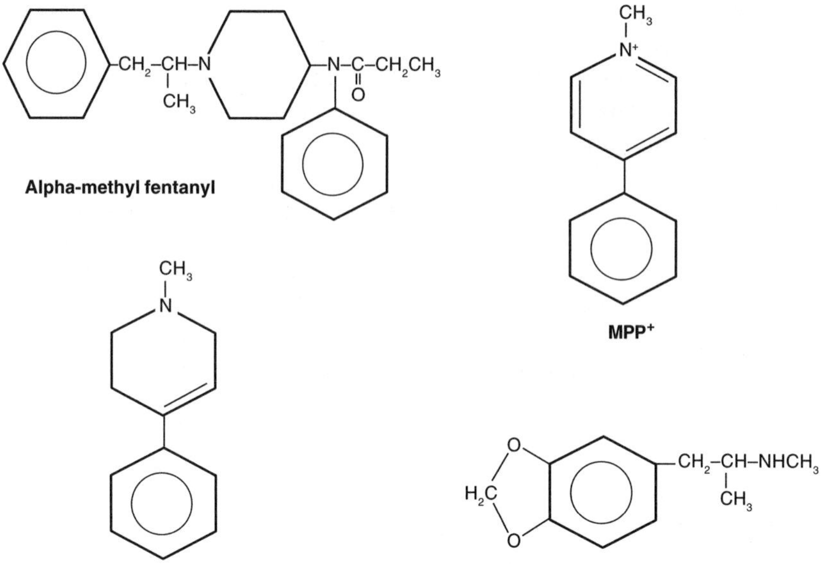

Fig. 13.4 Structure of some 'designer drugs' of misuse. Compare the structure of alpha-methyl fentanyl with that of fentanyl and MMP⁺ with that of pethidine (Fig. 13.2) and ecstasy with that of methamphetamine (Fig. 13.3).

reactions carry with them significant mortality and morbidity, while the neurotoxicity shown to occur in rodents, primates and now in humans suggests that they have a potential to cause permanent brain damage.

The structures of some of these 'designer drugs' are shown in Fig. 13.4. Their relationship to the amphetamines and opiates is apparent (see Figs 13.2 and 13.3).

Hallucinogens

Clinical effects

Many different classes of drugs can produce hallucinations when given in toxic doses (e.g. the anticholinergics, such as atropine and scopolamine), but such symptoms are generally associated with confusion and lack of sensory clarity. As such, hallucinations are a component of a toxic psychosis.

True hallucinogens, also called psychedelics or psychotomimetics, produce their effects without causing changes in levels of consciousness. Such effects are usually associated with a heightened sensory awareness

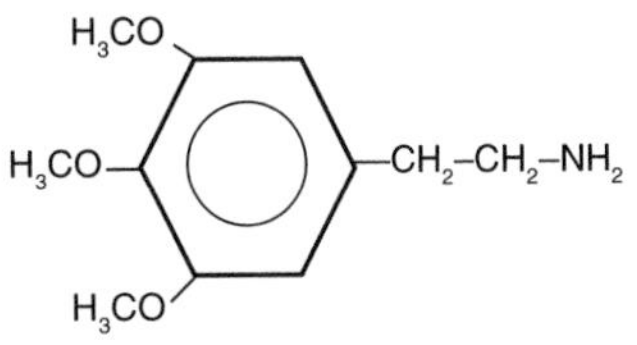

Mescaline*

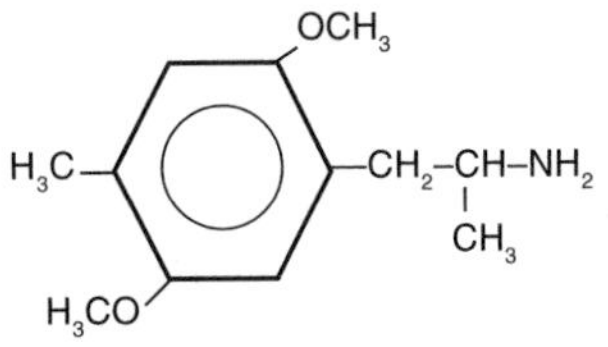

Dimethoxymethamphetamine (DOM, 'STP')

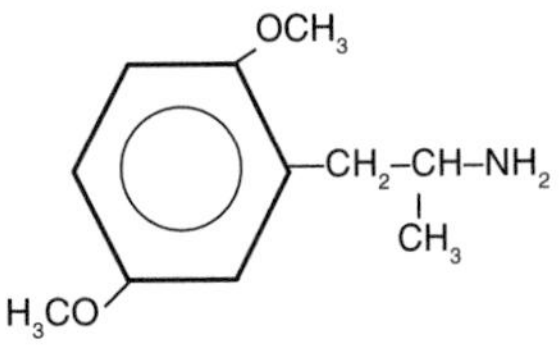

Dimethoxyamphetamine

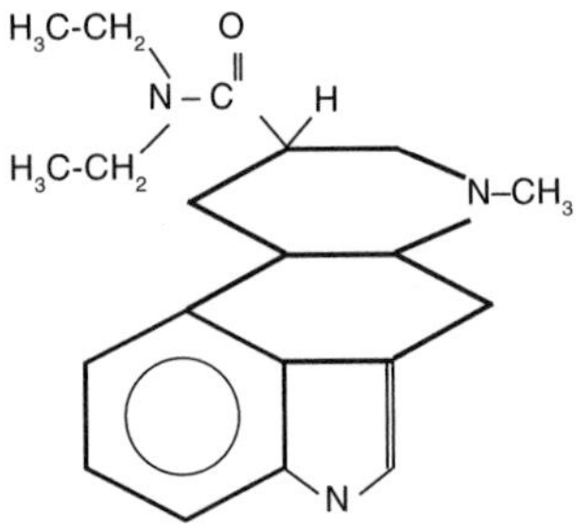

Lysergic acid diethylamide (LSD)

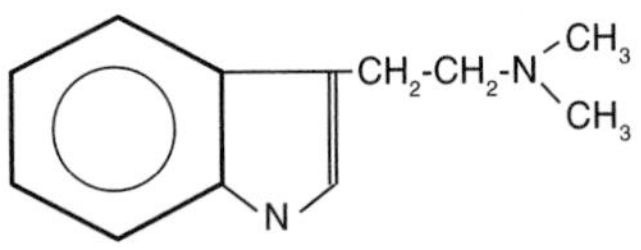

Dimethylamphetamine* (DMT)

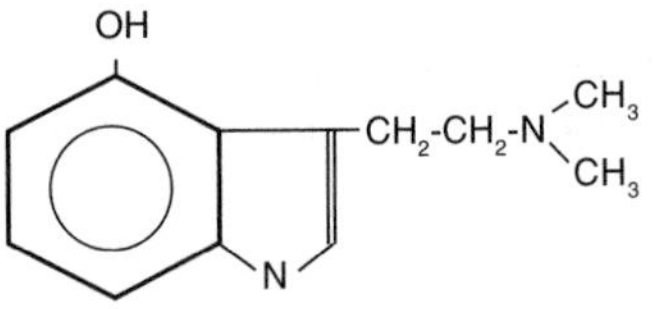

Psilocin*

Fig. 13.5 Structure of some naturally occurring (*) and synthetic hallucinogens.

but a diminished control of the incoming sensory impressions. Thus the individual frequently finds it impossible to differentiate between one sensory impression and another, which can lead to a feeling of being 'in union with mankind or the universe', a chemically induced equivalent of a religious experience (Falk & Feingold, 1987).

The drugs usually included among the hallucinogens are of the indolealkylamine type (such as lysergic acid diethylamide, LSD), the phenylethylamine (mescaline-like) type and the phenylisopropranolamine (amphetamine-like) type. Fig. 13.5 shows the structure of some of the more common hallucinogens.

Another method of classification is based on such criteria as a drug's subjective effects, the neurophysiological changes that it produces, and its ability to cause cross-tolerance with members of the same or a different chemical series. This has led to classification into the following:

(1) LSD-like drugs (e.g. LSD, psilocybin and psilocin)
(2) dimethoxyamphetamine (DMA), dimethoxymethylamphetamine (DOM), dimethyltryptamine (DMT) and related drugs
(3) drugs that lack the effects of LSD but which are hallucinogenic, such as the cannabinoids (e.g. delta-9-tetrahydrocannabinol from cannabis), bufotenin and phencyclidine.

The drug LSD was discovered accidentally by the Swiss chemist Hoffman in 1943 while he was trying to prepare oxytocin derivatives related to the ergot alkaloids. The profound visual hallucinations which LSD produces suggested that an understanding of the mechanism of action of such drugs may give some insight into the basis of psychotic disorders. Although drugs like LSD have had no lasting clinical application, they have been used illicitly for over three decades. However, while the illicit use of LSD has declined, particularly in the USA, in the UK its use seems to fluctuate with the dominant youth culture.

Mechanisms of action

Research into the action of the hallucinogens has largely concentrated on the serotonergic system, following the seminal hypothesis of Woolley & Shaw (1954) that LSD blocks serotonin receptors in the brain. It was subsequently found that the firing rate of dorsal Raphe neurons was specifically attenuated by low doses of LSD applied systemically or micro-iontophoretically. It is now known that such drugs stimulate the presynaptic serotonin receptors, thereby inhibiting the firing of the Raphe neurons; similar effects can be produced by applying serotonin. The net result is a decreased activity of serotonin terminals in the forebrain.

It would appear that the hallucinogens produce their effects by activating 5-HT_2-type receptors, effects that can be selectively blocked by the specific antagonist ritanserin. Most hallucinogens can also affect the activity of the locus ceruleus, again via the 5-HT_2 receptors located on the noradrenergic cell bodies. These receptors are linked to the phosphatidyl inositol second messenger system, and it has been observed that drugs like LSD have an effect on this system more like a partial than a full agonist. The rapid development of tolerance to the hallucinogenic effects of LSD-like drugs has been related to the rapid desensitisation of these receptors.

Pharmacological effects

Doses of 20–50 µg LSD in the normal adult can have pronounced effects on the brain but negligible changes in peripheral organs. Higher doses produce such peripheral sympathomimetic effects as pupillary dilatation, tachycardia, hypertension, hyper-reflexia, tremor, nausea, pilo-erection and hyperthermia. With slightly higher doses, the euphoriant effects tend to predominate initially, closely followed by visual hallucinations and peripheral changes after 2–3 hours; auditory hallucinations are rare.

The term 'synaesthesia' refers the phenomenon whereby sensory modalities overlap, so that music is 'seen' and colours 'heard'. This loss of sensory boundaries can be highly disturbing, and can lead to severe anxiety and even panic. At this stage, mood is often labile. After 4–5 hours, should the effects of a 'bad trip' not occur, the individual may become detached in thinking and behaviour. Doses of LSD in the range 1–16 μg/kg are associated with an accentuation of all these effects, which may last for 12 hours; the half-life of the drug is 3 hours. There is no evidence of long-term personality changes.

The pattern of effects of other hallucinogens is somewhat similar to that of LSD, but most of these drugs are less potent and often must be inhaled or injected because of their poor oral absorption. With the hallucinogenic amphetamines, such as DOM, low doses produce mild euphoria with hallucinations and enhanced self-awareness, while higher doses have LSD-like effects. These changes can be effectively blocked by selective serotonin antagonists, which suggests that all hallucinogens act via a common serotonergic pathway.

Tolerance and dependence

Tolerance to the effects of LSD can occur after only three or four daily doses, presumably because of desensitisation of the $5-HT_2$ receptors; the cardiovascular system shows a much slower development of tolerance.

Cross-tolerance occurs between LSD, mescaline and psilocybin, but not between this group and the amphetamine type of hallucinogens. This suggests that the latter must produce their effects by acting on other transmitter processes in addition to the serotonin system.

Unlike other drugs of misuse, the hallucinogens do not produce a pattern of regular use and they appear to be confined to occasional use. Abrupt withdrawal is not associated with any noticeable physical or psychological effects. The primary adverse effect of these drugs (a 'bad trip') is associated with severe anxiety and panic, which usually respond to anxiolytics. A recurrence of hallucinations when the user is not taking the drug, termed a 'flash-back', can occur in about 15% of former hallucinogen users. It is often precipitated by anxiety and may occur several years after the last administration of a hallucinogen.

In some people, the use of hallucinogens can precipitate a severe psychiatric disorder, such as depression or a schizophrenia-like psychosis.

Phencyclidine and related compounds

Phencyclidine (PCP) was first developed as a dissociative anaesthetic in the 1950s, but its use was mainly confined to veterinary anaesthesia after it had been established that it caused delirium and hallucinations in patients undergoing anaesthesia. However, a closely related congener, ketamine, is still used clinically, especially in children, as a dissociative anaesthetic, as such psychotomimetic effects are minimal. Both drugs produce intense analgesia, amnesia and finally anaesthesia after intravenous administration. Recovery from ketamine-induced anaesthesia is nevertheless often accompanied by nightmares and occasionally hallucinations, and many patients also experience delirium and excitement.

Phencyclidine has been an illicit drug of misuse for some 30 years, with the street names of 'PCP', 'angel dust' and 'crystal'.

The structure of phencyclidine and ketamine is shown in Fig. 13.6.

Both PCP and ketamine are arylcyclohexylamines with stimulant, depressant, hallucinogenic and analgesic properties. In humans, small doses produce signs of intoxication, as shown by staggering gait, slurred speech and nystagmus. Higher doses also cause sweating, a catatonic rigidity and disorientation; drowsiness and apathy may also be apparent. Such a state is sometimes accompanied by physical aggression. As such drugs are potent amnestic agents, the individual may be unaware of having performed violent acts on recovering from the effects of the drug. Increasing doses lead to anaesthesia and eventually coma. Heart rate and blood pressure are elevated and the individual shows hypersalivation, fever and muscular rigidity. Convulsions may

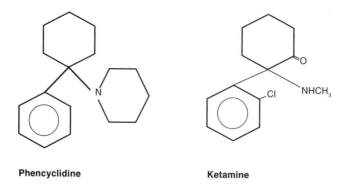

Phencyclidine   **Ketamine**

Fig. 13.6 Structure of the psychotomimetic compound phencyclidine and the structurally related dissociative anaesthetic ketamine.

occur at high doses. The effects of a single dose may last 4–6 hours; perceptual disturbances, disorientation and intense anxiety commonly occur.

Mode of action

Both PCP and ketamine bind with high affinity to a number of receptors in the brain, but it is now accepted that the primary target is the sigma PCP receptor site in the ion channel of the NMDA excitatory amino acid receptor complex. The precise function of this receptor in the brain is still the subject of debate. (It is now known that there are two distinct sigma receptor sites in the mammalian brain, σ_1 and σ_2, that are *not* associated with the NMDA receptor complex; haloperidol and the atypical antipsychotic remoxipride bind with high affinity to such sites, and it has been postulated that some typical and atypical antipsychotics may owe some of their pharmacological effects to their action on these receptors.)

Considerable attention is now being paid to the way in which PCP and ketamine block the ion channel controlled by the NMDA receptor. This prevents the movement of calcium ions in particular into the cell, which in the case of the NMDA receptors situated in the hippocampus inhibits long-term potentiation and thereby blocks memory formation. These drugs can also exhibit a neuroprotective effect against nerve cell damage arising from cerebral hypoxia. Such an action is of potential importance in the future development of drugs to prevent brain damage that arises as a consequence of stroke.

The pronounced effects of PCP on locomotor activity in both animals and humans, and the psychotomimetic effects in humans, may be a consequence of its facilitatory effects on dopaminergic transmission, particularly in mesolimbic regions of the brain. This is unlikely to be a direct effect of the drug on dopamine receptors, but is probably due to its action on NMDA heteroceptors on dopaminergic terminals in these brain regions.

After chronic use, the drug appears to have an extended half-life, of up to 3 days. This is due to the extensive enterohepatic circulation combined with the increased concentration of its metabolites, some of which are pharmacologically active.

Tolerance and dependence

Tolerance to the effects of PCP develops in both animals and humans. A slight physical dependence has been reported in humans, characterised by a craving for the drug, persistent amnesia, slurred speech and difficulty in thinking, which may last up to 1 year after discontinuation of the drug. Severe personality changes have also been reported.

Cannabis and the cannabinoids

Principal sources

The hemp plant, *Cannabis sativa*, has been used commercially as a source of hemp for the manufacture of rope, sacking and so on for well over 2000 years. The hemp seeds have been used as a source of oil, as an animal feed and for a form of soap, while the leaves were first used in China for the psychoactive ingredients they contain. From China, the use of hemp spread first to India and then to Europe via the Middle East in the 16th century.

All parts of the hemp plant contain psychoactive substances; some 60 active ingredients, the cannabinoids, have been isolated from the plant to date. In addition, over 300 non-cannabinoid compounds have been identified, which do not appear to contribute to the psychoactive properties of the plant. The highest cannabinoid concentrations are found in the flower heads.

There are three main types of cannabis preparation in use. *Herbal cannabis*, known as variously as 'grass', 'pot', 'joint' or 'marijuana' and so on, is prepared by collecting the flower heads or the upper leaves of the plant, allowing them to dry, and then removing the stems and stalks by rubbing the dried material. The resultant material is then rolled into cigarettes, or placed in a pipe, and smoked. The cannabinoid content of herbal cannabis varies according to the climate and growing conditions, but it comprises up to 8% cannabinoids.

Cannabis resin, an exudate secreted from the hairs on the leaves of the plant, is also collected from the upper leaves, and comprises up to 14% cannabinoids. The resinous material is powdered and usually compressed into a hard, brownish mass, which darkens in the air as a result of oxidation. This form of the drug is known as 'hash', 'resin' or 'charas'.

The purest form of the drug produced for illicit use is cannabis oil. This is prepared by solvent extraction of the resin followed by further purification to produce an oil that comprises up to 60% cannabinoids. Cannabis oil is generally added in small quantities to tobacco and smoked.

Cannabis in its various forms is still the most commonly used illicit drug in most countries. In the USA, more than 50% of young adults report the use of this drug on some occasion, although the prevalence of its casual use can fluctuate rather widely, for example from 37% in 1978 to about 18% ten years later. There is evidence that the smoke from the dried leaves contains potential carcinogens, together with carbon monoxide, and is therefore liable to affect the respiratory and cardiovascular systems adversely, in a similar manner to tobacco.

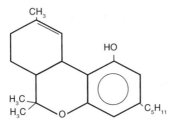

Fig. 13.7 Structure of delta-9-tetrahydrocannabinol (THC), the main psychoactive ingredient of the cannabis plant.

The main active ingredients of cannabis are cannabinol, cannabidiol and several isomers of tetrahydrocannabinol, of which delta-9-tetra-hydrocannabinol (THC) is probably responsible for most of the psychoactive effects of the various preparations. It is of interest to note that THC does not contain nitrogen in its three-membered ring system. The structure of THC is shown in Fig. 13.7.

Tetrahydrocannabinol and related compounds are very lipophilic and therefore readily absorbed from the lung and gastrointestinal tract. The bioavailability of oral THC varies from 4% to 12%, depending on the way in which it is delivered, whereas the availability of THC when smoked can be as high as 50%. Under optimal conditions, this could mean that a cigarette containing 1 g could lead to the delivery of up to 10 mg of THC to the circulation. The plasma concentration peaks after about 10 minutes, and the psychoactive effects reach a maximum after 20–30 minutes and last for about 2–3 hours. The time of peak effect and the duration of the pharmacological response are longer after oral administration.

Tetrahydrocannabinol is metabolised in the liver to form active metabolites; these are further metabolised to inactive polar compounds and excreted in the urine. Some metabolites are excreted into the bile and then recycled via the enterohepatic circulation. Because of their high lipophilicity, most active metabolites are widely distributed in fat deposits and the brain, from which sources they are only slowly eliminated. The half-life of elimination for many of the active metabolites has been calculated to be about 30 hours. Accordingly, accumulation occurs with regular, chronic dosing. Traces of the cannabinoids can be detected in the blood and urine of users many days after the last administration. There is some evidence of metabolic tolerance occurring after chronic use of the drug. THC and related cannabinoids readily penetrate the placental barrier and may possibly detrimentally affect foetal development.

Mechanisms of action

The high lipophilicity of THC and related compounds implies that these drugs are widely distributed throughout the brain, particularly in the grey matter; they appear to be taken up into neurons rather than the glia.

Understanding of the pharmacological properties of the cannabinoids has been greatly increased by the recent discovery and cloning of specific cannabinoid receptors in the mammalian brain, spleen and macrophages. In addition, possible endogenous candidates that act on these receptors have been identified. In the brain, the cannabinoids act on the CB1 type of receptor, which is distributed in regions of the brain concerned with motor activity and postural control (such as the basal ganglia and cerebellum), with emotion (e.g. the amygdala and hippocampus), with sensory perception (thalamus) and with autonomic and endocrine functions (hypothalamus, pons and medulla). The distribution of the CB1 receptors in the brain is similar to the distribution of THC and other cannabinoids, so it is not unreasonable to assume that they exert their pharmacological effects by activating the CB1 receptors. A second type of cannabinoid receptor, the CB2 receptor, has been detected on the surface of immune cells in the spleen and probably mediates the immunological effects of these drugs. Both types of receptor are present in peripheral tissues.

The first endogenous substance that was shown to interact with cannabinoid receptors was anandamide (from the Sanskrit work for bliss, *ananda*). This is a derivative of the polyunsaturated fatty acid arachidonic acid, namely arachidonyl ethanolamide. It appears that several other endogenous ligands also exist, including 2-arachidonyl-glycerol. Stimulation of neurotransmitter receptors appears to initiate the synthesis of these ligands. Thus it has been shown that anandamide release in the striatum is strongly enhanced by activation of dopamine D_2 receptors. Once released, anandamide activates CB1 or CB2 receptors or is accumulated in the adjacent cells by an energy- and sodium-dependent transport mechanism. Thus anandamide and 2-arachidonyl-glycerol can be released from neuronal and non-neuronal cells when the need arises, and utilise distinct receptor-mediated pathways from those used by conventional neurotransmitters. The non-synaptic release mechanisms and short half-lives of these endogenous cannabinoids suggest that they act near the sites of their synthesis to regulate the effects of primary neurotransmitters and hormones. A major implication of the discovery of the cannabinoid receptors is that it should be possible to develop selective cannabinoid agonists and antagonists for use either as therapeutic agents or as tools to unravel the precise physiological function of the cannabinoid system.

As the endogenous cannabinoids may serve important regulatory functions, it is not unreasonable to assume that they may have important therapeutic applications. Indeed, it would be surprising if the cannabinoid system, which appears to serve such an important function in the brain and peripheral system, did not facilitate the development of novel drugs in the near future. The following account summarises such possibilities.

Modulation of pain

Cannabinoids strongly reduce pain responses by interacting with CB1 receptors in the brain, spinal cord and peripheral sensory neurons. In the case of neuropathic pain, these drugs have been shown to be potent inhibitors of allodynia (pain from non-noxious stimuli) and hyperalgesia (increased sensitivity to noxious stimuli). In a rat model of neuropathic pain, the CB1 receptor agonist WIN552122 has been shown to attenuate such responses at doses that do not cause overt side-effects. These beneficial effects were antagonised by the CB1 antagonist SR141716A. In addition, CB1 receptor agonists have been shown to alleviate peripherally mediated pain, possibly via an effect on the gating mechanism, by enhancing the opioid peptides. The clinical impact of these advances is still modest but the development of novel cannabinoid receptor agonists may lead to the discovery of drugs to treat intractable conditions associated with neuropathic pain and multiple sclerosis.

Neuroprotection

CB1 receptor agonists inhibit both glutamatergic transmission and long-term potentiation, which suggests that the endogenous cannabinoids may play an important role in the regulation of excitatory transmission. In cultures of rat hippocampal neurons, the stimulation of glutamate release causes neuronal death. CB1 receptor agonists prevent this response but do not protect the neurons against the effects of exogenous glutamate. Similar protective effects of CB1 agonists have been shown to occur in *in vivo* models of cerebral ischaemia, these effects being blocked by CB1 receptor antagonists. Thus it seems possible that cannabinoids may be of potential value as neuroprotective agents.

Dopamine transmission, movement disorders and psychosis

CB1 receptors are densely expressed in the basal ganglia and cortex, a distribution that provides an anatomical substrate for the functional interaction between the cannabinoid system and ascending dopaminergic pathways. There is experimental evidence to show that anandamide modulates the dopamine-induced facilitation of psychomotor activity. In support of this hypothesis, 'knock-out' mice that lack the CB1 receptor show a profound decrease in locomotor activity. The therapeutic implications of this discovery have been shown by the finding that CB1 receptor agonists alleviate spasticity in various conditions, and tics in Tourette's syndrome.

With regard to psychosis, there is general consensus that heavy cannabis misuse can precipitate psychotic episodes in those with an underlying schizophrenic condition. It is possible that CB1 antagonists may therefore be of some therapeutic value in the treatment of psychotic disorders. CB1 agonists such as THC have, however, been shown to inhibit amphetamine-induced stereotypy in rodent models of psychosis. None the less, it has been shown that the chronic administration of cannabinoids causes an increase in the stimulant effects of amphetamine, which suggests that CB1 receptor desensitisation can exacerbate psychosis. Thus there is a need to investigate a wide variety of drugs which modulate the cannabinoid system.

Tolerance and dependence

Regular users of cannabis can take doses of THC that would be toxic to the naive user. This suggests that tolerance develops. While there is some evidence that metabolic tolerance may arise, it would appear that tissue tolerance is the most likely explanation for the effects observed. Tolerance develops to the drug-induced changes in mood, tachycardia, hyperthermia and decrease in intraocular pressure. Tolerance also develops to the effects of THC on psychomotor performance and changes on electroencephalography.

Cross-tolerance occurs between THC and alcohol, at least in animal studies, but this does not appear to occur between the cannabinoids and the psychotomimetics.

The abrupt withdrawal of very high doses of THC from volunteers has been associated with some withdrawal effects (irritability, insomnia, weight loss, tremor, changed sleep profile, anorexia), which suggests that both physical and psychological dependence may occasionally arise.

Pharmacological effects

Smoking a cigarette containing 2% THC adversely affects motor coordination, memory, cognition and sense of time. There is an enhanced sense of well-being and euphoria, accompanied by a feeling of relaxation and sleepiness. The intensity of these effects depends to some extent upon the environment in which the drug is taken. The effect upon short-term memory and the impairment of the ability to undertake memory-dependent, goal-directed behaviour is called 'temporal disintegration'. This process is correlated with a tendency to confuse the past, present and future, and to feel depersonalised. Such effects may last for several hours and may be intensified should the subject also consume alcohol.

Higher doses of THC are associated with hallucinations, delusions and paranoid ideas; the sense of depersonalisation also becomes more intense. The possibility that high doses of THC can trigger a schizo-phrenic episode in predisposed people is well recognised. 'Flash-backs' have been reported in those who have been exposed to high doses of the drug.

Many chronic cannabis users exhibit the 'amotivational syndrome', characterised by apathy, impaired judgement, memory defects and loss of interest in normal social pursuits. Whether chronic cannabis misuse leads to more permanent changes in brain function is uncertain, but it is known that chronic administration to animals results in permanent damage to the hippocampus. Regular use of cannabis by adolescents frequently predisposes them to other types of drug misuse later. This may reflect the social pressures placed upon them rather than the pharmacological consequences of misusing cannabis.

The most consistent effects of THC upon the cardiovascular system are tachycardia, increased systolic blood pressure and a reddening of the conjunctivae. As myocardial oxygen demand is increased, the chances of angina are enhanced in those who may be predisposed to this condition.

Pulmonary function is impaired in chronic cannabis smokers, despite the clear evidence that the acute use of the drug results in a significant and long-lasting bronchodilatation. However, it should be noted that the tar produced by cannabis cigarettes is more carcinogenic than that obtained from normal cigarettes, so that the risks of lung cancer and heart disease are increased in chronic cannabis smokers.

There are conflicting reports on the effects of chronic high doses of THC on human sexual function, but there is some evidence that spermatogenesis and testosterone levels are decreased. In women, a single cannabis cigarette can suppress release of luteinising hormone, so lack of ovulation frequently occurs in women who regularly misuse this drug. Lowered birth weight and increased chances of malformations have been reported in the offspring of women who misuse THC during pregnancy. It is also possible that in utero exposure to this drug causes behavioural abnormalities in childhood.

There are two features of the cannabinoids that may ultimately be of therapeutic importance. THC lowers intraocular pressure, which may be of benefit in the treatment of glaucoma. There is also evidence that THC is a moderately effective anti-emetic agent. Such a discovery has led to the development of nabilone, a synthetic cannabinoid, as an anti-emetic agent, but its use is limited because of the dysphoria, depersonalisation, memory disturbance and other effects that are associated with the cannabinoids. Whether the bronchodilator action of THC will ever find therapeutic application in the treatment of asthma remains an open question. Despite the widely held belief that the cannabinoids relieve some of the distressing symptoms associated with multiple sclerosis, objective studies of their efficacy are equivocal.

Conclusions

Whether a person will self-administer a drug depends on a number of factors in addition to its pharmacological properties, the dose administered and its route of administration. These factors include the environment in which the drug is taken and the nature of the previous experience following the administration of another drug with similar properties. With some exceptions, any mammal given continuous access to a drug of dependence will show a pattern of self-administration that is similar to that found in humans. This suggests that a pre-existing psychopathology is not a prerequisite for initial, or even continual, drug use, and that drugs of dependence have powerful reinforcing properties whether or not they cause physical dependence.

References

American Psychiatric Association (1990) *Benzodiazepine Dependence, Toxicity, and Abuse. A Task Force Report of the American Psychiatric Association.*Washington, DC: APA.

American Psychiatric Association (1994) *Diagnostic and Statistical Manual of Mental Disorders* (4th edn) (DSM–IV). Washington, DC: APA.

Falk, J. L. & Feingold, D. A. (1987) Environmental and cultural factors in the behavioural action of drugs. In *Psychopharmacology: A Third Generation of Progress* (ed. H. Meltzer), pp. 1503–1510. New York: Raven Press.

Hughes, J., Smith, T. W., Kosterlitz, H. W., *et al* (1975) Identification of two related pentopeptides from the brain with potent agonist activity. *Nature, 258,* 577.

Lader, M. H. (1983) Benzodiazepine withdrawal states. In *Benzodiazepines Divided* (ed. M. Trimble), pp. 17–32. Chichester: Wiley.

Nutt, E. (1986) Benzodiazepine dependence – the clinic: reason for anxiety? *Trends in Pharmacological Sciences, 7,* 457–460.

Sass, H., Soyka, M., Mann, K., *et al* (1996) Relapse prevention by acaprosate. Results from a placebo-controlled study on alcohol dependence. *Archives of General Psychiatry,* 53, 673–680.

Suzdak, P. D., Schwartz, R. D., Skolnick, P., *et al* (1986) Ethanol stimulates gamma-aminobutyric acid receptor mediated chloride transport in rat brain synaptosomes. *Proceedings of the National Academy of Sciences, USA,* **83,** 4071–4075.

Woolley, D. W. & Shaw, E. A. (1954) A biochemical and pharmacological suggestion about mental disorders. *Proceedings of the National Academy of Sciences, USA,* **40,** 228–235.

Further reading

Achte, K. & Tamminen, T. (eds) (2000) *Highlights of Modern Psychiatry.* Klaukkala: Recallmed.

Aiden, F., O'Connell, D. & Henry, D. (1995) Benzodiazepine use as a cause of cognitive impairment in elderly hospital inpatients. *Journal of Gerontology,* **50A,** M99–M106.

Baumgarten, H. G. & Göthert, M. (eds) (1999) *Serotoninergic Neurons and 5-HT Receptors in the CNS.* Berlin: Springer.

Benowitz, N. L. (1988) Pharmacological aspects of cigarette smoking and nicotine addiction. *New England Journal of Medicine,* **319,** 1315–1330.

British Medical Association (1997) *Therapeutic Uses of Cannabis.* London: Harwood Academic.

Busto, V., Sellers, E. M., Naranjo, C. A., *et al* (1986) Withdrawal reaction after long-term therapeutic use of benzodiazepines. *New England Journal of Medicine*, **313**, 854–859.

Chick, J. & Cantwell, R. (eds) (1994) *Seminars in Alcohol and Drug Misuse*. London: Gaskell.

Daws, L. C. & White, J. M. (1999) Regulation of opioid receptors by opioid antagonists: implications for rapid opioid detoxification. *Addiction Biology*, **4**, 391–397.

Dewey, W. L. (1986) Cannabinoid pharmacology. *Pharmacological Reviews*, **38**, 151–178.

Fischman, H. W. (1988) Behavioural pharmacology of cocaine. *Journal of Clinical Psychiatry*, **49**, 7–10.

Haynes, L. (1988) Opioid receptors and signal transduction. *Trends in Pharmacological Sciences*, **9**, 309–311.

Julien, J. L. & Leonard, B. E. (1989) Drugs acting as sigma and phencyclidine receptors: a review of their nature, function and possible therapeutic importance. *Clinical Neuropharmacology*, **12**, 353–374.

Lader, M. (1995) Clinical pharmacology of anxiolytic drugs: past, present and future. In *GABA Receptors and Anxiety: From Neurobiology to Treatment* (eds G. Biggio, E. Sanna & E. Costa), pp. 83–90. New York: Raven Press.

Littleton, J. (1989) Alcohol intoxication and physical dependence: a molecular mystery tour. *British Journal of Addiction*, **84**, 267–276.

Maldonado, R. (2003) (ed.) *Molecular Biology of Drug Addiction*. Totowa, NJ: Humana Press.

Maykut, M. D. (1989) Health consequences of acute and chronic marihuana use. *Progress in Neuro-psychopharmacology and Biological Psychiatry*, **9**, 209–238.

Nestler, E. J. & Aghajanian, G. (1997) Molecular and cellular basis of addiction. *Science*, **278**, 58–63.

Simonato, M. (1996) The neurochemistry of morphine addiction in the neocortex. *Trends in Pharmacological Sciences*, **17**, 410–415.

Spangel, R. & Weiss, F. (1999) The dopamine hypothesis of reward: past and current status. *Trends in Neurosciences*, **22**, 521–527.

Trimble, M. R. & Hindmarch, I. (2000) (eds) *Benzodiazepines*. Petersfield: Wrightson Biomedical Publishing.

Zernig, G., Saria, A., Kurz, M., *et al* (eds) (2001) *Handbook of Alcoholism*. Boca Raton, FL: CRC Press.

General reading

Bittar, E. E. & Bittar, N. (eds) (2000) *Biological Psychiatry*. Stamford, CT: JA Press.

Bloom, F. E. & Kupfer, D. J. (eds) (1995) *Psychopharmacology: The Fourth Generation of Progress*. New York: Raven Press.

Cooper, J. R., Bloom, F. E. & Roth, R. H. (1991) *The Biochemical Basis of Neuropharmacology* (6th edn). New York: Oxford University Press.

Feldman, R. S., Meyer, J. S. & Quenzer, L. F. (1997) *Principles of Neuropsychopharmacology*. Sunderland, MA: Sinauer Associates.

Leonard, B. E. (2003) *Fundamentals of Psychopharmacology* (3rd edn). Chichester: Wiley.

Schatzberg, A. F. & Nemeroff, C. B. (eds) (1998) *Textbook of Psychopharmacology* (2nd edn). Washington, DC: American Psychiatric Press.

Reviews and key publications

Burgess, C., O'Donohoe, A. & Gill, M. (2000) Agony and ecstasy: a review of MDMA effects and toxicity. *European Psychiatry*, **15**, 287–294.

Charney, D. S., Krystal, J. H., Delgade, P. L., *et al* (1990). Serotonin specific drugs for anxiety and depressive disorders. *Annual Review of Medicine*, **41**, 437–446.

Chuang, D. (1989) Neurotransmitter receptors and phosphoinositide turnover. *Annual Review of Pharmacology and Toxicology*, **29**, 71–110.

Di Chiara, G. (1999) Drug addiction as dopamine-dependent associative learning disorder. *European Journal of Pharmacology*, **375**, 13–30.

Feigner, J. P. & Boyer, W. F. (1991) *Selective Serotonin Reuptake Inhibitors*. Chichester: Wiley.

Haefely, W. (1990) The GABA–benzodiazepine interaction – 15 years later. *Neurochemical Research*, **15**, 169–174.

McGreer, E. G. (1989) Neurotransmitters. *Current Opinions in Neurology and Neurosurgery*, **2**, 520–531.

Meldrum, B. S. (1989) GABA-ergic mechanisms in the pathogenesis and treatment of epilepsy. *British Journal of Clinical Pharmacology*, **27**, 35–113.

Olney, J. W. (1989) Excitatory amino acids and neuropsychiatric disorders. *Biological Psychiatry*, **26**, 505–525.

Robbins, T. W. & Everitt, B. (1999) Drug addiction: bad habits add up. *Nature*, **398**, 567–571.

Schmidt, A. W. & Perontka, S. J. (1989) 5-hydroxytryptamine receptor 'families'. *FASEB Journal*, **3**, 2242–2249.

Spanagel, R. & Zieglgänsberger, W. (1997) Anti-craving compounds for ethanal: new pharmacological tools to study addictive processes. *Trends in Pharmacological Sciences*, **18**, 54–58.

Stolerman, I. (1992) Drugs of abuse: behavioural principals, methods and terms. *Trends in Pharmacological Science*, **13**, 170–176.

CHAPTER 14

Drug treatment of the personality disorders, premenstrual tension and erectile dysfunction, and male sexual suppressants

George S. Stein

Drug treatment of personality disorders

The treatment of personality disorders is a topic surrounded with much pessimism – many clinicians believe that these disorders are essentially untreatable and that most subjects with a personality disorder have little capacity for change. It is not surprising therefore that the benefits of drug treatment are usually quite modest. However, certain manifestations of these disorders, particularly behavioural dyscontrol, impulsivity, suicidal behaviour and brief psychotic episodes, require intervention, usually with short-term hospital admission and some drug therapy.

There are only three categories of personality disorder in DSM–IV (American Psychiatric Association, 1994, p. 654) that show some response to pharmacotherapy. These are borderline personality disorder, schizotypal personality disorder (both of which are classified as personality disorders) and a group of subjects suffering from inter-mittent explosive disorder (which is classified as one of the impulsive disorders). Other categories of personality disorder – such as dissocial, schizoid, paranoid, histrionic, dependent, avoidant, narcissistic and passive aggressive personality disorder – do not respond to pharmaco-therapy.

Borderline personality disorder is characterised by unstable mood, unstable interpersonal relationships and a disturbance of identity. Depression is common, with the predominant patterns being rapid and reactive shifts into depressions rather than a fixed continuous depression. The individual typically complains of boredom, intolerance of being alone, frustration and an unpleasant sense of emptiness. Impulsive behaviour such as binge eating, kleptomania, drug or alcohol misuse or other thrill-seeking behaviour may occur to alleviate the dysphoria. Anger and impulsivity may be turned inward and can lead to self-mutilation or repeated overdoses, which may occasionally result in an inadvertent death. Borderline subjects enter into ambivalent relationships that are often intense and characterised by a tendency to over-idealise or devalue their partner. At other times they may display manipulative or coercive behaviour to humiliate those who care for them. Aetiology is unclear, but family studies show that many relatives have personality disorders, affective disorder or occasionally bipolar disorder, and often there is a history of physical and sexual abuse in childhood. Over the longer term, the picture is one of unstable moods and unstable relationships, which tend to ameliorate with age. The DSM–IV criteria are shown in Box 14.1. Schizotypal personality disorder is classified under the personality disorders section in DSM–IV but together with the schizophrenias in ICD–10 (World Health Organization, 1992) because some subjects have a family history of schizophrenia and some go on to develop schizophrenia. The older term 'Kretschmer's sensitive personality type' is sometimes applied to this group. The disorder is uncommon and individuals tend to be aloof and isolated but they usually also have odd beliefs, referential ideas, magical thinking and suspiciousness (though not of delusional intensity). Unlike schizoid personality disorder, schizotypal personality disorder is associated with a degree of relatedness to the world, although some individuals do complain of feelings of estrangement and depersonalisation, and lead socially isolated lives. The diagnostic criteria are shown in Box 14.2. Many patients with severe personality disorder appear to have elements of both borderline personality disorder and schizotypal personality disorder.

Intermittent explosive disorder is classified as one of the impulse disorders in DSM–IV but as impulsive personality disorder in ICD–10. The essential feature of impulse control disorders is the failure to resist an impulse, drive or temptation to perform an act that is harmful to the individual or to others. In the case of intermittent explosive disorder, there is often a lifelong history of a failure to resist aggressive impulses that result in serious assaultive acts or destruction of property. The

---

Box 14.1 The DSM–IV criteria for borderline personality disorder

- Unstable or intense interpersonal relationships
- Impulsiveness, which may be self-damaging
- Affective instability
- Inappropriate or intense anger or temper
- Recurrent suicidal threats or self-mutilation
- Identity disturbance
- Chronic feelings of emptiness or boredom
- Frantic efforts to avoid real or imagined abandonment

Box 14.2   The DSM–IV features of schizotypal personality disorder

- Ideas of reference
- Excessive social anxiety
- Odd beliefs and magical thinking
- Unusual perceptual experience, such as illusions
- Odd or eccentric behaviour or experience
- No close relationships (or only one) apart from with first-degree relatives
- Odd speech, which may be impoverished, vague or abstract
- Inappropriate or constricted affect
- Suspiciousness or paranoid ideation

---

degree of aggressiveness is usually quite out of proportion to the trigger, which is often drug or alcohol misuse, irregular eating or sleeping habits or a psychosocial stressor. The electroencephalogram (EEG) is usually normal and attacks are sometimes accompanied by affective changes – increased energy and heightened mood before the episode, followed by depression, remorse, lack of energy or sleepiness afterwards. Some have suggested this represents a very brief manic episode. The diagnosis is made when this pattern is the dominant component of the clinical presentation, but these individuals often have other psychiatric disorders, particularly depression, substance misuse disorders (both drugs and alcohol), anxiety disorders and other personality disorders. However, the disorder can occur in isolation. There is often a history of other family members having a 'bad temper'. The DSM–IV criteria are shown in Box 14.3. It is of benefit to diagnose the condition because many subjects with a lifetime pattern of explosiveness may respond well to the selective serotonin reuptake inhibitors (SSRIs).

Personality disorders are both serious and common, whether they are deemed to be illnesses or not. The prevalence of borderline personality disorder is estimated to be 2% in the community, around 10% among psychiatric out-patients and 20% among psychiatric in-patients (who usually also have depression); around 75% of the subjects are women (American Psychiatric Association, 1994). The mortality rate among people aged 20–39 years admitted with a diagnosis of personality disorder is elevated sixfold and is similar to the rate found for schizophrenia and affective disorder. There is also a high suicide rate for both psychopathy and borderline personality disorder. Stone (1990) gives a figure of 8.5% for suicide for his group of subjects with borderline personality disorder in New York.

In the sections that follow, the use of each class of drugs (that is, antipsychotics, antidepressants, lithium and anti-epileptics) for people with personality disorders is reviewed. Brief overviews of suggested strategies for the use of these drugs, and of the use of stimulant drugs

> **Box 14.3** The DSM–IV criteria for intermittent explosive disorder
>
> - Several discrete episodes of failure to resist aggressive impulses that result in serious assaultive acts or destruction of property
> - The degree of aggressiveness is grossly out of proportion to any precipitating psychosocial stresses
> - Aggressive episodes are not better accounted for by another mental disorder (personality disorder, mania, psychosis, attention-deficit hyperactivity disorder, etc.)

in adult attention-deficit hyperactivity disorder (ADHD) are also given (although ADHD is not considered to be one of the personality disorders). A comprehensive list of all except the most recent drug studies in the literature is given by Soloff (2000).

Antipsychotic drugs

Because early theories on the aetiology of borderline personality disorder suggested a relationship with psychosis – for example, the term 'pseudo-neurotic schizophrenia' was used to describe such cases – it seemed logical to try antipsychotic drugs to treat it. The psychoanalyst Winkleman (1955) prescribed chlorpromazine to his borderline subjects during their psychotherapy and he observed diminished anxiety, improved reality testing and a diminution in 'id drives', which is presumably a psychoanalytic way of describing behavioural dyscontrol. Brinkley et al (1979) described five people with borderline personality disorder who had failed on previous drugs and made little progress in psychotherapy but who responded well to low doses of antipsychotics: 2–6 mg thiothixene in two patients, 10 mg perphenazine in one and 25 mg thioridazine in the two others. This was followed by other open-label studies, on pimozide, thioridazine and loxapine.

Although there have been only a few placebo-controlled trials of the use of antipsychotics in this personality disorder, these are highly informative. Cowdrey & Gardner (1988) used trifluoperazine as one of four active drugs in a well-designed complex cross-over trial and found benefits of this drug for subjects with depression, anxiety, rejection sensitivity and suicidality.

Soloff et al (1986) recruited subjects from the in-patient and out-patient departments of the Western Psychiatric Clinic in Pittsburgh and confirmed the diagnosis of borderline personality disorder with a standardised diagnostic interview. Sixty subjects were recruited, of whom 43% had borderline personality disorder, 6% had schizotypal personality disorder, and 51% had both borderline personality disorder and schizotypal personality disorder. Patients were randomised so that

20 patients received haloperidol (7.5 mg daily), 20 subjects received amitriptyline (mean 149 mg daily) and 20 subjects received placebo. Haloperidol emerged as superior to both amitriptyline and placebo for a variety of different symptoms (rated on the 90-item Hopkins Symptoms Check-List, HSCL-90), namely depression, anxiety, hostility, paranoid ideation and psychoticism, as well as on measures of behavioural dyscontrol. However, in a more recent trial the same authors compared haloperidol (4 mg) with placebo on a less severely morbid group of out-patients and were able to demonstrate benefits only for the symptoms of anger and depression on the HSCL-90 (Soloff et al, 1993). Even though haloperidol showed some limited value in both trials, once the trial was over 87.5% of those on haloperidol discontinued the drug, compared with 58% of those in the placebo group, which probably indicates that, from the patient's perspective, any therapeutic benefits of the drug were outweighed by its side-effects, a problem that may now also be appearing with the newer 'atypical' drugs.

Schulz et al (1999) reported on 11 subjects with borderline personality disorder, seven of whom also met criteria for schizotypal disorder. In an 8-week trial of olanzapine (mean dosage 7.5 mg daily) a large number of symptoms on the HSCL-90 improved and these included obsessive compulsivity, interpersonal sensitivity, depression, anxiety, anger–hostility, phobic anxiety, paranoia and psychoticism. No patient developed any movement disorder but there was a mean weight gain of around 4 kg during the trial, which four of the nine female patients found troublesome, and this led to a request for a change in medication during the continuation phase of the study. Patients titrated their own daily dosage of olanzapine using 2.5 mg tablets and the average dose emerged as 7.72 mg, which is around half the average dose when it is used to treat schizophrenia.

A placebo-controlled study of risperidone also showed substantial reductions in symptom scores, but in both the active drug and placebo arms of the trial, and at the end of the trial there were no significant differences between the active drug and placebo, which indicates that non-pharmacogenic factors are important in the therapy of the personality disorder (Cornelius et al, 1993).

There is also one report on the successful use of clozapine among seven subjects with borderline personality disorder and other psychiatric disorders (Chengappa et al, 1999). The comorbid condition was schizoaffective disorder in two cases, psychosis not otherwise specified in two cases, bipolar I disorder in one case, chronic paranoid schizophrenia in one case and impulse control disorder in one case. All the subjects had failed on multiple previous trials of other medication and all were prone to multiple episodes of extreme self-mutilation. Data were extracted from the case notes for the mirror image period (i.e. anchored to the clozapine start date) up to a maximum of 1 year for each subject and

STEIN

the results showed that clozapine led to major improvement and a significant reduction in the frequency and severity of self-mutilation, in the number of seclusion episodes (from a mean of 26 to 2.3 per patient) and in the number of injuries to staff and other patients (from a mean of 4.15 to 0.3 per patient). Clozapine can be prescribed only for psychotic disorders, but at the more severe end of the spectrum of borderline personality disorder there are a few individuals who have a psychosis in addition.

Antidepressant treatments

The SSRIs have proved to be an important advance in the management of borderline personality disorder. Even though they have little advantage in efficacy for the treatment of depression over the older, tricyclic antidepressants, they have three particular advantages in the management of borderline personality disorder:

(1) borderline personality disorder is a long-term disorder and because SSRIs are more easily tolerated than either tricyclics or antipsychotics, once a drug is found to be helpful the likelihood of it being discontinued is far less.
(2) SSRIs have proven efficacy in controlling impulsivity, and impulsive aggression is one of the most damaging features of borderline personality disorder
(3) SSRIs appear to be relatively safe in overdose, a common problem in this population.

Just occasionally the SSRIs may provoke increased aggressive and suicidal behaviours, possibly as part of a dysphoric adverse drug reaction, but the reason for this is obscure.

Coccaro & Kavoussi (1997) recruited 40 subjects who met DSM–III–R criteria for personality disorders who also had a history of impulsive aggression, but subjects with current major depression were excluded, as were those with a lifetime history of bipolar disorder, schizophrenia or drug misuse. Most of the patients had a personality disorder in the 'dramatic' cluster (borderline or antisocial). They entered a randomised double-blind trial which compared fluoxetine (20–40 mg daily) with placebo. Fluoxetine showed significant benefits over placebo on the Overt Aggressive Scale and measures of irritability, but there was no difference in depression scores, although these were low at the outset of the trial The effect of fluoxetine on aggression and irritability did not appear until week 4 and was unrelated to mood state or a current or lifetime history of any mood disorder. This study also has important implications for the management of intermittent explosive disorder because the central problem in this condition is also one of impulsivity and aggression.

534

Markowitz *et al* (1991) studied 17 patients with borderline personality disorder, nine of whom were on fluoxetine (doses ranging from 20 to 80 mg daily) and eight on placebo, for 14 weeks). Many of the subjects also had major depression. The patients on fluoxetine did significantly better than those on placebo on measures of anxiety and depression, but irritability was not measured.

Salzman *et al* (1995) conducted a 12-week trial of 22 well-functioning subjects with borderline personality disorder who were free of any other comorbid axis I or II diagnosis. Fluoxetine showed an advantage over placebo for the symptoms of anger, depression and global function, but because this group was functioning well at the start of the trial no subject improved more than 20% on any measure.

Of the SSRIs, only fluoxetine has been subjected to placebo-controlled evaluation, but there are numerous case reports and a few open-label studies of sertraline and venlafaxine, which also suggest useful clinical effects among subjects with borderline personality disorder and impulsive aggression.

Drug trials of the older antidepressants have demonstrated beneficial effects particularly for the monoamine oxidase inhibitors (MAOIs). In the cross-over trial by Cowdrey & Gardner (1988), tranylcypromine proved to be the most effective of all the four drugs used (trifluoperazine, carbamazepine, tranylcypromine, alprazolam and placebo) on a wide variety of measures. A history of childhood attention-deficit disorder was predictive of a therapeutic response, which suggests that the stimulant or amphetamine-like action of the MAOI may have been pharmacologically relevant. While MAOIs are still available and probably have some efficacy in borderline personality disorder, dietary restrictions associated with their use, their risks in overdose and when mixed with alcohol or other drugs (see Chapter 6) probably preclude their use in routine clinical practice in this risk-taking population. The SSRIs would be a safer alternative.

Tricyclic antidepressants have also been used in subjects with borderline personality disorder, but only a minority respond, and there has been only one controlled trial of their use. Thus Soloff *et al* (1986) compared 20 patients with borderline personality disorder or schizotypal personality disorder, or borderline personality disorder and schizotypal personality disorder combined, on amitriptyline (a mean of 149 mg daily) or placebo. Around half the patients improved, but the other half became worse – 57% worsened on a measure of hostile depression and 64% showed a deterioration on their schizotypal symptoms. Such paradoxical effects are sometimes seen in day-to-day clinical practice and clinicians should always be aware that patients with borderline personality disorder can sometimes be worsened by their medications.

Electroconvulsive therapy

Subjects with depression and personality disorder may show a good initial response to electroconvulsive therapy (ECT), but there is often a high early relapse rate. Zimmerman *et al* (1986) treated 25 patients with major depression, 10 of whom suffered from a variety of personality disorders as well (the other 15 had major depression only). The short-term response to ECT was good in both groups, but by 6 months five of the ten subjects with personality disorder had been readmitted, compared with only one out of 15 in the pure depression group.

A second, more subtle indication for ECT is the phenomenon of double depression. A patient with borderline personality disorder may suffer from a chronic, low-grade dysphoria with infrequent episodes of self-mutilation. Quite abruptly the condition deteriorates and there is severe regression, with daily or almost daily self-mutilation and suicidal actions. In these instances, an episode of major depression may have been superimposed on the low-grade dysphoria and the term 'double depression' has been applied. In these instances ECT can have a short-lived beneficial effect, which may occasionally be life-saving.

In general, ECT is not a useful intervention for the long-term management of the personality disorders and it should be used sparingly.

Lithium for aggressive personality disorders

In the USA in the 1970s, it was possible to conduct drug trials among seriously violent prisoners; such studies would not be permitted today. Tupin *et al* (1973) examined 27 male convicts who had a pattern of recurring, easily triggered violence. About half the subjects had explosive personality disorders and a few had schizophrenia and other miscellaneous disorders. They were treated with a rather high dose of lithium (1800 mg), but the mean plasma level was only 0.82 mmol/l. Fifteen of the subjects improved, four showed no change, and three became more aggressive while on lithium; two subjects became psychotic, possibly because of high serum lithium levels, although their aggression was well controlled, while the ratings for the remaining three subjects were insufficient to make any judgement. Of those who benefited, the lithium appeared to induce a state of reflective delay or, as one convict aptly put it, 'now I can think whether to hit him or not'.

In a larger, placebo-controlled study, Sheard *et al* (1976) examined a group of 66 subjects with various personality disorders who had committed serious aggressive offences, such as manslaughter, rape or assault, and who continued to show assaultive behaviour in prison. The frequency of major rule infraction (which generally meant an episode of violence that was punished by seclusion) was taken as a measure of drug response. By the third month, the rate of major infraction had dropped to zero among those taking lithium, but was unchanged in the placebo group. Once lithium was stopped there was an immediate rebound increase in the number of major infractions. Minor episodes of rule breaking were unchanged by lithium, which suggests that lithium lacked any general sedative effect.

These findings were confirmed in a more recent study, by Malone *et al* (2000), among a group of 40 conduct-disordered adolescents (mean age 12.5 years) whose aggressive behaviour was sufficiently severe to merit in-patient treatment. The diagnosis was ascertained rigorously by two child psychiatrists using a standardised interview, and cases of major depression and bipolar disorder were specifically excluded. Lithium was significantly superior to placebo on measures of aggression: 16 of 20 subjects (80%) responded to lithium, while only 6 of 20 (30%) responded to placebo, but nausea, vomiting and urinary frequency were troublesome side-effects among the lithium group.

Finally, Stone (1990) reported that around 8% of his large sample of subjects with borderline personality disorder subsequently developed bipolar II disorder, and some of these subjects showed a gratifying response to lithium.

Most patients with personality disorders do not respond to lithium: picking out the small minority of responders is like finding a needle in a haystack. Affective features, anger and aggression, brief periods of elation and a family history of classic affective disorder or alcoholism may be useful pointers. In some cases, particularly where there is severe and recurrent aggression, or a depression that has failed to respond to tricyclic antidepressants or SSRIs, a 2-month therapeutic trial of lithium may be indicated.

Lithium for self-mutilating and aggressive subjects with learning difficulties

A number of case reports in the 1960s and 1970s suggested that lithium may be helpful in the management of long-standing aggressive and self-mutilating behaviour in those with learning difficulties. An early, open study, by Dostal & Zvolsky (1970), showed that 11 out of 14 self-mutilating, hyperactive, phenothiazine-resistant, severely mentally deficient adolescents improved with respect to their aggressiveness, restlessness and undisciplined behaviour. Little improvement occurred when the subjects took small doses of lithium, and improvement seemed to occur only when the subjects took 1800 mg lithium a day, which gave them an average plasma level of 0.92 mmol/l. Unfortunately, while on this dosage, nine subjects experienced severe polydypsia and polyuria accompanied by enuresis, which rendered long-term lithium therapy impracticable.

Three double-blind placebo-controlled trials have confirmed these findings. In a trial of eight patients with non-bipolar aggression conducted by Worrall *et al* (1975) there was some improvement in aggression, but two patients showed signs of a progressive dementia, possibly as a result of lithium toxicity, and the authors cautioned against the use of lithium in brain-damaged subjects. Tyrer *et al* (1984) carried out a double-blind cross-over trial with 26 aggressive patients with learning disabilities aged between 14 and 50 years and 70% improved. Factor analysis showed that verbal and non-verbal aggression, destructiveness, self-mutilation and antisocial behaviour all improved. As hyperactivity and noisiness showed no difference between lithium and placebo, the authors concluded that the lithium did not have a tranquillising effect. In the third study, by Craft *et al* (1987), 73% of 42 adults with learning disabilities and self-mutilating behaviour improved, although 30% of the placebo group also improved, and lithium even led to increased aggression in a few patients.

There do not appear to be any more recent publications on the use of lithium in this population, which suggests that it may in fact be of limited use. Dangerous episodes of toxicity may be more frequent among this group, as they are perhaps less likely than others to report any intercurrent illness such as diarrhoea, while among subjects with pre-existing seizures or brain damage there may also be increased risks in using lithium.

Attention-deficit hyperactivity disorder in adults

Attention-deficit hyperactivity disorder (ADHD) in children and adolescents, which is described in Chapter 11, usually responds well to stimulant medication. In a meta-analysis of 56 studies covering 1700 childhood cases of ADHD, around a third persisted into adulthood (Spencer *et al*, 1998). Children with ADHD followed into adulthood have high levels of school failure, poor work histories, poor social interactions and sometimes low self-esteem. Persistent symptoms of inattention, disorganisation, distractibility and impulsiveness were associated with psychosocial dysfunction, school-related problems, work failure and psychiatric comorbidity (especially substance misuse and antisocial personality disorder). Weiss *et al* (1985) reported that employers of adults with ADHD reported poor levels of work performance, impaired task completion, lack of independent skills and poor relationships with supervisors. Studies of comorbidity have also revealed that adults with ADHD have high rates of substance misuse (27–46%), antisocial personality disorders (12–27%) and anxiety disorders (50%) (Morrison, 1980). The disorder should not be diagnosed in adulthood unless there is a good history of childhood ADHD. The key features of adult ADHD are shown in Box 14.4.

The treatment of adult ADHD has followed the same principles as the treatment of childhood ADHD – a combination of supportive

> **Box 14.4** Characteristics of adult attention-deficit hyperactivity disorder
>
> - Motor hyperactivity
> - Attention deficits
> - Affective lability
> - Hot temper
> - Emotional over-reactivity
> - Disorganisation and inability to complete tasks
> - Impulsivity
> - Comorbidity

psychotherapy and stimulants, usually methylphenidate (Ritalin) but sometimes dexamphetamine. However, as there is considerable concern about the use of potentially addictive drugs with this population, there are very few placebo-controlled trials. A number of earlier studies, mainly emanating from one centre in Utah, demonstrated benefits for methylphenidate, and for certain other dopaminergic-related drugs which had some stimulant properties. These included pargyline (an MAO-B inhibitor no longer marketed), selegiline, buproprion, L-dopa and precursors of L-dopa, phenylalanine and L-tyrosine (Spencer *et al*, 1998). Two double-blind studies have attempted to replicate some of these earlier findings with regard to methylphenidate. Mattes *et al* (1984) failed to demonstrate a favourable response to methylphenidate in 61 patients with loosely defined features of ADHD.

More recently, Spencer *et al* (1995) conducted a double-blind placebo cross-over trial in 23 adult patients (age range 18–60) using methylphenidate in doses of 1 mg/kg. All subjects had a DSM–IV diagnosis of ADHD by the age of 7, a chronic course from childhood to adulthood, and considerable functional impairment attributable to the ADHD. Using a specific ADHD rating scale to measure change, 18 of the 23 (78%) showed substantial improvement after 3 weeks on methylphenidate, compared with only 1 of the 23 (4%) while on placebo. Adverse effects were loss of appetite, insomnia and increased anxiety.

Subjects with a well-defined syndrome of ADHD and an authenticated history of childhood ADHD may benefit from stimulant therapy, but in the absence of such a history therapeutic benefits are unlikely. Methylphenidate is relatively short acting and the dose is 10–15 mg every 2–4 hours, up to a total of 40–90 mg daily. Some patients may also respond to dexamphetamine in doses of 5–15 mg every 3–4 hours, up to a total of 20–45 mg daily. Caution should be exercised before placing an adult patient on stimulants, particularly if the childhood history is equivocal, since some patients with comorbid personality disorders may misuse the drugs or inadvertently increase the dosage.

Anti-epileptic drugs

The most seriously disruptive symptoms of the personality disorders are episodes of impulsive aggression and behaviour dyscontrol. These take the form of rage reactions, assaults, self-mutilation (commonly wrist or body slashing), self-inflicted burns or drug overdoses. Monroe (1970) applied the term 'episodic dyscontrol disorder' to describe this phenomenon; its core feature was said to be 'an abrupt onset of intense dysphoric affects which interrupts the life flow of the individual'. The modern equivalent of this disorder in DSM–IV is intermittent explosive disorder (Box 14.3).

McElroy (1999) reported on a group of 27 patients (20 male, 7 female) with intermittent explosive disorder as defined in DSM–IV. Most of the subjects also had other psychiatric disorders, in particular anxiety and depression. Aggressive episodes were usually brief, with a mean duration of 22 minutes, but they were frequent, averaging 14 episodes per month. Around one-third of the subjects reported autonomic symptoms suggestive of panic disorder immediately before or during an episode and just under half the subjects reported pleasurable feelings during the outburst, although they regretted the damage afterwards. Using a criterion of a 50% reduction in symptom severity, around 50% of the subjects responded to an SSRI and 75% to a mood stabiliser – in this study sodium valproate.

Early controlled studies with some of the older anti-epileptics such as phenytoin failed to demonstrate any beneficial effects and some subjects actually worsened (Lefkowitz, 1969). A placebo cross-over trial of carbamazepine (600 mg daily) demonstrated a reduction in the frequency of severe episodes of behavioural dyscontrol compared with placebo (Cowdrey & Gardner, 1988), but these findings were not replicated in another 5-week placebo-controlled trial of carbemazepine in 20 in-patients with borderline personality disorder (De La Fuenta & Lotstra, 1994).

While the use of carbamazepine for the treatment of aggression has passed into some decline, there has been a rapid increase in the use of sodium valproate, particularly in the USA. A survey of the use of valproate in all New York state hospitals showed that in 1994, 15.5% of all in-patients received sodium valproate, and this had risen to a staggering 34.1% by 1996. The main uses for valproate were for aggressive outbursts in schizophrenia, bipolar disorder and dementia (Citrome et al, 1998).

Two preliminary open studies and one placebo-controlled trial on the use of valproate in subjects with cluster B personality disorders have given encouraging results. Stein et al (1995) conducted an 8-week trial of valproate monotherapy with blood levels in the 50–100 ng/ml range, in a group of in-patients with 'pure borderline personality disorder', that is, who did not have comorbid depression or bipolar disorder. There were significant reductions in anxiety, tension, time in seclusion and measures of aggression. Wilcox (1995) treated 30 in-patients who had borderline personality disorder; none had epilepsy but five had EEG abnormalities. The addition of divalproex sodium (Depakote) to the patients' drug regimen led to a reduction in global scores on the Brief Psychiatric Rating Scale, as well as scores for anxiety and tension, and time spent in seclusion. Finally, Hollander *et al* (2003) conducted a 12-week, double-blind, placebo-controlled trial of 96 patients who fulfilled DSM–IV diagnostic crieteria for cluster B personality disorders. The patients were randomised to take either placebo or divalproex sodium. The trial demonstrated that divalproex sodium was significantly better than placebo on measures of aggression, irritability and global severity.

Divalproex sodium may be useful even where other anti-aggressive remedies have failed. Kavoussi & Coccaro (1998) conducted an open-label study of ten subjects with personality disorder, five of whom had borderline personality disorder that had failed to respond to trials with fluoxetine (up to 60 mg for 8 weeks) and six out of the eight subjects who completed the trial reported improvement by the fourth week.

There is considerable speculation on the mode of action of valproate in aggressive disorders. Valproate has an enhancing effect on central levels of gamma-aminobutyric acid (GABA), a major neurotransmitter in the central nervous system (CNS). Valproate exerts its effect by inhibiting GABA transaminase, and the consequent increased levels of GABA can counteract increased dopaminergic activity in the mesolimbic and meso-prefontal cortical areas (Waseff *et al*, 1999). Valproate also enhances serotonergic transmission and this may underlie its anti-aggressive action in bipolar disorder. Finally, like any anti-epileptic, its effects may be mediated through its anti-kindling properties, which leads to suppression of subthreshold electrical impulses in the limbic system.

The latest anti-epileptic to be introduced into psychiatric practice is lamotrigine, a drug that has proven antidepressant action in subjects with bipolar depression (Calabrese *et al*, 1999). An open-label study of lamotrigine (300 mg daily) in eight patients with severe resistant borderline personality disorder who had failed on multiple previous drug trials was conducted by Pinto & Akiskal (1998). These authors reported an improvement in Global Assessment Form scores, from 40 to 80, during the trial, with impulsive, drug-taking and suicidal behaviours diminishing to the extent that subjects no longer met criteria for borderline personality disorder at the end of the trial. The lamotrigine was well tolerated by all except one patient, who developed a rash and dropped out (rashes due to lamotrigine can occasionally develop into the Stevens–Johnson syndrome, which can be lethal).

The pharmacology, pharmacokinetics and side-effects of the carbamazepine, sodium valproate and lamotrigine are described in Chapter 10.

A general strategy for selecting medications

Soloff (2000) has attempted to provide a general strategy for selecting drugs for patients with borderline personality disorder. He recommends a symptom-based approach. The dominant symptom at presentation may be cognitive perceptual distortions, affective dysregulation or impulsive behavioural dyscontrol.

Cognitive perceptual symptoms include suspiciousness, ideas of reference, illusions, eccentric thinking and transitory stress-related hallucinations, and irritability related to cognitive distortion. As a first choice Soloff recommends trying typical or atypical antipsychotics for presentations of this type, but most follow-up studies indicate that many subjects with borderline personality disorder either actively reject or simply cease taking antipsychotics over the long term, presumably because of their side-effects (motor side-effects with the older typical drugs, and weight gain with the atypicals).

Symptoms of affective dysregulation include depression, lability of mood, rejection sensitivity, 'mood crashes', intense anger, temper outbursts, anxiety, dysphoria and anhedonia. The SSRIs and related antidepressants such as venlaflaxine may be helpful in this group; if one drug does not work, a switch to another SSRI may be helpful or a lithium augmentation strategy may be attempted. The SSRIs are well tolerated when taken over the longer term and patients tend to continue using them without needing much prompting from their doctor. It is important to note that episodes of major depression may also occur in any person with any type of personality disorder. These should respond to standard antidepressive regimens and medication should not be withheld because a person has a diagnosis of personality disorder.

The third target group of symptoms, those that involve impulsive dyscontrol, includes self-mutilation, recurrent suicidal behaviour or threats, impulsive aggression, assaultiveness, binge behaviours with regard to drugs, alcohol, sex or food, and cognitive impulsivity (impulsive behaviour due to cognitive distortion). In these cases it is also helpful to initiate therapy with an SSRI, but if there is no response a mood stabiliser could be tried. Either lithium or one of the three anti-epileptics (i.e. carbamazepine, sodium valproate or lamotrigine) should be used. It has been suggested in the literature that for these drugs to be effective relatively high doses are required, which requires appropriate blood level monitoring. In the USA there has been dramatic increase in the use of divalproex sodium, a preparation of sodium valproate, but the reasons for this are unclear and may include intensive marketing.

Although such an algorithm may be helpful for the initiation of drug therapy, the clinician should be prepared to move flexibly from one group of medications to another, and to give each drug an appropriate trial until a safe and tolerable regimen is found. For many patients, perhaps the majority, some useful drug or drug combination may be found, but some patients do not respond to any medication, and some are worsened by it. 'Behavioural toxicity' may occur, that is, increased aggression with antipsychotics or tricyclics, aggression or suicidal behaviour with SSRIs, disinhibition and aggression with benzodiazepines, and depression with carbamazepine and beta-blockers. It is also important to withdraw medications that appear to be ineffective, as patients can end up taking a mixture of antipsychotics, antidepressants, lithium, a benzodiazepine and other drugs, none of which may be helping. In the treatment of a complex disorder such as borderline personality disorder, medication should be seen as providing only one arm of a comprehensive treatment programme; it cannot of itself change the patient's character, but by dampening down the swings of affective dysregulation it may permit better containment of the disorder and facilitate more prolonged psychotherapy.

Premenstrual syndrome

Around 20–40% of women experience some premenstrual symptoms but these are severe in only 3–5%. The condition was first recognised by R.T. Frank (1931), who described 15 women with severe symptoms, although Hippocrates had described women with mood changes occurring before menstruation. The observation that the premenstrual syndrome (PMS) does not occur before puberty or after the menopause, and the cyclical nature of the symptoms, has led to the suggestion that the hormones involved in ovulation are in some way responsible for the disorder. However, repeated studies have shown that the hormone levels are within the normal range and the cause appears to lie in a differential reactivity between women to normal hormone levels. Aetiology is unknown but there appears to be a definite genetic contribution, as demonstrated by twin studies (van den Akker *et al*, 1987; Kendler *et al*, 1998) and the association with affective disorder – around two-thirds of those presenting to PMS clinics also give a lifetime history of affective disorder (Halbreich & Endicott, 1985). There is commonly also a psychosocial contribution. For example, a high proportion of those presenting for treatment to PMS clinics also give a history of childhood sexual abuse (Golding *et al*, 2000). Most women presenting for treatment are over 30 years of age and the condition is most severe in the 5–10 years before the menopause, but it may be severe from the menarche onwards.

The main psychological symptoms of PMS are depression, irritability and lethargy, but a wide variety of other, mainly neurotic symptoms may also occur. The depression is usually labile, often associated with weeping, in contrast to the fixed, continuous low mood encountered in a depressive illness. A picture of atypical depression with hypersomnia, food craving and a reactive mood occurs in some cases, while in others there is agitation and hostility. Irritability is characteristic; husbands report increased anger or temper premenstrually in their wives.

There are premenstrual phase effects for school marks, the frequency of minor misdemeanours, suicide attempts and hospital admission rates for affective disorder but not schizophrenia. More somatic symptoms include painful swelling of the breasts (mastalgia), swelling of the abdomen, fingers or ankles, impaired efficiency in work tasks and sometimes clumsiness. Among those with a predisposition to migraine, premenstrual headache may be troublesome and premenstrual alcohol craving, heightened sexual urges and brief hypomanic episodes are all described.

For the diagnosis to be made, ICD–10 requires only a history of a single physical or mood symptom occurring on a cyclical basis without functional impairment. DSM–IV recognises a rather more severe variant, termed premenstrual dysphoric disorder (PMDD). The text includes this in an appendix entitled 'Criteria sets and axes for further study' and it is not in the main body of the book, which is an indication that PMDD is not fully accepted as an officially recognised psychiatric disorder but its status is still under consideration. The diagnostic criteria for PMDD are shown in Box 14.5.

To make the diagnosis of PMDD there should be a clear history of a premenstrual exacerbation with a resolution of the symptoms with onset of menstruation or shortly after, and the criteria should be confirmed by prospective daily ratings for at least two cycles. A small number of subjects also report an ovulatory exacerbation. There should also be a clear account that the symptom complex interferes with school, work, relationships or some of other aspect of daily living for a diagnosis of DSM–IV PMDD, but functional impairment is not necessary to diagnose PMS in the ICD–10 scheme. In addition the symptoms should not be due to a premenstrual exacerbation of some other condition such as depression (as sometimes occurs during or following an episode of postnatal depression), panic disorder or dysthymia.

A study of women in the UK, USA and France found that 3–11% of the 1045 women surveyed used a prescription medicine for their PMS, including analgesics, contraceptive pills, non-steriodal anti-inflammatory drugs (NSAIDs) or hormones, while a further 20–30% of the women used a variety of over-the-counter remedies purchased from their chemists, which included acetaminophen, aspirin, evening

---

Box 14.5 The DSM–IV criteria for premenstrual dysphoric disorder

- Clinically significant emotional and behavioural symptoms during the last week of the luteal phase, which remit with the onset of the follicular phase
- At least five of the following 11 symptoms, of which one symptom must be (1), (2), (3) or (4):
    (1) marked depressed mood
    (2) anxiety tension
    (3) anger, irritability, increased interpersonal conflict
    (4) affective lability
    (5) decreased interest
    (6) difficulty in concentrating
    (7) lethargy, lack of energy
    (8) overeating, specific food cravings
    (9) hypersomnia or insomnia
    (10) feeling overwhelmed or out of control
    (11) other physical symptoms, breast tenderness, headaches, muscle pain, feeling bloated.
- The condition should be of sufficient severity to cause marked impairment of social and occupational function
- The condition should have occurred in the majority of the menstrual cycles during the previous year
- The symptoms cannot be explained as an exacerbation of another disorder such as depression, panic disorder or personality disorder

---

primrose oil, vitamins, minerals and other preparations (Hylan *et al*, 1999).

Placebo-controlled trials that used strict inclusion criteria for PMDD have found that 30% of patients improve with placebo, which indicates that non-pharmacogenic remedies may help or that the condition has a fairly high rate of spontaneous remission. Patients presenting with a PMS-like syndrome should be given a full psychiatric evaluation, because the PMS may be no more than a cover for a host of other psychiatric or social difficulties.

Non-pharmacological remedies

These include dietary therapy, exercise, cognitive therapy and relaxation. Dietary recommendations are to increase complex carbohydrates and dietary fibre to 20–40 g daily, to reduce intake of refined sugar and salt, and to take frequent small meals, to lessen the tendency for blood sugar levels to fluctuate (Abraham & Rumley, 1987). However, frank hypoglycaemia has not been demonstrated in PMS. Some authors recommend a reduction in caffeine intake (tea and coffee), which is a generally helpful measure for any anxiety disorder. Exercise is recommended;

although there are no controlled studies, exercise is known to increase brain endorphin levels and in many subjects leads to a feeling of well-being. Twelve sessions of cognitive–behavioural therapy proved to be superior to a programme of group awareness and waiting-list controls, and cognitive therapy seems a promising approach, particularly in the light of its success in other psychiatric disorders (Kirby, 1994). Relaxation therapy is also superior to simply charting the symptoms and leisure reading (Goodale *et al*, 1990). Psycho-educational programmes have also proved helpful and a simple explanation of the origin of the symptoms should form a part of any treatment programme.

Vitamins and minerals

A recent large multi-centre trial of calcium supplements (1200 mg daily in two divided doses) showed that calcium was effective in 48% of cases, compared with 30% for placebo, in reducing all the emotional and physical symptoms of PMDD except for fatigue and insomnia (Thys-Jacobs *et al*, 1998). Magnesium supplements have also been marketed for some time, but a recent study suggested that the daily administration of 200 mg of magnesium was helpful only for reducing fluid retention and had little effect on emotional symptoms (Walker *et al*, 1998).

Vitamin B_6 has been in vogue for many years and comprises a group of compounds that includes pyridoxal and pyridoxamine. It is converted to pyridoxal phosphate, a coenzyme that is essential in the metabolism of most transmitters, including serotonin. Earlier reviews cast doubt on its efficacy, but a recent meta-analysis of nine controlled studies suggested weak beneficial effects for vitamin B_6 in doses of 50–100 mg daily, as well as a relative lack of neurotoxicity for the use of the vitamin at this dosage. However, Schaumberg *et al* (1983) described seven women on mega-dose vitamin therapy (2–6 g vitamin B_6 daily) who had unstable gait, numbness of the hands and peri-oral numbness.

Hormones and hormonal therapies

The fact that PMS is manifest only between the menarche and the menopause and is suppressed during pregnancy strongly suggests its association with ovulation. Strategies to suppress ovulation have therefore been used in its management and these include the use of gonadotrophin-releasing hormone (GnRH) agonists, oestrogen, progesterone and danazol.

Gonadotrophin-releasing hormone agonists

Gonadotrophin-releasing hormone is responsible for the release of the pituitary hormones: follicle-stimulating hormone (FSH), which primes the ovarian follicle; and luteinising hormone (LH), which causes the release of the ovum into the fallopian tube. GnRH agonists cause anovulation by chronic down-regulation of GnRH receptors in the hypothalamus and this leads to decreased secretion of FSH and LH, which in turn results in greatly lowered oestrogen and progesterone levels and anovulation. GnRH agonists (buserelin, leuprorelin acetate, triptorelin) need to be administered either by depot injection or, more commonly, by nasal spray, because oral preparations are metabolised by the liver. Several studies have now shown that these preparations reduce or even abolish the symptoms of PMS.

Although there is some theoretical interest in these preparations, they are difficult to use over the long term in clinical practice because they cause a profound fall in oestrogen levels, which can result in osteoporosis. To counteract this, oestrogen and progesterone can be added back to the regimen, but when this is done mood and anxiety symptoms recur. In a small, well-planned study, Schmidt *et al* (1998) compared a group of women with PMS to controls without PMS who had all been rendered anovulatory for 3 months through the use of monthly injections of the GnRH analogue leuprolide. The women with previous PMS experienced a resurgence of their mood and anxiety symptoms when either oestrogen or progesterone was reintroduced, but this did not happen to the control subjects. The authors suggest that women with PMDD appear to have some kind of intolerance to oestrogen and progesterone in replacement strategies.

Oestradiol

Gynaecologists use oestrogen implants to manage PMS because they suppress ovulation, although oestradiol can be effective without suppression of menstruation. However, by far the most frequent use of oestrogen is as hormone replacement therapy (HRT) for menopausal symptoms and a substantial number of women attending psychiatric clinics are taking HRT. A recent study from Finland reported that 27% of all women between 45 and 65 were taking oestrogen therapy (Hemminiki & Topo, 1997) and it is likely that similar high rates occur over most of the Western world. Thus, even if psychiatrists rarely initiate HRT, many patients in psychiatric clinics will be on it, and so it is important to have some knowledge of oestrogen preparations and their effects.

The major physiological metabolite of oestrogen is 17-β-oestradiol and this is produced in the ovaries. This is the most potent naturally occuring oestrogen, followed by oestrone and oestriol. Non-steroidal substances that have a similar stereochemistry, such as stilboestrol, can mimic the actions of oestrogen. Important physiological actions of oestrogen include stimulation of the secondary sexual characteristics at puberty, myometrial hypertrophy, proliferation of the endometrial lining during the follicular phase, and inhibition of gonadotrophin release. It also has a protective effect on osteoporosis (which is lost during states of oestrogen deficiency).

The unconjugated form of oestradiol is rapidly degraded in the liver, which makes its oral administration impracticable. It is therefore administered by injection, implant or transdermal patches. Side-effects are uncommon in the low doses used in clinical practice but sometimes occur with higher doses. These include nausea and vomiting, weight gain, breast enlargement, tenderness, withdrawal bleeding, sodium retention and occasionally jaundice, thrombosis, rashes, chloasma and depression (*British National Formulary*, 2001). Oestrogen is contra-indicated in pregnancy, oestrogen-dependent cancer, thrombo-embolism, sickle cell disease, undiagnosed vaginal bleeding, herpes gestationis and otosclerosis (as it may worsen the deafness).

The use of oestrogen unopposed by a progestin is associated with an increased risk of endometrial cancer among postmenopausal women, but not premenopausal women. This risk can be reduced by taking cyclical progestins as well. There is a small but definite increase in the risk of breast cancer. Baseline rates for breast cancer are 45/1000 women over a 20-year period. For subjects who use HRT for 5 years this figure rises by two extra cases per 1000, for those using it for 10 years there are six extra cases per 1000 and for those who use HRT for 15 years there are 12 extra cases per 1000 women (*British National Formulary*, 2001). Once breast cancer is diagnosed oestrogen should be stopped as some tumours are sensitive to oestrogen.

Gynaecologists have used oestrogen implants in the treatment of PMS for many years. Several studies show their efficacy in preventing premenstrual migraine. By suppressing ovulation they also appear to help reduce the symptoms of PMS, although a study by Magos *et al* (1984) revealed a very high rate of placebo responders. In that study implants of oestradiol (100 mg) were inserted into the subcutaneous fat of the lower abdominal wall and subjects were also given an oral progestion (5 mg norethysterone) to counteract the risk of unopposed oestrogen causing endometrial cancer.

Implants tend to lose effectiveness after 4–8 months and sometimes rebound depression or anxiety can occur when they do so.

Progesterone and progestins

Progesterone was once fashionable for the treatment of PMS but is no longer recommended, as several placebo-controlled double-blind trials have failed to demonstrate any efficacy for progesterone-based products, including the recently developed oral micronised progesterone. However, the continuous administration of high doses of progestins can cause anovulation. Medroxyprogesterone acetate (MPA) (Provera, or the injectable version, depot Provera) has had some success. Thus, in one trial, women who received 15 mg of MPA daily had a significant reduction in their symptoms compared with those taking either placebo or norethysterone. Ovulation was usually suppressed on this low dosage but breakthrough bleeding was a problem (West, 1990).

Other hormonal therapies

Danazol acts by inhibiting pituitary gonadotrophins. It is mainly anti-oestrogenic and anti-progestogenic and may suppress ovulation, but androgenic side-effects have limited its use. Oral contraceptives have also been investigated and although a few women report improvements others report worsening of symptoms; moreover, placebo-controlled trials show no efficacy. Androgens have also been used, more often for pre- and peri-menopausal symptoms, and it is suggested that they benefit women with decreased libido and fatigue. Dosage is restricted to a narrow therapeutic window in women because there is a risk of virilising side-effects with higher doses (Davis, 1999).

Antidepressants

Reduction in brain serotonin transmission is believed to be associated with poor impulse control, irritability and dysphoria, as well as increased carbohydrate craving, all of which are features of PMDD.

A special drink that results in acute tryptophan depletion lowers central serotonin levels by removing its precursor, L-tryptophan; this drink has been shown to aggravate the symptoms of premenstrual tension (Menkes et al, 1994). In addition, there is one placebo-controlled trial that shows that large doses of L-tryptophan (6 g daily) has a beneficial effect on the mood symptoms of PMDD, which again suggests a role for serotonin (Steinberg et al, 1999). Following a promising open study of small doses of clomipramine, Sunblad et al (1992) conducted a double-blind placebo-controlled trial of clomipramine (a mainly serotonergic tricyclic) in 40 women with PMDD who lacked major depression. They found that premenstrual irritability levels fell by 62% in the active drug group but by only 16% in the placebo group.

Trials of SSRIs, particularly fluoxetine, sertraline, paroxetene and citalopram, have proved to be even more beneficial. There are now over 30 reported studies, including 20 randomised trials involving more than 1100 patients, that show that these drugs are effective and mostly well tolerated in up to 70% of subjects with PMDD (Steiner & Pearlstein, 2000).

The first trial of an SSRI in PMS was described in Menkes et al (1992). They conducted a placebo cross-over trial in 16 women with PMS, 15 of whom improved while on fluoxetine, compared with only three on placebo, and all the women who improved on fluoxetine relapsed when the drug was withdrawn. A larger, more recent controlled trial compared 50–150 mg sertraline with desipramine and placebo in

189 subjects. Daily symptom scores for PMS fell by more than 50% among 65% of the patients who took sertraline but only 36% of those on desipramine and 29% in the placebo group; sertraline was significantly better than desipramine and placebo, with desipramine showing no advantage over placebo (Freeman *et al*, 1999).

Patients appear to respond fairly quickly to low doses of SSRIs and increasing the dosage only leads to more side-effects. Curiously, the somatic symptoms of PMS, such as breast pain, swelling and clumsiness, also improve with SSRI therapy. It is unclear whether this is due to a real decrease in these symptoms or merely a change in perception associated with the better mood. An interesting recent finding has been the demonstration that these drugs are just as effective if given during the luteal phase only (i.e. half-cycle treatment), and in one trial with citalopram intermittent dosing proved to be more effective than continuous dosing (Wikander *et al*, 1998).

The DSM–IV criteria for PMDD require the establishment of impairment of social function (Box 14.5) and one recent study that incorporated quality-of-life measures demonstrated beneficial effects of sertraline on social function (Yonkers *et al*, 1997). Open-label studies have shown these drugs can be used for 12–18 months, but it is important to note that not all patients can tolerate SSRIs over either the short or longer term.

Other medications

A variety of other medications have been used to treat PMS or particular symptoms in the PMS complex, and these have been reviewed by Pearlstein & Steiner (2000).

Diuretics were fashionable for many years to treat 'fluid retention', although direct weighing of subjects who claim to retain fluid reveals relatively small fluctuations in weight. Because thiazides can cause potassium loss, a potassium-sparing diuretic such as spironolactone may be preferable. Ammonium chloride is an old remedy and is combined with caffeine in the over-the-counter remedy Aquaban. Bromocriptine is useful for breast pain but is associated with vomiting and has other side-effects. Prostaglandin-related treatments such as the NSAIDs naproxen and mefaminic acid (although this drug is more commonly used for dysmenorrhoea) have shown some benefits, but the risk of more serious side-effects, such as gastrointestinal haemorrhage or agranulocytosis with mefaminic acid, probably preclude their use in a relatively benign condition such as PMS. Lithium is not effective in PMS but occasional patients with premenstrual hypomania or other exacerbations of bipolar affective disorder may benefit, and in one reported case there was a rise in plasma lithium levels premenstrually despite a constant lithium intake (Kukopulos *et al*, 1985). Other treatments that have been used include evening primrose oil, beta-blockers, calcium channel blockers, thyroxine, light therapy and sleep deprivation.

Among the more severe cases hysterectomy and oophorectomy may be curative because they abolish the menstrual cycle. Usually women who have some other indication for surgery, such as fibroids or endometriosis, but who have also been troubled by PMS for several years elect to have these operations, which must be followed with oestrogen replacement therapy. Cyclical mood changes can occasionally persist after hysterectomy.

Conclusion

Patients presenting with PMS may have a true cyclical disorder and if the symptoms are severe and persistent may qualify for a diagnosis of PMDD, as defined in DSM–IV. Quite commonly, however, women may offer a somatic presentation for other disorders, such as depression, marital disharmony, childhood sexual abuse, or other social pathology, which needs to be clarified before any programme of biological therapy is embarked upon. A useful schema suggested by Johnson (1998) is shown in Box 14.6.

Box 14.6 Selecting an appropriate treatment for premenstrual syndrome (after Johnson, 1998)

Non-pharmacological approaches
Regular meals: high in carbohydrate, low in sugar and salt
Regular aerobic exercises
Stress reduction, for example with cognitive–behavioural therapy

Around 25% respond to the above simple measures

Add an SSRI antidepressant
Initially luteal phase only
Later continuously (if no response)

Trial of ovulation suppression
High-dose oral MPA
Depot MPA every 3 months

Transdermal oestrogen patches with added cyclical progestin
Depot oestrogen preparations

Ovulation suppression (severe cases only)
GnRH agonists with add-back sex hormones (not that such treatments are very expensive)
Oophorectomy – with later HRT (rarely used solely for PMS)

A symptomatic approach is recommended for treatment, and women with the milder cases should be offered the non-pharmacological approaches such as diet, aerobic exercise, psycho-education and, where possible, stress reduction. Specific symptoms should be treated with particular therapies – for example, premenstrual migraine responds well to oestrogen implants, mastalgia to danazol, mood changes and irritability to serotonergic antidepressants. Women with more severe PMS should be offered hormonal therapy, in which ovulation is suppressed, or serotonergic antidepressants. Antipsychotic drugs and the benzodiazepines do not appear to be helpful in cases of PMS. The recent introduction of antidepressants in the treatment of PMS has considerably widened the available therapeutic options, since they can be readily prescribed by the patient's general practitioner or psychiatrist, and do not need to involve a gynaecological or endo-crinological referral.

Erectile dysfunction

Erectile dysfunction is a common disorder. The term refers to the inability to achieve an adequate erection, while the more colloquial 'impotence' covers a wider range of sexual dysfunctions, including loss of desire and ejaculatory disorders, and is less often used to describe erectile failure today. Over the past two decades the management of erectile dysfunction has been transformed, initially by the use of intracavernosal injections, which showed that the condition was amenable to pharmacotherapy, and more recently by the introduction of the oral preparation sildenafil (Viagra), a phosphodiesterase inhibitor, and this has led to a renewed interest in the pathophysiology of erections.

Epidemiology and aetiology of erectile dysfunction

Population surveys such as the Massachusetts Male Ageing Study (Feldman *et al*, 1994) have shown that around 10% of men aged 40–70 suffer from complete erectile dysfunction, 25% from moderate dysfunction and 17% have only minimal dysfunction. Increasing age leads to a decline in sexual activity in both sexes, but sexual activity often persists into old age. For example, Brecher (1984) found that 59% of men over 70 were still having regular coitus with their wives. Traditionally the cause of erectile dysfunction has been regarded as either psychological or organic but in fact an admixture of aetiologies is often present. Thus, in a study of over 400 subjects, psychological factors alone accounted for 29% of the cases and organic factors alone for 40%, while a combination of the two accounted for 25% and in the remainder the aetiology was unknown (Melman *et al*, 1988).

The main organic cause is diabetes mellitus. Thirty per cent of men with treated diabetes suffer from erectile dysfunction, and as many as 55% of those over 60. The direct cause in these cases is usually arteriolar disease or autonomic neuropathy, and this is often associated with ejaculatory disturbances.

Cardiovascular disease, particularly generalised atherosclerosis, may result in erectile dysfunction, while aorto-iliac disease may cause Leriche's syndrome, which comprises erectile dysfunction and intermittent buttock or leg claudication. Around 44% of those who have recently had a myocardial infarction may suffer from erectile dysfunction. Hypertension itself does not cause erectile dysfunction but predisposes to the development of atherosclerosis; moreover, many antihypertensive drugs cause erectile dysfunction. Venogenic erectile dysfunction is usually the result of smooth muscle dysfunction within the penis or rarely cavernoso-spongiosal shunts can cause venous leakage. Up to 85% of men who have had a stroke develop erectile dysfunction but a high proportion recover after 6–8 weeks.

Neurological disorders, particularly spinal cord injury or compression and lesions of the cauda equina (which carries the erectogenic parasympathetic nerves), may be associated with a complete or partial loss of erectile function. In multiple sclerosis there is loss of libido and 70–80% of men with the condition report erectile dysfunction. Other debilitating neurological disorders such as parkinsonism, Alzheimer's and temporal lope epilepsy are also associated with erectile dysfunction, although mechanisms are unclear.

Endocrine disorders such as hypogonadism of any cause may result in erectile dysfunction due to reduced testosterone levels. Hyperprolactinaemia may result in a syndrome of erectile dysfunction, reduced libido and galactorrhoea. This may be due to a prolactinoma but in psychiatric practice is more commonly the result of side-effects of antipsychotic drugs. Hyperthyroidism results in raised oestrogen levels and sex hormone binding globulins, while hypothyroidism results in reduced testosterone secretion, and both can result in erectile dysfunction. Almost any serious or debilitating medical disorder such as cancer or chronic renal failure may cause erectile dysfunction.

Alcohol is known to 'increase the desire but decrease the performance' and alcoholism causes erectile dysfunction through a variety of different mechanisms, including lowered testosterone and raised oestrogen levels, secondary mood disorders and alcoholic polyneuropathy. Cirrhosis itself is not associated with erectile dysfunction unless it is due to haemachromatosis. Smoking reduces penile blood flow, but epidemiological studies do not reveal an overall significantly lower rate of erectile dysfunction among smokers (9%) than among non-smokers (11%), although for men with pre-existing heart disease the rate of dysfunction is 56% for smokers and 21% for non-smokers (Feldman et al, 1994).

The most common cause of erectile dysfunction among those seen in a psychiatric clinic is the use of psychotropic drugs, particularly antidepressants of all classes. Individuals taking on antipsychotics complain less frequently (see below) but may still experience erectile dysfunction. Libido and sexual drive vary widely in the population and there are some men who have a low sex drive from early on, with the pattern showing little variation over a lifetime. Erectile function is normal in these men, but sexual intercourse is infrequently performed.

Psychological aetiologies are less clear-cut, but they may be more relevant for patients presenting to psychiatric clinics and they should be considered if there is an abrupt change in sexual function. Psychological factors should be suspected among physically fit and younger patients. Kaplan (1974) suggests that there are two groups of psychological causes: 'remote', relating to an abusive or dysfunctional childhood, and 'recent', referring to current stresses. Hawton (1985) has updated this scheme and classified significant factors as predisposing, precipitating and maintaining. Among the predisposing factors he includes a repressive (Victorian-type) upbringing, childhood sexual abuse of any type and poor sex education. The last may be associated with myths of harm that can arise out of sexual activity, or other irrational fears that sexual activity is dirty or debilitating, that sex can lead to maltreatment or that indulging in sexual fantasies is wrong. Dislike of a particular aspect of the sexual act, sexual deviations and an inhibited personality type may also contribute. Precipitating factors might include dysfunctional marital and family relationships, acute life stresses, any intercurrent physical or psychiatric disorder, or any break in sexual activity (e.g. after bereavement). Maintaining factors include relationship difficulties, poor communication, diminished feelings of attraction, fears of intimacy (which may relate to childhood problems) and lifestyle problems (e.g. preoccupation with work or financial worries). These factors may additionally give rise to performance anxiety.

Erectile dysfunction can have a significant effect on a relationship. One survey found that 21% of subjects with erectile dysfunction reported that their relationship had broken down and a further 9% reported relationship difficulties. Erectile dysfunction alone does not cause serious psychiatric disorder, such as major depression or schizophrenia, but it may be the result of such conditions or the drugs used to treat them; however, it is commonly associated with anxiety, mild depression and low self-esteem. The successful treatment of erectile dysfunction in such cases is associated with a marked improvement in the depression, for example (Seidman et al, 2000).

Physiology of erections

The physiology of normal erections is immensely complicated – it involves many different transmitters and biochemical mechanisms acting on trabecular smooth muscle in the corpora cavernosa penis, as well as central mechanisms. The subject is reviewed by Eardley & Sethia (1998), from which this account is drawn. Haemodynamic, neuronal and biochemical mechanisms are all involved and it is convenient to consider each separately.

Haemodynamic mechanisms

In the flaccid state, the arterioles of the penis are constricted and under dominant sympathetic influence. Blood flow to the penis is limited to around 15 ml/min and the trabecular smooth muscle is contracted, which keeps the sinusoids closed. Parasympathetic stimulation leads to arteriolar dilatation and blood flow rises to 30 ml/min; this is accompanied by relaxation of the trabecular smooth muscle, with resultant expansion and filling of the sinusoids. As the pressure in the corpora cavernosa rises, there is increasing pressure on the venous plexus below the tunica albuginea – the sub-tunical venous plexus – and this is gradually occluded and so venous outflow is blocked. Once intracavernosal pressure rises above diastolic blood pressure, blood enters only during the systolic phase and with outflow partially blocked the penis gradually elongates and becomes rigid, with intracavernosal pressure finally rising to around 90% of systolic blood pressure. This process is reversed during detumescence.

Neuronal mechanisms

The parasympathetic system, which governs the primary erectile mechanism, originates from the sacral spinal cord (S2, S3 and S4), passes in the cauda equina to the erigens nerves, to the pelvic plexus and then on the cavernosal nerves into the penis. Acetylcholine acting on M_2 and M_3 muscarinic receptors appears to be the main para-sympathetic neurotransmitter involved in this system, with receptors both on trabecular smooth muscle and on the arterioles.

The sympathetic system is more concerned with maintaining the flaccid state. It has its origins in the thoraco-lumbar cord (T11, T12, L1 and L2) and passes out of the spinal cord in the ventral roots to the hypogastric plexus, then to the pelvic plexus and in the cavernosal nerves into the penis. Available evidence suggests these are mainly α_1-noradrenergic pathways. Thus the intracavernosal injection of the α_1-adrenoreceptor antagonist phenoxybenzamine results in an erection, which can be reduced by metaraminol (an α-adrenoreceptor agonist) (the drug is in fact used to treat prolonged drug-induced erections). Intracavernosal injection of the specific α_1-receptor blocker moxisylyte is helpful for some men with erectile dysfunction, whereas the α_2-receptor blocker idazoxam has no tumescent effect. Although β-receptors, particularly β_2-receptors, are present in the penis, their role is unclear because injection of agonists such as salbutamol or antagonists such as propanolol have little effect.

The central control of erections is complex and depends on an intact hypothalamus, medial pre-optic nucleus and paraventricular nucleus. Projections from these nuclei descend in the spinal cord to the spinal nuclei that innervate the penis. Central noradrenaline, dopamine, serotonin, prolactin and melanocyte-stimulating hormone may also play a role. It is thought that the mesolimbic 'pleasure centre', which uses dopamine as the 'pleasure' neurotransmitter, may play a role. Thus drugs that boost dopamine, such as bupropion, methyphenidate, amphetamine and apomorphine, enhance sexual activity, whereas dopamine blockers such as the antipsychotics diminish sexual activity. Serotonin may block the release of dopamine and also, via the 5-HT$_2$ receptor, may block ejaculatory and orgasmic responses. Thus the SSRIs inhibit sex, but antidepressants that specifically block 5-HT$_2$ receptors, such as nefazodone and mirtazepine, do not cause these problems. As stated above, lesions to the brain, spinal cord or cauda equina may all also impair or abolish erectile function.

Erections are commonly considered to be of three types. Psychogenic erections occur in association with visual, imaginative or erotic stimuli and depend on an intact CNS and autonomic system. Their frequency decreases with age. Nocturnal and early-morning erections occur during rapid-eye-movement sleep, and their loss usually signifies some organic problem. Non-psychogenic reflex erections occur in response to tactile stimulation of the penis; they depend on an intact spinal cord but may still occur after some spinal cord damage.

Biochemical mechanisms

Smooth-muscle relaxation in the trabecular muscles of the penis permits the sinusoids to fill up with blood and enlarge, and this results in an erection. The most important substance inducing smooth-muscle relaxation is nitric oxide (NO), which is synthesised from its precursor L-arginine by the enzyme nitric oxide synthetase. Two subtypes of this enzyme exist, one in the parasympathetic nerve terminals and the other in the endothelium of the blood vessels and trabecular tissue. Nitric oxide is strongly lipophilic and so diffuses rapidly across cell membranes and enters the smooth-muscle cell. It has a half-life of around 5 seconds but once in the smooth-muscle cell it stimulates the enzyme guanylate cyclase, which converts guanosine triphosphate (GTP) into cyclic guanosine monophosphate (cGMP).

cGMP is the 'second messenger' and it stimulates an intracellular enzyme, protein kinase C, which simultaneously opens the potassium channels and closes off the L-type calcium channel. These electrolyte changes result in membrane depolarisation and smooth-muscle relaxation.

The activity of cGMP is then terminated by another group of enzymes, the phosphodiesterases (PDEs), which convert it to the inactive non-cyclic GMP. Sildenafil acts as a powerful inhibitor of one of these enzymes, PDE-5, and this results in a much slower breakdown of cGMP, and hence an enhanced action of NO and prolonged smooth-muscle relaxation.

Although these mechanisms probably explain in a simplified form the action of sildenafil, many other substances appear to have a direct or modulating role in promoting erections. These include a locally made peptide from the endothelium, various prostaglandins, including PGF_2a, PGE_2, PGI_2, thromboxane A_2, vasointestinal polypeptide, neuropeptide Y, angiotension, and arginine vasopressin, which is found in high concentrations in cavernosal tissue, but precise mechanisms have yet to be clarified.

Assessment

Patients with erectile dysfunction should be assessed for both psychological and organic factors; the latter should be suspected among older patients, particularly if there is a loss of nocturnal or early-morning erections. Among those attending psychiatric clinics, the history often reveals a high incidence of irrational fears concerning sexuality, relationship difficulties, deviancy, stresses and other causes outlined above, which sometimes respond to simple discussion.

Physical examination should focus on secondary sexual characteristics, distribution of body hair and fat, blood pressure, peripheral pulses, reflexes and peripheral sensation, particularly if the patient has diabetes, hepatomegaly or other stigmata of alcoholism. The size and shape of the penis should be checked to exclude Peyronie's disease. If indicated, prostrate examination may be required. All patients should have a blood sugar test, since diabetes is the commonest organic cause, and other endocrine tests should include plasma testosterone, prolactin and thyroid function, although abnormalities are uncommon. More specialised investigations fall into the province of the urologists and these include Doppler ultrasonography to measure systolic pulse pressure in the penile artery, to detect vascular disease, possibly followed by arteriography. Cavernosometry and cavernosography can detect venous leaks, while penile plethysmography and other tests of autonomic function may detect venous shunts or other causes and may be required if reparative surgery is being considered.

Psychological interventions

Psychotherapy or couple counselling should be offered to all patients, and should be first-line therapy for younger patients whose early-morning erections are preserved, as an organic aetiology is less likely in such cases. Where the history reveals difficulties early on in life or distorted or repressive ideas concerning sexuality, individual therapy may be helpful. More often the presentation is of distress associated with erectile dysfunction in a marriage in which the quality of communication is poor. Psychotherapy directed at improving the marriage may be helpful, but specific therapy usually revolves around the sensate focus technique. In this method the couple are initially banned from attempting sexual intercourse or touching the erogenous zones. Very gradually the couple are permitted to touch different areas and finally the erogenous zones, and when the couple feel confident enough they proceed to full sexual intercourse. The method is successful in around a third of cases. A more comprehensive account of psychological approaches is given by Crowe & Ridley (1990).

Oral treatments

Although a variety of local treatments and topical applications of drugs to the urethra were developed in the 1980s (see below), oral treatments are gradually superseding these in the management of both organic and non-organic cases. Sildenafil (Viagra) is a potent phosphodiesterase inhibitor which inhibits PDE-5 and has definite effects on erectile activity in humans. Phosphodiesterases are widely distributed and 11 homologous families situated on 22 genes, with a total of 45 types, have been isolated. Most involve the breakdown of cyclic adenosine monophosphate (cAMP) but a few involve the breakdown of cGMP. In the cavernosal smooth muscle PDE types 2, 3, 4 and 5 have been isolated, while type 6 is present in retinal photoreceptors. Theophylline and papaverine inhibit phosphodiesterases non-specifically, while dipyramidole, zipranast and sildenafil are specific PDE-5 inhibitors. Dipyramidole is a vasodilator but has no effect on erectile function, while zipranast has some erectile effects in the cat. Sildenafil is 100 times more potent as a PDE-5 inhibitor than either dipyramidole or zipranast and so it is not surprising that it has significant effects on erectile function. By increasing levels of cGMP it potentiates NO action in the penis and so prolongs the relaxation of smooth muscle and promotes or prolongs erections.

Large-scale trials have demonstrated efficacy for sildenafil for both organic and non-organic impotence. Thus, in one trial of 351 men with erectile dysfunction of no established cause, 89% of subjects responded to 50 mg sildenafil compared with 38% on placebo (Gingell *et al*, 1996).

Response rates among subjects with a known organic cause are somewhat lower; for example, 64% of a group of men with diabetes responded, compared with 10% of those on placebo (Boulton *et al*, 2001), while among a group of subjects with spinal cord injuries, where the erectile dysfunction was previously thought to be irreversible, sexual intercourse was successful in 55% of subjects on sildenafil compared to 0% on placebo (Guiliano *et al*, 1998).

Sildenafil

Sildenafil is available as 25, 50 and 100 mg tablets and dosage should be titrated to a clinically useful response. Peak plasma levels occur within 1 hour but in a semi-fasted patient may be reached in 30 minutes. The drug has a half-life of around 4 hours. It does not cause erections unless there is associated sexual stimulation and hence should be taken 30–60 minutes before sexual activity.

Its side-effects are predictable and include vasculogenic effects (e.g. dizziness and flushing) and around 5% of subjects also report dyspepsia, thought be due to the presence of PDE-5 at the gastro-oesophageal junction. Transient visual disturbance (e.g. an increased perception of bright light and the presence of a bluish tinge) are due to inhibition of PDE-6 on retinal photoreceptors. Because of its effects on NO metabolism, sildenafil is absolutely contraindicated for those taking nitrates (e.g. glyceryl trinitrate for angina) or with conditions in which vasodilatation or sexual activity is inadvisable. The manufacturer suggests it is contraindicated in Peyronie's disease, and in patients who have recently had a stroke or myocardial infarction, where blood pressure is below 90/50 mmHg, or among those with hereditary degenerative retinal disorders. In the UK at present the drug is available only from specialist centres within the National Health Service but it is available on private prescription and its use is increasing rapidly.

Sublingual apomorphine

Apomorphine, a dopamine (D_2) receptor agonist, was observed to cause occasional erections when used to treat Parkinson's disease and can produce erections in normal men. It acts in the paraventricular nucleus of the hypothalamus through dopaminergic stimulation via oxytocinergic pathways, but has no local effect on trabecular smooth muscle. Because it acts only in the CNS, it is effective only in the presence of some sexual stimulation. Without this it does not cause erections, nor does it increase libido. In a large phase III trial in subjects with diverse aetiologies of erectile dysfunction, 46% of subjects taking 2 mg responded, compared with 34% on placebo, and for the 3 mg tablet there was a response rate of 47%, compared with 32% on placebo.

Sublingual apomorphine (Uprima) is available as 2 mg and 3 mg tablets. It is rapidly absorbed – peak levels are attained in around 40–60 minutes. Side-effects include nausea, headache, dizziness, yawning, rhinitis, somnolence, pain, flushing, taste disorder and sweating. The drug is contraindicated for patients with angina, recent myocardial infarction or hypotension. It should be used with caution in the elderly or with other centrally acting dopaminergic agents or other treatments of erectile dysfunction. Because it has only just been introduced, its role in the treatment of erectile dysfunction has yet to be clarified.

Other oral agents

A number of other oral agents have some effects on erectile dysfunction but are now rarely used. Yohimbine was considered an aphrodisiac for more than a century. It is a reversible α_2-adrenoreceptor antagonist and sometimes helps psychogenic erectile dysfunction but has no effect on organic cases. Phentolamine is also an α-adrenoreceptor antagonist but has limited effects when taken orally and is more effective when given by intracavernosal injection (see below). Bromocriptine may be effective in cases of erectile dysfunction due to hyperprolactinaemia, provided testosterone levels are normal.

Androgen replacement therapy

Androgen replacement therapy is effective in cases of established hypogonadism but loss of sexual function will occur in hypogonadal men as soon as testosterone replacement therapy is withdrawn. However, the response rates for normal men who are found to have low testosterone levels is generally disappointing. Morales *et al* (1994) showed that only 9% of men responded to testosterone (10 mg three times a day); the best results were obtained by those with lowest initial testosterone levels.

Because testosterone is rapidly metabolised (it has a half-life of around 10 minutes), testosterone esters have been developed to delay its absorption. Thus the 17β-hydroxylated ester is given intramuscularly in an oil-based preparation as a pellet and this can last up to 3 months. Intramuscular injections of testosterone propionate or enanthate last around 3 weeks and recently acceptable skin patches have been developed. Side-effects of testosterone include weight gain due to sodium and water retention, a rise in haemoglobin, gynaecomastia, headache, anxiety, acne, hirsutism and various liver complications, including cholestatic jaundice, hepatitis, peliosis hepatis (cystic changes with bleeding) and, rarely, hepatocellular carcinoma. Testosterone preparations are contraindicated among subjects with prostate or breast cancer, ischaemic heart disease and hypercalcaemia.

Intracorporeal injection therapy

The introduction of intracorporeal injection therapy by Virag (1982) and Brindley (1983) revolutionised the treatment of erectile dysfunction in the 1980s. The first drug to be used was papaverine, a non-specific phosphodiesterase inhibitor, but it is less effective than some of the newer agents. Phenoxybenzamine, a non-selective α-blocker which reduces sympathetic tone, was also used in early trials but because of its prolonged half-life it had an unacceptably high rate of complications (penile pain, prolonged erection, priaprism and cavernous sinus thrombosis). Phentolamine is an $α_1$- and $α_2$-adrenoreceptor blocking agent that has little effect on its own but can be combined with other agents. Moxisylyte is a selective $α_1$-adrenoreceptor blocking agent associated with a low rate of side-effects and is widely used in France.

The most effective and widely used drug is prostaglandin E_1 (PGE_1, alprostadil). It acts on membrane receptors to stimulate the action of the enzyme adenylate cyclase, which converts adenosine triphosphate to cAMP, and this in turn opens calcium channels and the fall in intracellular calcium results in smooth-muscle relaxation.

These agents are sometimes combined together in an agent called Trimix, which is popular in the USA and consists of PGE_1, papaverine and phentolamine, which is claimed to maximise efficacy while minimising side-effects.

The technique of injection is relatively simple for the clinician but it needs to be taught to the patient for home use. The penis is drawn across the thigh and the injection is made around 1–2 cm from the base directly into the corpora cavernosa, with care being taken to avoid any veins. A small amount of blood is aspirated to ensure the needle is not in any major vein and then the drug is slowly injected. The penis is then gently massaged for approximately 30 seconds to distribute the drug and a typical response appears some 5–10 minutes later. A more detailed and illustrated account is given by Eardley & Sethia (1998).

Intracavernosal injection is undoubtedly effective and a meta-analysis (Junemann et al, 1996) found an efficacy of 45% for papaverine, 70% for papaverine and phentolamine, 75% for PGE_1 and 80% for Trimix. The main complications are penile pain, prolonged erection, priapism, bruising and corporeal fibrosis. If the drug enters the systemic circulation, hypotension and flushing may occur. The high drop-out rate from this technique led to a search for less invasive methods of applying drugs locally.

Topical applications

Glyceryl trinitrin, an NO donor, when applied topically to the skin of the penis can sometimes result in an erection. Unfortunately, topical creams are absorbed through the vagina and so side-effects such as headache may be experienced by both partners during sexual activity, which is hardly ideal. PGE_1 and minoxidil, a vasodilator claimed to reverse male-pattern baldness, have also been applied topically.

A substance called Triple Cream contains: 3% aminophylline, which is converted to theophylline, a non-specific PDE inhibitor; 0.25% isosorbide dinitrate, an NO donor; and 0.05% co-dergocine, an α-adrenergic blocker. It is claimed to be successful in 60% of cases, compared with only 8% for placebo (Gomaa *et al*, 1996). It should be applied in a thin layer to the glans and shaft of the penis 15 minutes before sex.

Inserting active agents into the urethra avoids the pain of injection and the risk of the partner absorbing the drug. The Medicated Uretheral System for Erection (MUSE) is a proprietary drug-delivery system for delivering PGE_1 (alprostadil) into the urethra. Although initial trials suggested a response rate of over 60%, a more recent study found a response rate of only 30%, and 80% of subjects discontinued treatment because of side-effects (Fulgam *et al*, 1998).

Vacuum devices

These devices consist of two components: a cylinder, which is placed over the penis; and a constriction ring, which is placed around the base of the penis. Air is pumped out of the cylinder to create a partial vacuum and the negative pressure on the skin of the penis results in blood being drawn into the corpora cavernosa, while the constriction ring helps to occlude venous outflow. There are conflicting reports as to how successful these devices are, with published reports claiming success in 26–80% of patients. Men who find these methods useful are able to continue using them for much longer than the more invasive techniques.

Surgery

Peyronie's disease is characterised by the formation of fibrotic plaques within the tunica albuginea of the penis. This results in pain and curvature of the penis during erections. It may be associated with Dupuytren's contracture, tympanosclerosis and thickening of the plantar fascia. Although it may occur at any age, it most commonly presents in the 40–60 age group, where its prevalence is between 0.4% and 1%. Physical examination reveals a lump on the penis, which can be excised; this is followed by reparative surgery with an appropriate graft.

Other indications for surgery include cavernoso-venous shunts, arterial disease, surgery for arterial disease and the insertion of a penile prosthesis. Surgery for the treatment of impotence alone is now rarely performed but operative techniques are described by Eardley & Sethia (1998).

Pharmacological treatment of the paraphilias: the use of male sexual suppressant drugs

Each year in the USA somewhere between 100 000 and 500 000 children are sexually molested by men. Those convicted are usually incarcerated for long periods, a strategy that has not been successful, but for which the costs were estimated to be a staggering $2 billion in 1990 (Bradford, 1998). The most serious of the paraphilias recognised in DSM–IV and ICD–10, because they which result in dangerous antisocial acts, are paedophilia and sexual sadism/sadomasochism (ICD–10). There is no established treatment for either disorder, but for a small number of subjects, particularly where there is associated hypersexuality, attempts have been made to treat patients with drugs that suppress androgen secretion and so abolish sexual desire and sexual fantasies.

In a recent review of the treatment of the paraphilias, Bradford (2001) draws parallels between the paraphilias and obsessive–compulsive disorder (OCD). He points out that sexual fantasies show some resemblence to obsessional thoughts, while compulsive rituals are similar to compulsive sexual behaviour, which can be paraphilic or non-paraphilic. In both OCD and sexual disorders there may be involvement of the serotonergic neurotransmission systems. Paraphilic behaviour may also sometimes appear in the spectrum of disinhibited behaviours associated with some organic brain disorders, such as temporal lobe epilepsy, Tourette's syndrome, frontal and temporal lobe lesions, septal lesions, post-encephalitic neuropsychiatric syndromes and multiple sclerosis. It is noteworthy also that the coprolalia and copropraxia of Tourette's syndrome usually have a sexual component. Compulsive sexual behaviours include masturbation, the use of pornography, promiscuity, telephone sex, dependence on sexual accessories and the use of drugs such as inhaled nitrate. Compulsive sexual behaviour is usually normal and only rarely of a paraphilic type. The observation that OCD responds well to the SSRIs stimulated an interest in the use of these drugs in the management of paraphilias.

Studies of comorbidity of patients with paraphilias have also high-lighted the importance of impulsivity and a history of ADHD. Kafka & Prentky (1998) found that around 50% of a group of patients with paraphilias (offenders and non-offenders) had a history of ADHD, but there was also a high prevalence of mood disorders (dysthymia 69%; major depression 48%; anxiety disorder 43%; panic disorder 12%). Although the authors did not specifically examine for adult ADHD, they observed a clustering of other axis I psychiatric morbidity among the subjects with ADHD, and suggested that the type of dysregulation found in ADHD also made a significant contribution to paraphilic behaviour.

Hypersexuality in men is poorly defined. Sex drive may normal, low or high and sexual behaviour may sometimes be compulsive with or without a paraphilia. Subjects who are hypersexual and have a compulsive, dangerous paraphilia such as paedophilia or sadomasochism pose a serious threat to society, and an important therapeutic challenge, particularly as the disorder may be lifelong. It is to this group that anti-androgen therapy is particularly directed.

The logic for using anti-androgen therapy for this group of subjects derives in part from studies of androgen replacement therapy in hypogonadal men, which have shown that as soon as testosterone is withdrawn all sexual behaviour, fantasies and desire disappear. This confirms the critical role of androgens in male sexual behaviour. The principal androgens in the human male are testosterone and dihydro-testosterone. Receptors for both these hormones are found in the brain, particularly in the septal region, the pituitary and hypothalamus; they are also located intracellularly. Testosterone may be aromatised to oestradiol in the hypothalamus and elsewhere, and this may also be related to sexual drive. Various other monoamine transmitters, particularly serotonin and dopamine, may also be involved, but precise mechanisms are unclear.

At a clinical level, sexual drive consists of several different components:

(1)   a psychological wish to engage in sexual activity (the sexual equivalent of hunger)
(2)   sexual fantasies, which may be paraphilic or non-paraphilic
(3)   a state of sexual arousal, which provides motivation for seeking out sexual activity
(4)   sexual activity itself, which generally results in an orgasm.

Pharmacological agents have been identified that can affect all four components of sexual drive and there are three main interventions, the SSRIs, the anti-androgen drugs and the GnRH analogues.

Selective serotonin reuptake inhibitors

Loss of sexual drive is one of the more prominent side-effects of the SSRIs, and this has been used with advantage to treat subjects with the milder paraphilias. In an open-label trial of sertraline (100 mg daily) for men with paraphilia and non-paraphilic hypersexuality, Kafka (1994) found significant reductions in deviant sexual fantasies, masturbation and both deviant and non-deviant sexual behaviour. Around 50% of the subjects improved and those who did not respond were offered fluoxetine, at a mean dosage of 51.1 mg daily. Of the sertraline non-responders, 60% showed some clinical improvement.

Greenberg *et al* (1996) reported a retrospective assessment of 58 subjects to whom sertraline, fluoxetine and citalopram had been given. They showed that the three SSRIs were equally effective in reducing deviant sexual fantasies and behaviours.

There has been a suggestion that SSRIs suppress of deviant sexuality more than they do the normal sexual response, which would make them the treatment of choice for subjects with the milder paraphilias and non-paraphilic hypersexuality.

Anti-androgens and hormonal agents

Oestrogens were the first hormones to be used in the treatment of the paraphilias but weight gain and feminising effects (e.g. the development of breasts) proved to be unacceptable side-effects. The two most commonly used drugs are medroxyprogesterone acetate (Provera), which is a progestogen, and cyproterone acetate (CPA), although the latter drug is unavailable in the USA.

Medroxyprogesterone acetate (MPA) blocks the secretion of gonado-trophins and it also induces the enzyme testosterone reductase, which decreases circulating levels of testosterone, but it does not compete with testosterone at the receptor level. Side-effects in men include weight gain, decreased sperm production, a tendency to precipitate diabetes, headache, deep-vein thrombosis, hot flushes, nausea and feminisation. Several open studies (for review see Bradford, 2001) have shown that weekly injections of 300–400 mg MPA significantly reduce sexual fantasies, and individual case studies using penile plethysmography show decreased nocturnal penile tumescence as well as decreased penile tumescence among paedophiles who have been shown erotic stimuli. The recidivism rate was also lower among a group of subjects who agreed to take MPA than among a group of treatment refusers (18% of those on active drug compared with 35% of treatment refusers), although pharmacological effects may not be the sole explanation for this finding.

Cyproterone acetate (CPA) is a competitive inhibitor of testosterone and dihydrotestosterone at androgen receptors throughout the body and it also blocks intracellular molecular testosterone receptors. Its main use in clinical medicine is in the treatment of prostratic cancer, which is often sensitive to testosterone. CPA has progestational activity and reduces levels of FSH and LH. The acetate radical is crucial for its action and cyproterone without the acetate has no anti-gonadotropic effects. Androgen receptor blockade results in a decrease in all types of sexual activity, including deviant and non-deviant sexual fantasies and behaviour, as well as erections. CPA can be given orally or by intra-muscular injection. Laschet & Laschet (1971) reported a series of 100 sexually deviant men, mainly exhibitionists and paedophiles, of whom around half were offenders. Subjects were given CPA either as a daily oral dose of 100 mg or as an intramuscular injection of 300 mg every 2 weeks. Most patients showed reductions in deviant sexual fantasies and behaviours but the treatment effects were not dramatic. For example, only 20% of exhibitonists showed a complete elimination of deviant sexual behaviour. Bradford & Pawlack (1993) conducted a placebo cross-over trial with a group of men who met DSM–III–R criteria for paedophilia and who had an average of 2.5 convictions for sexual offences. Sexual behaviour and sexual fantasies were significantly reduced, but the reduction in sexual arousal just failed to reach significance. One advantage of treatment with CPA appears to be that it is reasonably well tolerated, and some patients have been on the drug for up to 8 years.

Gonadotrophin agonists

Treatment with MPA or CPA does not always work because the suppression of testosterone is often incomplete. A more radical hormonal solution can be achieved with the use of an analogue of GnRH, which acts by inhibiting the secretion of LH and FSH. In a remarkable study, Rösler & Witzum (1998) gave a GnRH analogue, triptorelin, by monthly injections (of 3.75 mg) to a group of 30 men with severe paraphilias. All 30 had complained of uncontrollable sexual drives; 25 were paedophiles and the remainder had a variety of other sexual disorders. More than half the men had been in prison (3–8 times each) and the average number of episodes of abnormal sexual behaviour was around five per month. Some subjects had previously failed on CPA and others had failed on a variety of other psychotropic drugs, including the SSRIs. All the men volunteered for the study and were given supportive psychotherapy throughout the trial. A decision was made to exclude a placebo comparison, in case a subject in the placebo arm of the trial committed an offence.

The results were dramatic: almost all of the men had a prompt reduction in all paraphilic activity during therapy. The greatest decrease in the intensity of sexual desire and symptom scores occurred 3–10 months after therapy. Deviant sexual fantasies and urges disappeared completely and not a single offence against a child or any acts of exhibitionism, voyeurism or frotteurism were committed during the trial. Three patients who stopped treatment because of side-effects were given CPA instead, but all reoffended and were sentenced to prison for sex crimes. Six men also ceased treatment becaused they wished to father children (once the drug is stopped testosterone secretion rapidly increases) but in all cases there was a relapse of deviant sexuality.

These benefits were associated with quite severe side-effects. Serum testosterone fell from a mean of 545 ng/dl (normal range 280–870) to 26 ng/dl 6 months into the trial. Testicular volume decreased by 50% after 36 months, none of the men over 35 could maintain an erection or achieve intercourse, and in 11 of the 18 men (61%) who had measurements in the lumbar spine and femoral neck there was evidence of decreasing bone density/osteoporosis. These changes were treated with calcium and vitamin D supplements. The authors commented that non-compliance was not a problem in this study, even though none of the patients was legally bound to take the treatment. It is likely that they were aware from their own personal histories that without therapy reoffending and further periods of incarceration were a strong possibility.

Conclusions

Paraphilias vary in both type and severity, and drastic treatments are needed only for the more severe, persistent and dangerous cases. The aim in all cases is to reduce deviant sexual behaviour and fantasies, and so reduce the risk of recidivism and victimisation. Bradford (2001) proposes different levels of therapeutic intervention:

(1) At the lowest level, a simple cognitive–behavioural treatment and relapse prevention programme should be offered to all subjects.

(2) For mild to moderate paraphilias, treatment with an SSRI may be helpful, but if this does not work and the disorder is clinically significant an anti-androgen should be added to the regimen. A typical pharamacological regimen might be sertraline (200 mg daily) combined with oral MPA (50 mg daily) or CPA (50 mg daily).

(3) For the more severe cases, the full anti-androgen regimens would have to be instituted, usually doses of 50–300 mg MPA or 50–300 mg CPA. Where certainty that the drugs had been taken was deemed necessary, regimens based on intramuscular injections, for example weekly injections of 300 mg MPA or fortnightly injections of 200 mg CPA, would be required.

(4) For the most severe cases, complete suppression of androgen secretion with the use of a GnRH agonist could be offered to subjects. This is often, but not always, highly effective.

The use of such drug regimens should be confined to specialist forensic units with a particular interest in these disorders, and the more drastic regimens require full endocrinological support. There appears to be more interest in these regimens in the USA, Canada and some European countries such as The Netherlands and Germany – there is little published work from the UK.

References

Abraham, G. E. & Rumley, R. E. (1987) Role of nutrition in managing premenstrual tension syndromes. *Journal of Reproductive Medicine*, **32**, 405–422.

American Psychiatric Association (1994) *Diagnostic and Statistical Manual of Mental Disorders* (4th edn) (DSM–IV). Washington, DC: APA.

Boulton, A. J., Selam, J. L., Sweeney, M., *et al* (2001) Sildenafil citrate for the treatment of erectile dysfunction in men with type II diabetes mellitus. *Diabetologia*, **44**, 1296–1301.

Bradford, J. M. W. (1998) Treatment of men with paraphilia. *New England Journal of Medicine*, **338**, 464–465.

Bradford, J. M. W. (2001) The neurobiology, neuropharmacology, and pharmacological treatment of the paraphilias and compulsive sexual behaviour. *Canadian Journal of Psychiatry*, **46**, 26–33.

Bradford, J. M. W. & Pawlack, A. (1993) Double blind placebo crossover trial of cyproterone acetate in the treatment of the paraphilias. *Archives of Sexual Behaviour*, **22**, 383–402.

Brecher, E. M. (1984) *Love, Sex and Aging: A Consumers' Union Report*. Boston, MA: Little, Brown.

Brindley, G. S. (1983) Cavernosal alpha-blockade: a new technique for investigating and treating erectile impotence. *British Journal of Psychiatry*, **143**, 332–337.

Brinkley, J., Beitman, D. & Friedel, R. (1979) Low dose neuroleptic regimens in the treatment of borderline patients. *Archives of General Psychiatry*, **36**, 319–326.

British National Formulary (2001) *British National Formulary*. London: British Medical Association and Royal Pharmaceutical Society of Great Britain.

Calabrese, J. R., Bowden, C. L., Sachs, G. S., *et al* (1999) A double blind placebo-controlled study of lamotrigine monotherapy in outpatients with bipolar I depression. *Journal of Clinical Psychiatry*, **60**, 79–88.

Chengappa, K. N., Ebeling, T., Kang, J. S., *et al* (1999) Clozapine reduces self-mutilation and aggression in psychotic patients with borderline personality disorder. *Journal of Clinical Psychiatry*, **60**, 477–484.

Citrome, L., Levine, J. & Allingham, B. (1998) Utilization of valproate: extent of inpatient use in the New York State Office of Mental Health. *Psychiatric Quarterly*, **69**, 283–300.

Coccaro, E. F. & Kavoussi, R. J. (1997) Fluoxetine and impulsive–aggressive behaviour in personality disordered subjects. *Achives of General Psychiatry*, **54**, 1081–1088.

Cornelius, J. R., Soloff, P. H., Perel, J. M., *et al* (1993) Continuation pharmacotherapy of borderline personality disorder with haloperidol and phenelzine. *American Journal of Psychiatry*, **150**, 1843–1848.

Cowdrey, R. W. & Gardner, D. L. (1988) Pharmacotherapy of borderline personality disorder. Alprazolam, carbamazepine, trifluoperazine, and tranylcypromine. *Archives of General Psychiatry*, **45**, 111–120.

Craft, M., Ismail, I. A., Krishnamurti, D., *et al* (1987) Lithium in the treatment of aggression in mentally handicapped patients: a double-blind trial. *British Journal of Psychiatry*, **150**, 685–689.

Crowe, M. & Ridley, J. (1990) *Therapy with Couples: A Behavioural–Systems Approach to Marital and Sexual Problems*. Oxford: Blackwell.

Davis, S. R. (1999) Androgen treatment in women. *Medical Journal of Australia*, **172**, 46.

De La Fuenta, J. M. & Lotstra, F. (1994) A trial of carbamazepine in borderline personality disorder. *European Neuropsychopharmacology*, **4**, 479–486.

Dostal, T. & Zvolsky, P. (1970) Anti-aggressive effects of lithium salts in severely retarded adolescents. *International Pharmaco-psychiatry*, **5**, 203–207.

Eardley, I. & Sethia, K. (1998) *Erectile Dysfunction: Current Investigations and Management*. London: Mosby–Wolfe.

Feldman, H. A., Goldstein, I., Hatzichristou, D., *et al* (1994) Impotence and its medical and psychological correlates: results of the Massachusetts Male Ageing Study. *Journal of Urology*, **151**, 54–61.

Frank, R. T. (1931) The hormonal basis of premenstrual tension. *Archives of Neurology and Psychiatry*, **26**, 1053–1057.

Freeman, E. W., Rickels, K., Sondheimer, S. J., *et al* (1999) Differential response to antidepressants in women with premenstrual syndrome/premenstrual dysphoric disorder: a randomized controlled trial. *Archives of General Psychiatry*, **56**, 932–939.

Fulgam, P. F., Cochran, J. S., Denman, J. L., *et al* (1998) Disappointing initial results with transurethral alprostadil for erectile dysfunction in a urology practice setting. *Journal of Urology*, **160**, 2041–2046.

Gingell, J. C., Jardin, A., Olsson, A. M., *et al* (1996) UK-92, 480, a new oral treatment for erectile dysfunction: a double blind placebo-controlled, once daily dose response study. *Journal of Urology*, **155** (suppl.), 495A.

Golding, J. M., Taylor, D. L., Menard, L., *et al* (2000) Prevalence of sexual abuse history in a sample of women seeking treatment for premenstrual syndrome. *Journal of Psychosomatic Obstetrics and Gynaecology*, **21**, 69–80.

Gomaa, A., Shalaby, M., Osman, M., *et al* (1996) Topical treatment of erectile dysfunction: randomised double blind placebo controlled trial of cream containing aminophylline, isosorbide dinitrate and co-dergocrine mesylate. *BMJ*, **312**, 1512–1515.

Goodale, I. L., Domar, A. D. & Benson, H. (1990) Alleviation of premenstrual syndrome symptoms with the relaxation response. *Obstetrics and Gynaecology*, **75**, 649–655.

Greenberg, D. M., Bradford, J. M. W., Curry, S. , *et al* (1996) A comparison of treatment of paraphilias with three serotonin reuptake inhibitors. A retrospective study. *Bulletin of the Academy of Psychiatry and Law*, **24**, 525–532.

Guiliano, F., Hutting, C., El Masri, W. S., *et al* (1998) Sildenafil (Viagra): a novel oral treatment for erectile dysfunction (ED) caused by traumatic spinal cord injury (SCI). *International Journal of Impotence Research*, **10** (suppl. 3), A248.

Halbreich, U. & Endicott, J. (1985) Relationship of dysphoric premenstrual changes to depressive disorders. *Acta Psychiatrica Scandinavica*, **71**, 331.

Hawton, K. (1985) *Sex Therapy: A Practical Guide*. New York: Oxford University Press.

Hemminki, E. & Topo, P. (1997) Prescribing of hormone therapy in menopause and post menopause. *Journal of Psychosomatic Obstetrics and Gynaecology*, **18**, 145–157.

Hollander, E., Tracy, K. A., Swann, A. C., *et al* (2003) Divalproex in the treatment of impulsive aggression: efficacy in cluster B personality disorders. *Neuropsychopharmacology*, **28**, 1186–1197.

Hylan, T. R., Sundell, K. & Judge, R. (1999) The impact of premenstrual symptomatology on functioning and treatment-seeking behavior: experience from the United States, United Kingdom and France. *Journal of Women's Health and Gender-Based Medicine*, **8**, 1043–1052.

Johnson, S. R. (1998) Premenstrual syndrome therapy. *Clinical Obstetrics and Gynaecology*, **41**, 405–421.

Junemann, K. P., Manning, M., Krautschich, A., *et al* (1996) 15 years of injection therapy in erectile dysfunction. A review. *International Journal of Impotence Research*, **8**, A60.

Kafka, M. P. (1994) Sertraline pharmacotherapy for paraphilias and paraphilia related disorders: an open trial. *Annals of Clinical Psychiatry*, **6**, 189–195.

Kafka, M. P. & Prentky, R. A. (1998) Attentive deficit/hyperactivity disorder in males with paraphilia and paraphilia related disorders: a comorbidity study. *Journal of Clinical Psychiatry*, **59**, 338–396.

Kaplan, H. S. (1974) *The New Sex Therapy*. New York: Baillière Tindall.

Kavoussi, R. J. & Coccaro, E. F. (1998) Divalproex sodium for impulsive aggressive behaviour in patients with personality disorder. *Journal of Clinical Psychiatry*, **59**, 676–680.

Kendler, K. S., Karkowski, L. M., Corey, L. A., *et al* (1998) Longitudinal population-based twin study of retrospectively reported premenstrual symptoms and lifetime major depression. *American Journal of Psychiatry*, **155**, 1234–1240.

Kirkby, R. J. (1994) Changes in premenstrual symptoms and irrational thinking following cognitive–behavioral coping skills training. *Journal of Consulting and Clinical Psychology*, **62**, 1026–1032.

Kukopulos, A., Minnai, G. & Muller Oerlinghausen, B. (1985) The influence of mania and depression on the pharmacokinetics of lithium: a single case study. *Journal of Affective Disorders*, **8**, 159–166.

Laschet, U. & Laschet, L. (1971) Psychopharmacotherapy of sex offenders with cyproterone acetate. *Pharmakopsychiatrie Neuropsychopharmakologic*, **4**, 99–101.

Lefkowitz, M. (1969) Effects of diphenylhydantoin in disruptive behaviour: a study of male delinquents. *Archives of General Psychiatry*, **20**, 643–651.

Magos, A. L., Collins, W. P. & Studd, J. W. W. (1984) Management of premenstrual syndrome by subcutaneous implant of oestradiol. *Journal of Psychosomatic Obstetrics and Gynaecology*, **3**, 93–99.

Malone, R. P., Delaney, N. A. & Luebbert, J. F. (2000) A double blind placebo-controlled study of lithium in hospitalized aggressive children and adolescents with conduct disorder. *Archives of General Psychiatry*, **57**, 649–654.

Markovitz, P. J., Calabrese, J. R., Schulz, S. C., *et al* (1991) Fluoxetine in the treatment of borderline and schizotypal personality disorders. *American Journal of Psychiatry*, **148**, 1065–1067.

Mattes, J. A., Boswell, L. & Oliver, H. (1984) Methylphenidate effects on symptoms of attention deficit disorder in adults. *Archives of General Psychiatry*, **41**, 1059–1063.

McElroy, S. (1999) Recognition and treatment of DSM–IV intermittent explosive disorder. *Journal of Clinical Psychiatry*, **60** (suppl.15), 12–15.

Melman, A., Tiefer, L. & Pederson, R. (1988) Evaluation of the first 406 patients in a urology department based centre for male sexual dysfunction. *Urology*, **32**, 6–10.

Menkes, D. B., Taghavi, E., Mason, P. A., *et al* (1992) Fluoxetine treatment of severe premenstrual syndrome. *BMJ*, **305**, 346–347.

Menkes, D. B., Coates, D. C. & Fawcett, J. P. (1994) Acute tryptophan depletion aggravates premenstrual syndrome. *Journal of Affective Disorders*, **32**, 37–44.

Monroe, R. R. (1970) *Episodic Disorders*. Cambridge, MA: Harvard University Press.

Morales, A., Johnson, B., Heaton, J. W. P., *et al* (1994) Oral androgens in the treatment of hypogonadism in impotent men. *Journal of Urology*, 152, 1115–1118.

Morrison, J. R. (1980) Childhood hyperactivity in an adult psychiatric population: social factors. *Journal of Clinical Psychiatry*, **41**, 40–43.

Pearlstein, T. & Steiner, M. (2000) Non-antidepressant treatment of premenstrual syndrome. *Journal of Clinical Psychiatry*, **61** (suppl. 12), 22–27.

Pinto, O. C. & Akiskal, H. S. (1998) Lamotrigine as a promising approach to borderline personality: an open case series without concurrent DSM–IV major mood disorder. *Journal of Affective Disorders*, **51**, 333–343.

Rösler, A. & Witzum, E. (1998) Treatment of men with paraphilia with a long acting analogue of gonadotrophic releasing hormone. *New England Journal of Medicine*, **338**, 416–422.

Salzman, C., Wolfson, A. N., Schatzberg, A., *et al* (1995) Effect of fluoxetine on anger in symptomatic volunteers with borderline personality disorder. *Journal of Clinical Psychopharmacology*, **15**, 23–29.

Schaumberg, H., Kaplan, J., Windebank, A., *et al* (1983) Sensory neuropathy from pyridoxine abuse. A new megavitamin syndrome. *New England Journal of Medicine*, **309**, 445–448.

Schmidt, P. J., Nieman, L. K., Danaceau, M. A., *et al* (1998) Differential behavioral effects of gonadal steroids in women with and in those without premenstrual syndrome. *New England Journal of Medicine*, **338**, 209–216.

Schulz, C. S., Camlin, K. L., Berry, S. A., *et al* (1999) Olanzepine safety and efficiacy in patients with borderline personality disorder and comorbid dysthymia. *Biological Psychiatry*, **46**, 1429–1435.

Seidman, S. N., Rosen, R. C., Menza, M. A., et al (2000) Clinical trials report: sildenafil for erectile dysfunction in depression. *Current Psychiatry Reports*, **2**(3), 187.

Sheard, M. H., Marini, J. L., Bridges, C. I., et al (1976) The effect of lithium on unipolar aggressive behaviour in man. *American Journal of Psychiatry*, **133**, 1409–1413.

Soloff, P. H. (2000) Psychopharmacology of borderline personality disorder. *Psychiatric Clinics of North America*, **23**, 169–193.

Soloff, P. H., George, A., Nathan, S., et al (1986) Progress in pharmaco-therapy of borderline personality disorders. *Archives in General Psychiatry*, **3**, 691–697.

Soloff, P. H., George, A., Nathan, S., et al (1993) Efficacy of phenelzine and haloperidol in borderline personality disorder. *Archives of General Psychiatry*, **50**, 377–385.

Spencer, T., Wilens, T. E., Biederman, J., et al (1995) A double-blind crossover comparison of methylphenidate and placebo in adults with childhood-onset attention deficit hyperactivity. *Archives of General Psychiatry*, **52**, 434–443.

Spencer, T., Biederman, J., Wilens, T. E., et al (1998) Adults with attention deficit/ hyperactivity disorder: a controversial diagnosis. *Journal of Clinical Psychiatry*, **59** (suppl. 7), 59–68.

Stein, D. J., Simeon, D., Frenkel, M., et al (1995) An open trial of valproate in borderline personality disorder. *Journal of Clinical Psychiatry*, **56**, 506–510.

Steinberg, S., Annable, L., Young, S. N., et al (1999) A placebo controlled trial of L-tryptophan in premenstrual dysphoria. *Advances in Experimental Medicine and Biology*, **467**, 85–88.

Steiner, M. & Pearlstein, T. (2000) Premenstrual dysphoria and the serotonin system: pathophysiology and treatment. *Journal of Clinical Psychiatry*, **61** (suppl. 12), 17–21.

Stone, M. (1990) *The Fate of Borderline Patients*. New York: Guilford Press.

Sundblad, C., Modigh, K., Andersch, B., et al (1992) Clomipramine effectively reduces premenstrual irritablity and dysphoria: a placebo controlled trial. *Acta Psychiatrica Scandinavica*, **85**, 39–47.

Thys-Jacobs, S., Starkey, P., Bernstein, D., et al (1998) Calcium carbonate and the premenstrual syndrome: effects on premenstrual and menstrual symptoms. *American Journal of Obstetrics and Gynecology*, **179**, 444–452.

Tupin, J. P., Smith, D. B., Clanon, T. L., et al (1973) The long-term use of lithium in aggressive prisoners. *Comprehensive Psychiatry*, **14**, 311–317.

Tyrer, S. P., Walsh, A., Edwards, D. E., et al (1984) Factors associated with a good response to lithium in aggressive mentally handicapped subjects. *Progress in Neuro-psychopharmacology and Biological Psychiatry*, **8**, 751–755.

van den Akker, O. B., Stein, G. S., Neale, M. C., et al (1987) Genetic and environmental variation in menstrual cycle: histories of two British twin samples. *Acta Genetica Medica Gemellologica (Roma)*, **36**, 541–548.

Virag, R. (1982) Intracavernous injection of papaverine for erectile failure. *Lancet*, ii, 938.

Walker, A. F., De Souza, M. C., Vickers, M. F., et al (1998) Magnesium supplementation alleviates premenstrual symptoms of fluid retention. *Journal of Women's Health*, **7**, 1157–1165.

Waseff, A. A., Dott, S. G., Harris, A., et al (1999) Critical review of GABA-ergic drugs in the treatment of schizophrenia. *Journal of Clinical Psychopharmacology*, **19**, 222–232.

Weiss, G., Hechtman, L., Milroy, T., et al (1985) Psychiatric status of hyperactives as adults: a controlled prospective 15 year follow-up of 63 hyperactive children. *Journal of the American Academy of Child Psychiatry*, **24**, 211–220.

West, C. P. (1990) Inhibition of ovulation with oral progestins. Effectiveness in premenstrual syndrome. *European Journal of Obstetrics and Gynaecology and Reproductive Biology*, **34**, 119–128.

Wikander, I., Sundblad, C., Andersch, B., et al (1998) Citalopram in premenstrual dysphoria: is intermittent treatment during luteal phases more effective than continuous medication throughout the menstrual cycle? *Journal of Clinical Psychopharmacology*, **18**, 390–398.

571

Wilcox, J. A. (1995) Divalproex sodium as a treatment for borderline personality disorder. *Annals of Clinical Psychiatry*, **7**, 33–37.

Winkleman, N. W. (1955) Chlorpromazine in the treatment of neuropsychiatric disorders. *Journal of the Americal Medical Association*, **155**, 18–21.

World Health Organization (1992) *International Classification of Diseases* (10th revision) (ICD–10). Geneva: WHO.

Worrall, E. P., Moody, J. P. & Naylor, G. J. (1975) Lithium in non-manic–depressives: antiaggressive effect and red blood cell lithium values. *British Journal of Psychiatry*, **126**, 464–468.

Yonkers, K. A., Halbreich, U., Freeman, E., *et al* (1997) Symptomatic improvement of premenstrual dysphoric disorder with sertraline treatment: a randomised controlled trial. *Journal of the American Medical Association*, **278**, 983–988.

Zimmerman, M., Coryell, W., Pfohl, B., *et al* (1986) ECT response in depressed patients with and without a DSM–III personality disorder. *American Journal of Psychiatry*, **143**, 1030–1032.

CHAPTER 15

Unwanted effects of psychotropic drugs: 1. Effects on human physiological systems, mechanisms and methods of assessment

J. Guy Edwards

All drugs have unwanted as well as wanted effects, and in our day-to-day practice we therefore have to weigh the risks of adverse reactions against the anticipated benefits. Within any particular category of drugs there is usually no firm evidence that one drug is more effective than another, and our treatment choices are largely determined by side-effect profiles.

It is essential to study unwanted effects, not only so that we can give our patients the best tolerated and least toxic treatment, but also because research into the pathogenesis of adverse reactions could lead to an understanding of the mechanisms through which therapeutic effects are mediated; this in turn may throw light on the aetiology of the disorders being treated.

The effects of a drug result from highly complex interactions between the substance and the subject who takes them. Many effects are influenced not only by the subject's pathophysiological state, but also by psychological and social factors.

Adverse reactions are broadly categorised into those that are part of, or an extension of, the drug's known pharmacological profile and are thus dose-dependent, predictable and quantitatively abnormal (type A or augmented reactions) and those that are idiosyncratic, unpredictable and therefore qualitatively abnormal (type B or bizarre reactions). Type A reactions include such phenomena as oversedation and anticholinergic effects, while hypersensitivity or allergic dermatological reactions and blood dyscrasias are examples of type B reactions.

It is easy to fall into the trap of assuming that symptoms occurring during treatment are necessarily due to the medication. Difficulties in establishing a cause-and-effect relationship arise for several reasons: symptoms identical to minor side-effects occur in healthy people taking no medication; alleged adverse reactions may be manifestations of the disorder being treated, a concomitant physical illness or psychiatric disorder, or anxiety about treatment; and an unwanted effect may be due to some other drug being taken concurrently or that was recently discontinued.

Investigators who are overenthusiastic about specific effects may overdiagnose them, while checklists are more likely to elicit symptoms unrelated to treatment than are open-ended questions.

The assessment of a cause-and-effect relationship is also made more difficult because 'placebo side-effects' can occur. Most of these are non-specific symptoms, such as those that occur in a variety of physical and psychiatric illnesses. Severe placebo-induced effects have been reported, but they could be due to hypersensitivity reactions to excipients or additives.

A causal connection between a drug and an alleged effect is more likely to exist if:

(1)   there is a close temporal relationship between the effect and the taking of the drug
(2)   toxic levels of drug or active metabolites can be detected in body fluids
(3)   the effect differs from the manifestations of the disorder being treated or of any concurrent illness
(4)   no other substances are being taken or were recently withdrawn when the effect occurs
(5)   the reaction disappears when treatment is stopped
(6)   the effect reappears with a rechallenge test.

Unwanted effects can occur in any physiological system, although not surprisingly when dealing with psychotropic drugs most involve the central nervous system (CNS).

Neuropsychiatric effects

Cognitive and behavioural effects

Methods of assessing the psychomotor effects of drugs are dealt with by Hindmarch and McClelland in Chapter 3, while the effects of psychotropic drugs on sleep, tolerance, dependence and the problems of withdrawal have been discussed by Cooper in Chapter 5. They are therefore not described here.

The effects of psychotropic drugs on cognition and psychomotor performance are complex. They are influenced by many interrelated variables in the person and in the cognitive/psychomotor task being attempted. The subject's motivation, affective state, personality and demographic characteristics can all affect performance, as can the illness or illnesses being treated. The type of activity carried out is also important, with performance on repetitious, boring tasks, for instance, being different from that on interesting, challenging exercises. There may be differences between performance on laboratory tasks and real-life situations; in the latter, people are often able to use their experience to compensate for drug-induced decrements in functioning.

Knowledge of the cognitive and behavioural effects of psychotropic medication is limited by the fact that much of the research has been undertaken on small samples of normal volunteers, who were sometimes given only a single dose of a drug. Different researchers have used different tests (with different sensitivities) and different methods, which makes some comparisons between drugs difficult to interpret.

Despite these considerations, admirable attempts have been made to assess the effects of psychotropic drugs on higher cerebral functions, and a large body of knowledge on laboratory and simulation tests related to activities in the real world has accumulated. What are needed are more epidemiological data on actual performance and behaviour, particularly in potentially dangerous situations.

Different psychotropic drugs may affect cognition, memory, perception, mood and behaviour in different ways, although with some effects in common. Compounds such as some phenothiazines and tricyclic antidepressants can cause oversedation, with impairment of concentration, attention and intellectual functioning.

Benzodiazepines may cause memory impairment, mediated via their effects on attention, with failure to register events, or on the consolidation of registered events, with a resulting deficit in recall – that is, anterograde amnesia. Cognitive and behavioural effects occur more often, and are more marked when drugs are taken in high doses or in combination with other psychoactive agents, including alcohol, and when they are administered to susceptible people, such as elderly patients with pre-existing cerebral impairment.

Some of the behavioural effects of psychotropic drugs are not clinically obvious and may be detectable only by sensitive psychomotor tests. Alternatively, they may be more overt and vary in severity from mild to severe. When severe, they can cause such complications as falls, with the consequent possibility of injuries, especially fractures of the proximal femur (hip fractures), and hypostatic pneumonia – effects that are more likely to occur in elderly people. Occasionally, toxic confusional states occur, with fluctuating levels of consciousness, disorientation, perplexity, anxiety, fear, restlessness, hostility, illusions, delusions, hallucinations and subsequent fragmentary or total amnesia.

Psychomotor effects can influence complex skills, such as driving and working with industrial machinery, and are therefore potentially dangerous. Possible consequences include road vehicle crashes and threats to safety, decreased precision and lowered productivity in industry.

Unpleasant CNS effects can militate against therapeutic progress and contribute to non-compliance with treatment.

Some psychotropic drugs, for example fluphenazine decanoate and diazepam, have been alleged to cause depression, although critical reviews of the evidence have revealed that the low mood is more likely due to the disorders being treated. This holds true also for the 'paradoxical' depression that has been said to occur during treatment with anti-depressants. What does seem more likely, however, is the occurrence of increased anxiety as a CNS 'stimulant' effect during treatment with some selective serotonin reuptake inhibitors (SSRIs). Aggression and outbursts of rage have occurred during treatment with benzodiazepines, but these are thought to be the result of disinhibition, as occurs with alcohol, in potentially hostile personalities, rather than a specific effect arising *de novo*. It is likely that aggressive and suicidal behaviour allegedly caused by SSRIs is also related more to the personality of the patient and the disorders being treated than to the drug.

Convulsive seizures

Convulsive seizures have been reported during treatment with many psychotropic drugs. They are important to study because they are frightening and sometimes life-threatening; they may be particularly distressing to people already suffering from a mental illness, adding to their fears and sometimes undermining their confidence in treatment. This can lead to non-compliance with treatment and to relapse. The attacks may also cause concern to relatives. If the neurological investigations are prolonged, there may be a long, anxious wait for the results.

'Fits' and 'seizures' are words that are sometimes used inaccurately to describe non-epileptic behaviour – in fact, a wide range of physical and psychiatric disorders can cause loss or clouding of consciousness and other episodic phenomena, and this can lead to epilepsy being wrongly diagnosed. A detailed history from the patient and any witnesses to the attack and a thorough examination are the most important parts of the assessment. A single routine electroencephalogram (EEG) may be helpful in capturing a 'snapshot' of epileptiform spike activity, and is more likely to do so if techniques such as hyperventilation, photic stimulation, fasting or sleep deprivation are used to provoke the activity. But even in a population of patients with epilepsy, only about 50% of single EEGs show epileptiform activity, although repeated recordings will show it in 85% of cases.

Ambulatory EEG monitoring may be more helpful. Multichannel, battery-operated cassette systems, with small amplifiers mounted close to the recording electrodes to minimise artefacts, and a 24-hour recording capacity per cassette, are available. When the diagnosis remains in doubt, videotelemetry can be used. In this technique a patient's seizures are viewed on a television camera, and the EEG with time-locked recordings can be displayed simultaneously. It should be remembered, however, that epilepsy is a clinical diagnosis and EEG recordings, although helpful, are no substitute for a meticulous clinical assessment.

Seizures have been reported more often during treatment with anti-depressants than with other psychotropic drugs, but they also occur when antipsychotics (especially clozapine) are administered and when anxiolytics are abruptly withdrawn. Of the antidepressants, maprotiline appears to be a major offender, while the incidence with the newer drugs is low. The overall incidence during treatment with tricyclic antidepressants is about one per 1000 patients. With such a low incidence it is difficult to obtain accurate data from which the relative risk of seizures on different antidepressants can be determined.

Antidepressant-induced seizures are more likely to occur:

(1)   when high doses of antidepressants are used
(2)   in those who have had a change in medication during the previous week
(3)   in patients receiving concurrently other drugs capable of lowering the convulsive threshold
(4)   in those withdrawing from alcohol or anxiolytic sedatives
(5)   in patients with a relevant medical history, such as head injury, cerebrovascular disease and epilepsy itself
(6)   in first-born subjects, who may have a higher incidence of early brain damage.

Care should be taken in prescribing for vulnerable people and, if a seizure occurs, a switch should be made to a drug that is considered to have less epileptogenic potential.

The pathogenic mechanisms involved in convulsive seizures are not fully understood, but in the laboratory it has been shown that a range of cellular and synaptic processes in the cerebral cortex and hippo-campus give rise to epileptiform neuronal activity. In addition to the classic suppression of the inhibitory synaptic mechanism mediated by gamma-aminobutyric acid (GABA), *in vitro* studies in animal models of epilepsy and on human tissue suggest a prominent role for the N-methyl-D-aspartate (NMDA) subtype of excitatory amino acid receptors. Any mechanism that leads to the depolarisation of neurons is likely to result in facilitation of NMDA receptor involvement in excitatory neurotransmission, especially in the cortex and hippocampus, where the densities of the NMDA receptor are highest. It is possible that these are the processes that are involved in the pathogenesis of drug-induced seizures. Many believe that the anticholinergic properties of tricyclic antidepressants may also be involved.

Extrapyramidal effects

Extrapyramidal effects have been recognised since the introduction of antipsychotic drugs into clinical practice and, as they have caused so much concern, they have been studied in more detail than any of the other unwanted effects of neuroleptics. They can be distressing and disabling and, as a result, they are an important cause of non-adherence to treatment. The effects can be categorised into acute, early-onset syndromes, and chronic, late-onset disorders. The former include: muscle rigidity, bradykinesia, tremor and excessive salivation (Parkinsonian symptoms); acute dystonic reactions that can present in familiar ways, such as with oculogyric crises or trismus, or less familiar ways, for example with lingual dystonia or glossopharyngeal spasms; and akathisia. Late-onset disorders include tardive dyskinesia, tardive akathisia and tardive dystonia. Tardive dyskinesia is the best known of these. It can affect the mouth and face (orofacial dyskinesia) or the trunk and extremities with choreiform or choreo-athetoid movements. The severity of the involuntary movements in each of the syndromes is increased by stress and decreased by relaxation.

The clinical features of the various disorders present a challenging exercise in differential diagnosis and, because of the difficulty of treating the 'tardive syndromes', an even greater therapeutic challenge. Some of the manifestations may be mistaken for the symptoms and signs of the psychiatric illnesses for which the drugs were prescribed. For instance, bradykinesia may be wrongly diagnosed as a 'negative' or depressive symptom of schizophrenia, while akathisia may be regarded as pathological excitation or agitation. The late-onset disorders may be misdiagnosed as one or other of the various types of abnormal movements that have been observed in patients with schizophrenia since the pre-phenothiazine era. Further details concerning the differential diagnosis, the drugs more liable to cause extrapyramidal symptoms, predisposing factors, methods of assessment and treatment are discussed by King and Waddington (Chapter 9; Cunningham Owens, 1999).

Neuroleptic malignant syndrome

A particularly severe neuropsychiatric reaction to antipsychotics, which is usually categorised with the other extrapyramidal disturbances, is neuroleptic malignant syndrome. Its characteristic features are severe muscle rigidity and pyrexia. These are frequently accompanied by diaphoresis, dysphagia, tachycardia, tachypnoea, labile blood pressure and tremor. The patient may have a fluctuating level of consciousness and, in severe cases, this may progress to akinetic mutism or stupor (with or without waxy flexibility) or coma. The patient may become dehydrated and incontinent (most often of urine). There is frequently an increased level of creatine phosphokinase (CPK). The syndrome runs a rapid course and there is a high mortality.

Neuroleptic malignant syndrome may start any time (from hours to months) after exposure to the offending antipsychotic drug or after an increase in dose: at one extreme it has been reported three-quarters of an hour after the start of treatment and at the other extreme after 14 months of continuous exposure to the drug. The average time is about five days and 90% of cases start within 10 days. The syndrome occurs more commonly after drugs are given in high doses or by parenteral administration. Clinical features develop rapidly, over the course of 1–3 days, with the syndrome mostly being full blown by the third day. The syndrome typically lasts 5–10 days, although there has been a report of a case that lasted 7 weeks.

Before 1970, the mortality rate from neuroleptic malignant syndrome might have been as high as 76%. The subsequent death rate (up to the mid-1980s) was about 25%, while the rate during the following 5 years was about a half of this. It is unclear how much of the declining mortality is due to changes in the criteria used for the diagnosis of neuroleptic malignant syndrome and how much is due to improvements in supportive treatment. Death is usually due to respiratory arrest, cardiovascular collapse or renal failure. Of those who survive, few – only about 3% of patients – have permanent clinical sequelae.

There is some overlap between the clinical features of neuroleptic malignant syndrome and those of lethal catatonia (which is now rarely seen in Western communities) and it has been considered that the syndrome is an iatrogenic form of catatonia. However, in lethal catatonia, but not in neuroleptic malignant syndrome, there are usually several days of prodromal symptoms (especially excitation) and muscular rigidity is absent or intermittent. Other conditions that have to be considered in the differential diagnosis are organic brain syndromes, such as encephalopathy, malignant hyperthermia and heat stroke.

Essential components of management are the exclusion of other possible causes of the patient's symptoms and signs and discontinuation of the antipsychotic medication. There have been no well-controlled trials of treatments, but it is generally considered that supportive measures are crucial. These include the administration of oxygen, intravenous rehydration and lowering fever with the use of cooling blankets and antipyretic drugs. If the patient is on an anticholinergic drug, it should be continued while muscle rigidity persists. Other drugs have been tried but their contribution is unclear. The best known of these are dantrolene (a muscle relaxant), bromocriptine and amantadine (dopamine agonists to counter the dopamine antagonist effects of the antipsychotic) and benzodiazepines (because of their sedative and muscle-relaxant properties).

Neuroleptic malignant syndrome can be prevented by avoiding unnecessarily high doses of antipsychotics, careful monitoring and the early treatment of extrapyramidal symptoms. Particular care should be taken when administering the drugs to patients who may be dehydrated and those exposed to the high temperatures of the tropics.

Autonomic effects

The most familiar autonomic effects of psychotropic drugs are those due to their cholinergic and α-adrenergic blocking actions, but adrenergic, antiserotonergic and antihistaminic effects may also occur. Because of the complexity of their actions on neurotransmission, the clinical effects are difficult to predict.

Anticholinergic effects include dry mouth (that sometimes leads to polydipsia and can increase the risk of caries formation and oral candidiasis), dry skin, blurred vision (resulting from decreased accommodation), tachycardia (which may be experienced as palpitations) and constipation. More serious effects occur much less frequently; they are the precipitation or exacerbation of angle-closure glaucoma, urinary retention (mostly in patients with pre-existing genito-urinary pathology, especially prostatic hypertrophy), and paralytic ileus, which may be life-threatening.

The anti-adrenergic effects include nasal congestion, inhibition of ejaculation, and postural hypotension. A drop in blood pressure may be particularly hazardous in the elderly, as it can lead to: falls, fractures and other injuries; cerebrovascular ischaemia causing a toxic confusional state, loss of consciousness or a stroke; and myocardial ischaemia, which can result in a myocardial infarct. A patient with a phaeochromocytoma treated parenterally with a phenothiazine may have a sudden and severe drop in blood pressure followed by generalised circulatory failure.

Psychotropic drugs have central (hypothalamic) and peripheral anti-α-adrenergic effects on mechanisms regulating temperature, but these are usually important only after overdose. Other autonomic effects are referred to in the systems review that follows.

Autonomic effects are reported as being more troublesome during treatment with some drugs than others, particularly aliphatic and piperazine phenothiazines and the older tricyclic antidepressants. Symptoms such as dry mouth and constipation are particularly common, and do not attract as much medical attention as they should. To the sufferer, however, they can be a considerable source of distress, with dry mouth requiring regular mouth rinses and constipation needing treatment with laxatives. As with unwanted effects in other systems, consideration should be given to changing drugs if troublesome symptoms persist.

Cardiovascular effects

Psychotropic drugs, especially tricyclic antidepressants and anti-psychotics (such as thioridazine, which has a quinidine-like effect on the heart), cause various cardiovascular effects. Hypotension has already been referred to. Changes in the electrocardiogram (ECG), especially cardiac conduction defects and arrhythmias, also occur. Increased PR, QRS and QT intervals, depression of the ST segment, flattening or notching of the T waves, and the appearance of U waves may be observed. Various conduction defects, such as atrioventricular block and bundle branch block, have also been reported, as have a wide variety of arrhythmias, including atrial and ventricular extrasystoles, atrial flutter, ventricular tachycardia and ventricular fibrillation. Clinically important effects are most likely to occur when the drugs have been taken in overdose or when administered to patients with pre-existing heart disease, especially elderly people with atherosclerotic or hyper-tensive cardiac disease. If these predisposed subjects have left ventricular dysfunction, the drugs may precipitate congestive cardiac failure.

Serious arrhythmias and sudden unexpected death

Serious arrhythmias and sudden unexpected death have been reported during treatment with antipsychotic and antidepressant drugs since the 1960s, but more attention has been paid to these effects during recent years. Some antipsychotics have been incriminated to a greater extent than other psychotropic drugs. This has led to the restricted use of sertindole and thioridazine, and the withdrawal from the market of droperidol.

Over the years, various mechanisms have been considered as possible causes of sudden death. These include hyperpyrexia or aspiration resulting in asphyxiation in the case of phenothiazines, but the mechanism now thought to be the most likely is cardiac, mediated by prolongation of the QT interval. This interval represents the time between the onset of electrical depolarisation and the end of repolarisation of the ventricles. Prolongation of the QT interval is thought to increase the period of vulnerability of the myocardium during which ventricular arrhythmias – especially the polymorphic ventricular tachycardia known as *torsade de pointes* – may be precipitated by ventricular premature beats.

As the length of the QT interval is influenced by the heart rate, a rate correction is required to interpret the length. One of the most widely used corrections (the QTc) is calculated using Bazett's formula (QT/$\sqrt{RR}$ interval). Suggested normal values for this QTc are <450 ms in women and <430 ms in men. Prolonged values are >470 ms and >450 ms, respectively, with intermediate values being categorised as borderline.

It should be stressed, however, that conventional ECGs recorded at the usual paper speed of 25 mm/s do not allow for accurate measurements of the QT interval. A recording made at a minimum of 50 mm/s is required, and measurements are most accurate if they are made on lead 2, V2 and V3 recordings.

Prolongation of the QT interval may be congenital or acquired. The former is determined by mutations of genes that encode for specific components of cardiac ion channels. Of specific interest is the rapid component of the delayed rectifier potassium current, IK_r, responsible for repolarisation following an action potential. The gene that encodes a major component of the protein responsible for IK_r has been cloned and is called the 'human ether-a-go-go-related gene' (HERG). Antipsychotics bind to this HERG channel and thereby decrease the outward movement of potassium, which is responsible for ventricular repolarisation. Some antipsychotics – notably droperidol, pimozide, sertindole and thioridazine – have a greater capacity than others to cause IK_r blockade. The administration of these compounds to people who already have prolonged repolarisation adds to the risk of arrhythmias.

Serious arrhythmias and sudden unexpected death can be prevented by avoiding high doses of antipsychotics and by carefully monitoring the treatment of vulnerable patients. Vulnerable patients include: those with pre-existing heart disease, such as ischaemic heart disease and ventricular dysfunction or hypertrophy; patients who have previously had *torsade de pointes*; patients with ECG abnormalities (including a prolonged QT interval), bradycardia, ventricular extrasystoles or heart block; those with hepatic or renal failure; and patients with low serum levels of potassium, calcium or magnesium, including that caused by taking diuretics. It should be noted also that there is a higher incidence of *torsade de pointes* in women, elderly people, and alcohol-dependent subjects with liver disease. It is crucial to avoid prescribing drug combinations that can result in an increase in the QT interval (see Chapter 16, Appendices 16.3–16.6). A prolonged QT interval should always be suspected in vulnerable subjects who present with an acute onset of palpitations, dizziness and/or syncope. Failure to diagnose and treat the disorder can have fatal consequences.

The newer antidepressants have less effect on the cardiovascular system than the older tricyclics and should therefore be prescribed for patients with severe heart disease. The newer drugs are also safer in overdose.

Respiratory effects

In therapeutic doses, psychotropic drugs have few clinically important effects on the respiratory system, although they may on rare occasions precipitate bronchospasm in susceptible patients. Similarly, β-adreno-ceptor blocking agents (used in the treatment of somatic symptoms of anxiety) can exacerbate obstructive airways disease and lead to complications in patients with pulmonary insufficiency or asthma.

In overdose, most psychotropic drugs, especially if taken in combination with other CNS depressant drugs, can cause respiratory depression.

Gastrointestinal effects

Gastrointestinal symptoms, such as nausea, vomiting, abdominal discomfort and bowel dysfunction, are so commonly encountered in clinical practice that it is often difficult to relate them to the use of psychotropic drugs. Nevertheless, such symptoms are well-known unwanted effects of psychotropic drugs, especially lithium and the SSRIs – often limiting treatment with the latter.

Constipation occurs during treatment with tricyclic antidepressants; it may be particularly troublesome in the elderly and require treatment with laxatives. Pre-existing disorders in the alimentary tract, such as peptic ulceration, coeliac disease and ulcerative colitis, may make the patient more vulnerable to gastrointestinal effects and add to the difficulty of establishing a cause-and-effect relationship between drug and effect.

Reference has already been made to anticholinergic effects; it is likely that α-adrenergic and especially serotonergic mechanisms are also involved in the pathogenesis of gastrointestinal symptoms. Nausea and vomiting may occur after abrupt withdrawal of phenothiazines. This is thought to be due to a 'rebound' increase in either cholinergic or dopaminergic activity, or a combination of these effects.

Elderly patients receiving antidepressants with a high potency for inhibiting the reupatke of serotonin are at increased risk of upper gastrointestinal haemorrhage. This is probably due to decreased uptake of serotonin from the blood by platelets, which leads to decreased platelet aggregation. The effect is considered to be of clinical importance in patients at high risk of bleeding, notably octogenarians, those with a past history of upper gastrointestinal bleeding and patients receiving concurrently other substances that increase the risk of bleeding, such as aspirin and other non-steroidal anti-inflammatories (NSAIDs) (see Blood dyscrasias, p. 592).

Hepatic dysfunction

The liver, being the principal organ involved in the detoxification of drugs, is particularly vulnerable to adverse reactions, although the effects may not be overt because of the liver's large functional reserve.

In general, the occurrence and severity of hepatic effects depend on the blood flow, oxygenation and enzyme activity in the liver; these may be adversely affected by liver disease and the concomitant use of other potentially hepatotoxic substances. Mild hepatic reactions may show themselves as abnormalities only in the results of liver function tests. It is often difficult to relate these abnormalities, and indeed more severe reactions, to drug treatment, especially in patients who have a history of alcohol or drug misuse, infectious diseases or nutritional deficiencies.

Hepatic reactions may be predictable or unpredictable, occurring in susceptible people with an immunological defect or inherent abnormality of liver enzymes. The damage that results can be categorised as cholestatic, diffuse hepatic, or of mixed type. Certain drugs tend to produce one type of reaction, but variations occur.

Cholestatic jaundice is a well-documented reaction to chlorpromazine, but other antipsychotics, tricyclic antidepressants and benzodiazepines have also been alleged to cause it on rare occasions. The clinical picture is that of an acute-onset obstructive-type jaundice, while laboratory investigations may show: hyperbilirubinaemia; increased levels of serum alkaline phosphatase, aspartate aminotransferase (AST, previously known as serum glutamic oxalacetic transaminase) and alanine amino-transferase (ALT, previously referred to as serum glutamic pyruvic transaminase); eosinophilia; and bile in the urine. Liver biopsy shows centrilobular cholestasis, with little or no parenchymal damage, and eosinophils in the portal tracts.

Spontaneous recovery usually occurs (sometimes during continued treatment with the suspect drug, although it should have been discontinued because of the danger), although a significant number of cases have biochemical and histological evidence of liver cell damage and necrosis. Rarely, jaundice is prolonged and the patient develops features of chronic liver disease, including hepatosplenomegaly and xanthomas. Hypersensitivity mechanisms have been incriminated, because cholestatic jaundice is not dose related, occurs after a latent period of 2–4 weeks and may be accompanied by other allergic phenomena, such as a rash and eosinophilia.

Jaundice due to liver cell disease has been reported during treatment with monoamine oxidase inhibitors (MAOIs), tricyclics and other antidepressants. It mostly occurs after about 4 weeks of treatment; the clinical picture mimics viral hepatitis, although fever is rare and the disorder is often of greater severity. The similarity suggests the possibility of a coincidental viral infection or aggravation of a pre-existing infection. Despite these considerations, the disease does not spread from one person to another and the mortality from severe drug-induced hepatitis (due to hepatic necrosis) is higher than from viral hepatitis. It is thought that a biochemical sensitivity reaction occurs – due either to covalent binding to hepatocyte fractions or an immunological attack on a metabolite–liver cell complex – and results in liver cell damage.

It is apparent from what has been said that the diagnosis of drug-induced hepatic dysfunction, like that of other adverse reactions, is not as straightforward as it seems. Apart from viral hepatitis (including that transmitted by the intravenous use of illegal drugs), the effects of any concurrent disease, poor diet, alcohol and other substances all have to be considered. When a hepatic reaction occurs – especially if accompanied by jaundice – the suspect drug should be withdrawn and, unless there is an urgent need for continued treatment, a 'drug holiday' is advisable. If the severity of the underlying mental illness requires continued treatment or when it becomes necessary to reintroduce pharmacotherapy, a switch to a different type of drug should be made. In the case of phenothiazine-induced jaundice, it is common practice to substitute haloperidol, although this drug itself has been alleged to cause hepatic reactions on rare occasions. During recovery from a hepatic reaction (with or without a change of drug), careful monitoring of liver function is crucial, and whenever there is any concern about the patient's clinical progress, the advice of a physician with a specialised knowledge of liver disease should be sought.

Renal effects

The renal effects of psychotropic drugs that have caused most concern – and stimulated a vast amount of research – are those of lithium. This substance has been known to be nephrotoxic for 50 years, and polyuria and polydipsia have been observed since the early days of treatment. These symptoms were regarded as benign and reversible until histological changes were found in renal biopsy specimens in the late 1970s. These were initially seen only in patients who had had lithium toxicity, but later they were observed in patients whose serum lithium levels had been within the normal range. The biopsies revealed focal nephron atrophy (glomerular sclerosis and tubular atrophy) and interstitial fibrosis. However, concern over the risk of clinically significant irreversible renal damage during treatment with lithium has diminished over the years and it is important to see the risk of significant damage in relation to the considerable benefit that the drug has had for so many patients. Lithium is discussed in detail in Chapter 7.

Polyuria results from inability of the kidney to concentrate urine. owing to inhibition by lithium of the action of antidiuretic hormone (ADH) on the distal tubule, a process mediated by intracellular adenylate cyclase. The degree to which lithium does this is related to the duration of treatment, total cumulative dose of the drug and possibly high trough plasma concentrations. The impairment of concentrating ability increases with continued treatment, even after adjustment for the expected age-related decrease. It exposes the patient to an increased risk of dehydration and lithium toxicity. Frank nephrogenic diabetes insipidus occurs only occasionally. On stopping treatment polyuria decreases and urine-concentrating ability recovers. Polyuria may also occur in the presence of normal tubular responsiveness to ADH – when it is due to polydipsia caused by a dry mouth (an anticholinergic effect of concomitant antidepressant medication), a high fluid intake recommended by a physician or psychogenic polydipsia.

The risk of renal complications in patients on long-term treatment with lithium can be minimised by assessing renal function annually. The most frequently used measure of glomerular function is the serum creatinine concentration. This, however, is an insensitive measure, as there can be up to a 50% reduction in the glomerular filtration rate before the serum creatinine concentration exceeds the normal range. It is therefore important to use a formula or nomogram to predict the creatinine clearance from the serum creatinine level, taking into account the sex and age of the patient. If the predicted clearance is low, the glomerular filtration rate should be measured using a radiolabelled marker, such as ^{51}Cr-labelled ethylenediaminetetra-acetic acid (EDTA) (see suggested scheme for monitoring renal function in Box 15.1). Tubular function is best measured by estimating the urine osmolality of a morning specimen (this is a measure of the solute content determined by the degree to which the freezing point of water is depressed). If the osmolality is consistently low, it is recommended that the maximum osmolality (max U_{osm}) achieved following the administration of desamino-D-arginine vasopressin (DDAVP) be measured (Box 15.1).

Difficulty in micturition has already been mentioned as an anticholinergic effect of psychotropic drugs. It may lead to retention of urine, particularly in elderly men with pre-existing genito-urinary disease, such as prostatic hypertrophy. In chronic cases retention may be associated with vesicular atonicity, thought to be due to competitive antagonism of acetylcholine at the neuromuscular junction within the detrusor. Incomplete emptying of the bladder, distention with overflow and even permanent loss of bladder tone (caused by damage to smooth muscle, elastic and collagenous tissue) may result.

When urinary difficulty occurs during treatment with a drug known to have marked anticholinergic effects, it is advisable to change to a compound that has less anticholinergic effect, for example from a tricyclic antidepressant to an SSRI. When retention occurs, referral to a genito-urinary surgeon is crucial.

Sexual and genital effects

Sexual and genital dysfunction caused by psychotropic drugs has been investigated to a much lesser extent than most of the effects discussed

---

Box 15.1 Monitoring of renal function during treatment with lithium

Before treatment
- Estimate the serum creatinine level and predict creatinine clearance from serum creatinine (using formula below).
- If predicted clearance <70 ml/min, measure GFR using a radio-labelled marker such as ^{51}Cr-EDTA or ^{99m}Tc-DTPA.
- If GFR <60 ml/min confirmed, refer to physician and reconsider using lithium. If GFR <30 ml/min avoid lithium treatment.

At 12-monthly intervals during treatment
- Monitor serum creatinine and predicted creatinine clearance.
- If progressive impairment of glomerular function is confirmed, consider stopping lithium.
- Measure osmolality of early morning specimen of urine in patients with polyuria.
- If osmolality consistently <300 mosmol/kg measure max U_{osm} after DDAVP.
- If max U_{osm} after DDAVP does not exceed 300 mosmol/kg and progressive impairment of tubular function confirmed, reconsider continuing treatment with lithium.

GFR = glomerular filtration rate; EDTA = ethylenediaminetetra-acetic acid; DTPA = diethylenenetriamine penta-acetate; DDAVP = desamino-D-arginine vasopressin.

Formula for calculating creatinine clearance (ml/min/70kg) from serum creatinine:

men: $\dfrac{(140 - \text{age in years}) \times \text{weight in kg}}{\text{plasma creatinine in } \mu\text{mol/l}} \times 1.23$

women: $\dfrac{(140 - \text{age in years}) \times \text{weight in kg}}{\text{plasma creatinine in } \mu\text{mol/l}} \times 1.03$

---

above. Furthermore, such dysfunction is encountered so often in clinical practice that here too there is difficulty in relating it to treatment. Sexual problems may be associated with: the disorder being treated; a concomitant psychiatric or physical illness; the drugs used to treat a concurrent illness; and substance misuse (for a list of possible aetiological factors see Box 15.2). They may also be secondary to other unwanted effects, such as oversedation, antipsychotic-induced parkinsonism or excessive weight gain.

The size of the problem is not known, because doctors do not ask their patients about sexual side-effects as often as they should and because the reporting of such effects varies with the knowledge, experience, attitude and interview technique of the doctor. The problem is likely to be larger than often realised.

Box 15.2 Sexual dysfunction: factors involved in aetiology

Patient
- Personality
- Relationships
- Social stresses

Illness
- Psychiatric disorder
- Concomitant illnesses
- Alcohol/substance misuse

Treatment
- Psychotropic drugs
- Drugs for concurrent illness
- Type of drug, dose, duration of treatment, interactions

Neurotransmitters possibly involved
- Dopamine
- Noradrenaline
- Serotonin
- Acetylcholine
- Gamma-aminobutyric acid
- Oxytocin
- Arg-vasopressin
- Angiotensin II
- Gonadotrophin-releasing hormone
- Nitric oxide
- Substance P
- Neuropeptide Y
- Cholecystokinin-8

There are suggestions from individual trials and observational studies that sexual side-effects are more likely with some psychotropic drugs than others of the same class. For example, it was reported in one trial that sexual dysfunction occurred more often during treatment with sertraline than fluvoxamine, and a prescription event-monitoring study suggested that impotence and ejaculatory failure occurred more often with paroxetine than fluoxetine, fluvoxamine and sertraline. By contrast, a meta-analysis of SSRIs failed to reveal any significant differences between the drugs. Notwithstanding these seemingly conflicting results, the limited data available from these and other studies suggest that paroxetine may be the SSRI most likely to cause sexual dysfunction and fluvoxamine the least likely (Anderson & Edwards, 2001).

Laboratory tests are limited in the light they throw on adverse sexual and genital effects of drugs because of differences between animal species, the sexes, and the central and peripheral actions of the compounds. The number of patients included in clinical reports is often too small to allow for meaningful conclusions and the results are sometimes inconsistent, as exemplified above. The many neurotransmitters that affect sexual function create formidable difficulty in trying to explain the mechanism of action of the offending drugs.

While acknowledging these difficulties, decreased libido has been encountered during treatment with various psychotropic drugs, including phenothiazines and butyrophenones. The mechanism for this, like that of other sexual effects, is not fully understood, but the problem could be related to dopamine blockade or changes in gonadotrophins, oestrogen, progesterone or other hormones. Tricyclic antidepressants may decrease libido or cause difficulty obtaining or maintaining an erection because of α-adrenoceptor blockade.

Various antipsychotics (particularly thioridazine) may cause ejaculatory failure or retrograde ejaculation, which could be related to α-adrenoceptor blocking or anticholinergic effects. Anorgasmia or delayed orgasm may also occur during treatment with antipsychotics, especially phenothiazines, and antidepressants, including SSRIs. The effect has at different times been attributed to α-adrenergic, anticholinergic and serotonergic effects. Persistent priapism has been encountered rarely during treatment with antipsychotics and antidepressants, including trazodone; it is possibly mediated by peripheral adrenoceptor blockade.

Amenorrhoea is a common unwanted effect of various psychotropic drugs. It is uncertain whether it is the result of a non-specific toxic effect or a specific inhibitory effect on the endocrine system related to changes in oestrogen, follicle-stimulating hormone (FSH) or luteinising hormone (LH). Its occurrence with galactorrhoea supports the possibility that it may be a hypothalamic–pituitary effect mediated (at least in the case of antipsychotic drugs) via hyperprolactinaemia.

Psychotropic drugs may affect the sperm count, although this may also be decreased by stress and disease. In contrast to MAOIs, which may decrease the sperm count, amitriptyline may increase it.

Many psychological and pharmacological treatments for sexual side-effects have been proposed. The psychological treatments include counselling, brief supportive psychotherapy, couple therapy and group therapy. The pharmacological treatments are:

(1) waiting for tolerance to the drug to develop
(2) delaying dosing until after sexual intercourse
(3) dose reductions
(4) drug holidays
(5) drug substitution
(6) the use of adjunctive agents.

Examples of switching drugs that have been claimed to result in improvement include substituting desipramine and nortriptyline for imipramine, and nefazadone for various other antidepressants. A variety of adjunctive agents have been used; they include dopamine agonists (amantidine, dexamphetamine and pemoline); the 5-HT$_{1A}$ partial agonist buspirone; adrenergic antagonists (e.g. yohimbine); cholinergic antagonists (such as neostigmine); and the serotonin antagonist cyproheptidine. Priapism should be regarded as a medical emergency and urgent referral to a genito-urinary surgeon should be made if permanent sexual dysfunction is to be prevented.

Unfortunately, most reports of sexual dysfunction in association with psychotropic drugs are anecdotal or based on small sample sizes. Few controlled trials looking specifically at the incidence of sexual dysfunction have been carried out. There have been a number of good reviews on the subject. These are useful in bringing together animal and human data from various sources, summarising the possible mechanisms of production of the adverse effects and listing treatment options. However, the reviews provide little in the way of weighting of the evidence or step-by-step practical guidelines to management. The usual conclusion is the familiar 'more research is required'.

Metabolic effects

Seen from the broadest perspective, all adverse reactions are mediated via biochemical processes and can therefore be regarded as metabolic effects. However, the effect on metabolism that is of most concern is weight gain. An increase or decrease in weight, mostly related to age and changes in appetite, diet and activity, frequently occurs in psychiatric disorders and may therefore be difficult to relate to drug treatment.

It is widely accepted, nevertheless, that antipsychotics (especially chlorpromazine, clozapine and olanzapine), antidepressants (particularly tricyclics, irreversible MAOIs and mirtazapine) and lithium are liable to cause weight increase, mostly during the early months of treatment. By contrast, SSRIs – notably fluoxetine – may cause an initial weight loss. In the case of tricyclics, the weight increase is often associated with a craving for carbohydrates, but in general the mechanisms involved in weight change are poorly understood. Possible processes involved (which may vary with the drug) include: histamine, serotonin and dopamine antagonism; the development of insulin resistance; and increased secretion of leptin (a polypeptide produced by adipose cells that is involved in the production of further adipose tissue).

Phenothiazines, especially high doses of chlorpromazine, have long been thought to inhibit insulin secretion and thereby cause hyper-glycaemia and glycosuria. Antipsychotic-induced changes in glucose tolerance were thought to precipitate overt diabetes mellitus in patients with latent diabetes and to cause instability in the control of established diabetes in patients receiving antidiabetic treatment. However, in some of the early studies the alleged effects on glucose metabolism are difficult to interpret because of a high prevalence of diabetes in the populations studied (or in their families) and because the research was carried out in older and more obese subjects (subjects who are more prone to diabetes). Furthermore, there is some evidence of an independent association between schizophrenia and an increased risk of diabetes.

More recently some case reports have suggested an association between newer antipsychotic drugs (especially clozapine) and diabetes mellitus. Earlier epidemiological studies, in which adjustments were made for comorbidity, did not confirm the association. However, a more recent large-scale nested case-controlled study carried out in primary care revealed a significant association between treatment with olanzapine and an increased risk of diabetes. There was also an increased risk in patients treated with risperidone, but this did not reach statistical significance.

The association between antipsychotic drug treatment and diabetes has not been fully established and is likely to remain uncertain until the results of well-controlled, large-scale, long-term prospective studies are available. As the association is in doubt, it is not surprising that the mechanism of the alleged association is also doubtful. However, it has been suggested that the abnormality could be mediated by disrupted glucose metabolism and weight gain, with the possible involvement of serotonin antagonism, changes in β-adrenergic transmission and/or increased leptin secretion.

The increased thirst that occurs during treatment with lithium may lead to an increased intake of high-calorie drinks. Water retention may occur during treatment with antidepressants, lithium and anti-psychotics, and this can cause problems for patients with incipient congestive cardiac failure or oedema from other causes.

Endocrine effects

Psychotropic drugs have various effects on endocrine function. Antipsychotic drugs, for example, stimulate the release of prolactin, melanocyte-stimulating hormone (MSH) and ADH, and suppress adreno-corticotrophic hormone (ACTH), growth hormone (GH), thyrotrophin-stimulating hormone (TSH), FSH and LH. The effects may be mediated by actions on hypothalamic releasing and inhibiting hormones and factors. The clinical relevance of the effects is not known, although antipsychotic-induced hyperprolactinaemia may be associated with galactorrhoea and amenorrhoea (or oligomenorrhoea).

The release of prolactin is kept under tonic inhibition by dopamine, some less important neurotransmitters, and small peptides of unknown chemical sequence, collectively known as prolactin inhibitory factor (PIF). Prolactin enhances the release of PIF and hence controls its own release, but in addition to this negative feedback mechanism it is also influenced by other releasing factors. Antipsychotic drugs increase plasma prolactin levels by decreasing the availability of dopamine at its receptor. As a result, inappropriate lactation has been reported during treatment with antipsychotics, with reported incidences ranging from 10% to 80%, depending on the drug, the investigator's awareness of the effect, whether or not the breasts were examined specifically for galactorrhoea, and the concomitant use of other drugs, such as oral contraceptives. Hyperprolactinaemia has also been reported during treatment with tricyclic antidepressants, MAOIs and benzodiazepines.

The possible endocrine involvement in ocular and cutaneous pigmentation is described below, while the endocrine effects on sexual function were referred to above. Miscellaneous effects include the syndrome of inappropriate secretion of ADH and false-positive pregnancy tests during treatment with antipsychotic drugs. Treatment with lithium may cause hypothyroidism and sometimes a goitre, but it has also been suspected as a cause of hyperthyroidism. The mechanism of these effects is not known, although lithium may inhibit thyrotrophin-stimulated adenylcyclase activity and block the biosynthetic pathway leading to the production of thyroid hormone.

Blood dyscrasias

Psychotropic drugs have been purported to cause many haematological reactions. These range from minor, mainly quantitative white cell abnormalities, such as eosinophilia and neutropenia, to more serious and potentially life-threatening conditions, such as agranulocytosis, thrombocytopenia and aplastic anaemia. The allegations are commonly anecdotal and the evidence for causation is often purely circumstantial.

Selective serotonin reuptake inhibitors inhibit the uptake of serotonin by platelets and thereby decrease the storage of serotonin in them. As the release of serotonin increases platelet aggregation, SSRIs are thought to cause a variety of bleeding disorders. In support of this, there have been published case reports suggesting an association between excessive bruising, petechiae and ocular and cerebral haemorrhages. There is a link between the use of SSRIs and gastrointestinal bleeding, although the risk is small in patients under 80 years of age and in those with no past history of gastrointestinal bleeding (see Gastrointestinal effects, p. 583). SSRIs should be avoided or used with caution in these patients and also in those receiving aspirin and other NSAIDs.

Agranulocytosis is the most serious dyscrasia. It is defined as the absence of circulating blood neutrophils, although concern should be expressed when the cell count is $<1.0 \times 10^9/l$ (and especially $<0.2 \times 10^9/l$). Drug-induced agranulocytosis is an idiosyncratic reaction which is more common in the elderly and in females; chlorpromazine-related agranulocytosis appears to be confined to individuals of Afro-Caribbean ethnic origin.

The clinical presentations of agranulocytosis include fever, sore throat and mouth ulceration. Life-threatening sepsis is a significant risk and patients should be referred for expert haematological advice and care, to support them until neutrophil recovery occurs. Withdrawal of the causative agent mostly results in complete recovery. Blood abnormalities persisting after withdrawal require a thorough investigation, as they may have an alternative, unrelated cause.

Many published cases of agranulocytosis seen in psychiatric practice have occurred during treatment with phenothiazines. Chlorpromazine is toxic to bone marrow *in vitro*. Marrow from patients who have recovered from chlorpromazine-induced agranulocytosis does not grow as well as that from normal controls, in either the presence or absence of chlorpromazine. The significance of this finding is not clear but it may indicate that some individuals are intrinsically more susceptible to a direct toxic effect of the drug. By contrast, it is thought that immune mechanisms are involved in the pathogenesis of agranulocytosis induced by various other (non-psychotropic) drugs, and possibly also clozapine, although the evidence for this is conflicting.

It is important to differentiate toxic from immune (hypersensitivity) reactions, as patients can be re-treated with drugs that caused the former, so long as they are administered in a lower dose, while there is a high morbidity rate in those exposed to drugs that previously caused an immunological reaction. In a toxic reaction, neutropenia usually develops gradually, and there may be abnormalities of other blood constituents, such as red cells or platelets. On the other hand, hypersensitivity reactions develop rapidly, especially if the patient is re-exposed to the offending agent; other features of hypersensitivity, such as rash and eosinophilia, may occur, and blood counts are more likely to show that the reduction is confined to neutrophils.

Laboratory investigations of the cause can be carried out only after the patient has recovered from agranulocytosis. Ideally, serum should be collected and frozen at the time of the dyscrasia. Toxic mechanisms are usually investigated in bone-marrow cultures to which the suspect drug and, if possible, its metabolites are added. If the metabolites are not known or are not available, the serum or urine of a healthy person who has taken the drug can be used, as it will contain the metabolites. Immunological mechanisms can be postulated when there are antibodies that react with the myeloid precursor cells in the marrow, circulating blood neutrophils, or both. Such mechanisms have also been suspected because of suppression of myelopoiesis, shown by a decreased number of colonies in marrow cultured in the presence of the drug and serum extracted at the time of the neutrophilia, compared with the number in non-sensitive subjects. Antibodies against neutrophils or precursor cells may be demonstrated by the use of immunofluorescent techniques that detect hapten formation (that is, a drug or metabolite becoming immunogenic by combining with a protein or other large molecule), immune complexes and auto-antibodies. The deposition of immuno-globulin or immune complex on the surface of the cell is detected using fluorescence-labelled antihuman immunoglobulin, the amount deposited being proportional to the amount of membrane fluorescence measured.

Dermatological reactions

Psychotropic drugs have been alleged to cause many different types of cutaneous reactions, although here, too, there is often difficulty in establishing a cause-and-effect relationship. Unrelated conditions, such as normal sunburn, acne vulgaris, neurodermatitis and allergic reactions to other drugs and chemicals, have been wrongly attributed to psychotropic drugs. In general, there are few dermatological symptoms and signs that cannot be caused by medication, but most fall into familiar patterns.

Although individual drugs tend to produce a limited range of reactions, they are capable of causing many different types. By far the most common reaction, however, is an exanthematic reaction, such a rash, this having been reported during treatment with most drugs. It may resemble an infectious disease and be referred to as, for instance, a morbilliform or scarlatiniform rash, but more often it shows itself as a diffuse, maculopapular eruption with no close resemblance to any particular infective exanthem. Cross-sensitivity with chemically related drugs may occur.

Other cutaneous reactions allegedly caused by psychotropic drugs (most of them rare) are listed in Table 15.1.

Some rashes are photosensitive, either phototoxic or photoallergic. Drugs that have phototoxic effects increase the reactivity of the skin to ultraviolet or visible light. The reaction has no immunological basis and often occurs on first exposure to the sensitising agent. Photoallergic reactions, on the other hand, involve immunological mechanisms. The two types of reaction may be clinically indistinguishable, and resemble normal sunburn. They may be induced by fluorescent lighting.

Skin pigmentation occasionally follows prolonged treatment with high doses of phenothiazines. It occurs more often in women than in men. It is sometimes confined to those parts of the skin that have been exposed to sunlight, and it may be associated with corneal and lenticular opacities (see below). Pigmentary deposits also occur throughout the reticulo-endothelial system and in the parenchymal cells of internal organs.

Melanin is formed in the cytoplasmic organelles of melanocytes by oxidation of the amino acid tyrosine in the presence of the enzyme tyrosinase. Its production is under hormonal and neural control. The

Table 15.1 Some alleged dermatological reactions to commonly used psychotropic drugs

Type of reaction	Drugs alleged to cause reaction[1]
Acneiform eruptions	Lithium Maprotiline
Alopecia	Haloperidol Lithium Tricyclic antidepressants
Erythema multiforme	Chlorpromazine Chlordiazepoxide Lithium Mianserin Trazodone
Exanthematous reaction	Imipramine Phenothiazines
Exfoliative dermatitis	Chlorpromazine Imipramine Lithium Trazodone
Fixed eruptions	Chlordiazepoxide Lormetazepam Temazepam Trifluoperazine
Lichenoid eruption	Phenothiazines
Lupus erythematosus-like syndrome	Chlorpromazine Lithium
Onycholysis	Phenothiazines
Photosensitivity reaction	Benzodiazepines Phenothiazepines Tricyclic antidepressants
Pigmentation	Diazepam Imipramine Nitrazepam Phenothiazines

Table continues overleaf

most important darkening factors are α-MSH, oestrogen and thyroid hormones. Lightening factors include adrenaline, noradrenaline, serotonin and, most importantly, melatonin present in the pineal gland and peripheral nerves. Although the mechanism is uncertain, it has been suggested that phenothiazines disturb the balance between darkening and lightening factors, as a result of which there is a relative excess of MSH and overproduction of melanin.

Table 15.1 *Continued*

Type of reaction	Drugs alleged to cause reaction[1]
Pseudolymphomatous eruptions	Amitriptyline Benzodiazepines Fluoxetine Lithium Phenothiazines
Psoriasiform eruptions	Lithium[2] Trazodone
Subcutaneous nodules (at injection site)	Fluspirilene
Toenail dystrophy	Lithium
Toxic epidermal necrolysis	Chlorpromazine Phenothiazines
Urticaria	Chlordiazepoxide Fluoxetine Tricyclic antidepressants
Vasculitis	Fluoxetine Maprotiline Phenothiazines Trazodone Tricyclic antidepressants

1. The listing of a drug class (eg phenothiazines) means that some but not all members of the class have been incriminated.
2. Lithium may also aggravate existing psoriasis, make it resistant to treatment, and/or convert it to a pustular type.

Ophthalmic effects

Most of the effects of psychotropic drugs on the eye are part of a more generalised reaction. An allergic skin reaction, for instance, may affect the eyelids and conjunctiva, while a drug's antimuscarinic effect may cause cycloplegia (paralysis of the ciliary muscle, causing loss of accommodation) and mydriasis. Similarly, extrapyramidal disturbances may include oculogyric crises.

Mydriasis can cause the peripheral part of the iris, especially in those with narrow irido-corneal angles, to occlude access of aqueous humour to the drainage canals, thereby impeding its outflow and increasing intra-ocular pressure. Although glaucoma precipitated by drugs is not common, caution is advised when drugs with marked anticholinergic effects are administered to patients at risk. The main risk factor for angle-closure glaucoma is longsightedness, although glaucoma can occur in normal or even shortsighted subjects. Elderly patients, particularly those with advanced cataracts, are also at increased risk. Symptoms of angle closure are blurred vision and pain in the eye, which is sometimes preceded by episodes of seeing coloured rings (halos) around lights. The oblique illumination test is helpful in diagnosis. In dimmed light the beam of a flashlight is directed from the temporal side of the eye tangentially towards the pupil. In the normal eye the nasal and temporal parts of the iris are equally well illuminated, but in those with narrow irido-corneal angles the nasal part of the iris is in shadow. Whenever there is a doubt, the patient should be referred to an ophthalmologist for tonometry and gonioscopy (assessment of the irido-corneal angle).

Phenothiazines cause pigmentation in the eye as well as in the skin (see above). Its appearance depends on the dose of drug, duration of treatment, sex of the patient, climate and amount of exposure to light. Pigmentation occurs in exposed parts of the bulbar conjunctiva and cornea, while specks of pigmentation can be seen in the lens; these become aggregated and form star-shaped opacities, but usually they do not affect vision. Pigmentary retinopathy may also occur following treatment with phenothiazines, especially thioridazine in doses exceeding 800 mg per day. The clinical picture resembles retinitis pigmentosa, with decreased visual acuity, night blindness and transient scotomas, confined to the central part of the field of vision. In most cases vision improves on stopping treatment.

The blood–eye barrier resembles the blood–brain barrier, and the ability of a drug to enter the eye depends on its chemical structure, water and lipid solubility, polarity and ionic charge. In some animals phenothiazines reach concentrations in uveal tissue 50 times the mean distribution levels. It is thought that chlorpromazine or one of its metabolites, acting as a photosensitising agent, interacts with lens protein to cause denaturation and flocculation; this in turn results in the lenticular opacities.

Treatment and prevention of adverse reactions

Treatment

Many minor unwanted effects disappear spontaneously, while tolerance to others may develop rapidly. Decreasing the dose or stopping treatment usually leads to the disappearance of adverse reactions. Sometimes reintroducing the offending drug or substituting a related compound does not lead to a recurrence, which is not surprising when we consider the many uncertainties and large number of variables involved. Adverse effects may also respond to symptomatic treatment and some even respond to placebo.

Serious adverse reactions call for specialist assessment and treatment, while less serious effects should be managed by the psychiatrist who initiated the treatment. Included among the former are glaucoma, blood dyscrasias and urinary retention. Treatment of extrapyramidal reactions is an integral part of psychiatric care, and psychiatrists should know how to manage a potentially dangerous reaction, such as a drug-induced hypertensive crisis, with an intravenous α-adrenergic receptor blocking agent or intramuscular chlorpromazine.

Prevention

Many adverse reactions can be prevented if psychotropic drugs are used with caution or avoided altogether in conditions where pathological disturbances of tissue sensitivity or pharmacokinetics are likely to lead to exaggerated reactions. Depending on the drug, these predisposing conditions include: organic brain disorders; cardiac, hepatic and renal diseases; blood dyscrasias; and a predisposition to allergy. Particular care should be taken when prescribing psychotropic drugs for children and elderly people, especially those who are debilitated. Psychoactive drugs should be used with great care in patients who drive or who work in dangerous situations.

The greater the number of patients that are exposed to drugs, the greater will be the prevalence of untoward effects. Avoiding the unnecessary administration of drugs and adhering to sound principles of prescribing are therefore important preventive measures. Drug combinations that are not essential should be avoided, particularly in the elderly. Polypharmacy increases the incidence of adverse reactions and interactions, and using more than one drug of the same class (e.g. antipsychotics or antidepressants) is rarely justified.

Acknowledgement

I should like to express my appreciation to colleagues in the medical specialties related to the physiological systems reviewed for their helpful comments and to Althea Edwards for her secretarial assistance.

Further reading

Anderson, I. M. & Edwards, J. G. (2001) Guidelines for choice of selective serotonin reuptake inhibitor in depressive illness. *Advances in Psychiatric Treatment*, 7, 170–180.

Baldessarini, R. J. (2001) Drugs and the treatment of psychiatric disorders. Depression and anxiety disorders. In *Goodman & Gilman's The Pharmacological Basis of Therapeutics* (10th edn) (eds J. G. Hardman, L. E. Limbird & A. G. Gilman), pp. 447–483. New York: McGraw-Hill.

Baldessarini, R. J. (2001) Drugs and the treatment of psychiatric disorders. Psychosis and mania. In *Goodman & Gilman's The Pharmacological Basis of Therapeutics* (10th edn) (eds J. G. Hardman, L. E. Limbird & A. G. Gilman), pp. 485–520. New York: McGraw-Hill.

Baldwin, D. & Mayers, A. (2003) Sexual side-effects of antidepressant and antipsychotic drugs. *Advances in Psychiatric Treatment*, **9**, 202–210.

Baldwin, D. S., Thomas, S. C. & Birtwistle, J. (1997) Effects of antidepressant drugs on sexual function. *International Journal of Psychiatry in Clinical Practice*, **1**, 47–58.

Barnes, T. R. E. & Edwards, J. G. (1993) The side-effects of antipsychotic drugs. 1. CNS and neuromuscular effects. In *Antipsychotic Drugs and Their Side Effects* (ed. T. R. E. Barnes), pp. 213–247. London: Academic Press.

Barnes, T. R. E. & Harvey, C. (1992) Sexual side effects of psychotropic drugs. In *Sexual Pharmacology* (eds A. Riley, T. Wilson & M. Peet), pp. 176–196. Oxford: Oxford University Press.

Beutler, E., Lichtman, M. A., Coller, B. S., *et al* (eds) (2001) *Williams' Hematology* (6th edn). New York: McGraw-Hill.

Breathnach, S. M. (1998). Drug reactions. In *Textbook of Dermatology* (6th edn) (eds R. H. Champion, J. L. Burton, D. A. Burns, *et al*), vol. 4, pp. 3349–3517. Oxford: Blackwell.

Cohen, L. S., Friedman, J. M., Jefferson, J. W., *et al* (1994) A reevaluation of risk of in utero exposure to lithium. *Journal of the American Medical Association*, **271**, 146–150.

Cunningham Owens, D. G. (1999) *A Guide to the Extrapyramidal Side-effects of Antipsychotic Drugs*. Cambridge: Cambridge University Press.

Davis, K. L., Charney, D., Coyle, J. J., *et al* (2002) *Neuropsychopharmacology: The Fifth Generation of Progress*. Philadelphia, PA: Lippincott, Williams & Wilkins.

Dickey, W. (1991) The neuroleptic malignant syndrome. *Progress in Neurobiology*, **36**, 425–436.

Dollery, C. (ed.) (1999) *Therapeutic Drugs* (2nd edn), vols 1 and 2. Edinburgh: Churchill Livingstone.

Dukes, M. N. G. (1975–96) *Meyler's Side Effects of Drugs* (8th–13th edns). Amsterdam: Elsevier.

Dukes, M. N. G. (ed.) (1977–91) *Side Effects of Drugs Annuals*, vols 1–15. Amsterdam: Elsevier.

Dukes, M. N. G. & Aronson, J. K. (eds) (1992–2000) *Side Effects of Drugs Annuals*, vols 16–23. Amsterdam: Elsevier.

Dukes, M. N. G. & Aronson, J. K. (2000) *Meyler's Side Effects of Drugs* (14th edn). Amsterdam: Elsevier.

Edwards, J. G. (1981) Unwanted effects of psychotropic drugs and their mechanisms. In *Handbook of Biological Psychiatry, Part VI. Practical Applications of Psychotropic Drugs and Other Biological Treatments* (eds H. M. van Praag, M. H. Lader, O. J. Raphelson, *et al*), pp. 1–38. New York: Marcel Dekker.

Edwards, J. G. (1981) Adverse effects of antianxiety drugs. *Drugs*, **22**, 495–514.

Edwards, J. G. (1986) The untoward effects of antipsychotic drugs: pathogenesis and management. In *The Psychopharmacology and Treatment of Schizophrenia* (eds P. B. Bradley & S. R. Hirsch), pp. 403–441. Oxford: Oxford University Press.

Edwards, J. G. (1989) Drug-related depression: clinical and epidemiological aspects. In *Depression: An Integrated Approach* (eds K. Herbst & E. Paykel), pp. 81–110. Oxford: Heinemann.

Edwards, J. G. & Anderson, I. (1999) Systematic review and guide to selection of selective serotonin reuptake inhibitors. *Drugs*, **57**, 507–533.

Edwards, J. G. & Barnes, T. R. E. (1993) The side-effects of psychotropic drugs. II. Effects on other physiological systems. In *Antipsychotic Drugs and Their Side Effects* (ed. T. R. E. Barnes), pp. 249–275. London: Academic Press.

Edwards, J. G., Long, S. K. & Sedgwick, E. M. (1986) Antidepressants and convulsive seizures: clinical, electroencephalographic and pharmacological aspects. *Clinical Neuropharmacology*, **9**, 329–360.

Geddes, J., Freemantle, N., Harrison, P., *et al*, for the National Schizophrenia Guideline Development Group (2000) Atypical antipsychotics in the treatment of schizophrenia: systematic overview and meta-regression analysis. *BMJ*, **321**, 1371–1376.

Glassman, A. H. & Bigger, J. T. (2001) Antipsychotic drugs: prolonged QTc interval, torsade de pointes, and sudden death. *American Journal of Psychiatry*, **158**, 1774–1782.

Haddad, P. M. & Anderson, I. M. (2002) Antipsychotic-related QTc prolongation, torsade de pointes and sudden death. *Drugs*, **62**, 1649–1671.

Hall, R. L., Smith, A. G. & Edwards, J. G. (2003) Haematological safety of antipsychotic drugs. *Expert Opinion in Drug Safety*, **2**, 395–399.

Johnson, D. A. W. (1986) Depressive symptoms in schizophrenia: some observations on the frequency, morbidity and possible causes. In *Contemporary Issues in Schizophrenia* (eds A. Kerr & P. Snaith), pp. 451–458. London: Gaskell.

King, D. J. (1986) Drug-induced psychiatric disorders. In *Iatrogenic Diseases* (3rd edn) (eds P. F. D'Arcy & J. P. Griffin), pp. 651–670. London: Oxford University Press.

Kohen, D. & Bristow, M. (1996) Neuroleptic malignant syndrome. *Advances in Psychiatric Treatment*, **2**, 151–157.

Koro, C. E., Fedder, D. O., L'Italien, G. L., *et al* (2002) Assessment of independent effect of olanzapine and risperidone on risk of diabetes among patients with schizophrenia: population based nested case-control study. *BMJ*, **325**, 243–245.

Lee, G. R., Foerster, J. & Lukens, J. (eds) (1999) *Wintrobe's Clinical Hematology* (9th edn). Philadelphia: Lea & Febiger.

Litt, J. Z. (1999) *Drug Eruption Reference Manual 1999*. London: Parthenon.

Nutt, D. J. (ed.) (1992) Symposium on Methods of Assessing Unwanted Effects of Psychotropic Drugs. *Journal of Psychopharmacology*, **6**, 191–229.

Read, A. E. (1992). The liver and drugs. In *Wright's Liver and Biliary Disease* (3rd edn) (eds G. H. Millward-Sadler, R. Wright & M. J. P. Arthur), vol. 2, pp. 1233–1261. London: W. B. Saunders.

Rosen, R. C., Lane, R. M. & Menza, M. (1999) Effects of SSRIs on sexual function: a critical review. *Journal of Clinical Psychopharmacology*, **19**, 67–85.

Shiloh, R., Nutt, D. & Weizman, A. (1999) *Atlas of Psychiatric Pharmacotherapy*. London: Martin Dunitz.

Speight, T. M. & Holford, N. H. G. (1997) *Avery's Drug Treatment* (4th edn). Auckland: Adis International.

Stahl, S. M. (2000) *Essential Psychopharmacology. Neuroscientific Basis and Practical Applications* (2nd edn). Cambridge: Cambridge University Press.

Stern, R. S. & Wintroub, B. U. (1999) Cutaneous reactions to drugs. In *Fitzpatrick's Dermatology in General Medicine* (5th edn) (eds I. M. Freedberg, A. Z. Eisen, K. Wolff, *et al*), vol. 1, pp. 1633–1642. New York: McGraw-Hill.

Taylor, D. M. (2003) Antipsychotics and QT prolongation. *Acta Psychiatrica Scandinavica*, **107**, 85–95.

van Walraven, C., Mamdani, M. M., Wells, P. S., *et al* (2001) Inhibition of serotonin reuptake by antidepressants and upper gastrointestinal bleeding in elderly patients: retrospective cohort study. *BMJ*, **323**, 655–658.

Waller, D. G. & Edwards, J. G. (1989) Lithium and the kidney: an update. *Psychological Medicine*, **19**, 825–831.

Warrington, S. J., Padgham, C. & Lader, M. (1989) The cardiovascular effects of antidepressants. *Psychological Medicine* (monograph suppl. 16), 1–40.

CHAPTER 16

Unwanted effects of psychotropic drugs: 2. Drug interactions, effects during pregnancy and breast-feeding, pharmaco-vigilance and medico-legal considerations

J. Guy Edwards

The untoward effects of psychotropic drugs on various physiological systems that are of clinical relevance are discussed in Chapter 15. This chapter discusses adverse interactions between these drugs and describes their effects on the unborn and newborn. It goes on to give an account of methods of drug safety monitoring and ends with a discussion of the medico-legal aspects of drug treatment in psychiatry.

Drug interactions

If two or more drugs are administered at the same time they may produce their effects independently or they may interact. The interactions may be mediated via pharmacokinetic or pharmacodynamic mechanisms. Like other unwanted effects, the interactions may be predictable or unpredictable. They are more likely to be predictable if the pharmacokinetics and mechanism of action of the substances are known.

Most interactions are harmless and are only of theoretical interest. Some may even be beneficial and be employed, for instance, in augmentation therapy. Clinically important adverse interactions occur in only a small proportion of those treated with drug combinations, and even then the severity of the interaction varies from patient to patient. However, the potential seriousness of these interactions should not be underestimated. Drugs with a small therapeutic ratio and substances that require careful control of dosage are those most often responsible for hazardous interactions. The patients most at risk include the elderly and subjects with impaired hepatic or renal function.

Pharmacokinetic interactions

Pharmacokinetic interactions occur when one compound alters the absorption, distribution, metabolism or excretion of another and thereby increases or decreases the concentration of drug available to produce its pharmacological effects. If such interactions occur with one compound, it cannot be assumed that they will occur with a related substance, but they are more likely to if it has a similar chemical structure or if its pharmacological properties are similar.

Delayed absorption resulting from an interaction is not of clinical importance unless high peak plasma concentrations are required, as in the case of analgesics or antibiotics. In such cases, a decrease in the total amount of drug absorbed may result in ineffective treatment. After being absorbed, drugs are bound to plasma proteins, but the protein-binding sites are non-specific. One drug can displace another, thereby increasing the proportion of drug free to diffuse from the plasma to its site of action. This produces a detectable increase in effect only if the drug is extensively bound (>90%) and is not widely distributed through the body. Even then displacement rarely produces more than transient potentiation because the raised concentration of free drug increases the rate of elimination.

Many drugs are metabolised in the liver. Induction of the hepatic micro-enzymal system by one substance can increase the rate of metabolism of another and so decrease its effect. On discontinuing treatment with the inducer, the plasma concentration of the drug whose metabolism had been accelerated increases and toxicity may occur. Conversely, when one drug inhibits the metabolism of another, higher plasma concentrations are produced, with the risk of toxicity.

Drugs are eliminated through the kidney by glomerular filtration and active tubular secretion. Competition occurs between substances that share active transport mechanisms in the proximal tubule.

During recent years much interest has been shown in the cytochrome (CYP) P450 enzymes. These are widespread throughout the animal kingdom and are involved in the oxidation of xenobiotics and drugs in people. They are located mainly in the membranes of the smooth endoplasmic reticulum of hepatocytes but also in the gut mucosa, lungs, kidney, brain and skin. Fourteen families of the enzymes have been identified by molecular biological techniques. These are further categorised into sub-families according to the degree of similarity of their amino acid sequences. Each is encoded by a separate gene. Each of the enzymes is given the prefix CYP(cytochrome)450 followed by a number for the family, a letter for the sub-family and a number for the individual enzyme within the sub-family.

There are four cytochrome enzymes of importance in psychotropic drug metabolism and interactions: CYP1A2, CYP2C, CYP2D6 and

CYP3A4 (see Table 16.1). These four respectively make up 10–15%, 20%, <5% and 25% of the P450 enzyme content of the liver. P450 enzymes of different families have at least 35% similarity in their amino acid composition. Those of different sub-families have different degrees of similarity. Each enzyme is influenced by genetic, constitutional and environmental factors to a different extent.

The differences in amino acid composition are reflected in differences in the substrates on which the enzymes act. Although many drugs have a high affinity for one particular P450 enzyme, most drugs are oxidised by more than one P450 enzyme. Furthermore, an individual enzyme is able to oxidise several drugs. There is therefore considerable overlap between the substrate specificities (see Table 16.1).

The quality of the evidence for specific interactions varies. Some interactions have been demonstrated in animals only, while the evidence for others is based on *in vitro* studies with hepatic microsomal enzyme preparations, isolated case reports or small-scale studies, many of which were uncontrolled or produced conflicting results. The evidence for yet other interactions is circumstantial, being purely based on the fact that two (or more) drugs are substrates for the same enzyme. Table 16.1 does not contain a comprehensive list of substrates, but only those listed in the tables of interactions, produced as Appendices 16.1–16.6 to this chapter.

The interactions shown in Appendices 16.1–16.7 are those thought to be of clinical relevance to psychotropic drug treatment by the expert advisers to the *British National Formulary* (BNF). Some of the processes involved in the interactions have been incorporated into the tables but, as there is currently much uncertainty about the relative role of different enzymes and as new knowledge of enzyme activity is rapidly accumulating, these tables (like Table 16.1) should be regularly updated. Before prescribing a new drug combination, it is also prudent to check for any new interactions reported in the latest edition of the BNF.

It should be stressed that interactions are only one of many factors that influence the response to drug combinations. Other factors include: the doses of the drugs; diet, age and genetic make-up of the patient; and any concurrent illnesses. Thus, for example, an interaction involving a P450 enzyme is no different to the effect of administering the drug to someone with a genetic deficiency of the particular enzyme – as in the case of CYP2D6 oxidation, which is deficient in 5–10% of the population.

Interactions are of special importance in:

(1) patients with concomitant illnesses receiving polypharmacy, especially when treatment is not carefully monitored
(2) polydrug misusers, particularly those who take drugs of unknown strength (often with unknown substances added)

Table 16.1   Cytochrome P450 enzymes, substrates, inducers and inhibitors

Psychotropic substrates	Other substrates	Inducers	Inhibitors
CYP1A2			
Citalopram	Propranolol	Carbamazepine	Cimetidine
Chlorpromazine	Theophylline	Omeprazole	Clarithromycin
Clozapine	Verapramil	Phenobarbital	Erythromycin
Diazepam	Warfarin	Phenytoin	Fluvoxamine
Fluvoxamine		Rifampicin	Isoniazid
Haloperidol		Ritonavir	Ketaconazole
Mirtazapine			Mirtazapine
Olanzapine			Moclobemide
Thioridazine			Nefazodone
Tricyclics, tertiary			Omeprazole
Trifluoperazine			Sertraline
Zotepine			
CYP2C9/19			
Barbiturates	Omeprazole	Carbamazepine	Amiodarone
Citalopram	NSAIDs	Phenobarbital	Carbamazepine
Diazepam	Phenytoin	Phenytoin	Cimetidine
Fluoxetine	Warfarin	Rifampicin	Fluconazole
Moclobemide			Fluoxetine
Tricyclics, tertiary			Fluvoxamine
			Ketonazole
			Moclobemide
			Omeprazole
			Sertraline
			Tranylcypromine
CYP2D6			
Chlorpromazine	Amphetamines	Carbamazepine	Amiodarone
Citalopram	Antiarrhythmics	Phenobarbitone	Chlorpromazine
Desipramine	Beta-blockers	Phenytoin	Cimetidine
Fluoxetine	Flecainide	Rifampicin	Citalopram
Flupentixol	Galantamine	Ritonavir	Diltiazem
Fluphenazine	Opioids		Flecainide
Fluvoxamine	Propranolol		Fluphenazine
Haloperidol			Fluoxetine
Mirtazapine			Fluvoxamine
Nefazodone			Haloperidol
Olanzapine			Methadone
Paroxetine			Metoclopramide
Perphenazine			Mirtazapine
Risperidone			Moclobemide

Table continues opposite

Table 16.1 *Continued*

Psychotropic substrates	Other substrates	Inducers	Inhibitors
Sertindole			Nefazodone
Thioridazine			Quinidine
Trazodone			Paroxetine
Tricyclics,			Perphenazine
secondary and			Propranolol
tertiary			Ritonavir
Venlafaxine			Sertraline
			Thioridazine
			Trifluoperazine
			Tricyclics
			Venlafaxine
CYP3A4			
Benzodiazepines	Amiodarone	Barbiturates	Amiodarone
Buspirone	Antihistamines	Carbamazepine	Cimetidine
Carbamazepine	Calcium channel	Phenytoin	Citalopram
Citalopram	blockers	Rifampicin	Clarithromycin
Clozapine	Carbamazepine	Primidone	Diltiazem
Fluoxetine	Diltiazem		Erythromycin
Mianserin	Disapyramide		Fluoxetine
Mirtazapine	Indinavir		Fluvoxamine
Nefazodone	Itraconazole		Indinavir
Pimozide	Ketaconazole		Itraconazole
Quetiapine	Macrolidines		Ketraconazole
Reboxetine	Omeprazole		Macrolidines (some)
Risperidone	Progesterone		Mirtazapine
Sertraline	Quinidine		Nefazodone
Sertindole	Rifampicin		Omeprazole
Tricyclics, tertiary	Ritonavir		Paroxetine
Venlafaxine	Terfanadine		Retinavir
Zolpidem	Verapamil		Sertraline
Zopiclone			Sertindole
Zotepine			Trazodone
			Tricyclics
			Verapamil
			Venlafaxine

Substrates listed may be partly or fully metabolised by the CYP enzyme.

Both weak and powerful, competitive and non-competitive, inhibitors are listed.

From the table actual and potential interactions can be predicted.

Onset and effect of inhibition depends on half-life and time to steady state of inhibitor and drug metabolised.

Because some drugs are metabolised by several enzymes, if one is inhibited others may compensate.

(3)   patients receiving high doses of medication in the management of drug-resistant disorders

(4)   developing countries in which there is a high prevalence of dangerous self-medication and irresponsible dispensing by unqualified or unethical pharmacists.

In the Appendices, both drug categories and individual compounds are shown. The listing of a drug group means that all or many of the substances within the group have been implicated in the drug interaction. But even when only an individual drug is considered responsible for the interaction, clinicians should be vigilant for the possible occurrence of the same or a similar interaction with related compounds. Some of the 'query' interactions listed are theoretical possibilities based on laboratory experiments, isolated case reports or the fact that the drugs are substrates for the same enzyme.

Hazardous interactions, such as extreme sedation and respiratory depression brought about by the inhibition of metabolism of benzodiazepines by retinavir and ventricular arrhythmias produced by the inhibition of metabolism of terfenadine produced by the selective serotonin reuptake inhibitors (SSRIs), are shown in italics in the Appendices. Central nervous system (CNS) toxicity, another serious reaction caused, for instance, by the combined use of SSRIs and other drugs acting through serotonergic mechanisms, may present with a wide range of neuropsychiatric symptoms. These include: excitation and restlessness; pyrexia with sweating and flushing; fluctuating vital signs; tremor, rigidity and myoclonus; delirium; and, rarely, coma and death. In the case of interactions where only some CNS toxic effects have been observed, such as agitation and nausea occurring during treatment with an SSRI and tryptophan, only the reported individual symptoms are shown.

Most of the pharmacokinetic interactions listed are due to altered metabolism. Inhibition of metabolism causes an increase in plasma drug concentration, which in turn produces an increase in the dose-related adverse effects discussed in the previous chapter. By contrast, accelerated metabolism brought about by enzyme induction (see Table 16.1) lowers the plasma drug concentration and this can lead to a subtherapeutic response.

Pharmacodynamic interactions

Most pharmacodynamic interactions can be predicted from the known pharmacological properties of the relevant drugs. The most common effects are due to summation. The CNS depressant effects of psychotropic drugs may be added to those of other drugs that depress the nervous system, including alcohol and over-the-counter medication (particularly antihistamines). Similarly, the anticholinergic effects (described under 'Autonomic effects' in the section 'Neuropsychiatric effects' in Chapter 15) may summate, as may the adrenoceptor blocking effects (leading to hypotensive episodes) and antidopaminergic effects (resulting in an increase in extrapyramidal disturbance). It will be recalled that CNS depressant and hypotensive effects cause particular problems for the elderly.

Another group of pharmacodynamic interactions result from inhibition of monoamine oxidase in the gut wall and liver. This results in increased levels of circulating pressor amines – the mechanism responsible for the well-known 'cheese reaction'. Inhibition of monoamine oxidase can also cause increased levels of drugs that would normally be metabolised by the mixed hepatic oxidases, while inhibition of presynaptic mitochondrial monoamine oxidase increases the availability of noradrenaline in the synaptic vesicles. The clinical results of such interactions are shown in the Appendices.

Reference was made in Chapter 15 to serious cardiac arrhythmias and the increased chance of these occurring in subjects with a prolonged QT interval. Administering more than one drug with the potential to increase the QT interval increases the risk of an arrhythmia and therefore the possibility of sudden unexpected death.

A possible interaction that has caused much concern in everyday psychiatric practice is that between haloperidol and lithium, but detailed critical reviews of the evidence show that the risk has been exaggerated. There are no good reasons why the two drugs cannot be prescribed together but, to err on the side of safety, it is advisable to keep serum lithium levels below 1 mmol/l and to discontinue treatment with both drugs if pyrexia occurs in the presence of extrapyramidal symptoms.

Prevention of interactions

It is particularly important to prevent the serious interactions listed in italic in the Appendices. Drug combinations that cause these inter-actions should be avoided wherever possible. On the rare occasions when it is essential to use the combined treatment, careful supervision and monitoring of the patient should be carried out.

Some of the interactions can be prevented by delaying the start of treatment. For instance, when it is necessary to prescribe selegiline for patients who have been on fluoxetine or sertraline, the dopaminergic should be withheld until 5 weeks after stopping fluoxetine or 2 weeks after stopping sertraline. Similarly, each of these SSRIs should be withheld until 2 weeks after stopping selegiline. Other potentially hazardous interactions can be prevented by prescribing a lower dose of one of the interacting drugs, for example half of the usual dose of theophylline when given with fluvoxamine.

The interactions that matter in clinical practice involve drugs that cause severe toxic effects and those with a low therapeutic ratio. Particular attention should be paid to the drug combinations listed in the Appendixes, but this in itself is not enough. The cytochrome enzymes responsible for biotransformation are known in only about 20% of marketed drugs, because many of the compounds were developed at a time when current knowledge of the enzymes and the technology for quantifying them did not exist. We therefore owe it to our patients to make detailed enquiry into all the substances they are taking (including over-the-counter medication and illegal drugs), to keep abreast of rapidly evolving knowledge of interactions, and to report suspected adverse interactions – in the UK to the Committee on Safety of Medicines (CSM).

Effects on the unborn and newborn

Lessons from thalidomide

During the early 1960s, confidence in medicine and the pharmaceutical industry was shaken by an epidemic of one of the most horrendous and tragic adverse drug reactions ever described. This was the thalidomide disaster, which has had the most profound effect on the development and licensing of new drugs and our thinking about prescribing medication for pregnant women. Within three years of the launch of the hypnotic thalidomide on to the (then) West German market, 477 cases of phocomelia and other mesodermal abnormalities were encountered. Phocomelia – the bilateral absence of a large part of an arm, leg or all four limbs – is normally a very rare congenital abnormality that most paediatricians hardly ever see. In the German epidemic at least half of the mothers of the children with phocomelia and related malformations, but none of a control group, remembered taking thalidomide during the early stages of pregnancy.

The drug was not prescribed to the same extent in Britain, but even so at least 349 children with thalidomide-induced damage survived long enough to be recorded in a national survey carried out in 1962. Worldwide, thousands of malformed babies were born to mothers who had taken the drug. It was found that the British epidemic began nine months after the drug was supplied to wholesalers and ceased when it was withdrawn from the market.

Despite the lessons that have been learnt from the thalidomide disaster and the many warnings that have since been issued, many women take drugs while pregnant or become pregnant while taking drugs, including those whose teratogenic potential is not known. This exposes their unborn babies to the risk of intra-uterine damage. What is even more worrying is that thalidomide is currently being used in Third World countries to treat the leprosy reaction, erythema nodosum leprosum (ENL type II lepra reaction), controls are not being exercised as stringently as they should be, and new cases of phocomelia are still being encountered.

Principles of teratogenicity

Psychotropic drugs are prescribed during pregnancy not only for the treatment of psychiatric disorders but also to treat complications of pregnancy, such as hyperemesis gravidarum. Most drugs cross the placental barrier to some extent, the rate of transfer being dependent on:

(1)   the concentration gradient between mother and foetus
(2)   the thickness and surface area of the placental membrane
(3)   the blood flow in the intervillous space
(4)   placental enzyme activity
(5)   the molecular weight, configuration, polarity, protein-binding capacity and lipid solubility of the drug.

Drugs (or other chemical substances) that have an adverse effect on the embryo or foetus are called teratogens. In the past a teratogen was defined as a substance that produced congenital structural abnormalities. During recent years, however, the definition has been extended to embrace all substances that, through a direct or indirect effect *in utero*, cause functional as well as structural abnormalities in the foetus or in the child after birth. This may include abnormalities that do not manifest themselves until late in development. Thus, at various stages a teratogen can cause:

(1)   chromosomal abnormalities
(2)   failure of implantation of the foetus
(3)   resorption of the embryo
(4)   an abortion
(5)   structural malformations – dysmorphogenesis
(6)   retardation of intra-uterine growth
(7)   death of the foetus
(8)   neonatal functional impairment
(9)   abnormal behaviour at a later stage
(10) learning disability.

The last three of these are examples of 'behavioural teratogenicity'. Other potential hazards are transplacental carcinogenicity, mutogenesis and the effects of paternal exposure to a drug, although such reactions have not been specifically related to the use of psychotropic drugs.

Factors influencing teratogenicity

Factors that influence teratogenicity include the type of drug, dose, timing of exposure, synergic effect of other substances and genetic predisposition.

During the pre-embryonic period (up to 17 days after conception) the undifferentiated blastocyst is totipotent. Cells damaged by a drug during this period may be replaced by extra divisions of the other cells and normal development may occur. However, if the toxic damage is extensive, the embryo will not be implanted in the uterus or, if it is, a spontaneous abortion may occur. If a drug with a short half-life that is completely excreted has been taken for only a month after the last menstrual period and the pregnancy continues, there may not be an increased risk to the foetus because of this 'all or nothing' principle.

Foetal development can be affected at any time during gestation, although the foetus is most vulnerable during periods of rapid growth – between implantation and the completion of organogenesis, that is, between the first and ninth weeks of pregnancy, and the growth spurt during the second half of pregnancy. Individual organs are most susceptible at times of maximum differentiation. For some drugs there is thus a period of maximum risk.

Drugs administered after the fourth month of pregnancy do not cause structural teratogenesis; they reach concentrations in the foetus similar to those in the mother but may produce exaggerated adverse effects because of the immaturity of the foetus's metabolic and enzyme system. A drug given to the mother that is present in the infant at birth may cause predictable effects and such effects may also occur when a drug known to cause dependence is being withdrawn from the mother during delivery.

There is a threshold dose – a no-effect level (NEL) – below which a teratogen has no known effect. Above this threshold the dose–response curve is steep and there is a narrow margin between the no-effect and lethal doses. There is evidence (e.g. from studies of anti-epileptics) that the teratogenic effect of a drug may be enhanced by a second drug, or even by environmental chemicals, although this could partly be explained by the severity of the disease being treated. Although teratogenicity is influenced by the genetic predisposition of the foetus, it is not known how this influence is mediated, the extent to which it interacts with environmental factors or how it affects the pharmacokinetics and metabolism of the offending agents.

To put the chances of drug-induced foetal damage in perspective, it should be noted that a half of human conceptions end in a very early spontaneous abortion. A further 8–15% of recognised pregnancies end in early spontaneous abortion due to defects in implantation and abnormalities in early development. When pregnancy continues, major defects may be diagnosed and an abortion may be carried out. In addition to these risks, 1–2% of newborn babies have major congenital abnormalities, while 5–9% have minor abnormalities.

Teratogenic effects of specific drugs

Teratogenesis is difficult to assess. Few conclusions can be drawn from animal experiments because of differences between species. Voluntary reporting systems are dependent on the doctor's knowledge and initiative in reporting and are therefore prone to reporting bias; such systems are also uncontrolled. Retrospective studies have compared populations of subjects who have had a particular drug with those who have not had the drug (cohort-controlled studies). Other studies have compared the drugs taken by mothers who have had babies with congenital abnormalities with the drugs taken by mothers who have had normal babies (case-controlled studies). In both types of study the results are influenced by recall bias and problems in matching.

Some research has suggested a possible association between the use of barbiturates and minor foetal abnormalities, although this has not been confirmed. Similarly, the suggested association between treatment with diazepam and cleft lip (with or without cleft palate) has not been proven. There is no known risk associated with the use of antidepressants, but there is a significant (albeit small) risk of an increased incidence of abnormalities associated with phenothiazines.

The international Register of Lithium Babies revealed a 7.8% incidence of abnormalities, with a fivefold increase in cardiovascular malformations (e.g. mitral and tricuspid valve atresia, aortic coarctation and patent ductus arteriosus) and a 400-fold increase in the rare Ebstein anomaly (tricuspid valve distortion and displacement into the right ventricle). The period of maximum vulnerability appeared to be 20–45 days post-conception. However, the apparently high incidence of abnormalities could have been due to an ascertainment bias and a prospective case-controlled study of treatment with lithium in 148 women during the first trimester found no difference in the rates of malformations, spontaneous abortion, prematurity or stillbirth. However, there is still sufficient concern about lithium to justify stopping treatment during the first trimester. If, in the interests of the mother, treatment has to be continued, the lowest therapeutic dose should be used.

Most prospective surveys, cohort-controlled and case-controlled studies have not shown that psychotropic drugs are teratogenic, but until it can be shown beyond all reasonable doubt that a drug does not produce harmful effects, it should not be prescribed during pregnancy unless it is absolutely essential for the well-being of the mother. To do otherwise is at best unenlightened and at worst exposes helpless young humans to unethical, uncontrolled experimentation. If it is necessary to prescribe during pregnancy, newer psychotropic drugs should not usually be chosen, because less is known about their teratogenic potential. Women of child-bearing age receiving treatment with newer drugs should be advised to take adequate contraceptive precautions.

Effects on the newborn

As discussed above, newborn babies may be affected by psychotropic drugs received through the placenta. The newborn child (especially if born prematurely) is susceptible to the drug's effects because of his or her low protein-binding capacity, deficiencies in the immature liver and kidney of drug-metabolising enzymes, and limited renal clearance. Immaturity of the glucuronyl transferase system is one of the most important of these.

Benzodiazepines given to pregnant women have been said to cause a delay in the initiation of respiration, drowsiness, lethargy, diminished responsiveness, feeding difficulties, hypotonia, hypothermia, attacks of apnoea and a low Apgar score. Cardiac and respiratory distress, neuromuscular symptoms and urinary retention have been described following treatment with tricyclic antidepressants. Phenothiazines may lead to extrapyramidal symptoms, respiratory depression, hypothermia and hypotension in the newborn, while lithium has been reported as a cause of hypotonia, poor sucking and respiratory difficulties. Such associations are based on isolated case reports, but when the mother is not at serious risk of a relapse of mental illness, consideration should be given to reducing the dose of psychotropic drug given to the mother during the last four weeks of pregnancy.

Withdrawal phenomena may also occur, particularly in the newborn babies of drug-dependent women. Withdrawal from opiates may cause irritability, tremor, a shrill cry, sneezing, yawning, fever, sweating, scratching of the face, respiratory distress (with dyspnoea and cyanosis), convulsions and, rarely, death. As these phenomena cannot be successfully treated with other drugs, opiates may have to be administered to the neonate.

Effects during breast-feeding

Most drugs are excreted in breast milk. The concentration reached in the breast-fed infant depends on: the dose of drug and duration of treatment; the drug's lipid solubility, protein-binding properties and degree of ionisation; the pharmacokinetics in the mother (which are influenced by her hepatic and renal function); the volume, pH, protein, lipid and other constituents of the milk; and other factors.

Little research has been carried out into the effects on the newborn of psychotropic drugs excreted in breast milk. In the case of SSRIs, for instance, there are published reports on maternal breast milk concentrations, maternal and infant plasma concentrations, and possible toxic effects in only 30 infants whose mothers were on fluoxetine, 26 on sertraline, and two each on fluvoxamine and paroxetine (there were no reports for citalopram). Published reports of suspected adverse reactions to psychotropic drugs are anecdotal. The reactions include lethargy, weight loss and an increase in fast-wave activity in the EEG of a breast-fed infant of a mother receiving diazepam, and crying, irritability and colic in the child of a mother on fluoxetine.

The use of psychotropic drugs in lactating mothers requires us to balance risks that are unquantifiable in the light of available evidence. As there is so little knowledge of the effects on a developing infant, psychotropic drugs should be prescribed only when there are un-equivocal indications. At such times the drugs chosen should be those on which most data are available. In the case of SSRIs, for example, there is a larger body of information on fluoxetine and sertraline, although fluoxetine has the potential disadvantage of causing a more prolonged effect because of its long half-life and that of its major metabolite (norfluoxetine).

Delay in recognition of unwanted effects

The beneficial effects of drugs can be demonstrated fairly quickly with relatively small samples of patients, but it may take many years and many patients may have to be exposed to a drug before an uncommon adverse reaction is discovered. To encounter a reaction occurring with a frequency of one in 1000 cases, 3000 patients would have to be screened for the reaction, occurring only once, to be detected with 95% confidence. For a reaction with a frequency much less than this in a population with an appreciable background incidence of the reaction, hundreds of thousands, if not millions, of patients would have to be studied for the effect to be detected with the same confidence.

Delay in recognition is partly the result of failure to report unwanted effects to drug regulatory authorities, and it has been estimated that, in the UK, only about 10% of cases of all adverse reactions are reported to the CSM. Unfortunately, hints of danger sometimes go unheeded, especially when suspected reactions are atypical or unusual. This happened, for instance, before the discovery of the 'cheese reaction'. Observations made by medical practitioners and the comments of a drug firm's representative were laughed at and the reactions were labelled 'hysterical'. The pressor properties of tyramine (a name derived from *tyros* – the Greek word for cheese) had been known for decades and the effects of ingesting pressor amines while receiving MAOIs were foreseeable, yet it was not until years later that the phenomenon was properly investigated and the reaction became common knowledge.

Withdrawal from the market

Since the thalidomide disaster, many psychotropic drugs have been launched commercially, although many of them have been 'me-too' substances. Relatively few novel compounds have been introduced into practice, but it is of concern that a sizeable proportion of these new drugs have been withdrawn from use.

There has been no consistent pattern to withdrawal from the market. The products that have been withdrawn have different chemical structures and different pharmacological properties. Psychotropic examples include:

(1)   anxiolytic/hypnotic substances – methaqualone and triazolam
(2)   antidepressants – zimeldine and nomifensine
(3)   antipsychotic drugs – droperidol and remoxipride.

Clozapine and L-tryptophan were temporarily withdrawn. Clozapine was given a reprieve and reintroduced into practice when it was shown that, with careful monitoring, its benefits in drug-resistant schizophrenia outweighed the risks. Its use is now restricted to patients who are unresponsive to, or intolerant of, conventional antipsychotics and are registered with the Clozaril Patient Monitoring Service. L-tryptophan was re-employed when it was shown that it was a contaminant, not the drug itself, that was responsible for the untoward effects that had occurred.

There was also a 'near miss'. Concern was expressed over the occurrence of agranulocytosis during treatment with mianserin, but the risk of suspension was halted when its benefits were considered to exceed the risk. More recently sertindole and thioridazine were taken out of general use in the UK because of an association with serious cardiac arrhythmias. Sertindole and thioridazine are now available only for patients who have not responded to, or who are intolerant of, other antipsychotics, and in the case of sertindole, those enrolled in clinical trials.

The aforementioned drugs were withdrawn or their use was restricted for various reasons – blood dyscrasias in the case of clozapine, nomifensine and remoxipride; misuse, dependence and toxicity in overdose (due to a low therapeutic ratio) resulting from treatment with methaqualone; the Guillain–Barré syndrome following the administration of zimeldine; the eosinophilia–myalgia syndrome due to L-tryptophan's contaminant; ventricular arrhythmias associated with the use of droperidol, pimozide, sertindole and thioridazine; and alleged behavioural toxicity occurring during treatment with triazolam.

It took different periods of time to establish the possible, probable or proven causal connection between the drugs and the adverse reactions and to determine that the risks were beyond acceptable limits – under 3 years in the case of remoxipride and zimeldine; 9 years for nomifensine; and 13 years in the case of triazolam. The longer delays in particular underline the importance of reporting cases to the CSM (in the UK) – even when the events do not appear to be clearly drug related – and the need for improved methods of pharmaco-vigilance (see below). These steps are the least that can be taken for our patients. Unless the appropriate measures are put into effect, we must be prepared to face public, legal and media criticism – with media reporting often being sensational, alarming and damaging to patients, doctors and the pharmaceutical industry on which we depend for new treatments.

Reporting and monitoring adverse reactions

All existing systems of assessing, recording and monitoring adverse reactions have their strengths and their weaknesses (see Tables 16.2 and 16.3). Voluntary reporting of single cases – which are sometimes the earliest signals of unwanted effects – is dependent on the awareness, vigilance and initiative of the practitioner. Adverse reactions may be unrecognised or not reported, and even when they are reported, it is difficult to relate them to the drug.

Unwanted effects are more likely to be identified if they occur during a clinical trial, but even in trials the methods of eliciting adverse reactions and relating them to the drug usually leave much to be desired. Most trials are carried out with relatively small numbers of patients and are of short duration; they therefore do not allow for the recognition of rare effects and reactions that occur after prolonged treatment. Some of the weaknesses of trials can be overcome by carrying out a meta-analysis in which all relevant trials of sufficient quality are reviewed. The pooling of data increases the power and the analysis provides a summary quantifiable outcome measure.

In some larger-scale methods of drug safety monitoring, researchers compare retrospectively the frequency of exposure to a drug in patients who have experienced a particular effect with that in subjects who have not had the reaction. Other methods compare prospectively the incidence of unwanted effects in patients exposed to a drug with that in a control group who do not receive the drug. Yet others investigate prospectively the frequency of all adverse reactions in patients exposed to a wide variety of drugs.

615

Table 16.2 Methods of identifying unwanted effects: strengths

Methods	Strengths
Case reports	May draw attention to hitherto unrecognised unwanted effects
Controlled clinical trials	Randomisation and blinding minimises bias Likely to identify more common unwanted effects Provides comparative data
Meta-analysis of controlled trials	Attempts to identify all relevant trials by systematic review (although analysis limited to controlled trials) Pooling of data increases power Provides comparative data Provides a summary, quantified outcome measure
CSM's 'yellow card' system	Nationwide system that monitors all drugs in use throughout their lives Has potential for • all practitioners to report suspected reactions • all reactions in all patients to be reported Allows for monitoring in real world of general practice and hospital Provides a means of detecting rare adverse reactions Allows for comparisons of drugs with similar indications in similar patient populations during similar market lives Provides for research large subsamples of patients with uncommon or rare adverse reactions
PEM	Non-interventional observational design reflecting practice in real world Nationwide in scope Provides larger cohort within short time of drug's launch on to market than any other system Monitors events not just suspected adverse reactions Provides quantitative data on events as seen from perspective of GP Helps to identify events with incidence of 1 or more per 3000 patients Allows for identification of delayed adverse events Allows for comparisons of drugs with similar indications in similar patient populations Provides subsamples of patients who have had specific events (eg convulsions, pregnancy, death) for in-depth studies Provides pharmacoepidemiological data on prescribing practices

CSM = Committee on Safety of Medicines.
PEM = Prescription event monitoring.
Adapted from J. G. Edwards & I. Anderson (1999) Systematic review and guide to selection of selective serotonin reuptake inhibitors. *Drugs*, **57**, 507–533.

Table 16.3 Methods of identifying unwanted effects: weaknesses

Methods	Weaknesses
Case reports	Cause-and-effect relationship with drug cannot be established
Controlled clinical trials	Small sample sizes Unrepresentative patients Heterogeneity of patients Uncertainty over blinding Lack of information on compliance Difficulty relating less-common effects to drug Lack of inter-rater reliability in multicentre studies
Meta-analysis of controlled trials	Same weaknesses as for individual controlled trials Cannot eliminate publication/reporting bias Pooling of data, may be invalidated by heterogeneity of trials; may require simplification of outcome measures of individual trials Tendency to overinterpretation and sense of false certainty
CSM's 'yellow card' system	Under-reporting[a] of suspected adverse reactions and reactions not clearly drug related Biases in reporting • ease of recognition of reaction • severity and seriousness of reaction • novelty of drug • extent of use of drug • promotion of and publicity given to drug, side-effects and/or reporting of suspected adverse reactions. Cause-and-effect relationship with drug cannot be established Does not allow for assessment of incidence because • number of reactions and number of patients who received (and took) drug not known • difficulties in relating reaction to drug
PEM	Relatively low response rate (return of 'green forms')[b] Lack of data on patients of practitioners who do not return 'green forms' Lack of information on compliance Uncertainty over precise nature of some recorded events, e.g. mania Confined to general practice; not yet fully implemented in hospitals

[a]Estimated at about 10% of total.
[b]About 60%; likely to be due to variables in practitioner rather than drug or events.
CSM = Committee on Safety of Medicines.
PEM = Prescription event monitoring.
Adapted from J. G. Edwards & I. Anderson (1999) Systematic review and guide to selection of selective serotonin reuptake inhibitors. *Drugs*, **57**, 507–533.

Committee on Safety of Medicines

The best-known method of recording adverse drug reactions in the UK is the 'yellow card' system of the CSM. Pharmaco-vigilance is carried out by the Medicines and Healthcare Products Regulatory Agency, which uses this information together with data from other sources, including worldwide spontaneous reporting of suspected adverse reactions, published reports, post-marketing safety studies, record-linkage databases, pharmaceutical companies and drug regulatory authorities. Data from these sources are entered into a specialised computer system, the Adverse Drug Reactions On-line Information Tracking (ADROIT), to facilitate their rapid processing and analysis.

The CSM system is invaluable in contributing to the early recognition of previously unrecognised untoward effects and as a means of obtaining large cohorts of patients with uncommon or rare reactions for further research. Because of its limitations, however, it is not possible to assess the incidence of unwanted effects, although reports to the CSM can serve as signals of possible risk. Its limitations include not only underreporting but variations in rates of reporting for different drugs and types of reactions, and the fact that reported rates for individual drugs tend to decrease with time. Unfortunately, many doctors think that, as a reaction is well known, it need no longer be reported. This can result in an unfair comparison between an older drug and one more recently introduced into clinical practice. Another limitation is that certain drugs may be used preferentially in a particular group of patients at risk. If, for instance, a compound is thought to be less cardiotoxic than others, it may be used more often in patients with cardiovascular disease, and this can result in a distorted profile of alleged adverse drug reactions.

Prescription event monitoring

Prescription event monitoring, as carried out by the Drug Safety Research Unit (DSRU) in Southampton, is also able to survey large populations. About 70% of the general practitioners (GPs) in England provide data on patients, for post-marketing surveillance. The total population surveyed is 10 times larger than that in any other system in the world. Patients receiving a drug and the GPs who prescribed it are identified by the Prescription Pricing Authority, and legible prescriptions are selected for the study. The names and addresses of the practitioners are checked against the DSRU register of doctors, and large cohorts of patients who receive particular drugs (mostly those newly marketed) are identified.

Six months after the first prescription is written, the GPs are sent 'green form' questionnaires, on which they are asked to report any events that have occurred since treatment was started, including any new diagnosis, any reason for a referral to a consultant or admission to hospital, and any suspected drug reaction. The doctor is not required to decide whether there is a cause-and-effect relationship between the event and the drug. Pre-existing diseases are not recorded as events unless an exacerbation occurs. Up to the year 2002, prescription event monitoring of 15 psychotropic drugs (including one anxiolytic, two hypnotics, eight antidepressants and four antipsychotics) had been carried out. It is hoped that all new psychotropic drugs launched on to the British market in future will be studied in the way described.

Other systems

The aforementioned systems of monitoring are the most important in Britain. Other developed countries have their own systems. One of the better known of these is the Boston Collaborative Drug Surveillance Program. In this, large cohorts of in-patients and out-patients are monitored, and as the number of patients receiving treatment is known, the system allows for a measure of the incidence of adverse reactions.

Medico-legal considerations

Psychiatrists have to practise in an increasingly litigious climate. It is crucial therefore for us to be aware of our duties and responsibilities, not just as we see them but also from the perspective of the law. Patients can sue for injuries allegedly due to psychotropic drugs, but even though an injury occurs during treatment, it does not necessarily mean that anyone is responsible, because side-effects are an accepted risk of taking any medication. Nevertheless, those injured may seek redress, and the doctor who prescribes the drug, as well as the manufacturer (and sometimes even health and regulatory authorities), may be the targets of litigation. The apportionment of any responsibility for the injury should be objectively, legally and morally determined, but in general there is a tendency to seek to hold the wealthiest and best-insured party (usually the manufacturer) liable in the first instance. Here, only the duties and responsibilities of the doctor are discussed.

The duty to use drugs restrictively

This duty requires the doctor to justify the type of treatment administered in relation to the benefit–risk balance and, where that balance could be unfavourable, to consider alternative treatments.

The duty of careful choice

The doctor then has a duty to choose carefully an appropriate drug and dosage regimen. This is usually based on widely accepted recommendations, such as those in the *BNF*. Practitioners may deviate from these recommendations and be defensible in so doing, but if they do not follow the advice given, they take much legal responsibility on themselves.

The duty to consult and obtain consent

The doctor has a duty to discuss with the patient the benefits and risks of treatment, and to obtain informed consent for the treatment. The greater the risk, the more explicit the consent should be. In everyday practice consent to most treatments is not formally requested, but is implied by the acceptance of the treatment recommended.

The duty to explain

The doctor has a duty to explain how the treatment should be used, when it should be taken, and what concomitant treatment should be avoided to prevent interactions. Any relevant precautions or warnings of possible adverse effects should be spelt out.

The duty to record with care

Although this duty is self-evident, deficiencies in record keeping can lead to problems for the court in apportioning any liability for damage.

The duty to administer with skill

Doctors should administer treatment with due care and to a standard of skill reasonably expected of them. Here, too, they should heed the advice and warnings given by the manufacturers. Failure to do this could expose them to the risk of being considered negligent.

The duty to terminate treatment

Doctors readily prescribe a drug but do not always know how long it should be continued, because for some disorders there is no consensus on the required length of treatment. Nevertheless, practitioners have a duty to terminate treatment that has served its purpose and whose continuation could lead to injury. Failure to do so could expose the clinician to the risk of litigation.

For each of these duties of care, the standard against which a clinician would be judged in law is that which would be exercised by a responsible body of practitioners practising at the time of the alleged negligence (the Bolam test). It is accepted that there are many uncertainties in the practice of medicine, so the level of proof of drug-induced injury required is based on the balance of probabilities.

Conclusions

It is clear from what has been reviewed in this chapter that in considering unwanted effects of psychotropic drugs, we have to extend our horizons beyond the effect of the substances on specific physiological systems. We have to consider the effects of the drugs when prescribed in a world in which, for sound or flimsy reasons, patients are given ever changing polypharmacy or take psychotropics together with over-the-counter medication or illegal substances, or both. Such combinations carry recognised risks and probably risks yet to be discovered.

And then, more importantly, we have to accept the troublesome fact that, when we prescribe psychotropic drugs for women of childbearing age, a proportion of them may be, or may become, pregnant. This means that we inadvertently administer substances about which we have much to learn to helpless young humans. Fortunately, what we know to date provides grounds for cautious optimism, but as there are many more unanswered than answered questions, we must keep an open mind about the possibility of at least subtle behavioural teratogenic effects.

We must remain vigilant not only with regard to interactions and effects *in utero* but also with regard to adverse effects in general. We owe it to patients being treated now, and those who will be treated in the future, to report suspected untoward effects to the drug regulatory authorities more often than we do and to cooperate more conscientiously with major non-promotional pharmaco-vigilance projects such as prescription event monitoring.

We all condemn frivolous litigation and are aware of the problems of practising defensive medicine. But at the same time we have to accept that mistakes will inevitably be made from time to time, especially when working in the UK's under-resourced National Health Service. Those injured as a result should be fairly compensated for the pain, suffering and losses they endure, but more important than compensation is prevention. Much medical negligence can be prevented, or at least kept to a minimum, by practising evidence-based medicine and adhering to sound principles of prescribing.

Acknowledgements

I thank Derek Waller for his advice on the mechanisms of drug interactions, Karen Brackley and Michael Vickers for theirs on terato-genic effects, and Althea Edwards for her secretarial assistance.

Further reading

Aranda, J. V., Edwards, D. J., Hales, B. F., *et al* (2002) Developmental pharmacology. In *Neonatal–Perinatal Medicine. Diseases of the Fetus and Infant* (7th edn) (eds A. A. Fanaroff & R. J. Martin), vol. 1, pp. 145–166. St Louis: Mosby.

British Medical Association & Royal Pharmaceutical Society of Great Britain (2003) *British National Formulary*, 45. Oxford and London: Pharmaceutical Press and BMJ Books.

Brøsen, K. (1996) Are pharmacokinetic drug interactions with SSRIs an issue? *International Clinical Psychopharmacology*, **11** (suppl. 1), 23–27.

Davis, S. & Raine, J. M. (2002) Spontaneous reporting – UK. In *Pharmacovigilance* (eds R. D. Mann & E. B. Andrews), pp. 195–207. Chichester: Wiley.

Dukes, M. N. G. & Swartz, B. (1988) *Responsibility for Drug Induced Injury*. Amsterdam: Elsevier.

Edwards, J. G. (1997a) Withdrawal of psychotropic drugs from the market. I. From thalidomide to zimeldine. In *Human Psychopharmacology: Measures and Methods* (eds I. Hindmarch & P. D. Stonier), vol. 6, pp. 199–224. Chichester: Wiley.

Edwards, J. G. (1997b) Withdrawal of psychotropic drugs from the market. II. From nomifensine to remoxipride. In *Human Psychopharmacology: Measures and Methods* (eds I. Hindmarch & P. D. Stonier), vol. 6, pp. 215–233. Chichester: Wiley.

Edwards, J. G. & Anderson, I. (1999) Systematic review and guide to selection of selective serotonin reuptake inhibitors. *Drugs*, **57**, 507–533.

Elhatton, P. R. (1999) Principles of teratogenicity. *Current Obstetrics and Gynaecology*, **9**, 163–169.

Jacobson, S. J. (1992) Prospective multicentre study of pregnancy outcome after lithium exposure in first trimester. *Lancet*, **339**, 530–533.

Kennedy, I. & Grubb, A. (eds) (2000) *Medical Law* (3rd edn). London: Butterworths.

King, D. (2000) Drug interactions. In *Schizophrenia and Mood Disorders. The New Drug Therapies* (eds P. F. Buckley & J. L. Waddington), pp. 223–233. Oxford: Butterworth Heinemann.

Koren, G., Pastuszak, A. & Ito, S. (1998) Drugs in pregnancy. *New England Journal of Medicine*, **338**, 1128–1137.

Mann, R. D. & Andrews, E. B. (eds) (2002) *Pharmacovigilance*. Chichester: Wiley.

Nemeroff, C. B., DeVane, C. L. & Pollock, B. G. (1996) Newer antidepressants and the cytochrome P450 system. *American Journal of Psychiatry*, **153**, 311–320.

Pons, G., Rey, E. & Matheson, I. (1994) Excretion of psychoactive drugs into breast milk. Pharmacokinetic principles and recommendations. *Clinical Pharmacokinetics*, **27**, 270–289.

Rawlins, M. D. (1988a) Spontaneous reporting of adverse reactions. I: The data. *British Journal of Clinical Pharmacology*, **26**, 1–5.

Rawlins, M. D. (1988b) Spontaneous reporting of adverse reactions. II: Uses. *British Journal of Clinical Pharmacology*, **26**, 7–11.

Shakir, S. A. W. (2002) PEM in the UK. In *Pharmacovigilance* (eds R. D. Mann & E. B. Andrews), pp. 333–344. Chichester: Wiley.

Spina, E. & Perucca, E. (1994) Newer and older antidepressants. A comparative review of drug interactions. *CNS Drugs*, **2**, 479–497.

Stephens, M. D. B., Talbot, J. C. C. & Routledge, P. A. (eds) (2000) *Detection of New Adverse Drug Reactions* (4th edn). Basingstoke: Macmillan.

Stockley, I. H. (1999) *Drug Interactions. A Source Book of Drug Interactions, Their Mechanisms, Clinical Importance and Management* (5th edn). London: Blackwell.

Strom, B. L. (ed.) (2000) *Pharmacoepidemiology* (3rd edn). Chichester: Wiley.

Trixler, M. & Tenyi, T. (1997) Antipsychotic use in pregnancy. What are the best treatment options? *Drug Safety*, **16**, 403–410.

Wood, S. M. & Coulson, R. (1993) Adverse Drug Reactions On-line Information Tracking (ADROIT). *Pharmaceutical Medicine*, **7**, 203–213.

Worsley, A. J. (2000) Psychiatric disorders. In *Therapeutics in Pregnancy and Lactation* (1st edn) (eds A. Lee, S. Inch & D. Finnegan). Oxford: Radcliffe Medical Press.

Yoshida, K., Smith, B. & Kumar, R. (1999) Psychotropic drugs in mothers' milk: a comprehensive review of assay methods, pharmacokinetics and safety of breast-feeding. *Journal of Psychopharmacology*, **13**, 64–80.

Appendix 16.1 Interactions with anxiolytics and hypnotics

Anxiolytics/ hypnotics	Interact with	To produce	Mechanism
All or several	Alcohol	Enhanced sedation	Summation
	Anaesthetics	Enhanced sedation	Summation
	Analgesics opioids	Enhanced sedation	Summation
	Antidepressants	Enhanced sedation	Summation
	Anti-emetic nabilone	Enhanced sedation	Summation
	Anti-epileptic clonazepam	Impaired control of epilepsy	Increased metabolism → decreased plasma concentration of clonazepam
	Antihistamines	Enhanced sedation	Summation
	Antihypertensives	Enhanced hypo-tension	Summation
	alpha-blockers	Enhanced sedation	Summation
	moxonidine	Enhanced sedation	Summation
	Antipsychotics	Enhanced sedation	Summation
	Antiviral ritonavir	? Increased side-effects of anxiolytic/ hypnotic	? Inhibition of CYP3A4 → decreased metab-olism → increased plasma concentration of some anxiolytics and hypnotics
	Cannabinoid nabilone	Enhanced sedation	Summation
	Drug for opioid withdrawal lofexidine	Enhanced sedation	Summation
	Muscle relaxants baclofen tizanidine	Enhanced sedation	Summation

Table continues opposite

Anxiolytics/ hypnotics	Interact with	To produce	Mechanism
Alprazolam	Antidepressant nefazodone	Increased side-effects of alprazolam	Inhibition of CYP3A4 → decreased metabolism → increased plasma concentration of alprazolam
	Antivirals amprenavir indinavir ritonavir	*Increased risk of prolonged sedation* *Extreme sedation, respiratory depression*	Inhibition of CYP3A4 → decreased metabolism → increased plasma concentration of alprazolam
Benzodiazepines	Antidepressant fluvoxamine	Increased side-effects of some benzodiazepines	Decreased metabolism → increased plasma concentration of benzodiazepine
	Anti-epileptic phenytoin	Increased side-effects or impaired control of epilepsy	? Decreased metabolism or displacement from binding sites → increased or decreased plasma concentration of phenytoin
	Dopaminergic levodopa	Antagonism of effect of levodopa	? Mechanism
	Drug for alcohol dependence disulfiram	Enhanced sedation	Inhibition of metabolism → increased plasma concentration of benzodiazepine
	Ulcer-healing drug cimetidine	Increased side-effects of benzodiazepines	Decreased metabolism → increased plasma concentration of benzodiazepines
Buspirone	Antibacterial erythromycin	Increased side-effects of buspirone	Decreased metabolism → increased plasma concentration of buspirone

Table continues overleaf

Anxiolytics/ hypnotics	Interact with	To produce	Mechanism
	Antidepressants MAOIs	Increased blood pressure	? Mechanism
	Antifungal traconazole	Increased side-effects of buspirone	Decreased metabolism → increased plasma concentration of buspirone
	Antipsychotic haloperidol	Increased side-effects of haloperidol	Decreased metabolism → increased plasma concentration of haloperidol
	Calcium-channel blockers diltiazem verapamil	Increased side-effects of buspirone	Inhibition of CYP3A4 → decreased metabolism → increased plasma concentration of buspirone
Chloral hydrate	Anticoagulants acenocoumalol arfarin	Transient increase in anticoagulant effect	? Displacement from protein binding sites
Clomethiazole	Ulcer-healing drug cimetidine	Increased side-effects of clomethiazole	Inhibition of CYP1A2 → decreased metabolism → increased plasma concentration of clomethiazole
Clorazepate	Antivirals amprenavir ritonavir	*Extreme sedation, respiratory depression*	Inhibition of CYP3A4 → decreased metabolism → increased plasma concentration of clorazepate
	Diuretic furosemide (parenteral)	Decreased thyroid function	Displacement of thyroid hormone from binding site
Diazepam	Antibacterials isoniazid	Increased side-effects of diazepam	Decreased metabolism → increased plasma concentration of diazepam

Table continues opposite

626

Anxiolytics/ hypnotics	Interact with	To produce	Mechanism
	rifampicin	Decreased therapeutic effect of diazepam	Increased metabolism → decreased plasma concentration of diazepam (and ? other benzodiazepines and zaleplon)
	Anti-epileptics clonazepam	Increased risk of seizures	Increased metabolism → decreased plasma concentration of clonazepam
	phenytoin	Increased side-effects of phenytoin or impaired control of epilepsy	Decreased metabolism or displacement from plasma protein sites → increased or decreased plasma concentration of phenytoin
	Antipsychotic zotepine	Increased side-effects of zotepine	Decreased metabolism → increased plasma concentration of zotepine
	Antivirals amprenavir ritonavir	*Extreme sedation, respiratory depression*	Inhibition of CYP3A4 → decreased metabolism → increased plasma concentration of diazepam
	Ulcer-healing drugs cimetidine	Increased side-effects of diazepam	Decreased metabolism → increased plasma concentration of diazepam
	esomeprazole omeprazole	Increased side-effects of diazepam	? Decreased metabolism → increased plasma concentration of diazepam
Flurazepam	Antivirals amprenavir ritonavir	*Extreme sedation, respiratory depression*	Inhibition of CYP3A4 → decreased metabolism → increased plasma concentration of flurazepam

Table continues overleaf

627

Anxiolytics/ hypnotics	Interact with	To produce	Mechanism
Midazolam	Antibacterials clarithromycin erythromycin quinupristin/ dalfopristin telithromycin	*Profound sedation*	Inhibition of CYP3A4 → decreased metabolism → increased plasma concentration of midazolam
	Antifungals fluconazole itraconazole ketoconazole	*Prolonged sedation*	Inhibition of CYP3A4 → decreased metabolism → increased plasma concentration of midazolam
	Antivirals amprenavir efavirenz indinovir nelfinavir saquinovir ritonavir	Prolonged sedation *Extreme sedation, respiratory depression*	Inhibition of CYP3A4 → decreased metabolism → increased plasma concentration of midazolam
	Calcium-channel blockers diltiazem verapamil	Increased sedation	Inhibition of CYP3A4 → decreased metabolism → increased plasma concentration of midazolam
Temazepam	Drug for alcohol dependence disulfiram	Increased side-effects of temazepam	Decreased metabolism → increased plasma concentration of temazepam
Triclofos	Anticoagulants (oral)	Transient increase in anticoagulant effect	? Displacement from protein binding sites
Zaleplon	Ulcer-healing drug cimetidine	Increased side-effects of zaleplon	Inhibition of CYP3A4 → decreased metabolism → increased plasma concentration of zaleplon
Zolpidem	Antiviral ritonavir	*Extreme sedation, respiratory depression*	Inhibition of CYP3A4 → decreased metabolism → increased plasma concentration of zolpidem

Table continues opposite

Anxiolytics/ hypnotics	Interact with	To produce	Mechanism
Zopiclone	Antibacterials erythromycin quinupristin/ dalfopristin	Increased side-effects of zopiclone	Inhibition of CYP3A → decreased metabolism → increased plasma concentration of zopiclone

Potentially hazardous interactions are shown in italics.

The listing of a drug category does not mean all compounds in the group are implicated in the interactions.

Some of the '?' interactions are theoretical possibilities suspected from pre-clinical experiments and/or isolated case reports.

Knowledge of interactions is advancing rapidly; it will be necessary to keep up to date.

Only data of clinical relevance are reported in the Mechanism column.

Many mechanisms are uncertain, unknown or inconsistently reported; knowledge concerning them is rapidly changing and evolving; mechanisms other than those listed may be involved in the interactions.

Appendix 16.2 Interactions with monoamine oxidase inhibitors (MAOIs)

MAOIs Interact with	To produce	Mechanism
Alcohol some alcoholic and de- alcoholised beverages containing tyramine	*Hypertensive crisis*	Inhibition of MAO → increased absorption of tyramine
(beverages without tyramine)	*(Hypotension)*	Summation of vasodilatation
α_2-adrenoceptor stimulants apraclonidine brimonidine	Hypertension	Inhibition of MAO → increased effects of biogenic amines
Analgesics nefopam pethidine ?other opioids	*CNS excitation or depression (Hypertension or hypotension)*	Decreased metabolism → increased plasma concentra- tion of analgesic
Anaesthetics	*Ventricular arrhythmias* Hypotension	Increased effects of biogenic amines Summation
Antagonist for central nervous and respiratory depression doxapram	Increased effects of doxapram	Decreased metabolism → increased plasma concentration of doxapram
Antibacterial linezolid	*CNS toxicity*	Summation Linezolid is a reversible non-selective MAOI
Antidepressants MAOIs, other SSRIs	*CNS toxicity* *CNS toxicity*	Summation Increased effects of biogenic amines
tricyclics and related antidepressants	*CNS toxicity* *Hypertension*	Inhibition of MAO → increased effects of biogenic amines
tryptophan	*CNS toxicity*	Inhibition of MAO → increased effects of biogenic amines
Antidiabetics insulin metformin sulphonylureas	Increased effect of antidiabetic drug	? Mechanism Inhibition of metabolism → increased plasma concentra- tion of antidiabetics
Anti-epileptics	*Impaired control of epilepsy*	Lowered convulsive theshold

Table continues opposite

MAOIs Interact with	To produce	Mechanism
Antihistamines	Increased sedation Increased muscarinic effects	Summation Summation
Antihypertensives	*Increased hypo-tension*	Summation
Antimalarials artemether with lumefantrine	Ventricular arrhythmias	Increased effect on QT interval
Antimuscarinics	Increased anti-muscarinic effects	Summation
Antineoplastic altretamine	*Severe postural hypotension*	?Mechanism
Antipsychotics clozapine	*CNS toxicity*	Increased effects of biogenic amines
Anxiolytic buspirone	Hypertension	?Increased effects of biogenic amines
Appetite suppressant sibutramine	*CNS toxicity*	Increased effects of biogenic amines

Dopaminergics
  entacapone
  L-dopa
  selegiline
	Hypertensive crisis
	
	Hypotension
		Increased effects of biogenic amines
		
		Summation of vasodilatation

Drug for cigarette smoking buproprion (amfebutamone)	*Hypertension*	Increased effects of biogenic amines

5-HT$_1$ agonists
  rizatriptan
  sumatroptan
  zolmitripton
	CNS toxicity	Increased serotonergic effects

Respiratory stimulant doxapram	*Hypertension*	Increased effects of biogenic amines

Table continues overleaf

MAOIs Interact with	To produce	Mechanism
Sympathomimetics	*Hypertensive crisis*	Increased effects of biogenic amines
Tetrabenazine	*CNS toxicity* *Hypertension*	Increased effects of biogenic amines

See footnote to Appendix 16.1.

Appendix 16.3   Interactions with selective serotonin reuptake inhibitors

SSRIs	Interact with	To produce	Mechanism
All or several	Alcohol	*Increased sedation*	Summation
	Analgesics aspirin NSAIDs tramadol	Increased risk of bleeding *CNS toxicity*	Decreased uptake of serotonin by platelets → decreased platelet aggregation
	Anticoagulants acenocoumaral warfarin	*Increased effect of anticoagulant*	Inhibition of CYP2C9 → inhibition of metab- olism → increased plasma concentration of anticoagulant
	Antidepressants MAOIs	*CNS toxicity*	Increased effects of biogenic amines
	St John's wort	*CNS toxicity*	Increased effects of biogenic amines
	tricyclics	Increased side- effects of some tricyclics	Inhibition of CYP1A2 and 2D6 → decreased metabolism → increased plasma concentration of tricyclics
	tryptophan	Agitation, nausea	Increased effect of serotonin
	Anti-epileptics	*Decreased control of epilepsy*	Lowered convulsive threshold
	Antimalarial artemether with lumefantrine	*Ventricular arrhythmias*	Inhibition of CYP2D6 → increased plasma concentration of anti- malarial → increased QT interval
	Antimanic lithium	*CNS toxicity*	Increased effect of biogenic amines
	Antiviral ritonavir	*Increased side- effects of SSRI*	Inhibition of CYP2C19, 2D6 and 3A → decreased metabolism → increased plasma concentration of SSRI

Table continues overleaf

SSRIs	Interact with	To produce	Mechanism
	Appetite suppressant sibutramine	*CNS toxicity*	Increased effects of biogenic amines
	Antimanic lithium	*CNS toxicity*	? Increased effects of biogenic amines
	5-HT$_1$ agonist sumatriptan	*CNS toxicity*	Increased effects of serotonin
	Opioid analgesic tramadol	*? Increased risk of convulsions*	? Lowered convulsive threshold
	Sympathomimetic methylphenidate	*Increased side-effects of SSRIs*	Increased effects of biogenic amines
Citalopram	Antihistamine terfenadine	*Ventricular arrhythmias*	Inhibition of CYP3A4 → decreased metabolism → increased plasma concentration of terfenadine → increased QT interval
Fluoxetine	Anti-arrhythmic flecainide	Increased side-effects of flecainide	Inhibition of CYP2D6 → decreased metabolism → increased plasma concentration of flecainide
	Antidepressant nefazodone	Increased side-effects of nefazodone	Inhibition of CYP3A4 → decreased metabolism → increased plasma concentration of nefazodone
	Anti-epileptics carbamazepine phenytoin	Increased side-effects of anti-epileptics	Inhibition of CYP3A4 and 2C9, respectively, → decreased metabolism → increased plasma concentration of anti-epileptic

Table continues opposite

634

SSRIs	Interact with	To produce	Mechanism
	Antihistamine terfenadine	*Ventricular arrhythmias*	Inhibition of CYP3A4 → decreased metabolism → increased plasma concentration of terfenadine → increased QT interval
	Antipsychotics clozapine haloperidol risperidone sertindole zotepine	Increased side-effects of antipsychotics	Inhibition of CYP1A2 and 2D6 → decreased metabolism → increased plasma concentration of antipsychotics
	Dopaminergic selegiline	*Hypertension CNS toxicity*	Increased effects of biogenic amines
Fluvoxamine	Anaesthetic ropivacaine	Increased side-effects of ropivacaine	Inhibition of CYP1A2 → decreased metabolism → increased plasma concentration of ropivacaine
	Analgesic methadone	Increased side-effects of methadone	Inhibition of CYP2D6 → decreased metabolism → increased plasma concentration of methadone
	Anti-epileptics carbamazepine phenytoin	*Increased side-effects of anti-epileptics*	Inhibition of CYP3A4 and 2C9, respectively → decreased metabolism → increased plasma concentration of anti-epileptics
	Antihistamine terfenadine	*Ventricular arrhythmias*	Inhibition of CYP3A4 → decreased metabolism → increased plasma concentration of terfenadine → increased QT interval

Table continues overleaf

635

SSRIs	Interact with	To produce	Mechanism
	Antipsychotics clozapine olanzapine	*Increased side-effects of antipsychotics*	Inhibition of CYP1A2 → decreased metabolism → increased plasma concentration of antipsychotics
	Benzodiazepines (some)	Increased side-effects of benzodiazepines	Inhibition of CYP2C and 3A4 → decreased metabolism → increased plasma concentration of benzodiazepines
	Beta-blocker propranolol	Increased side-effects of propranolol	Inhibition of CYP1A2 and 2DC → decreased metabolism → increased plasma concentration of propranolol
	Bronchodilator theophylline	*Increased side-effects of theophylline*	Inhibition of CYP1A2 → decreased metabolism → increased plasma concentration of theophylline
	5-HT$_1$ agonist zolmitriptan	*Increased side-effects of zolmitriptan*	Inhibition of CYP1A2 → decreased metabolism → increased plasma concentration of zolmitriptan
Paroxetine	Anti-epileptics phenytoin ? others	Decreased therapeutic effect of of paroxetine	Induction of CYP2D6 and 3A4 → increased metabolism → decreased plasma concentration of paroxetine
	Antimuscarinic procyclidine	Increased side-effects of procyclidine	? Mechanism
	Antipsychotics clozapine sertindole thioridazine	Increased side-effects of antipsychotics *Ventricular arrhythmias*	Inhibition of CYP1A2 → decreased metabolism → increased plasma concentration of antipsychotics

Table continues opposite

SSRIs	Interact with	To produce	Mechanism
	Dopaminergic selegiline	Hypertension *CNS toxicity*	Increased effects of biogenic amines
	Parasympatho-mimetic galantamine	*Increased side-effects of galantamine*	Inhibition of CYP2D6 → decreased metabolism → increased plasma concentration of galantamine
Sertraline	Antipsychotic clozapine	Increased side-effects of clozapine	Inhibition of CYP1A2 → decreased metabolism → increased plasma concentration of clozapine
	Dopaminergic selegiline	*Hypertension CNS toxicity*	Increased effects of biogenic amines
	Ulcer-healing drug cimetidine	*Increased side-effects of sertraline*	Inhibition of CYP2D6 and 3A4 → decreased metabolism → increased plasma concentration of sertraline

See footnote to Appendix 16.1.

Appendix 16.4   Interactions with tricyclic and related antidepressants

Antidepressants interact with:	To produce	Mechanisms
Alcohol	*Increased sedation*	Summation

α$_2$-adrenoceptor stimulants
  apraclonidine
  brimonidine
	Hypertension	Summation

Anaesthetics	Hypotension Ventricular arrhythmias	? Summation

Analgesics
  nefopam
 	
  opioids
  tramadol
	? Increased side-effects of nefopam
	Increased sedation
	CNS toxicity
		? Mechanism
		
		Summation
		? Increased effects of biogenic amines

Anti-arrhythmics
  amiodarone
  disopyramide
  procainamide
  propafenone
  quinidine
	Ventricular arrhythmias	Increased effect on QT interval

Antibacterial rifampicin	Decreased effectiveness of antidepressant	Induction of CYP1A2, 2C19 and 3A → increased metabolism → decreased plasma concentration of some tricyclics

Antidepressants
  MAOIs
  SSRIs
	CNS toxicity
	Hypertension
	Increased side-effects of some tricyclics
		Increased effects of biogenic amines
		Inhibition of CYP1A2, 2D6 and 3A4 → decreased metabolism → increased plasma concentration of tricyclics

Anti-epileptics	*Impaired control of epilepsy* Decreased effectiveness of some tricyclics	Lowered convulsive threshold Induction of CYP1A2 and 2C9 → increased metabolism → decreased plasma concentration of tricyclic

Table continues opposite

Antidepressants interact with:	To produce	Mechanisms
Antihistamines	Increased anti-muscarinic effects	Summation
	Increased sedation	Summation
terfenadine	*Ventricular arrhythmias*	Inhibition of CYP3A → inhibition of metabolism → increased plasma concentration of terfenadine → increased QT interval
Antihypertensives	*Increased hypotension*	Summation
adrenergic neuron blockers	Decreased hypotensive effect	Competitive inhibition at receptor site
clonidine	Decreased hypotensive effect	Opposing effects on central monoamine concentrations
	Increased risk of hypertension on withdrawal of clonidine	Rebound noradrenergic effect
Antimalarial artemether with lumefantrine	*Ventricular arrhythmias*	Inhibition of CYP2D6 → decreased metabolism → increased plasma concentration of antimalarial → increased QT interval
Antimuscarinics	Increased anti-muscarinic effects	Summation
Antipsychotics phenothiazines ? clozapine	Increased side-effects of tricyclics	Inhibition of CYP1A2 and 2D6 → decreased metabolism → increased plasma concentration of tricyclics
pimozide thioridazine	*Ventricular arrhythmias*	Inhibition of CYP1A2 and 2D6 → decreased metabolism → increased plasma concentration of antipsychotic → increased QT interval
Antiviral ritonivar	? Increased side-effects of tricyclics	? Inhibition of CYP2C9, 2D6 and 3A4 → decreased metabolism → increased plasma concentration of tricyclics
Anxiolytics/ hypnotics	Increased sedation	Summation

Table continues overleaf

Antidepressants interact with	To produce	Mechanisms
Beta-blocker sotalol	*Ventricular arrhythmias*	Summation of effects on cardiac conduction
Calcium-channel blockers diltiazem	? Increased side-effects of imipramine and ? other tricyclics	Inhibition of CYP3A4 → decreased metabolism → increased plasma concentration of tricyclics
Diuretics	Postural hypotension	Summation
Dopaminergics entacapone selegiline	*CNS toxicity*	Increased effects of biogenic amines
Drug for alcohol dependence disulfiram	Increased side-effects of tricyclics Increased disulfiram–alcohol reaction with amitriptyline	Inhibition of hepatic enzymes → decreased metabolism → increased plasma concentration of tricyclics
Muscle relaxant baclofen	Increased relaxant effect	? Mechanism
Nitrates	Reduced effect of sublingual nitrate	Anticholinergic effect of tricyclics → dry mouth → decreased absorption of nitrate
Oestrogens/ progestogens oral contraceptives	Decreased anti-depressant effect Increased side-effects of tricyclics	? Depressogenic effect of contraceptives Decreased metabolism → increased plasma concentration of tricyclics
Sympathomimetics adrenaline noradrenaline methylphenidate	*Hypertension* *Ventricular arrhythmias* *Hypertension* *Increased side-effects of tricyclics*	Summation Inhibition of metabolism → increased plasma concentration of tricyclics
Ulcer-healing drug cimetidine	Increased side-effects of tricyclics	Inhibition of CYP3A → decreased metabolism → increased plasma concentration of tricyclics

See footnote to Appendix 16.1.

Appendix 16.5 Interactions with other antidepressants

Drug	Interacts with	To produce	Mechanism
Mianserin	Alcohol	Increased sedation	Summation
	α_2-adrenoceptor stimulants apraclonidine brimonidine	Hypotension	Summation
	Anti-epileptics carbamazepine phenytoin	Impaired control of epilepsy Decreased anti-depressant effect	Lowered convulsive threshold Induction of CYP3A4 $\rightarrow$ increased metabolism $\rightarrow$ decreased plasma concentration of mianserin
	Antimalarial artemether with lumefantrine	? *Ventricular arrhythmias*	? Concomitant effects on CYP3A4 $\rightarrow$ decreased metabolism $\rightarrow$ increased plasma drug concentration $\rightarrow$ effect on QT interval
	Anxiolytics/ hypnotics	Increased sedation	Summation
	Appetite suppressant sibutramine	*CNS toxicity*	Increased effect of biogenic amines
Mirtazapine	Alcohol	Increased sedation	Summation
	α_2-adrenoceptor stimulants apraclonidine brimonidine	Hypotension	Summation
	Antidepressants	(Effects as for tricyclics – Appendix 16.4)	
	Antimalarial artemether with lumefantrine	? *Ventricular arrhythmias*	? Concomitant effects on CYP3A4 $\rightarrow$ decreased metabolism $\rightarrow$ increased plasma drug concentration $\rightarrow$ effect on QT interval

Table continues overleaf

Drug	Interacts with	To produce	Mechanism
	Anxiolytics/ hypnotics	Increased sedation	Summation
	Appetite suppressant sibutramine	*CNS toxicity*	Increased effect of biogenic amines
Moclobemide	Analgesics dextromethorpean pethidine ? fentanyl ? morphine and other opioids	*CNS excitation or depression Hypertension or hypotension*	Increased effect of biogenic amines
	Anorectics	(Effects as for other MAOIs – Appendix 16.2)	
	Antidepressants	(Effects as for other MAOIs – Appendix 16.2)	
	Antimalarials artemether with lumefantrine	*? Ventricular arrhythmias*	? Concomitant effects on CYP3A4 and 2D6 → decreased metabolism → increased plasma drug concentrations → effect on QT interval
	Dopaminergics L-dopa selegiline	*Increased side-effects of dopaminergics*	Potentiation of pressor effects of tyramine ? due to simultaneous inhibition of MAO-A and B
	Appetite suppressant sibutramine	*CNS toxicity*	Increased effect of biogenic amines
	Drug for cigarette smoking bupropion (amfebutamone)	*Increased risk of seizures*	Lowered convulsive threshold
	5-HT$_1$ agonists rizatriptan sumatriptan zolmitiptan	*CNS toxicity*	Increased serotonergic effect
	Sympathomimetic	(Effects as for other MAOIs – Appendix 16.2)	

Table continues opposite

Drug	Interacts with	To produce	Mechanism
	Ulcer-healing drug cimetidine	Increased side-effects of moclobemide	Inhibition of CYP2C → decreased metabolism → increased plasma concentration of meclobomide
Reboxetine	Anti-arrhythmics	? Increased risk of ventricular arrhythmias	Increased effect on QT interval
	Antibacterial macrolides	*Ventricular arrhythmias*	Increased effect on QT interval
	Antidepressants fluvoxamine MAOIs	*CNS toxicity*	Increased effects of biogenic amines
	Antifungals imidazoles triazoles	*Increased side-effects of reboxetine*	Inhibition of CYP3A4 → decreased metabolism → increased plasma concentration of reboxetine
	Antimalarial artemether with lumefantrine	*? Ventricular arrhythmias*	? Concomitant effects on CYP3A → decreased metabolism → increased plasma drug concentrations → effect on QT interval
	Antimigraine ergometrine	? Hypertension	? Increased effects of biogenic amines
	Appetite suppressant sibutramine	*CNS toxicity*	Increased effects of biogenic amines
	Diuretics loop diuretics thiazides	? Increased risk of hypokalaemia	? Mechanism
	Immuno-suppressant ciclosporin	Hypertension	? Mechanism

Table continues overleaf

643

Drug	Interacts with	To produce	Mechanism
St John's wort	Antibacterial telithromycin	*Decreased antibacterial effect*	Increased metabolism → decreased plasma concentration of telithromycin
	Anticoagulant warfarin	*Decreased anticoagulant effect*	Increased metabolism → decreased plasma warfarin
	Antidepressants SSRIs	*CNS toxicity*	Increased serotonergic effect
	Anti-epileptics barbiturates carbamazepine phenobarbitone phenytoin brimidone	*Increased risk of convulsions*	Increased metabolism → decreased plasma concentration of anti-epileptic
	Antiviral protease inhibitors efavirenz nevirapine	*Decreased antiviral effect*	Increased metabolism → decreased plasma concentration of antiviral
	Bronchodilator theophylline	*Decreased bronchodilator effect*	Increased metabolism → decreased plasma concentration of theophylline
	Cardiac glycoside digoxin	*Decreased therapeutic effect of digoxin*	Increased metabolism → decreased plasma concentration of digoxin
	5-HT$_1$ agonists	*CNS toxicity*	Summation of serotonergic effects
	Immuno-suppressant ciclosporin	*Decreased immuno-suppressant effect*	Increased metabolism → decreased plasma concentration of ciclosporin

Table continues opposite

Drug	Interacts with	To produce	Mechanism
	Oral contra-ceptives	*Decreased contra-ception effect*	Increased metabolism → decreased plasma oestrogens and progestogens
Trazodone	Alcohol	Increased sedation	Summation
	α_2-adrenoceptor stimulants apraclonidine brimonidine	Sedation Hypotension	Summation
	Antidepressants	(Effects as for tricyclics – Appendix 16.4)	
	Anti-epileptics	*Increased risk of convulsions*	Antagonism of anti-convulsant effect
	Antimalarial artemether with lumefantrine	*? Ventricular arrhythmias*	? Concomitant effect on CYP3A → decreased metabolism → increased plasma drug concen-tration → increased effect on QT interval
	Anxiolytics/ hypnotics	Increased sedation	Summation
	Appetite suppressant sibutramine	*CNS toxicity*	Increased effect of biogenic amines
Tryptophan	Antibacterial linezolid	*CNS toxicity*	Increased effect of biogenic amines
	Antidepressants MAOIs	CNS toxicity	Increased effect of biogenic amines
	SSRIs	Agitation, nausea	Increased serotonergic effect
	Antimalarial artemether with lumefantrine	*? Ventricular arrhythmias*	Increased effect on QT interval

Table continues overleaf

645

Drug	Interacts with	To produce	Mechanism
	Appetite suppressant sibutramine	*CNS toxicity*	Increased effect of biogenic amines
Venlafaxine	Antibacterial linezolid	*CNS toxicity*	Increased effect of biogenic amines
	Anticoagulant warfarin	*? Increased anti-coagulant effect*	Decreased metabolism → increased plasma concentration of warfarin
	Antimalarial artemether with lumefantrine	*? Ventricular arrhythmias*	? Concomitant effect on CYP3A4 → decreased metabolism → increased plasma drug concentration → increased effect on QT interval
	Antipsychotic clozapine	Increased side-effects of clozapine	Decreased metabolism → increased plasma concentration of clozapine
	Appetite suppressant sibutramine	*CNS toxicity*	Increased effect of biogenic amines
	Dopaminergic entacapone	CNS toxicity	Increased effects of biogenic amines

See footnote to Appendix 16.1.

Appendix 16.6 Interactions with antipsychotic drugs

Antipsychotics	Interact with	To produce	Mechanism
All or several	Alcohol	Increased sedation	Summation
	Anaesthetics	*Increased hypotension*	Summation
	Analgesics opioids	*Increased sedation* *Increased hypotension*	Summation
	tramadel	*Increased risk of convulsions*	
	Anti-epileptics	*Impaired control of epilepsy*	Lowered convulsive threshold
	Antihypertensive methyldopa	Increased hypotensive effect Increased risk of extrapyramidal effects	Summation
	Antimalarial artemether with lumefantrine	*? Ventricular arrhythmias*	? Concomitant effect on CYP3A4 → decreased metabolism → increased plasma drug concentration → increased effect on QT interval
	Antivirals	Increased side-effects of anti-psychotics	Inhibition of CYP2D6 → decreased metabolism → increased plasma concentration of antipsychotics
	Anxiolytics/hypnotics	Increased sedation	Summation
	Appetite suppressant sibutramine	*CNS toxicity*	Increased effects of biogenic amines
	Calcium-channel blockers	Increased hypotensive effect	Summation
	Dopaminergics apomorphine bromocriptine	Decreased anti-Parkinsonian effect	Competition at receptor site → antagonism of dopaminergic effect

Table continues overleaf

647

Antipsychotics	Interact with	To produce	Mechanism
	cabergoline L-dopa lisuride pergolide pramipexol rapinirol		
	Drug for dementia memantine	Decreased therapeutic effect of memantine	? Mechanism
	Drug for movement disorder tetrabenazine	Increased risk of extrapyramidal effects	Summation
	Drug for nausea and vertigo metoclopramide	Increased risk of extrapyramidal effects	Summation
	Drugs affecting renin–angiotensin system ACE inhibitors angiotensin II antagonists	Increased hypotension	Summation
	Sympathomimetics	Decreased pressor effect	Antangonism at receptor site
Amisulpride	Anti-arrhythmics amiodarone disopyramide quinidine procainamide	*Ventricular arrhythmias*	Summation of effect on QT interval
	Antibacterial erythromycin (parenteral)	*Ventricular arrhythmias*	Summation of effect on QT interval
	Antimanic lithium	*Increased risk of extrapyramidal effects*	? Mechanism
	Beta-blocker sotalol	*Ventricular arrhythmias*	Summation of effect on QT interval

Table continues opposite

Antipsychotics	Interact with	To produce	Mechanism
	Diuretics	*Ventricular arrhythmias*	Hypokalaemia
	Dopaminergic L-dopa	Decreased therapeutic effect of L-dopa	Antagonism of dopaminergic effect
	Drugs for pneumocystis pneumonia pentamidine isetionate	*Ventricular arrhythmias*	? Increased effect on QT interval
Chlorpromazine	Analgesic levacetyl-methadol	*Ventricular arrhythmias*	Summation of effects on QT interval
	Antihypertensives adrenergic neuron blockers	Antagonism of hypotensive effect by high doses of chlorpromazine	Competition at receptor site
	Beta-blocker propranolol	Increased side-effects of both drugs	Inhibition of CYP2D6 → decreased metabolism → increased plasma concentration of both drugs
	Ulcer-healing drug cimetidine	Increased side-effects of chlorpromazine (? and other antipsychotics)	Inhibition of CYP2D6 → decreased metabolism → increased plasma concentration of chlorpromazine
Clozapine	Antibacterials erythromycin	*Increased risk of convulsions*	Inhibition of CYP3A4 → decreased metabolism → increased plasma concentration of clozapine
	rifampicin	Decreased antipsychotic effect	Induction of CYP1A2 → increased metabolism → decreased plasma concentration of clozapine

Table continues overleaf

Antipsychotics	Interact with	To produce	Mechanism
	Antidepressants SSRIs MAOIs tricyclics venlaxafine	*Increased side-effects of clozapine*	Inhibition of CYP2D6 → decreased metabolism → increased plasma concentration of clozapine
		? Increased CNS effects of MAOIs	Summation
		Increased side-effects of tricyclics	Inhibition of CYP1A2 and 2D6 → decreased metabolism → increased plasma concentration of tri-cyclics
		Increased side-effects of clozapine	Inhibition of CYP1A2 and 2DC → decreased metabolism → increased plasma con-centration of clozapine
		? Increased anti-muscarinic effects	Summation
		Increased side-effects of venlafaxine	Inhibition of CYP2D6 → decreased metabolism → increased plasma concentration of venlafaxine
	Anti-epileptics carbamazepine phenytoin	Decreased thera-peutic effect of clozapine	Induction of CYP1A2 → increased metabolism → decreased plasma concentration of clozapine
	Antimanic lithium	Increased risk of extrapyramidal effects and ? CNS toxicity	? Mechanism
	Antimuscarinics	Increased anti-muscarinic effects of clozapine	Summation
	Antipsychotics, long-acting depot	*Increased myelo-suppressive potential*	? Mechanism

Table continues opposite

Antipsychotics	Interact with	To produce	Mechanism
	Antivirals ritonavir ? amprenavir	*Increased side-effects of clozapine*	Inhibition of CYP2D6 → decreased metabolism → increased plasma concentration of clozapine
	Myelosuppressives	Increased risk of agranulocytosis	Summation
	Ulcer-healing drug cimetidine	*Increased side-effects of clozapine*	Inhibition of CYP2D6 → decreased metabolism → increased plasma concentration of clozapine
Haloperidol	Analgesics indomethacin levacetyl-methadol	Severe drowsiness *Ventricular arrhythmias*	Summation Summation of effects on QT interval
	Anti-arrhythmic amiodarone	*Ventricular arrhythmias*	Summation of effects on QT interval
	Antibacterial rifampicin	Decreased therapeutic effects of haloperidol	Induction of CYP1A and 2D6 → increased metabolism → decreased plasma concentration of haloperidol
	Antidepressants fluoxetine nefazodone	Increased side-effects of haloperidol	Inhibition of CYP1A2 and 2D6 → decreased metabolism → increased plasma concentration of haloperidol
	Anti-epileptics carbamazepine phenobarbitone	Decreased therapeutic effect of haloperidol	Induction of CYP1A2 → increased metabolism → decreased plasma concentration of haloperidol
	Antihypertensives adrenergic neuron blockers	Antagonism of hypotensive effect	Competition at receptor site

Table continues overleaf

Antipsychotics	Interact with	To produce	Mechanism
	Antimanic lithium	Increased risk of extrapyramidal effects ? CNS toxicity	? Mechanism
	Anxiolytic buspirone	Increased side-effects of haloperidol	Inhibition of CYP2D6 → inhibition of metabolism → increased plasma concentration of haloperidol
Olanzapine	Antidepressant fluvoxamine	*Increased side-effects of olanzapine*	Decreased metabolism → increased plasma concentration of olanzapine
	Anti-epileptics carbamazepine	Decreased therapeutic effect of olanzapine	Induction of CYP2D6 → increased metabolism → decreased plasma concentration of olanzapine
	valproate	Increased risk of neutropenia	? Mechanism
Oxypertine	Antidepressants MAOIs	*CNS excitation Hypertension*	? Increased effects of biogenic amines
Phenothiazines	Antacids and ? kaolin	Decreased therapeutic effect of phenothiazine	Decreased absorption → decreased plasma concentration of phenothiazine
	Antidiabetics sulphonylureas	? Antagonism of hypoglycaemic effect	? Mechanism
	Antidepressants tricyclics	*Increased side-effects of tricyclics*	Inhibition of CYP2D6 → decreased metabolism → increased plasma concentration of tricyclic
		Increased anti-muscarinic effects	Summation

Table continues opposite

Antipsychotics	Interact with	To produce	Mechanism
	Antimanic lithium	Increased risk of extrapyramidal effects ? CNS toxicity	? Mechanism
	Antimuscarinics	Increased anti-muscarinic effects (but decreased plasma concentration of phenothiazines)	Summation
	Beta-blocker sotalol	*Ventricular arrhythmias*	Summation of effects on cardiac conduction
Pimozide	Analgesic levacetyl-methadol	*Ventricular arrhythmias*	Summation of effects on QT interval
	Anti-arrhythmics amiodarone disopyramide quinidine procainamide	*Ventricular arrhythmias*	Inhibition of CYP3A4 → decreased metabolism → increased plasma concentration of pimozide → increased effect on QT interval
	Antibacterials clarithromycin ? erythromycin telithromycin	*Ventricular arrhythmias*	Inhibition of CYP3A4 → decreased metabolism → increased plasma concentration of pimozide → increased effect on QT interval
	Antidepressants tricyclics	*Ventricular arrhythmias*	Summation of effects on QT interval
	Antifungals imidazoles triazoles	*Ventricular arrhythmias*	Inhibition of CYP3A4 → decreased metabolism → increased plasma concentration of pimozide → increased effect on QT interval

Table continues overleaf

Antipsychotics	Interact with	To produce	Mechanism
	Antihistamine terfenadine	*Ventricular arrhythmias*	Summation of effects on QT interval
	Antimalarials mefloquine quinine	*? Ventricular arrhythmias*	Summation of effects on QT interval
	Antipsychotics phenothiazines	*Ventricular arrhythmias*	Summation of effects on QT interval
	Antivirals ritonavir ? other protease inhibitors	*Ventricular arrhythmias*	Inhibition of CYP3A4 → decreased metabolism → increased plasma concentration of pimozide
	Beta-blocker sotalol	*Ventricular arrhythmias*	Summation of effects on cardiac conduction
	Diuretics	*Ventricular arrhythmias*	Hypokalaemia → increased effect on QT interval
Prochlorperazine and levo-mepromazide/ methotimeprazine	Desferrioxamine	*Transient metabolic encephalopathy → prolonged unconsciousness*	? Mechanism
Quetiapine	Antibacterials macrolidines	Increased side-effects of quetiapine	Inhibition of CYP3A4 → decreased metabolism → increased plasma concentration of quetiapine
	Anti-epileptics carbamazapine phenytoin	Decreased therapeutic effect of quetiapine	Induction of CYP3A4 → increased metabolism → decreased plasma concentration of quetiapine
Risperidone	Antidepressant fluoxetine	*Increased side-effects of risperidone*	Inhibition of CYP3A4 → decreased metabolism → increased plasma concentration of risperidone

Table continues opposite

Antipsychotics	Interact with	To produce	Mechanism
	Anti-epileptic carbamazepine	Decreased therapeutic effect of risperidone	Induction of CYP3A4 → increased metabolism → decreased plasma concentration of risperidone
Sertindole	Anti-arrhythmias amiodarone disopyramide procainamide quinidine	*Ventricular arrhythmias*	Inhibition of CYP2A and 3A4 → decreased metabolism → increased plasma concentration of sertindole → increased effect on QT interval
	Antibacterials erythromycin ? other macrolidines	*Ventricular arrhythmias*	Inhibition of CYP3A4 → decreased metabolism → increased plasma concentration of sertindole → increased effect on QT interval
	Antidepressants fluoxetine paroxetine	*Increased side-effects of sertindole*	Inhibition of CYP2D6 and 3A4 → decreased metabolism → increased plasma concentration of sertindole
	Anti-epileptics carbamazepine phenytoin	Decreased therapeutic effect of sertindole	Induction of CYP2D6 and 3A4 → increased metabolism → decreased plasma concentration of sertindole
	Antifungals itraconazole ketoconazole ? other imipazoles and triazoles	*Ventricular arrhythmias*	Inhibition of CYP3A4 → decreased metabolism → increased plasma concentration of sertindole → increased effect on QT interval
	Antihistamine terfenadine	*Ventricular arrhythmias*	Inhibition of CYP3A4 → decreased metabolism → increased plasma concentration of sertindole → increased effect on QT interval

Table continues overleaf

655

Antipsychotics	Interact with	To produce	Mechanism
	Antimanic lithium	Increased risk of extrapyramidal effects	? Mechanism
	Antivirals amprenavir indinavir retinovir ? other protease inhibitors	*Ventricular arrhythmias*	Inhibition of CYP3A4 → decreased metabolism → increased plasma concentration of sertindole → increased effect on QT interval
	Beta-blocker solatol	*Ventricular arrhythmias*	Inhibition of CYP2D6 → decreased metabolism → increased plasma concentration of sertindole → increased effect on QT interval
	Diuretics	*Ventricular arrhythmias*	Hypokalaemia → increased effect on QT interval
	Ulcer-healing drug cimetidine	*Ventricular arrhythmias*	Inhibition of CYP2D6 → decreased metabolism → increased plasma concentration of sertindole → increased effect on QT interval
Sulpiride	Antacids	Decreased therapeutic effect of sulpiride	Decreased absorption of sulpiride
	Antimanic lithium	Increased risk of extrapyramidal effects	? Mechanism
	Ulcer-healing drug sucralfate	Decreased therapeutic effect of sulpiride	Decreased absorption → decreased plasma concentration of sulpiride

Table continues opposite

Antipsychotics	Interact with	To produce	Mechanism
Thioridazine	Analgesic levacetyl- methadol	*Ventricular arrhythmias*	Increased effect on QT interval
	Anti-arrhythmics amiodarone disopyramide procainamide quinidine	*Ventricular arrhythmias*	Inhibition of CYP2D6 → decreased metabolism → increased plasma concentration of thioridazine → increased effect on QT interval
	Antidepressants tricyclics	*Ventricular arrhythmias*	Summation of effects on QT interval
	paroxetine	*Increased side- effects of thioridazine*	Inhibition of CYP2D6 → decreased metabolism → increased plasma concentration of thioridazine
	Antihistamine terfenadine	*Ventricular arrhythmias*	Summation of effects on QT interval
	Antimalarial quinine	Increased side-effects of thioridazine	Inhibition of CYP2D6 → decreased metabolism → increased plasma concentration of thioridazine
	Antipsychotics amisulpride phenothiazines (other) pimozide sertindole	*Ventricular arrhythmias*	Summation of effects on QT interval
	Antivirals amrenavir indinavir retonavir ?other protease inhibitors	*Ventricular arrhythmias*	Inhibition of CYP3A4 → decreased metabolism → increased plasma concentration of thioridazine → increased effect on QT interval

Table continues overleaf

657

Antipsychotics	Interact with	To produce	Mechanism
	Diuretics	*Ventricular arrhythmias*	Hypokalaemia → increased effect on QT interval
	Drugs for pneumo-cystitis pneumonia pentamidine isetionate	*Ventricular arrhythmias*	? Mechanism
Zotepine	Antidepressant fluoxetine	Increased side-effects of zotepine	Inhibition of CYP2D6 → decreased metabolism → increased plasma concentration of zotepine
	Anxiolytic diazepam	Increased side-effects of zotepine	Inhibition of CYP1A2 → decreased metabolism → increased plasma concentration of zotepine

See footnote to Appendix 16.1.

Appendix 16.7   Interactions with lithium

Lithium interacts with	To produce	Mechanism
Antacid sodium bicarbonate	Decreased therapeutic effect of lithium	Increased excretion of lithium → decreased plasma concentration of lithium
Anti-arrhythmic amiodarone	Increased risk of hypothyroidism	Summation of antithyroid effect
Antibacterial metronidazole	Lithium toxicity ? renal damage	Decreased excretion of lithium
Antidepressants SSRIs	*CNS toxicity* *Lithium toxicity*	? Mechanism
Antidiabetics	Impaired glucose tolerance	? Mechanism

Anti-epileptics
  carbamazepine
  phenytoin
	CNS toxicity	? Mechanism

Antihypertensive methyldopa	*CNS toxicity*	? Mechanism

Antipsychotics
  amisulpride
  sertindole
  thioridazine
	Ventricular arrhythmias	Summation of CNS toxicity ? due to combined effects on basal striatal adenylase cyclase

clozapine
  haloperidol
  phenothiazines
  sulpiride
	Increased risk of extrapyramidal effects
	? neurotoxicity
		? Mechanism

Bronchodilator theophylline	Decreased therapeutic effect of lithium	Increased renal blood flow → increased excretion of lithium → decreased plasma concentration of lithium

Calcium-channel blockers
  diltiazem
  verapamil
	CNS toxicity	? Mechanism

Table continues overleaf

Lithium interacts with	To produce	Mechanism
Diuretics		
acetazolamide	Decreased therapeutic effect of lithium	Increased excretion of lithium → decreased plasma concentration of lithium
potassium-sparing diuretics thiazides	*Lithium toxicity*	Decreased excretion of lithium → increased plasma concentration of lithium
Drugs affecting the renin–angiotensin system		
ACE inhibitors	*Lithium toxicity*	Decreased excretion of lithium → increased plasma concentration of lithium
Muscle relaxants		
baclofen	Enhanced muscle relaxant effect	Summation
	? Hyperkinesis	? Mechanism
Non-steriodal anti-inflammatory drugs azaproprazone diclofenac ibuprofen indomethacin kerorolac mefanamic acid naproxen parecoxib piroxicam rofecoxib ? others	*Lithium toxicity*	? Inhibition of renal prostaglandins (PGE2) → decreased renal blood flow → decreased excretion of lithium → increased plasma concentration of lithium
Parasympathomimetics neostigmine pyridostigmine	Decreased effect of parasympathomimetics	Antagonistic effect at neuro-muscular junction

See footnote to Appendix 16.1.

Index

Complied by Caroline Sheard

661